EMERGENCY NURSING PROCEDURES

FOURTH EDITION

Jean A. Proehl, RN, MN, CEN, CCRN, FAEN

Emergency Clinical Nurse Specialist
Dartmouth-Hitchcock Medical Center
Lebanon, New Hampshire

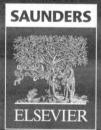

SAUNDERS

ELSEVIER

SAUNDERS
ELSEVIER

11830 Westline Industrial Drive
St. Louis, Missouri 63146

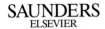
Emergency Nursing Procedures   ISBN: 978-1-4160-4098-9

Notice

Knowledge and best practice in this field are constantly changing. As new research and experience broaden our knowledge, changes in practice, treatment, and drug therapy may become necessary or appropriate. Readers are advised to check the most current information provided (i) on procedures featured or (ii) by the manufacturer of each product to be administered, to verify the recommended dose or formula, the method and duration of administration, and contraindications. It is the responsibility of the practitioner, relying on their own experience and knowledge of the patient, to make diagnoses, to determine dosages and the best treatment for each individual patient, and to take all appropriate safety precautions. To the fullest extent of the law, neither the Publisher nor the Authors assume any liability for any injury and/or damage to persons or property arising out or related to any use of the material contained in this book.

The Publisher

Previous editions copyrighted 1993, 1999, 2004

Library of Congress Control Number: 2007940904

Managing Editor: Maureen Iannuzzi
Senior Developmental Editor: Jennifer Ehlers
Editorial Assistant: Mary Ann Zimmerman
Publishing Services Manager: Jeff Patterson
Project Manager: Jeanne Genz
Design Direction: Julia Dummitt

Working together to grow
libraries in developing countries

www.elsevier.com | www.bookaid.org | www.sabre.org

ELSEVIER   BOOK AID International   Sabre Foundation

Printed in the United States of America

Last digit is the print number: 9   8   7   6   5   4   3   2   1

For my husband, Jeff; my children, Christopher and Madeline; and my parents, John and Betty Brewer.

And, for emergency nurses who use their heads, hearts, and hands to provide care and comfort every hour of every day, everywhere.

Contributors

Tamara Bleak, RN, BSN
Neonatal Coordinator
Intermountain Life Flight Children's Services
Primary Children's Medical Center
Salt Lake City, Utah

Andrew J. Bowman, RN, MSN, CEN, CTRN, CCRN-CMC, BC, CVN-I, FAACN, NREMT-P
Staff Nurse/Clinical Educator
Witham Health Services
Emergency Department
Lebanon, Indiana

Lori Carpenter, RRT
Respiratory Therapist Team Leader
Life Flight
Intermountain Health Care
Salt Lake City, Utah

Garrett K. Chan, APRN,BC, PhD, CEN
Assistant Clinical Professor
University of California-San Francisco
San Francisco, California
Lead Advanced Practice Nurse
Clinical Decision Area
Emergency Department
Stanford Hospital and Clinics
Stanford, California

Donna York Clark, RN, MS, CFRN, CMTE
Senior Account Manager
Golden Hour Data Systems
Indianapolis, Indiana

Joni Hentzen Daniels, MSN, RN, CEN, CRRN
Regional Director
Clinical Services
EmCare, Inc.
Dallas, Texas

Patricia A. DeWitt, RN, MSN
Practice and Education Associate
Office of Professional Nursing
Dartmouth-Hitchcock Medical Center
Lebanon, New Hampshire

Andrew A. Galvin, APRN,BC, CEN
Emergency Nurse Practitioner
Montgomery Regional Hospital
Blacksburg, Virginia

Reneé Semonin Holleran, RN, PhD, CEN, CCRN, CFRN, CTRN, FAEN
Nurse Manager
Adult Transport Services
Intermountain Life Flight
Salt Lake City, Utah

Patricia Kunz Howard, PhD, RN, CEN
Operations Manager
Emergency and Trauma Services
University of Kentucky
Chandler Medical Center
Lexington, Kentucky

K. Sue Hoyt, RN, PhD, FNP, APRN,BC, CEN, FAEN
Emergency Nurse Practitioner
St. Mary Medical Center
Long Beach, California

Margo E. Layman, MSN, RN, RNC, CN-A
Assistant Professor/Clinical Educator
University of Texas Health Science Center
San Antonio, Texas
Emergency Department Nurse and Educator
McKenna Memorial Hospital
New Braunfels, Texas

Kyle Madigan, RN, BSN, CEN, CFRN, CCRN
Chief Flight Nurse
Dartmouth-Hitchcock Advanced Response Team
Dartmouth-Hitchcock Medical Center
Lebanon, New Hampshire

Mike D. McMahon, RN, BSN
Clinical Analyst
Patient Care Information Services
University of Washington Medical Center
Seattle, Washington

Jean A. Proehl, RN, MN, CEN, CCRN, FAEN
Emergency Clinical Nurse Specialist
Dartmouth-Hitchcock Medical Center
Lebanon, New Hampshire

Maureen T. Quigley, MS, ARNP
Nurse Practitioner
Bariatric Surgery Program
Dartmouth-Hitchcock Medical Center
Lebanon, New Hampshire

Ruth Altherr Rench, MS, RN, FAHA
Genentech
Senior Clinical Specialist
Indianapolis, Indiana

Lucinda W. Rossoll, RN, MSN, CCRN, CEN
Unit Leader
Emergency Department
Dartmouth-Hitchcock Medical Center
Lebanon, New Hampshire

Michael Rouse, MSN, CRNA
Nurse Anesthestist
University Hospital
Cincinnati, Ohio

Ruth L. Schaffler, RN, PhD, ARNP, CEN
Assistant Professor of Nursing
Pacific Lutheran University
Family Nurse Practitioner
Pacific Lutheran University Wellness Clinic
Tacoma, Washington

Robin A. Scott, RN, ND
Clinical Nurse Educator
Emergency Department
University of Colorado Hospital
Denver, Colorado

Daun A. Smith, RN, MSN
Professor
Department of Nursing
New Hampshire Community Technical College
Claremont, New Hampshire
Clinical Nurse
Emergency Department
Dartmouth-Hitchcock Medical Center
Lebanon, New Hampshire

June F. Stacey, RN, BSN, CEN
Unit Leader
Emergency Department
Dartmouth-Hitchcock Medical Center
Lebanon, New Hampshire

Deborah A. Upton, MSN, ARNP-BC, CEN
Critical Care Nurse Practitioner
Dartmouth-Hitchcock Medical Center
Lebanon, New Hampshire

Teresa L. Will, MSN, RN, CEN
Education Specialist
Community Hospitals Indianapolis
Indianapolis, Indianapolis

Reviewers

Kirstine Buchan, PN
International SOS
Johannesburg, South Africa

Karen Crouse, EdD, APRN, FNP (BC), CEN
Western Connecticut State University
Danbury, Connecticut

Susan C. Czarnecki, RN, MSN, MDiv
Pastor
United Methodist Church of the Good Shepherd
Philadelphia, Pennsylvania

**Joyce Forseman-Capuzzi, BSN, RN, CEN,
CPN, CTRN, EMT-P**
Temple University Health System
Temple Health System Transport Team
Philadelphia, Pennsylvania

Thom Hodges, RN, MN
Clinical Nursing Instructor
Pierce College
Puyallup, Washington

Tammy Camille Killough, RN, BSN
Louisiana Technical College, Westside Campus
Plaquemine, Louisiana

David Pickham, RN, MN (AdvPrac)
Department of Physiological Nursing
University of California-San Francisco
San Francisco, California

Preface

Emergency nurses see it all. There is no other specialty that cares for such a wide variety of patients. We see all comers, from the worried well to the critically ill; from birth to death; and with conditions involving all parts of the mind, body, and spirit; from brain trauma to ingrown toenails. Our patients come from every stratum of society with one common denominator—they have a problem that they feel needs immediate attention, and they trust us to care for them.

Caring for such a wide variety of patients is no easy task, and, with ongoing advances in care, it is impossible to retain the vast amount of knowledge and skill that is needed for every possible situation. This book is intended to help you by serving as a ready resource at the bedside. Every effort has been made to make this a comprehensive reference for practicing emergency nurses. Novices will find the basic procedures a helpful review; experienced emergency nurses will appreciate information about new or infrequently performed procedures. The focus is clear, pertinent information to help you perform or assist with procedures. Research findings have been incorporated whenever possible to provide a scientific basis for practice.

Jean A. Proehl

Introduction

This book presents essential information in a standard format about a wide variety of procedures. It is assumed that the reader possesses basic nursing knowledge, and, accordingly, some information is not included in procedures because it is assumed to be part of standard nursing practice. These components of standard nursing practice include, but are not limited to:

- Attending to life-, limb-, or vision-threatening emergencies first
- Verifying the patient's identity according to institutional policy
- Introducing yourself
- Washing your hands and maintaining aseptic/sterile technique when indicated
- Protecting yourself with personal protective equipment as indicated
- Obtaining an appropriate history and physical examination
- Providing age-appropriate care
- Explaining the procedure in lay terminology to the patient
- Providing emotional support
- Obtaining verbal or written consent, or both, as indicated by institutional policy
- Draping the patient to provide privacy and warmth
- Placing the patient in a position of comfort when possible
- Participating in a "time out" or moment of truth prior to invasive procedures according to institutional policy
- Documenting assessment findings and interventions and the patient's response to them
- Including the family and significant others in explanations, follow-up teaching, and emotional support
- Teaching the patient about home care, including prescribed medications

Nursing practice varies from state to state and institution to institution. An asterisk (*) has been used throughout the book to indicate portions of a procedure usually performed by a physician or an advanced practice nurse. Some of these tasks are also performed by paramedics, physician's assistants, and nurses in extended roles such as air or ground transport. The use of the asterisk is not intended to prescribe nursing or medical practice, but rather to indicate the usual role delineation in the experience of the editor and contributors. The information about nonnursing components of a procedure helps the nurse anticipate needs and expedite safe patient care.

This text describes the use of many commercial products; no endorsement of these products is intended. Likewise, omission of products does not imply lack of endorsement. Products are included if they are commonly in use in emergency care based on the experience of the editor and contributors.

Jean A. Proehl

Acknowledgments

I would like to gratefully acknowledge the generosity of numerous authors, publishers, and manufacturers who shared illustrations for this book. Good illustrations are essential for explaining procedures, and this book would not be so richly illustrated without the contributions of these individuals and companies. The manufacturers of products provided gratis illustrations and, in some cases, reviewed the content for accuracy as it pertains to their products.

I would also like to acknowledge the contributions of authors to the previous editions; they provided a strong foundation upon which to build and expand for the fourth edition.

Jean A. Proehl

Contents

Section 5: Suctioning

Section 6: Ventilation

Section 7: Inhalation Therapy

Section 8: Pleural Decompression

Section 9: Circulation Procedures

Section 10: Vascular Access

Section 11: Blood Product Administration

Section 12: Electrical Therapy

Section 13: Cardiac Pacing

Section 14: Invasive Hemodynamic Monitoring

Section 15: Neurologic Procedures

Section 16: Abdominal and Genitourinary Procedures

Section 17: Musculoskeletal Procedures

Section 22: Nasal Procedures

Section 23: Dental and Throat Procedures

Section 24: Medication Administration

Section 25: Miscellaneous Procedures

Assessment Procedures

Primary Assessment

Jean A. Proehl, RN, MN, CEN, CCRN, FAEN

INDICATION

1. To rapidly assess and intervene for life-threatening conditions in critically ill or injured patients.

CONTRAINDICATIONS AND CAUTIONS

1. The presence of an environmental hazard, such as fire, noxious fumes, or explosion risk, that mandates immediate evacuation of the area takes priority over the primary assessment.
2. Do not proceed to the next assessment step until interventions for life-threatening conditions have been implemented.

EQUIPMENT

Towel rolls, foam blocks, or other head-support devices
Stethoscope
Flashlight
Other equipment as indicated for resuscitative procedures

PROCEDURAL STEPS

1. Assess airway patency while simultaneously maintaining cervical spine alignment with manual stabilization. Airway patency is assessed by looking for chest rise and fall and by listening and feeling for air movement from the nose and mouth. If the airway is partially or completely obstructed, implement the appropriate intervention. Potential interventions include the following and are described elsewhere in this text:
   Procedure 3—Airway Positioning
   Procedure 4—Airway Foreign Object Removal
   Procedure 5—Oral Airway Insertion
   Procedure 6—Nasal Airway Insertion
   Procedure 7—Laryngeal Mask Airway
   Procedures 8–12—Endotracheal Intubation
   Procedure 14—Combitube Airway
   Procedure 15—Cricothyrotomy
   Procedure 16—Percutaneous Transtracheal Ventilation
   Procedure 17—Tracheostomy
   Procedure 29—Pharyngeal Suctioning
2. If the patient is at risk for cervical spine injury, have an assistant manually stabilize the head until the primary and secondary assessments are complete and more definitive immobilization can be instituted (see Procedure 111). In the absence of an assistant, towel rolls or foam blocks set alongside the head

will help maintain alignment and remind a conscious patient not to move. Do not tape down the head and blocks until the patient is fully strapped to a backboard. Cervical spine immobilization should be maintained until the neck is cleared by x-ray or clinical examination.

3. Assess breathing adequacy by observing the respiratory rate, depth, and difficulty. Briefly auscultate breath sounds bilaterally. Implement pulse oximetry monitoring for all seriously injured or ill patients (see Procedure 21). If respirations are absent or abnormal, implement appropriate interventions. Potential interventions include the following and are described elsewhere in this text:

    Procedure 18—Positioning the Dyspneic Patient
    Procedure 25—General Principles of Oxygen Therapy and Oxygen Delivery Devices
    Procedures 29–31—Suctioning
    Procedure 32—Bag-Mask Ventilation
    Procedure 38—Emergency Needle Thoracentesis
    Procedure 39—Chest-Tube Insertion

Use a flutter valve (occlusive dressing taped on three sides) for open pneumothorax (sucking chest wound).

4. Assess circulation by evaluating the radial or carotid pulse for rate and strength. Observe and palpate the skin for warmth, color, and moisture. Check for exsanguinating external hemorrhage and, if present, apply direct pressure to the site. If the circulation is absent or altered, implement appropriate interventions, including chest compressions, as indicated. If an assistant is available, institute electrocardiographic monitoring (see Procedure 55). Other potential interventions include the following and are described elsewhere in this text:

    Procedure 48—Positioning the Hypotensive Patient
    Procedure 53—Pericardiocentesis
    Procedure 54—Emergency Thoracotomy and Internal Defibrillation
    Procedures 60–67—Vascular Access
    Procedure 81—Defibrillation
    Procedure 82—Synchronized Cardioversion
    Procedure 85—Transcutaneous Cardiac Pacing

5. Evaluate the neurologic status to determine whether the patient is alert (A), responds to verbal stimuli (V), responds to painful stimuli (P), or is unresponsive to all stimuli (U). Assess pupil size, equality, and reaction to light.

AGE-SPECIFIC CONSIDERATIONS
Pediatric

1. *Airway:* Young infants are obligate nose breathers. Nasal flaring is an indication of respiratory distress. Nasal suctioning is a high-priority intervention in an infant with nasal secretions. Infants also have a proportionately larger tongue, which may obstruct their airway.

2. *Breathing:* The ribs and sternum are more cartilaginous in children; therefore, retractions are common during respiratory distress. Infants rely heavily on diaphragmatic breathing because of poorly developed intercostal muscles; for this reason, an upright posture is preferred for children in respiratory distress. Because the chest wall of infants and small children is thin,

auscultation of breath sounds may be misleading—that is, breath sounds may be transmitted from the opposite side, leading to "equal breath sounds," even in the presence of right mainstem intubation or pneumothorax.

3. *Circulation:* Assess a brachial pulse in infants. Capillary refill is an important circulatory assessment in infants and young children. Assess it in a central area, such as the child's forehead or chest. Normal capillary refill is less than 2 seconds.

4. *Neurologic status:* In infants and preverbal children, level of consciousness is more difficult to assess. During the primary assessment, response to handling or painful procedures and the presence of spontaneous movements should be noted. At the completion of the secondary assessment (see Procedure 2) assess neurologic status using an appropriate pediatric coma scale.

Geriatric

1. *Airway:* Displaced dentures may cause airway obstruction.

2. *Breathing:* A supine position may be poorly tolerated and cause respiratory distress in elderly patients, especially those with significant preexisting pulmonary or cardiac disease.

3. *Circulation:* Capillary refill time increases as part of the aging process and is not a reliable indicator of systemic perfusion in adults.

4. *Neurologic status:* Altered mental status in elderly patients should be assumed to be a new finding unless a history of prior dementia is known. Elderly patients who are hard of hearing may appear to be confused if they attempt to respond to a question that they did not hear correctly.

COMPLICATIONS

1. Failure to recognize and intervene appropriately for life-threatening conditions before progressing to the next assessment step may result in patient deterioration.

2. Intervening for noncritical conditions, such as extremity fractures, before correcting life-threatening conditions may result in patient deterioration.

PATIENT TEACHING

Do not move until a spinal injury has been ruled out.

Secondary Assessment

Jean A. Proehl, RN, MN, CEN, CCRN, FAEN

INDICATIONS

1. To rapidly and systematically assess injured patients from head to toe to identify all injuries.
2. To rapidly and systematically assess critically ill patients in whom the etiology of signs and symptoms is unclear.

CONTRAINDICATIONS AND CAUTIONS

1. Do not begin the secondary assessment until the primary assessment has been completed and resuscitation procedures have been initiated as indicated (see Procedure 1).
2. Continue to monitor airway, breathing, circulatory, and neurologic status during the secondary assessment, and interrupt the secondary assessment to initiate interventions for life-threatening conditions as indicated.
3. Prioritize and initiate interventions for injuries or conditions discovered in the secondary assessment after the entire head-to-toe examination is complete.

EQUIPMENT

Trauma scissors to cut clothing, if necessary
Stethoscope
Pulse oximeter
Cardiac monitor
Blood pressure cuff or noninvasive blood pressure monitor
Thermometer
Blanket

PROCEDURAL STEPS

1. Maintain cervical spine alignment for trauma patients as initiated in the primary assessment.
2. Remove all clothing to facilitate a complete patient assessment. Cover the patient to preserve the body temperature.
3. Obtain blood pressure, pulse, and respirations. Temperature determination may be deferred until the secondary assessment is completed, but it should be performed as quickly as possible in the very old, the very young, and those with potential hypothermia or hyperthermia.
4. Initiate cardiac (see Procedure 55) and pulse oximetry (see Procedure 21) monitoring.
5. If the patient is conscious, obtain information about painful areas by instructing him or her to report any tenderness elicited by palpation. Obtain a brief history of the mechanism of the injury; the history of the present illness; any chronic diseases, allergies, or pertinent immunizations; current medications

(prescription, over the counter, and herbal); and any recent use of alcohol or illicit drugs.

6. Inspect the head and face for wounds, deformities, discolorations, or bloody/serous drainage from the nose or ears. Palpate the entire head and face for wounds, deformities, or tenderness. In the conscious and cooperative patient, evaluate extraocular movements, gross vision, and dental occlusion. Note any unusual odors, for example, gasoline, fruity breath, or ethanol.

7. If necessary, remove the anterior portion of the cervical collar while another person maintains manual immobilization of the head and neck. Inspect the anterior neck for wounds, jugular venous distention, discolorations, or deformities. Palpate the anterior neck for deformities, crepitus, tenderness, or tracheal deviation (best palpated in the notch above the manubrium). Gently palpate the posterior neck from the base of the skull to the upper back for wounds, deformities, tenderness, or muscle spasm.

8. Inspect the anterior and lateral chest for wounds, deformities, discolorations, respiratory expansion, symmetry, and paradoxical movement. Palpate the anterior and lateral chest for deformities, tenderness, or crepitus. Auscultate breath sounds to determine whether they are present and equal bilaterally, and note any abnormal sounds, such as crackles and wheezes. Auscultate heart sounds to determine whether they are clear or muffled.

9. Inspect the abdomen for wounds, discolorations, or distention. Auscultate all quadrants for the presence of bowel sounds. Gently palpate the abdomen for tenderness, guarding, rigidity, or masses (palpate the areas that are known to be painful last).

10. Inspect the pelvic area and genitalia for wounds, deformities, discolorations, or bleeding from the urinary meatus, vagina, or rectum. Palpate for pelvic tenderness, crepitus, or instability by gently pressing in on the anterosuperior iliac crests bilaterally and pushing down on the pubic symphysis. Palpate femoral pulses for presence and equality.

11. Inspect all extremities for wounds, deformities, or discolorations. Palpate all extremities for tenderness, deformities, muscle spasm, and distal pulses. If the patient is conscious, determine gross motor and sensory function by having the patient wiggle the toes and fingers and asking whether he or she can feel your touch.

12. In the injured patient, obtain assistance to maintain cervical spine alignment and support injured extremities while logrolling the patient to the side. Avoid rolling the patient onto an injured extremity if possible. In some patients, it may be necessary to roll the patient to both sides to assess the posterior surfaces adequately. Inspect the posterior surfaces for wounds, deformities, or discolorations. Palpate all posterior surfaces for wounds, deformities, or muscle spasm.

13. *In male trauma patients, perform a rectal examination to assess sphincter tone, prostate position, and stool for occult blood. In female trauma

---

*Indicates portions of the procedure that are usually performed by a physician or an advanced practice nurse.

TABLE 2–1
NORMAL PEDIATRIC VITAL SIGNS BY AGE

Age	Heart Rate (beats per minute)	Respiratory Rate (breaths per minute)
0-3 months	90-180	30-60
3-6 months	80-160	30-60
6-12 months	80-140	25-45
1-3 years	75-130	20-30
6 years	70-110	16-24
10 years	60-90	14-20

From Warren, D, Jarvis, A., & LeBlanc, L. (2001). Canadian paediatric triage and acuity scale: Implementation guidelines for emergency departments, *Canadian Journal of Emergency Medicine* 3(4 Suppl), S1–S27.

patients, perform a rectal examination to assess sphincter tone and stool for occult blood.

AGE-SPECIFIC CONSIDERATIONS

1. Infants and young children have immature thermoregulatory capability and are susceptible to iatrogenic hypothermia. Elderly patients may have less subcutaneous fat and lose body heat easily. Keep both groups of patients covered and provide warming as indicated.
2. The normal range for vital signs in children varies by age (Table 2–1). The heart and respiratory rates may be altered by fear, pain, and anxiety, in addition to physiologic problems such as hypoxia and hypovolemia. In children, blood pressure may be maintained in the presence of significant hypovolemia. Therefore, other assessments of circulatory status (heart rate, capillary refill, skin color, and so forth) should be monitored closely. In older patients, the decreased sensitivity of baroreceptors, decreased response to beta stimulation, and medications may prevent a compensatory tachycardia in response to decreased systemic perfusion.
3. Pediatric patients should be weighed as soon as possible because medication doses, fluid resuscitation, and other interventions are influenced by the child's size. If obtaining a weight is not feasible, a length-based resuscitation tape can be used to estimate weight.

COMPLICATIONS

1. Failure to recognize and intervene appropriately for life-threatening conditions that develop or worsen during the secondary assessment may result in patient deterioration.
2. In the injured patient, failure to maintain spinal alignment and immobilization throughout the secondary assessment may result in trauma to the spinal cord.
3. Failure to complete the secondary assessment and prioritize interventions before initiating them may result in patient deterioration.
4. Intervening for noncritical problems, such as extremity fractures, before correcting life-threatening conditions may result in patient deterioration.

PATIENT TEACHING

Do not move until spinal injury has been ruled out.

Airway Procedures

Airway Positioning

Donna York Clark, RN, MS, CFRN, CMTE

INDICATION

1. To establish and maintain a patent airway or to relieve a partial or total airway obstruction due to displacement of the tongue into the posterior pharynx and/or the epiglottis at the level of the larynx. These positions are indicated for unconscious patients who do not have an adequate airway.

CONTRAINDICATIONS AND CAUTIONS

1. In an unconscious trauma patient or a patient with a known or suspected neck injury, the head and neck should be maintained in a neutral position without neck hyperextension. Use the jaw-thrust or chin-lift maneuver to open the airway in this situation. In resuscitation, maintaining a patent airway is a priority; the head-tilt/chin-lift maneuver may be used if the jaw thrust does not open the airway (AHA, 2005).
2. Positioning alone may be insufficient to achieve and maintain an open airway. Additional interventions, such as suctioning, oral/nasal airway insertion, and intubation, may be indicated.

PROCEDURAL STEPS

1. Place the patient in a supine position.
2. For the head-tilt/chin-lift maneuver, lift the chin forward to displace the mandible anteriorly while tilting the head back with a hand on the forehead (Figure 3-1). This maneuver results in hyperextension of the neck and is contraindicated when a neck injury is suspected or known to be present.
3. If the head-tilt/chin-lift maneuver is unsuccessful or contraindicated, use either the jaw-thrust or the chin-lift maneuver.
   a. *Jaw-thrust maneuver:* Lift the mandible forward with your index fingers while pushing against the zygomatic arches with your thumbs (Figure 3-2). Your thumbs provide counterpressure to prevent movement of the head when the mandible is pushed forward.
   b. *Chin-lift maneuver:* Place one hand on the forehead to stabilize the head and neck. Grab the mandible between the thumb and index finger of the other hand. Lift the mandible forward (Figure 3-3).
4. Reassess airway patency after any maneuver.

AGE-SPECIFIC CONSIDERATIONS

1. For the head-tilt/chin-lift maneuver in the infant or child, place one hand on the patient's forehead and tilt the head gently back into a neutral position. The neck should be slightly extended. This is known as the "sniffing position." Hyperextension of an infant's neck may cause airway compromise or

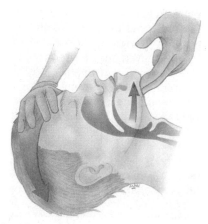

FIGURE 3-1 Head-tilt/chin-lift maneuver. (From Sanders, M. [2003]. *Mosby's paramedic textbook* [2nd ed]. St. Louis: Mosby, p. 397.)

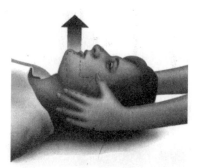

FIGURE 3-2 Jaw thrust. (From Emergency Nurses Association. [2002]. *Trauma nursing core course: Provider manual* [5th ed]. Des Plaines, IL: Author, p. 364.)

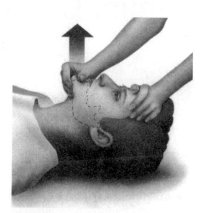

FIGURE 3-3 Chin lift. (From Emergency Nurses Association. [2002]. *Trauma nursing core course: Provider manual* [5th ed]. Des Plaines, IL: Author, p. 364.)

obstruction due to the relative flexibility of their trachea. Place fingers under the bony part of the lower jaw at the chin and lift the mandible upward and outward. Use caution not to close the mouth or push on the soft tissues under the chin because these maneuvers may obstruct the airway.

2. All children should be allowed to maintain a position of comfort. This is particularly important in children presenting with symptoms of epiglottitis, such as high fever, drooling, and respiratory distress. Forcing them into a supine position could obstruct the airway. Allow the child to maintain a position of comfort until definitive airway management is available.

COMPLICATIONS

1. If the airway remains obstructed, suctioning should be completed, and then an oropharyngeal or nasopharyngeal airway should be inserted. (See Procedures 5, 6, and 29.)
2. Injury to the spinal cord may occur if the head and/or neck is moved in patients with cervical spine injuries.
3. If your fingers press deeply into the soft tissue under the chin, blood vessels or the airway could be obstructed.

REFERENCE

American Heart Association (AHA). (2005). *Basic life support for healthcare providers*. Dallas: Author.

PROCEDURE 4

Airway Foreign Object Removal

Donna York Clark, RN, MS, CFRN, CMTE

Abdominal thrusts are also known as the *Heimlich maneuver.*

INDICATION

To relieve upper airway obstruction caused by foreign objects. Signs and symptoms of airway obstruction are characterized by some or all of the following:

1. Sudden inability to speak or cry
2. Poor or no air exchange

3. Universal sign for choking: clutching the neck (AHA, 2005a)
4. Noisy airflow (high-pitched sounds) during inspiration
5. Accessory muscle use during respiration and increasing work of breathing
6. Weak or ineffective cough or an inability to cough
7. Absence of spontaneous respirations or cyanosis
8. Infants or children with a sudden onset of respiratory distress associated with coughing, gagging, stridor, or wheezing (AHA, 2005a)

CONTRAINDICATIONS AND CAUTIONS

1. In the conscious patient, a voluntary cough generates the greatest airflow and may relieve the obstruction. Do not interfere with the patient's attempts to cough up the obstruction.
2. Chest thrusts should not be used in the patient who has a chest injury, for example, flail chest, cardiac contusion, or sternal fractures.
3. In the advanced stages of pregnancy or in the markedly obese, chest thrusts are recommended (AHA, 2005b).
4. Correct hand placement is essential to avoid injury to underlying organs during the delivery of abdominal thrusts.

EQUIPMENT

Oral suction, if available
Magill or Kelly forceps and laryngoscope (optional for the removal of a foreign object that can be visualized in the upper airway)

PATIENT PREPARATION

1. The patient may be sitting, standing, or supine.
2. Suction any blood or mucus you can visualize in the patient's mouth.
3. Remove broken or loose-fitting dentures.
4. Be prepared to perform more definitive airway management, such as cricothyrotomy (see Procedure 15).
5. Before performing abdominal thrusts on a conscious adult or child, ask the person if he or she is choking. If the victim nods yes and cannot talk, communicate that you are going to help.

PROCEDURAL STEPS (ADULT OR CHILD OLDER THAN AGE 1)

1. Stand or kneel behind the victim and wrap your arms around the victim's waist.
2. Make a fist with one hand and place the thumb side of your fist against the abdomen of the victim, just above the navel but below the xiphoid process.
3. Grasp your fist with your other hand and press into the victim's abdomen with a quick upward thrust (Figure 4-1).
4. Thrusts should be repeated, each as a separate, distinct movement, until the object is expelled or the victim becomes unresponsive.
5. For the pregnant or obese patient, the chest thrust may be performed. The patient may be supine, sitting, or standing. Put one hand directly over the other and position the bottom hand at the midsternal area above the xiphoid process (mid-nipple line, the same position used in external cardiac massage). Thrust straight down toward the spine. If necessary, repeat chest thrusts several times to relieve airway obstruction (Figure 4-2).

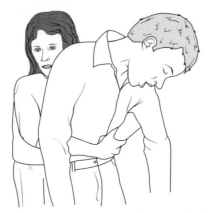

FIGURE 4-1 Abdominal thrusts for the standing or sitting victim of choking.

6. If the victim becomes unresponsive, open the airway, remove any object you can see, and begin cardiopulmonary resuscitation (CPR). Each time the airway is opened for breaths, assess for an object and remove it if seen. If nothing is seen, continue with CPR (AHA, 2005c) (Figure 4-3).
7. *For complete obstruction in an unconscious patient, where thrusts are ineffective, use Magill forceps with direct laryngoscopy before ventilation to facilitate removal of the obstruction (Walls, 2004) or surgical cricothyroidotomy.

---

*Indicates portions of the procedure usually performed by a physician or an advanced practice nurse.

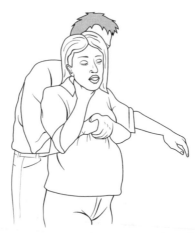

FIGURE 4-2 Chest thrusts for the pregnant or obese victim of choking.

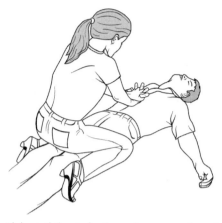

FIGURE 4-3 Abdominal thrusts for the supine, unconscious victim of choking.

AGE-SPECIFIC CONSIDERATIONS
Infant (Younger Than Age 1 Year)
1. Kneel or sit with the infant in your lap, and hold the infant prone with the head slightly lower than the chest. Support the infant's head and jaw with your hand (Figure 4-4).
2. Deliver up to five forceful back slaps between the shoulder blades using the heel of your hand.
3. Turn the infant supine, supporting the head and neck and keeping the infant's head lower than the trunk.
4. Give up to five quick downward chest thrusts in the same location as for chest compressions, just below the nipple line. Thrusts should be delivered at

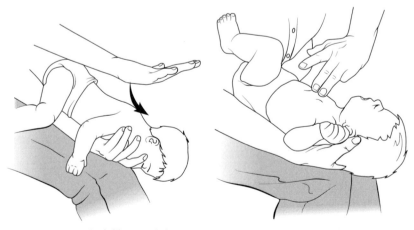

FIGURE 4-4 Back blows and chest thrusts for foreign body obstruction in an infant.

a rate of about one per second with enough force to dislodge the foreign body (AHA, 2005b, 2002c; ACEP and AAP, 2004).

5. Steps 1 through 4 are continued until the object is expelled or the infant loses consciousness.

6. If the infant becomes unresponsive, open the airway, remove any object you can see, and begin CPR. Each time the airway is opened for breaths, assess for an object and remove it if seen. If nothing is seen, continue with CPR (AHA, 2005a).

7. *For complete obstruction in which ventilation is not possible, use Magill forceps with direct laryngoscopy to facilitate removal of the obstruction (ACEP and AAP, 2004) or perform a cricothyroidotomy (see Procedure 15).

COMPLICATIONS

1. Abdominal pain, ecchymosis
2. Nausea, vomiting
3. Fractured ribs
4. Injury to underlying abdominal or chest organs

---

*Indicates portions of the procedure usually performed by a physician or an advanced practice nurse.

REFERENCES

American College of Emergency Physicians (ACEP) and American Academy of Pediatrics (AAP). (2004). *APLS: The pediatric emergency medicine resource* (4th ed.). Boston: Jones and Bartlett Publishers.

American Heart Association (AHA). (2005a). *Advanced pediatric life support: Instructors manual.* Dallas: Author.

American Heart Association (AHA). (2005b). *Basic life support for healthcare providers.* Dallas: Author.

American Heart Association (AHA). (2005c). *ACLS provider manual.* Dallas: Author.

Walls, R. (2004). Foreign body in the adult airway. In R. Walls, M. Murphy, R. Luten, & R. Schneider (Eds.), *Manual of emergency airway management* (2nd ed., pp. 307-311). New York: Lippincott Williams & Wilkins.

Oral Airway Insertion

Donna York Clark, RN, MS, CFRN, CMTE

The oral airway is also known as an *oropharyngeal airway, OPA, Guedel airway,* or *Berman airway.*

INDICATIONS

To maintain airway patency for patients in the following situations:
1. An unconscious spontaneously breathing patient with an airway obstruction caused by an impaired gag reflex and a loss of tone to the submandibular muscles.
2. Unsuccessful airway opening by other maneuvers, such as the head tilt, the chin lift, and the jaw thrust.
3. A patient ventilated by a bag-mask device. The oral airway elevates the soft tissues of the posterior pharynx, easing ventilation and minimizing gastric insufflation.
4. An orally intubated patient who bites/clenches the endotracheal tube; the oral airway is used as a bite block.
5. An unconscious patient during suctioning, to facilitate the removal of a patient's oral secretions (AHA, 2005).

CONTRAINDICATIONS AND CAUTIONS

1. Insertion of an oral airway in a conscious or semiconscious patient stimulates the gag reflex and may stimulate airway spasm or cause the patient to retch and to vomit (AHA, 2005).
2. Incorrect placement of an oral airway may compress the tongue into the posterior pharynx and cause further obstruction (Vrocher & Hopson, 2004).
3. An airway that is too small may push the tongue into the oropharynx and cause an obstruction, and an airway that is too large may obstruct the trachea (Vrocher & Hopson, 2004).
4. Failure to clear the oropharynx of foreign material before insertion of the airway may result in aspiration.
5. To avoid vomiting and aspiration, the oropharyngeal airway should be removed immediately after the patient regains a gag reflex.

EQUIPMENT

Oropharyngeal suction equipment
Oropharyngeal airway
Tongue blade

TABLE 5-1
ORAL AIRWAY SIZING BY AGE

Age	Oral Airway Size
Premature infant	000
Neonate	00
Full-term infant	0
1-3 yr	1
3-8 yr	2
Large child, small adult	3
Medium adult	4
Large adult	5, 6

PATIENT PREPARATION

1. Place the patient in a supine position.
2. Suction blood, secretions, or other foreign material from the patient's oropharynx.
3. Select the appropriately sized oropharyngeal airway. Table 5-1 lists usual airway sizes by age. Align the tube on the side of the patient's face, so the airway extends from the level of the central incisors with the bite block portion parallel to the hard palate. The tip of the appropriate size airway will meet the angle of the jaw (AAP, 2006).

PROCEDURAL STEPS

1. Use a tongue blade to depress and displace the tongue forward. Insert the airway with the curve pointing up, and advance it over the tongue into the oropharynx (Figure 5-1).

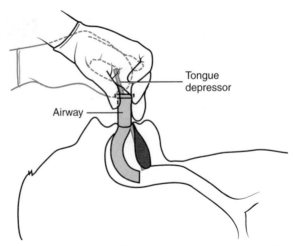

FIGURE 5-1 Correct placement of oropharyngeal airway using a tongue blade to displace the tongue.

2. As an alternative procedure for adults and adolescents, insert the airway upside down (with the curve pointing toward the back of the patient's head) into the mouth. As the tip of the airway reaches the posterior wall of the pharynx, rotate the airway 180 degrees to the proper position.
3. The distal tip of the airway should lie between the base of the tongue and the back of the throat. The flange of the tube should sit comfortably on the lips.
4. Reassess the airway patency, and auscultate the lung for equal and clear breath sounds during ventilation.

AGE-SPECIFIC CONSIDERATION

For pediatric patients, depress and displace the tongue forward with a tongue blade and insert the airway (described in step 1 above). Do not insert an upside-down airway and then rotate it (described in step 2 above), because this technique may injure the soft tissue of the oropharynx (AAP, 2006).

COMPLICATIONS

1. Trauma to the lips, tongue, teeth, and oral mucosa
2. Vomiting and aspiration (Vrocher & Hopson, 2004)
3. Complete airway obstruction (AHA, 2005)

REFERENCES

American Academy of Pediatrics (AAP). (2006). *Pediatric education for prehospital professionals* (2nd ed.). Boston: Jones and Bartlett.
American Heart Association (AHA). (2005). *Textbook of advanced cardiac life support*. Dallas: Author.
Vrocher, D. & Hopson, L. (2004). Basic airway management and decision-making. In J. R. Roberts, & J. R. Hedges (Eds.), *Clinical procedures in emergency medicine* (4th ed., pp. 53-68). Philadelphia: Saunders.

PROCEDURE 6

Nasal Airway Insertion

Donna York Clark, RN, MS, CFRN, CMTE

Nasal airways are also known as *nasopharyngeal airways* and *nasal trumpets*.

INDICATIONS

The nasal airway is indicated in the following situations:
1. There is a question of patency of the posterior nasopharynx with intact upper airway reflexes.

2. Bag-mask ventilation is ineffective because of difficulty maintaining a patent airway; use of a nasopharyngeal airway may facilitate ventilation. The nasal airway may be used in combination with the oropharyngeal airway in this setting.
3. Insertion of an oropharyngeal airway is technically difficult or impossible because of massive trauma around the mouth, such as mandibulomaxillary wiring.
4. To decrease soft tissue trauma when frequent nasotracheal suctioning is necessary (AHA, 2005; Vrocher & Hopson, 2004).

CONTRAINDICATIONS AND CAUTIONS

1. The insertion of a nasal airway may stimulate the gag reflex and cause the patient to vomit.
2. If the tube is too long, it may enter the esophagus and cause gastric insufflation and hypoventilation (AHA, 2005).
3. Epistaxis may occur and may lead to aspiration of blood.
4. Nasal airways should not be used in patients who have extensive facial trauma or a basilar skull fracture.

EQUIPMENT

Nasopharyngeal suction equipment
Water-soluble lubricant or anesthetic jelly
Nasopharyngeal airway

PATIENT PREPARATION

1. Place the patient in a supine position or high Fowler's position.
2. Select the nostril that appears to be the largest and most open. Assess the nasal passages for trauma, foreign body, septal deviation, or polyps.
3. Prepare suction equipment for use.

PROCEDURAL STEPS

1. Select an appropriately sized nasal airway. Use the largest airway that will pass easily through the naris. Sizing is labeled by a number indicating the inside diameter in millimeters, and sizes are available for neonates through adults. An endotracheal tube can be used if the correct size nasopharyngeal airway is not available. Measure the length of the nasopharyngeal airway from the tip of the nose to the tragus of the ear (ENA, 2004).
2. Vasoconstriction of the mucous membranes may be indicated. Agents commonly prescribed for this purpose include phenylephrine (Neo-Synephrine) or cocaine spray or liquid (Vrocher & Hopson, 2004).
3. Lubricate the tube with water-soluble gel or anesthetic jelly.
4. Pass the airway along the floor of the nostril with the bevel facing the nasal septum (Figure 6-1). Direct the airway posteriorly and rotate it slightly toward the ear until the flange rests against the nostril. Note that all nasal airways have a bevel that is angled for insertion into the right naris. The airway may be used in the left naris. Place the airway in the left naris with the bevel facing the nasal septum. The nasopharyngeal airway curvature will be opposite of the natural nasal curvature. Once the airway tip has reached the correct position, rotate the airway 180 degrees.

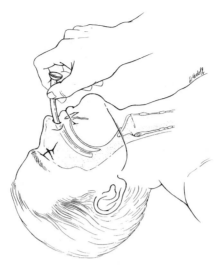

FIGURE 6-1   Correct placement of nasopharyngeal airway. (Courtesy of P. Rosen, MD.)

5. If resistance is met, a slight rotation of the tube may facilitate passage as the device reaches the hypopharynx. Insertion should never be forced.
6. Reassess the airway patency.

COMPLICATIONS

1. Epistaxis
2. Aspiration
3. Hypoxia secondary to aspiration or improper placement
4. Contraindications include suspected basilar skull fracture, facial trauma, or nasal obstruction that prevents easy insertion of airway (ENA, 2004).

REFERENCES

American Heart Association (AHA). (2005). American Heart Association Guidelines for cardio-pulmonary resuscitation and emergency cardiovascular care. *Circulation, 112*(suppl. IV).

Emergency Nurses Association (ENA). (2004). *Emergency nursing pediatric course provider manual* (3rd ed.). Des Plaines, IL. Author.

Vrocher, D. & Hopson, L. (2004). Basic airway management and decision-making. In J. R. Roberts, & J. R. Hedges (Eds.), *Clinical procedures in emergency medicine* (4th ed., pp. 53-68). Philadelphia: Saunders.

Laryngeal Mask Airway

Donna York Clark, RN, MS, CFRN, CMTE

The laryngeal mask airway (LMA) resembles an endotracheal tube with a spoon-shaped mask at one end. The spoon-shaped mask has an inflatable collar that forms a seal around the larynx (Murphy, 2004; Walls, 2006) (Figure 7-1).

The LMA provides a reliable and more secure means of ventilation than the face mask. Training in the insertion of the LMA is less complex than that for endotracheal intubation, and there may be advantages over intubation in the prehospital setting, where access to the patient is limited. Although some risk of aspiration is present, studies have shown that emesis is more likely with mask ventilation than with the LMA (Walls, 2006).

The LMA is manufactured solely by Laryngeal Mask Company Limited (San Diego, CA). Four types of LMA devices are produced: the LMA Classic (a reusable LMA), the LMA Unique (a disposable LMA designed like the classic), the LMA Fastrach (designed to facilitate tracheal intubation with an endotracheal tube), and the LMA ProSeal (LMA, 2003).

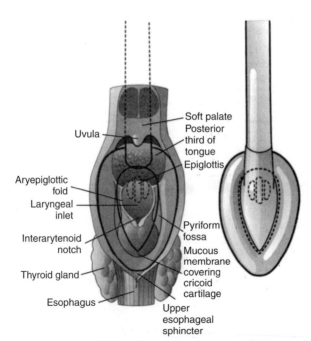

FIGURE 7-1 Dorsal view of the laryngeal mask airway (LMA) showing position in relation to pharyngeal anatomy. (Courtesy of LMA North America, Inc.)

The LMA ProSeal is designed to do the following (Brain, Verghese, and Strube, 2000; LMA, 2006; Vrocher & Hopson, 2004):

- Improve the laryngeal seal without increasing mucosal pressures
- Separate the respiratory and alimentary tracts
- Provide higher airway seal pressures for use with positive-pressure ventilation

However, the ProSeal is intended for use in the operating room, and the procedure for the placement and use of this product is beyond the scope of this chapter.

INDICATIONS

1. The LMA is used as an alternative to a face mask during manual ventilation. The LMA is not intended to be used instead of intubation for continued ventilation (LMA North America, 2005; Murphy, 2004; Urocher and Hopson, 2004; Walls, 2006). It may be used in the operating suite for short procedures when lighter anesthesia levels are preferred.
2. In an emergency, the LMA may serve as a temporary route for gas exchange in failed intubation scenarios until definitive airway control is achieved (Murphy, 2004; Pollack, 2001; Walls, 2006). A laryngoscope is not required and the insertion technique allows the user to rapidly obtain an airway for ventilation. Studies have shown that the LMA provides equivalent ventilation compared with the endotracheal tube (AHA, 2005).

CONTRAINDICATIONS AND CAUTIONS

1. The patient must have absent glossopharyngeal and laryngeal reflexes and be unresponsive.
2. The LMA does not constitute definitive airway control. It does not protect the airway from gastric content aspiration and should be used only in a patient with an empty stomach.
3. The LMA is not indicated for patients with decreased pulmonary compliance, because the low-pressure seal that is formed around the larynx may not allow adequate ventilation (Murphy, 2004).
4. Obstructive or abnormal lesions of the oropharynx.

EQUIPMENT

LMA (Table 7-1 provides sizing information.)
Water-soluble lubricant
Syringe
Tonsil-tip suction
Bag ventilation system
Oxygen source and connecting tubing
Tape or securing device
For intubating LMA (Fastrach): accompanying silicone-tipped endotracheal tube

PATIENT PREPARATION

1. Preoxygenate the patient with bag-mask ventilation.
2. If necessary, administer sedation, as prescribed. Deep sedation or an unconscious state is required for LMA use (Murphy, 2004).

TABLE 7-1
LARYNGEAL MASK AIRWAY SIZING AND CUFF INFLATION VOLUMES

Patient Weight	Recommended LMA Size	Maximum Cuff Inflation Volume
Less than 5 kg	1	Up to 4 ml
5-10 kg	1.5	Up to 7 ml
10-20 kg	2	Up to 10 ml
20-30 kg	2.5	Up to 14 ml
Greater than 30 kg	3	Up to 20 ml
Normal-size and large adults	4	Up to 30 ml
Large adults	5	Up to 40 ml

Modified from LMA North America (2005). *Laryngeal mask airway instruction manual.* San Diego: Author.

3. Position the patient with the head extended and the neck flexed (except in patients with potential cervical spine injury). During LMA insertion, it may be helpful to push the patient's head from behind to maintain this position.

PROCEDURAL STEPS
LMA Classic, LMA Unique
1. *Inflate the cuff to check for leaks and deflate it to form a spoon shape (Figure 7-2).
2. *Coat the posterior surface of the LMA with a water-soluble lubricant.
3. *Grasp the LMA by positioning your index finger in the crease between the airway tube and the laryngeal mask.
4. *Insert the LMA with the cuff tip gliding against the posterior pharyngeal wall.
5. *Using your index finger to push the LMA, apply slight backward (toward the ears) pressure and follow the anatomic curve.
6. *Advance the mask until resistance is noted at the hypopharynx (Figure 7-3).
7. *Remove the index finger while applying slight pressure to the airway tube for the prevention of dislocation (Figure 7-4).
8. *Inflate the cuff with air; the volume varies with the LMA size (see Table 7-1). During inflation, release the LMA to ensure that placement is maintained as the cuff expands.

---

*Indicates portion of the procedure usually performed by a physician or an advanced practice nurse.

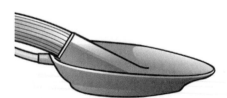

FIGURE 7-2 LMA cuff properly deflated for insertion. (Courtesy of LMA North America, Inc.)

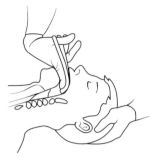

FIGURE 7-3 Maintaining pressure with the finger on the tube in the cranial direction, advance the mask until definite resistance is felt at the base of the hypopharynx. (Courtesy of LMA North America, Inc.)

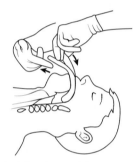

FIGURE 7-4 Hold the outer end of the airway while removing the index finger. (Courtesy of LMA North America, Inc.)

   9. Assess the LMA placement. The following signs indicate an appropriate placement:
     a. A slight outward movement of the airway tube with cuff inflation
     b. A slight swelling at the cricoid region
     c. No visible cuff in the oral cavity
     d. Equal bilateral breath sounds and chest rise and fall
     e. Pulse oximetry readings that indicate adequate oxygenation
10. Ventilate the patient with a bag-valve and supplemental oxygen.
11. Secure the LMA with tape or a securing device; a bite block may be used (LMA, 2005).

Intubating LMA (Fastrach)
1. *Deflate the cuff of the mask and apply a water-soluble lubricant to the posterior surface. Distribute the lubricant over the anterior hard palate.
2. *Place the curved metal tube in contact with the chin and the mask tip flat against the palate before advancing.

---

*Indicates portion of the procedure usually performed by a physician or an advanced practice nurse.

3. *Rotate the mask into place with a circular motion, maintaining pressure against the palate and the posterior pharynx.
4. *Inflate the mask. Without holding the tube or handle, inflate cuff to a pressure of 60 cm H_2O (Murphy, 2004).

Intubating through the intubating LMA (Fastrach)
(LMA, 2005; Murphy, 2004)

LMA North America educational literature states that the Fastrach should be used in situations when blind intubation is anticipated. The *LMA Instruction Manual* states the success rate using the LMA Classic varies from 20% to 100% depending on the person's skill and experience (LMA North America, 2005).

1. *Validate endotracheal tube (ETT) cuff integrity.
2. *Deflate the ETT cuff, lubricate the ETT, and pass it through the intubating LMA tube. Rotate and move the ETT up and down to ensure adequate distribution of water-soluble lubricant.
3. *Advance the ETT to the 15-cm depth indicator. This position signifies passage of the tip of the ETT through the epiglottic opening of the LMA.
4. *Use the handle to gently lift the device 2 to 5 cm. A slight resistance is felt as the ETT is advanced.
5. *Advance until intubation is complete.
6. Inflate the ETT cuff and confirm intubation (see Procedure 8).
7. *Remove the LMA. Remove the ETT connector, and gently ease the intubating LMA out over the ETT into the oral cavity while using the stabilizer rod to hold ETT in position as the LMA is pulled over the tube.
8. *Remove the stabilizer rod and hold onto the ETT at the level of the incisors.
9. *Remove the LMA completely.
10. Replace the ETT connector.
11. Confirm tube placement (see Procedure 8).

---

*Indicates portion of the procedure usually performed by a physician or an advanced practice nurse.

AGE-SPECIFIC CONSIDERATIONS

An appropriately sized LMA is effective for use in infants and children of all weights (see Table 7-1) (LMA, 2006; Luten and Kissoon, 2004). When intubation of the pediatric patient is not possible, the LMA is acceptable for use by skilled providers (AHA, 2005) and LMAs are used routinely with pediatric patients in the surgery suite.

COMPLICATIONS (LMA, 2003; Vrocher & Hopson, 2004; Walls, 2006)

1. Air leak
2. Laryngospasm
3. Desaturation
4. Severe hypercarbia
5. Regurgitation, aspiration
6. Sore throat

7. Laryngeal hematoma
8. Hypoglossal nerve injury

REFERENCES

American Heart Association (AHA). (2005). American Heart Association guidelines for cardio-pulmonary resuscitation and emergency cardiovascular care. *Circulation, 112*(suppl. IV). Available on-line at www.circulationaha.org

Brain, A. I. J., Verghese, C. & Strube, P. J. (2000). The LMA ProSeal: A laryngeal mask with an oesophageal vent. *British Journal of Anaesthesia, 84*(5), 650-654.

LMA North America (2005). *Airway instruction manual.* Retrieved December, 13, 2006, from http://www.lmana.com/prod/components/education_center/instructions_for_use.html

Luten, R. & Kissoon, N. (2004). Pediatric airway management. In R. Walls, M. Murphy, R. Luten, & R. Schneider (Eds.), *Manual of emergency airway management* (2nd ed., pp. 212-227). Philadelphia: Lippincott Williams & Wilkins.

Murphy, M. (2004). Laryngeal mask airway. In R. Walls, M. Murphy, R. Luten, & R. Schneider (Eds.), *Manual of emergency airway management* (2nd ed., pp. 97-109). Philadelphia: Lippincott Williams & Wilkins.

Pollack, C. (2001). The laryngeal mask airway: A comprehensive review for the emergency physician. *Journal of Emergency Medicine, 20*(1), 53-66.

Vrocher, D. & Hopson, L. (2004). Basic airway management and decision-making. In J. R. Roberts, & J. R. Hedges (Eds.), *Clinical procedures in emergency medicine* (4th ed., pp. 53-68). Philadelphia: Saunders.

Walls, R. M. (2006). Airway. In J. A. Marx, R. S. Hockberger, & R. M. Walls (Eds.), *Rosen's emergency medicine: Concepts and clinical practice* (6th ed., pp. 2-26). Philadelphia: Mosby.

PROCEDURE 8

General Principles of Endotracheal Intubation

Donna York Clark, RN, MS, CFRN, CMTE

Endotracheal intubation refers to the procedure of inserting a tube directly into the trachea. The endotracheal (ET) tube (ETT) may be placed through the nose or the mouth. Methods of insertion include visual (using laryngoscopy), blind (through the nose), digital (also blind), or facilitated using a flexible fiberoptic bronchoscope, the Eschmann tracheal tube introducer, a gum elastic bougie, or a lighted stylet. Details of oral and nasal intubation procedures are included in Procedures 10 and 11.

INDICATION

The purpose of intubation is to secure a patent and effective airway. Intubation is the preferred means of airway control because it has the following benefits:

1. Protects the trachea and lungs from aspiration of gastric contents, saliva, or blood and fluid into the upper airway (Vrocher & Hopson, 2004).
2. Provides an airway for mechanical ventilation in the presence of failure of ventilation or oxygenation (Walls, 2004).
3. Allows direct access to the lungs for removal or suctioning of secretions (Walls, 2004).
4. Allows tracheal administration of emergency medications for rapid absorption through the pulmonary tree (AHA, 2005).

CONTRAINDICATIONS AND CAUTIONS

1. There are no absolute contraindications to endotracheal intubation; however, the procedure should be considered carefully when it is performed in a patient with any of the following (Lutes & Hopson, 2004; Vrocher & Hopson 2004; Walls, 2004):
   a. Intact gag reflex
   b. Potential or actual cervical spine injury
   c. Head trauma, increased intracranial pressure, or both
   d. Facial fractures
2. Epiglottitis complicates any intubation attempt because of the potential for laryngospasm and complete airway obstruction. Ideally, intubation of the patient with epiglottitis should be performed in the most controlled setting with the most skilled intubator. Contingency planning should include set-up for the performance of a surgical airway.
3. Specific precautions exist for each method of endotracheal intubation. These are discussed in the procedures devoted to nasal and oral intubation.

EQUIPMENT

Endotracheal tubes
  • 2.5 to 5 mm, uncuffed; 4.5 to 9 mm, cuffed
Laryngoscope handle
Laryngoscope blades
  • Curved (sizes 2 to 4)
  • Straight (sizes 1 to 4)
Stylets to fit each size of endotracheal tube
10-ml syringe for inflating the cuff of the tube
Lubricating or lidocaine jelly for nasal intubation
Benzocaine, cocaine, or phenylephrine hydrochloride (Neo-Synephrine) drops or spray for nasal intubation (optional)
Medications as prescribed for paralysis and sedation (see Procedure 9)
Tube-securing device (commercially manufactured device or tape)
Stethoscope
Adjuncts as indicated, e.g., bronchoscope, lighted stylet, or elastic gum bougie

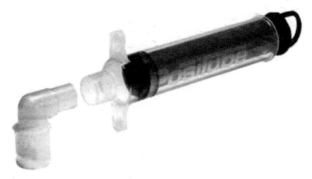

FIGURE 8-1 Flotec Esophageal Detector Device. (Courtesy of Flotec, Inc, Indianapolis, IN.)

Bag-mask device with reservoir connected to 100% oxygen
Additional supportive equipment:
- Suction, complete with tonsil and catheter tips
- Extra laryngoscope bulbs and batteries
- End-tidal carbon dioxide detector for tube position confirmation (optional)
- Esophageal detector device for tube position confirmation (optional) (Figure 8-1)
- Pulse oximeter to monitor oxygen saturation during intubation and to help confirm tube placement (optional)
- Limb restraints (optional)

PATIENT PREPARATION
1. Preoxygenate the patient with 100% oxygen by using a nonrebreather oxygen mask or a bag-mask device as indicated.
2. Administer sedatives, paralytic agents, or topical anesthesia as prescribed (see Procedure 9, Rapid Sequence Intubation).
3. Restrain the patient as indicated to prevent inadvertent extubation.

PROCEDURAL STEPS
Intubate
The specific steps of intubation depend on the method of insertion used. See Procedures 10 and 11 for specific directions for oral and nasal intubation.

Confirm Tube Placement
No single confirmation technique is completely reliable; therefore, both clinical assessment and other methods should be used to assess appropriate tube placement immediately after insertion as well as after moving the intubated patient (AHA, 2005; Walls, 2004).
1. *Epigastric sounds/chest rise:* With the first ventilation, auscultate over the epigastric area while observing for chest rise (AHA, 2005). The presence of burping sounds over the epigastrium in the absence of chest rise suggests esophageal placement. Remove the tube immediately, and reoxygenate the patient before attempting intubation again.

2. *Breath sounds:* Auscultate the right and left axilla, and then the right and left anterior chest for equal bilateral breath sounds. Unilaterally absent or decreased breath sounds (usually on the left) suggest that the tube was advanced into a mainstem bronchus. Withdraw the tube slightly and reassess until breath sounds are equal bilaterally.

3. *End-tidal carbon dioxide detection and/or monitoring* also helps confirm tube placement (see Procedure 24). These devices are recommended as a secondary technique of tube confirmation in patients with adequate perfusion (AHA, 2005). If the patient is poorly perfused or in cardiac arrest, there may be minimal CO_2 expiration even when the tube is properly placed.

4. *Esophageal detector devices:* These devices are attached to the ETT, and suction is applied with a bulb or syringe device. If the ETT is in the esophagus, the tissue will collapse around the tube when suction is applied and there will be resistance to filling of the bulb or syringe. If the ETT is in the trachea, the bulb or syringe will fill with air easily. These devices are recommended for secondary confirmation of tube placement for the adolescent or adult patient in cardiac arrest (AHA, 2005).

5. *Direct visualization* of the tube passing through the cords with the laryngoscope.

6. *Bag compliance:* Ventilation of the stomach is easier than ventilation of the lungs, whereas tube obstruction, bronchospasm, or tension pneumothorax makes ventilation more difficult.

7. *Condensation in the ETT* on exhalation suggests that the tube is positioned in the trachea.

8. *Transillumination of the neck using a lighted stylet:* If the neck glows after intubation with the lighted stylet, the tube is placed correctly in the trachea (Murphy & Hung, 2004).

9. *Pulse oximetry:* Maintenance of adequate oxygen saturation helps confirm tube placement.

10. *Presence of gastric contents in the ETT:* Material resembling food present in the tube may indicate esophageal intubation.

11. *Cuff palpation* may be used to verify the appropriate placement within the trachea in reference to the carina and the bronchi. After the cuff is inflated, and with the patient's head in a neutral position, gently palpate at the suprasternal notch while holding the pilot balloon in your other hand. Advance or withdraw the tube slightly. When the pilot balloon is maximally distended in response to pressure at the suprasternal notch, the tube is appropriately positioned within the trachea (Kaur & Heard, 2003; Pollard & Lobato, 1995).

12. *Chest radiographic* documentation of the tube location in the trachea just above the carina.

Secure the Endotracheal Tube

To prevent inadvertant extubation, the ETT must be secured carefully. Although several techniques can be used for this maneuver, many principles apply to all of them:

1. A bite block or oral airway should be inserted after oral intubation to prevent the patient from biting the tube and occluding the airway.

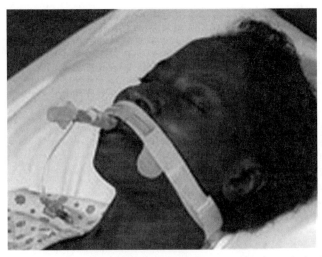

FIGURE 8-2   Dale Stabilock endotracheal tube holder. (Courtesy of Dale Medical, Plainville, MA.)

2. To allow suctioning and mouth care, the mouth must not be completely occluded by tape or other devices.
3. The method used should prevent the inadvertant advancement or withdrawal of the tube.
4. When possible, the method used should minimize pressure points on the skin to prevent long-term complications.
5. When tape is used, it should encircle the head completely for maximum security.
6. When possible, the markings on the tube should be noted at the patient's teeth and documented so that movement of the tube can be checked visually.
7. The commonly used methods include commercial tube-securing devices (follow the manufacturer's directions) or tape (Figure 8-2). Apply tape as follows:
   a. Tear off approximately 24 inches of 1-inch adhesive tape.
   b. Split the tape in half for the last 4 inches at each end.
   c. Slide the tape under the middle of the neck, adhesive side up.
   d. Bring each end of the tape alongside the patient's head and wrap the split ends securely around the tube. Split the tape farther if necessary.
8. Reconfirm the tube position after it has been secured.

AGE-SPECIFIC CONSIDERATIONS

1. Several methods exist for estimating the correct tube size (Table 8-1), usually based on age and weight. Other methods include the following:
   a. Estimates based on the size of the patient's little finger: Men usually require a 7.5- to 9-mm tube, whereas women usually require a 7- to 8-mm tube. Nasal intubation generally requires a tube that is 0.5 to 1 mm smaller than the tube used for oral intubation (Lutes & Hopson, 2004).

TABLE 8-1
USUAL ENDOTRACHEAL TUBE SIZE BY AGE AND WEIGHT

Age	Weight (kg)	Endotracheal Tube Size (internal diameter)
Premature	1.5-2	3
Newborn-3 months	3–6	3.5
6-12 months	7–10	4
2 years	12	5
4 years	16	5.5
6 years	20	6
8 years	25	6.5
10 years	34	6.5
12 years	40	6.5-7
14 years	50	7

   b. The following formula may be used to calculate the appropriately sized ETT for children aged 2 years or older (Cole, 1957; Luten & Kissoon, 2004):

$$(16 + \text{age in years})/4 = \text{ETT size}$$

2. The depth to which the ETT should be advanced into the trachea varies with the age and size of the patient. Adult women require an average depth (from the central incisors) of 21 cm, and adult men require 23 cm (Lutes & Hopson, 2004). The following formula estimates the required length of the oral tracheal tube from lip to midtrachea for children (Luten & Kissoon, 2004):

   Tracheal tube depth (cm) = Internal diameter of the tube $\times 3$

3. Oral intubation is the preferred method for intubation in the pediatric population (Luten & Kissoon, 2004).

4. Children younger than age 8 are generally intubated with uncuffed ETTs (Luten & Kissoon, 2004). The narrowest region of the airway in children is the cricoid cartilage. This area forms a physiologic cuff around the uncuffed ETT (Luten & Kissoon, 2004). In the hospital setting, cuffed tubes may be used in infants beyond the newborn period and in young children. The cuff pressure should be kept at less than 20 cm H2O. In the pediatric patient with poor lung compliance or high airway resistance, the cuffed tube may be necessary in order to provide adequate ventilation (AHA, 2005).

5. In infants and small children, transmittal of breath sounds across the chest may result in "equal" breath sounds, even in the presence of mainstem bronchus intubation or pneumothorax. A chest radiograph is indicated to help ascertain appropriate position of the tube.

6. Take care to maintain neutral head position in intubated infants and toddlers. Because the airway is shorter and the tubes are uncuffed in this population, head movement may result in significant tube movement. Flexion may

withdraw the tube, resulting in extubation. Extension may advance the tube into the right mainstem bronchus.

7. Esophageal detector devices are unreliable in children less than 1 year old, morbidly obese patients, and patients in late pregnancy. There is insufficient evidence to support their use in children younger than age 1 at this time (AHA, 2005).

8. In infants and children with a perfusing rhythm, assessing end-tidal CO_2 via a colorimetric device or capnography should be used to confirm tube placement. Appropriately sized colorimetric devices can be used on any patient weighing over 2 kg (AHA, 2005).

COMPLICATIONS

1. Esophageal intubation: This is a serious complication, because the patient's lungs are not ventilated and gastric distention may occur. Gastric distention increases the risk of vomiting and may decrease the tidal volume.

2. Dislodgment of the tube: Frequent reassessment of the tube position is necessary, especially after the patient is moved.

3. Damage to teeth, nasal mucosa, posterior pharynx, or larynx (depending on the method of insertion) may occur.

PATIENT TEACHING

1. You will not be able to speak while the tube is in place.
2. Swallowing may help diminish gagging.
3. Do not move or manipulate the tube in any way.

REFERENCES

American Heart Association (AHA). (2005). American Heart Association guidelines for cardiopulmonary resuscitation and emergency cardiovascular care. *Circulation, 112*(suppl. IV).

Cole, F. (1957). Pediatric formulas for the anesthesiologist. *American Journal of Disease in Children, 94*, 472.

Kaur, S. & Heard, S. O. (2003). Airway management and endotracheal intubation. In R. S. Irwin, & J. M. Rippe (Eds.), *Irwin and Rippe's intensive care medicine* (5th ed., pp. 4-16). Philadelphia: Lippincott Williams & Wilkins.

Luten, R. C. & Kissoon, N. (2004). Approach to the pediatric airway. In R. Walls, M. Murphy, R. Luten & R. Schneider (Eds.), *Manual of emergency airway management* (2nd ed., pp. 212-227). Philadelphia: Lippincott Williams & Wilkins.

Lutes, M. & Hopson, L. R. (2004). Tracheal intubation. In J. R. Roberts, & J. R. Hedges (Eds.), *Clinical procedures in emergency medicine* (4th ed., pp. 69-99). Philadelphia: Saunders.

Murphy, M. & Hung, O. (2004). Lighted stylet intubation. In R. Walls, M. Murphy, R. Luten, & R. Schneider (Eds.), *Manual of emergency airway management* (2nd ed., pp. 120-126). Philadelphia: Lippincott Williams & Wilkins.

Pollard, R. J. & Lobato, E. B. (1995). Endotracheal tube location verified reliably by cuff palpation. *Anesthesia and Analgesia, 81*, 135-138.

Vrocher, D. & Hopson, L. (2004). Basic airway management and decision-making. In J. R. Roberts, & J. R. Hedges (Eds.), *Clinical procedures in emergency medicine* (4th ed., pp. 53-68). Philadelphia: Saunders.

Walls, R. (2004). The decision to intubate. In R. Walls, M. Murphy, R. Luten, & R. Schneider (Eds.), *Manual of emergency airway management* (2nd ed., pp. 1-7). Philadelphia: Lippincott Williams & Wilkins.

Rapid Sequence Intubation

Donna York Clark, RN, MS, CFRN, CMTE

The information in this procedure should be used in conjunction with the information in Procedures 8 and 10.

Rapid sequence intubation is also known as *RSI, crash intubation, paralytic intubation,* and *neuromuscular blockade intubation.*

INDICATIONS

1. To facilitate intubation of a critically ill or injured patient when the ability of the patient to protect his or her airway is in question and trismus or a gag reflex is present (Walls, 2004).
2. To augment intubation of combative head-injured patients (Semonin-Holleran, 2003).
3. To minimize the risk of aspiration in non-fasting patients with complex airway emergencies (Walls, 2004).

CONTRAINDICATIONS AND CAUTIONS

1. Neuromuscular blocking agents (NMBAs) are the foundation of emergency airway management. They allow placement of the oral endotracheal tube while minimizing potential complications, such as aspiration. There are two classes of NMBAs. One class is the noncompetitive depolarizing agents, of which succinylcholine is the most common. The second class is the competitive, nondepolarizing NMBAs, which is made up of two categories of agents: benzylisoquinolone compounds and aminosteroid compounds. Benzylisoquinolone compounds include atracurium and mivacurium, and aminosteroid compounds include vecuronium, pancuronium, and rocuronium (Schneider & Caro, 2004b).
2. The most common method of RSI uses succinylcholine. Succinylcholine is absolutely contraindicated in patients who have a family history of malignant hyperthermia, burn injuries that are greater than 24 hours old, or crush injuries greater than 7 days old. These patients are at risk for developing life-threatening hyperkalemia (Schneider & Caro, 2004b). There are many other conditions in which succinylcholine must be given with care, if at all. Consult a pharmacist or medication reference material for details.
3. Penetrating eye injuries are considered relative contraindications to RSI because of the increased intraocular pressure resulting from some of the medications; alternatives may need to be considered (Schneider & Caro, 2004b; Kelly et al., 1993).
4. RSI requires rapid administration of several medications. Keeping the medications, needles, and syringes together in a kit facilitates rapid administration. Box 9-1 lists a sample kit inventory.

BOX 9-1
SAMPLE LIST OF RSI CONTENTS

MEDICATIONS
- Atropine 1-mg prefilled syringe
- Lidocaine 100-mg prefilled syringe
- Succinylcholine 200-mg vial
- Vecuronium 10-mg vial
- Sterile water 10-ml vial
- Rocuronium 50-mg vial
- Etomidate 40-mg vial
- Normal saline 10-ml vial

SYRINGES/NEEDLES
- 5-ml syringes with attached needle
- 10-ml syringes
- 18-G needles
- Syringe caps

MISCELLANEOUS
- Alcohol wipes
- Medication labels for each medication
- RSI worksheets

Courtesy of Dartmouth-Hitchcock Medical Center Emergency Department, Lebanon, NH.

EQUIPMENT (Walls, 2004; Schneider & Caro, 2004a; Schneider & Caro, 2004b; Schneider & Caro, 2004c)

Endotracheal intubation and ventilation supplies (see Procedure 8)

Cricothyrotomy supplies (see Procedure 15)

Syringes and needles

Premedication(s) (Schneider & Caro, 2004a):
- Lidocaine (1.5 mg/kg) 3 minutes before induction
- Fentanyl (3 mcg/kg) 3 minutes before intubation in all who will be negatively impacted by the systemic catecholamine release caused with the intubation
- Atropine (0.02 mg/kg) 3 minutes before induction for all children 10 years of age or younger
- Some sources suggest a defasciculating dose of a competitive neuromuscular blocking agent; e.g., 10% of the paralyzing dose of vecuronium, pancuronium, or rocuronium 3 minutes prior to induction in patients who will be receiving succinylcholine except in children

Induction agent(s) (Schneider & Caro, 2004b):
- Thiopental (3–6 mg/kg)
- Midazolam (0.2–0.3 mg/kg)
- Etomidate (0.3 mg/kg)
- Methohexital (1–3 mg/kg)

Neuromuscular blocking agent(s) (Schneider & Caro, 2004c):
- Succinylcholine (1.5–2 mg/kg)
- Vecuronium (0.15 mg/kg)
- Rocuronium (1 mg/kg)

PATIENT PREPARATION

1. Complete a brief neurologic assessment.
2. Maintain the patient in a supine position with spinal stabilization, if indicated.
3. Preoxygenate the patient with 100% oxygen. Deliver assisted ventilation in coordination with patient efforts. Avoid vigorous bag-mask ventilation to

prevent gastric distention, which increases the risk of vomiting and aspiration.
4. Initiate an intravenous line (see Procedure 60).
5. Attach oxygen saturation and cardiac monitors (see Procedures 21 and 55).
6. Draw up all pharmacologic agents in individual syringes and label clearly. A worksheet can help with dosing and sequencing of medications. See Figure 9-1 for a sample worksheet.

PROCEDURAL STEPS (Walls, 2004; Hopson & Dronen, 2004)
1. Administer premedications as prescribed:
   a. Give lidocaine to attenuate the increase in intracranial pressure associated with intubation. Lidocaine is usually used in patients with head injuries (Walls, 2004). Administer the lidocaine approximately 3 minutes before administering succinylcholine.
   b. Give atropine to minimize the bradycardic impact of succinylcholine for children younger than 10 years of age (Schneider & Caro, 2004a) or bradycardic adults.

Rapid Sequence Intubation Worksheet

Estimated Patient Weight_____
All medications are given IV.

Pre-treatment Agents
3 minutes before induction

Lidocaine (1.5 mg/kg)	_____mg
Fentanyl (3 mcg/kg)	_____mcg
Atropine (0.02 mg/kg)	_____mg

Patients younger than age 10 undergoing RSI with succinylcholine

Defasciculating dose _____mg
10% of the paralytic dose of a non-depolarizing agent vecuronium, rocuronium or pancuronium. Not used in children.

Sedation

Thiopental (3-6 mg/kg)	_____mg
Midazolam (0.2-0.3 mg/kg)	_____mg
Etomidate (0.3 mg/kg)	_____mg

Not studied in children younger than age 10

| Ketamine (1-2 mg/kg) | _____mg |
| Methohexital (1-3 mg/kg) | _____mg |

Paralysis

Succinylcholine (1.5-2 mg/kg)	_____mg
Vecuronium (0.15 mg/kg)	_____mg
Rocuronium (1 mg/kg)	_____mg

FIGURE 9-1 RSI worksheet. (Courtesy of Dartmouth-Hitchcock Medical Center Emergency Department, Lebanon, NH.)

    c. Give vecuronium or another nondepolarizing paralytic agent at one tenth of the paralytic dose. This is a defasciculating dose and may be used for adolescent and adult patients when succinylcholine is the prescribed paralytic.

2. As soon as the defasciculating dose is administered or the patient begins to lose consciousness (Hopson & Dronen, 2004), apply cricoid pressure, that is, the Sellick maneuver.

    a. Cricoid pressure is applied by placing your thumb and index finger on the cricoid cartilage.

    b. Firmly press the cricoid cartilage backward to occlude the esophagus. This helps prevent regurgitation and may improve visualization of the vocal cords.

    c. Maintain cricoid pressure throughout the procedure until the endotracheal tube placement is verified and the cuff is inflated.

3. Administer the induction agent of choice.

4. Administer the neuromuscular blocking agent of choice.

5. *Perform laryngoscopy and intubate the trachea.

6. Verify the endotracheal tube placement, inflate the cuff, and ventilate the patient with 100% oxygen while manually maintaining the tube placement (see Procedure 8).

7. Release the cricoid pressure. Have suction immediately available in case of regurgitation when the cricoid pressure is released.

8. Secure the endotracheal tube.

9. Assure adequate sedation/analgesia in conjunction with NMBAs.

10. Decompress the stomach with a gastric tube (see Procedure 98).

11. If intubation is unsuccessful and an alternative airway must be established, consider a laryngeal mask airway (see Procedure 7), needle cricothyrotomy (see Procedure 16), or surgical cricothyrotomy (see Procedure 15) (Murphy, 2004).

AGE-SPECIFIC CONSIDERATIONS

1. Most sources recommend that children younger than age 11 receive premedication with atropine to prevent bradycardia associated with intubation and the administration of RSI agents (Schneider & Caro, 2004a; Luten & Kissoon, 2004).

2. A defasciculating dose of a nondepolarizing paralytic agent is not used in children because dosing errors may result in earlier than intended paralysis.

3. Uncuffed endotracheal tubes are recommended for children younger than age 8 in many sources (Luten & Kissoon, 2004). In the 2005 AHA/AAP Pediatric Advanced Life Support guidelines, cuffed endotracheal tubes are suggested for children age 1 and older in hospital settings provided that the tube cuff pressure is maintained at less than 20 cm H_2O (AHA, 2005).

4. Surgical cricothyrotomy is not recommended in children younger than age 12 because of the small size of the cricothyroid membrane; needle cricothyrotomy is the procedure of choice (Vissers & Bair, 2004).

---

*Indicates portions of the procedure usually performed by a physician or an advanced practice nurse.

COMPLICATIONS

Complications are related to the medications administered or to the intubation procedure (see Procedure 8). Vasodilation results from many of the medications and may result in profound hypotension, especially in the hemodynamically unstable patient.

PATIENT TEACHING

1. We have given you medications that relax your muscles temporarily so the machine can breathe for you. We are here to take care of you and keep you safe.
2. Reassure the family that the patient's paralysis and any new decrease in level of consciousness the desired effect of the medications.
3. See Procedure 8.

REFERENCES

American Heart Association. (2005). Guidelines for cardiopulmonary resuscitation (CPR) and emergency cardiovascular care (ECC) of pediatric and neonatal patients. *Pediatrics, 117,* 989-1004.

Hopson, R. L. & Dronen, S. (2004). Pharmacologic adjuncts to intubation. In J. R. Robert, & J. R. Hedges (Eds.), *Clinical procedures in emergency medicine* (4th ed., pp. 100-114). Philadelphia: Saunders.

Kelly, R. E., et al. (1993). Succinylcholine increases intraocular pressure in the human eye with extraocular muscles detached. *Anesthesiology, 79,* 948-952.

Luten, R. & Kissoon, N. (2004). The difficult pediatric airway. In R. Walls, M. Murphy, R. Luten, & R. Schneider (Eds.), *Manual of emergency airway management* (2nd ed., pp. 236-244). Philadelphia: Lippincott Williams & Wilkins.

Murphy, M. (2004). Laryngeal mask airways. In R. Walls, M. Murphy, R Luten, & R. Schneider (Eds.), *Manual of emergency airway management* (2nd ed., pp. 97-109). Philadelphia: Lippincott Williams & Wilkins.

Schneider, R. & Caro, D. A. (2004a). Pretreatment agents. In R. Walls, M. Murphy, R. Luten, & R. Schneider (Eds.), *Manual of emergency airway management* (2nd ed., pp. 181-188). Philadelphia: Lippincott Williams & Wilkins.

Schneider, R. & Caro, D. A. (2004b). Sedatives and induction agents. In R. Walls, M. Murphy, R. Luten, & R. Schneider (Eds.), *Manual of emergency airway management* (2nd ed., pp. 189-198). Philadelphia: Lippincott Williams & Wilkins.

Schneider, R. & Caro, D. A. (2004c). Neuromuscular blocking agents. In R. Walls, M. Murphy, R. Luten, & R. Schneider (Eds.), *Manual of emergency airway management* (2nd ed., pp. 200-211). Philadelphia: Lippincott Williams & Wilkins.

Semonin-Holleran, R. (2003). *Air and surface patient transport: Principles and practice* (3rd ed). St. Louis: Mosby.

Vissers, R., & Bair, A. (2004). Surgical airway techniques. In R. Walls, M. Murphy, R. Luten, & R. Schneider (Eds.), *Manual of emergency airway management* (2nd ed., pp. 158-182). Philadelphia: Lippincott Williams & Wilkins.

Walls, R. (2004). Rapid sequence intubation. In R. Walls, M. Murphy, R. Luten, & R. Schneider (Eds.), *Manual of emergency airway management* (2nd ed., pp. 22-31). Philadelphia: Lippincott Williams & Wilkins.

Oral Endotracheal Intubation

Donna York Clark, RN, MS, CFRN, CMTE

The information in this procedure should be used in conjunction with the information found in Procedure 8.

INDICATIONS

To place an endotracheal tube (ETT) via the mouth. The oral route is usually used for comatose, apneic, sedated, or chemically paralyzed patients. Indications include the following:
1. To maintain an adequate, patent airway
2. To facilitate mechanical ventilation
3. To provide a route for pulmonary secretion evacuation
4. To provide a route for medication administration for a patient in cardiac arrest

CONTRAINDICATIONS AND CAUTIONS

There are no absolute contraindications to oral intubation; however, the procedure should be considered carefully if performed when the patient has either of the following:
1. An intact gag reflex.
2. Potential or actual cervical spine injury. Laryngoscopy is known to cause spinal movement (Aprahamian et al., 1984). Many studies have examined the impact of orotracheal intubation on cervical spine movement and resulting neurologic sequelae. No conclusive data have been published that clearly state the safety of endotracheal intubation in the presence of a cervical spinal injury, but there is literature supporting the safety of this procedure (Schneider & Murphy, 2004).

EQUIPMENT

See Procedure 8.

PATIENT PREPARATION

1. Place the patient in the supine position with the head in the sniffing position unless there is a potential cervical spine injury. Provide manual stabilization of the head if spinal movement is contraindicated.
2. If necessary for an apneic or hypoventilating patient, initiate oxygenation with 100% oxygen using a bag-mask (see Procedure 33).
3. Apply cardiac and oxygen saturation monitors (see Procedures 21 and 55).
4. Administer sedative, paralytic agents, or topical anesthesia as prescribed (see Procedure 9).

5. Restrain the patient as indicated to prevent inadvertent extubation (see Procedure 190).

PROCEDURAL STEPS

1. Ensure that all larnygoscopic equipment is in appropriate working order. Inflate the ETT cuff to test for air leaks and deflate after testing.
2. Insert the stylet into the ETT and apply a water-soluble lubricant to allow easy advancement of the tube. Confirm appropriate placement of the stylet within the ETT. Ensure that the stylet has not been advanced beyond the end of the tube.
3. Turn on the suction and place the tonsil-tip suction next to the patient's head.
4. *Insert the laryngoscope with the left hand. The patient's tongue should be swept to the left side and the laryngoscope inserted and lifted up and away from the intubator (Figure 10-1). Do not rock the laryngoscope against the patient's teeth or gums. Advance the laryngoscope blade under the epiglottis when using a straight blade or into the vallecula when using a curved blade.
5. *Visualize the epiglottis and the vocal cords (Figure 10-2).
6. If the cords are not visible, downward cricoid pressure (also known as the Sellick maneuver) may move the glottis into view (Schneider & Murphy, 2004). This maneuver is performed by placing the index finger and thumb on the cricoid membrane and applying posterior pressure to occlude the esophagus. The cricoid pressure may also prevent aspiration of emesis by occluding the esophagus during intubation (Sellick, 1961). If applied, cricoid pressure should be maintained until tube placement is verified and the cuff inflated.
7. *Using the right hand, pass the ETT through the cords. The tube should be advanced until the cuff moves forward 1 to 2 cm through the cords.
8. *Remove the laryngoscope while maintaining a grip on the ETT to keep it in place.
9. *Remove the stylet.
10. The gum elastic bougie is an aid for oral intubation, especially if difficulty is encountered during the initial attempts with a laryngoscope.
    a. The bougie is a solid or hollow, partially malleable stylet that serves as an introducer for the ETT. The bougie helps the intubator manipulate the ETT when the larnyx cannot be visualized during laryngoscopy (Rosenblatt, 2006).
    b. The ETT is threaded over the bougie and advanced into the trachea. The bougie extends beyond the ETT and is more easily manipulated to enter the trachea.
    c. Once the bougie is placed between the vocal cords, the ETT is advanced and positioned normally.
    d. Once the ETT is in position, the bougie is then removed and the tube assessed and secured as usual.

---

*Indicates portions of the procedure usually performed by a physician or an advanced practice nurse.

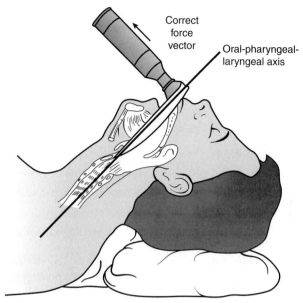

FIGURE 10-1 The laryngoscope is lifted up and away from the intubator to align the airway structures.

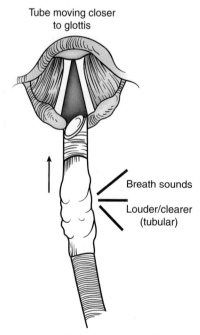

FIGURE 10-2 After the cords are visualized, the tube should be advanced through the cords until the cuff disappears.

11. Verify correct ETT placement, and secure the tube as described in Procedure 8.
12. Inflate the cuff and instill air until an adequate seal is attained; 10 to 15 ml of air is usually required. Ventilate the patient with 100% oxygen.

AGE-SPECIFIC CONSIDERATION

Oral intubation is the preferred method of intubation in the pediatric population (Luten & Kissoon, 2004).

COMPLICATIONS

See Procedure 8.

PATIENT TEACHING

See Procedure 8.

REFERENCES

Aprahamian, C., et al. (1984). Experimental cervical spine injury model: Evaluation of airway management and splinting techniques. *Annals of Emergency Medicine, 13*, 584-587.

Luten, R. C. & Kissoon, N. (2004). Approach to the pediatric airway. In R. Walls, M. Murphy, R. Luten, & R. Schneider (Eds.), *Manual of emergency airway management* (2nd ed., pp. 212-235). Philadelphia: Lippincott Williams & Wilkins.

Rosenblatt, W. H. (2006). Airway management. In P. G. Barash, B. F. Cullen, & R. K. Stoelting (Eds.), *Clinical anesthesia* (5th ed., pp. 596-642). Philadelphia: Lippincott Williams & Wilkins.

Schneider, R. E. & Murphy, M. (2004). Bag/mask ventilation and endotracheal intubation. In R. Walls, M. Murphy, R. Luten, & R. Schneider (Eds.), *Manual of emergency airway management* (2nd ed., pp. 43-69). Philadelphia: Lippincott Williams & Wilkins.

Sellick, B. A. (1961). Cricoid pressure to control regurgitation of stomach contents during induction of anesthesia. *Lancet, 2*, 404-408.

PROCEDURE 11

Nasotracheal Intubation

Donna York Clark, RN, MS, CFRN, CMTE

The information in this procedure should be used in conjunction with the information in Procedure 8.

Nasotracheal intubation is also known as *blind nasotracheal intubation* or *BNT*.

INDICATION

To place an endotracheal tube (ETT) via the nose in a patient with spontaneous respirations. Nasotracheal intubation is becoming obsolete and is being replaced by other emergency airway management techniques that result in higher success rates and fewer complications (Murphy, 2004). Alternate emergency airway management strategies include using supraglottic adjuncts such as the Combitube and the laryngeal mask airway or orotracheal intubation facilitated by neuromuscular blockade (Godwin, 2004).

CONTRAINDICATIONS AND CAUTIONS

The only absolute contraindication to blind nasotracheal intubation is apnea. Relative contraindications include the following:

1. Suspected facial, nasal, or basilar skull fractures. Many sources cite head trauma as a contraindication to nasal intubation because of concerns that the ETT will pass through the cribriform plate into the brain (Reichman, 2005). However, there is only one documented case of ETT penetration into the brain (Horellou et al., 1978).
2. Concurrent coagulopathy, anticoagulant therapy, or thrombolytic therapy, which increases the risk of epistaxis (Murphy, 2004).
3. Obstructions of the nose or posterior nasopharynx, including trauma, tumor, and foreign body (Murphy, 2004; Skouteris et al., 2002).

EQUIPMENT

See Procedure 8; note that no laryngoscope or stylet is used with this technique.

PATIENT PREPARATION

1. Place the patient in the supine position, with the head in the sniffing position unless there is a potential cervical spine injury. Provide manual stabilization of the head if spinal movement is contraindicated.
2. Initiate preoxygenation with 100% oxygen via nonrebreather mask or bag-mask (see Procedures 25 and 33). Avoid bag-mask ventilation when spontaneous ventilations are ample because air may be forced into the stomach and increase the risk of regurgitation (Godwin, 2004; Reichman, 2005).
3. Apply cardiac and oxygen saturation monitors (see Procedures 21 and 55).
4. Administer sedatives or topical anesthesia as prescribed.
5. Restrain the patient as indicated to prevent inadvertant extubation (see Procedure 190).

PROCEDURAL STEPS

1. Ensure that equipment is in appropriate working order. Inflate the ETT cuff to test for air leaks and deflate after testing. Liberally apply a water-soluble lubricant to the ETT.
2. Turn on the suction and place the tonsil-tip suction next to the patient's head.
3. *Insert the ETT through the naris with the bevel facing the septum. Advance the tube along the floor of the nasal passage, directing it toward the bottom of the ear. Resistance will be felt at the posterior pharyngeal wall. Rotate the tube a quarter turn to place the short aspect of the bevel in the superior position. Gentle pressure should facilitate entry to the posterior

---

*Indicates portions of the procedure usually performed by a physician or an advanced practice nurse.

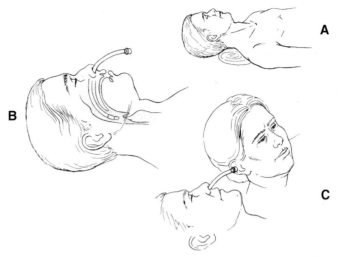

FIGURE 11-1 A, Place the patient in the sniffing position. **B,** Advance the tube along the floor of the nasal cavity. Continue advancing until the glottis is reached. **C,** Listen to the respiratory pattern; the tube is advanced on inspiration. (Courtesy of P. Rosen, MD.)

oropharynx. Advance the tube until it reaches the glottis, usually heralded by a cough or gag. Retract the tube slightly (Godwin, 2004; Reichman, 2005) (Figure 11-1).

4. *Listen to the breath sounds to develop a sense of timing and rhythm. Advance the tube through the glottis on inspiration while applying cricoid pressure (Reichman, 2005).

5. *Continue to listen for breath sounds through the tube. If breath sounds are clearly audible and air movement is felt, hold the tube in position. If breath sounds are absent through the tube and no air movement is felt, you may assume the tube has entered the esophagus. Retract the tube to the posterior pharynx and reattempt intubation.

6. Verify the appropriate ETT placement and secure the tube as described in Procedure 8.

7. Inflate the cuff and instill air until an adequate seal is obtained; 10 to 15 ml of air is usually required. Ventilate the patient with 100% oxygen.

8. Neuromuscular blockade must **not** be administered until tracheal tube placement is confirmed. Most references state that the most reliable method of correct placement is by end-tidal carbon dioxide detection (Godwin, 2004) (see Procedure 24).

AGE-SPECIFIC CONSIDERATION

Nasotracheal intubation is not a method of choice for the pediatric patient; because of the small size of the nasal passages, the procedure is difficult, and

---

*Indicates portions of the procedure usually performed by a physician or an advanced practice nurse.

the small size often prevents the placement of an ETT that is large enough to be effective (Luten & Kissoon, 2004).

COMPLICATIONS

See Procedure 8. Complications specific to the nasotracheal route include the following (Murphy, 2004):
1. Nasal bleeding during the intubation procedure or after extubation
2. Turbinate disruption or retropharyngeal perforation
3. Laryngeal injury or spasm
4. Sinusitis

PATIENT TEACHING

See Procedure 8.

REFERENCES

Godwin, S. A. (2004). Blind intubation techniques. In R. Walls, M. Murphy, R. Luten, & R. Schneider (Eds.), *Manual of emergency airway management* (2nd ed., pp. 90-96). Philadelphia: Lippincott Williams & Wilkins.

Horellou, M. D. (1978). A hazard of naso-tracheal intubation. *Anaesthesia, 33*, 73-74.

Luten, R. C. (2004). Approach to the pediatric airway. In R. Walls, M. Murphy, R. Luten, & R. Schneider (Eds.), *Manual of emergency airway management* (2nd ed., pp. 212-227). Philadelphia: Lippincott Williams & Wilkins.

Murphy, M. (2004). Applied functional anatomy of the airway. In R. Walls, M. Murphy, R. Luten, & R. Schneider (Eds.), *Manual of emergency airway management* (2nd ed., pp. 33-42). Philadelphia: Lippincott Williams & Wilkins.

Reichman, E. F. (2005). Airway procedures. In A. B. Wolfson, G. W. Hendey, P. L. Hendry, C. H. Linden, C. L. Rosen, J. Schaider, G. O. Sharieff, & J. R. Suchard (Eds.), *Harwood-Nuss' Clinical practice of emergency medicine* (4th ed., pp. 13-27). Philadelphia: Lippincott Williams & Wilkins.

Skouteris, C. A, Mylonas, A. I. & Galanaki, E. J. (2002). Acute bronchial obstruction after nasotracheal intubation: Report of a case. *Journal of Oral and Maxillofacial Surgery, 60*, 1188-1192.

PROCEDURE 12

Retrograde Intubation

Donna York Clark, RN, MS, CFRN, CMTE

The information in this procedure should be used in conjunction with the information in Procedure 8.

Retrograde intubation (RI) is also known as *retrograde transtracheal intubation (RTI), retrograde guide for endotracheal intubation, guided blind oral intubation,* and *translaryngeal guided intubation.* RI is performed by puncturing the cricothyroid membrane, feeding a wire retrograde between the vocal cords, and exiting through the nose or the mouth. The tube is passed over this guide wire and advanced through the glottis (Rosenblatt, 2006).

INDICATIONS

1. To facilitate emergent intubation when visualization of the vocal cords is not possible because of anatomic alterations, secretions, or blood (Reichman, 2005).
2. To facilitate intubation in patients with restricted range of motion of the head or neck because of anatomic variance or trauma (Kaur & Heard, 2003, Williams & Shani, 2001).
3. To facilitate tracheal intubation when other routes have failed or significant difficulty is anticipated (Reichman, 2005).

CONTRAINDICATIONS AND CAUTIONS

1. Infection at the area of insertion is an absolute contraindication.
2. Relative contraindications include the following (Rosenblatt, 2006):
   • Apneic patient not able to be effectively ventilated with a bag-valve device
   • Unfavorable anatomy
   • Laryngotracheal disease
   • Coagulopathies

EQUIPMENT

1 Extra stiff wire guide: 110 cm long
1 Radiopaque catheter
1 Syringe (10 to 20 ml)
1 18-G introducer needle
1 Catheter introducer needle
(Prepackaged kits with the equipment listed above are available.)
Scissors
Laryngoscope
Magill forceps
Bag-mask system
Oxygen source/delivery system
Suction with tonsil-tip adapter

PATIENT PREPARATION

1. Place the patient in the supine position with the neck extended and maintain the neck in the neutral position. Provide manual stabilization of the head if spinal movement is contraindicated.
2. Initiate preoxygenation with 100% oxygen via a nonrebreather mask or bag-mask (see Procedures 25 and 33). Administer oxygen via nasal cannula throughout the procedure.
3. Apply cardiac and oxygen saturation monitors (see Procedures 55 and 21).
4. Administer sedatives as prescribed.

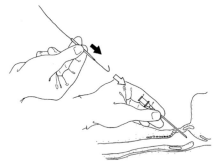

FIGURE 12-1 Insertion of needle and guide wire in cephalad direction. (From Mariani, P. [1992]. Endotracheal intubation. In M. S. Jastremski, M. Dumas, & L. Peñalver [Eds.]: *Emergency procedures* [p. 84]. Philadelphia: Saunders.)

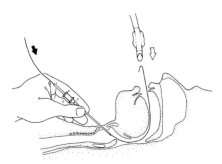

FIGURE 12-2 Advance the endotracheal tube over the wire. (From Mariani, P. [1992]. Endotracheal intubation. In M. S. Jastremski, M. Dumas, & L. Peñalver [Eds.], *Emergency procedures* [p. 85]. Philadelphia: Saunders.)

5. Restrain the patient as indicated to prevent inadvertent extubation (see Procedure 190).

PROCEDURAL STEPS

1. *Palpate the cricothyroid membrane.
2. *Infiltrate the cricothyroid area with local anesthetic if indicated.
3. *Puncture the cricothyroid membrane with the introducer needle and direct it cephalad.
4. *Insert the wire through the introducer needle and direct it cephalad (Reichman, 2005; Rosenblatt, 2006) (Figure 12-1).
5. *Advance the wire through the vocal cords and into the oropharynx (Reichman, 2005; Rosenblatt, 2006) (Figure 12-2).
6. *Use a laryngoscope to visualize the wire.

---

*Indicates portions of the procedure usually performed by a physician or an advanced practice nurse.

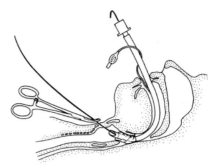

FIGURE 12-3 Advance the endotracheal tube into the airway. (From Mariani, P. [1992]. Endotracheal intubation. In M. S. Jastremski, M. Dumas, & L. Peñalver [Eds.], *Emergency procedures* [p. 85]. Philadelphia: Saunders.)

7. *Use the Magill forceps to grasp the wire and draw it out through the mouth.
8. *Insert the cephalad end of the wire through the Murphy eye (side hole) of the endotracheal tube (outside to inside) and out the proximal end of the tube.
9. *Place slight tension on the wire and advance the endotracheal tube through the glottic opening (Reichman, 2005; Rosenblatt, 2006) (Figure 12-3).
10. *After the advancement of the endotracheal tube to the level of the cricothyroid membrane, cut the wire at the skin (be sure to retain a grasp on the wire as it is being cut) or pull the wire through and advance the tube into the trachea (Reichman, 2005) (Figure 12-4).
11. Verify the appropriate endotracheal tube placement and secure the tube as described in Procedure 8.
12. Inflate the cuff and instill air until an adequate seal is obtained; 10 to 15 ml of air is usually required. Ventilate the patient with 100% oxygen.

AGE-SPECIFIC CONSIDERATIONS

Airway management in the pediatric patient is challenging because of immature structures. Little current literature is available addressing the efficacy of retrograde intubation in the pediatric population. Orotracheal intubation is still the procedure of choice in children (Luten & Kissoon, 2004).

COMPLICATIONS

Complications specific to retrograde intubation include the following:
1. Bleeding of the nasopharynx and oropharynx
2. Localized subcutaneous emphysema (Powell & Ozdil, 1967)
3. Guide wire breakage requiring surgical removal of the broken segment of wire
4. Pneumothorax
5. Trigeminal nerve damage

---

*Indicates portions of the procedure usually performed by a physician or an advanced practice nurse.

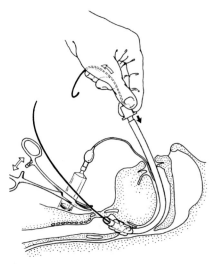

FIGURE 12-4 Retract the wire while maintaining mild forward force on the tube. Alternatively, cut the wire at skin level. (From Mariani, P. [1992]. Endotracheal intubation. In M. S. Jastremski, M. Dumas, & L. Peñalver [Eds.], *Emergency procedures* [p. 87]. Philadelphia: Saunders.)

PATIENT TEACHING

See Procedure 8.

REFERENCES

Kaur, S. & Heard, S. O. (2003). Airway management and endotracheal intubation. In R. S. Irwin, & J. M. Rippe (Eds.), *Irwin and Rippe's intensive care medicine* (5th ed., pp. 4-18). Philadelphia: Lippincott Williams & Wilkins.

Powell, W. & Ozdil, T. (1967). A translaryngeal guide for tracheal intubation. *Anesthesia and Analgesia, 46*, 231-234.

Rosenblatt, W. H. (2006). Airway management. In P. G. Barash, B. F. Cullen, & R. K. Stoelting (Eds.), *Clinical anesthesia* (5th ed., pp. 596-642). Philadelphia: Lippincott Williams & Wilkins.

Reichman, E. F. (2005). Airway procedures. In A. B. Wolfson, G. W. Hendey, P. L. Hendry, C. H. Linden, C. L. Rosen, J. Schaider, G. Q. Sharieff, & J. R. Suchard (Eds.), *Harwood-Nuss' clinical practice of emergency medicine* (4th ed., pp. 13-27). Philadelphia: Lippincott Williams Wilkins.

Williams, J. B. & Sahni, R. (2001). Performance of retrograde intubation in a multiple-trauma patient. *Prehospital Emergency Care, 5*(1), 49-51.

Extubation

Donna York Clark, RN, MS, CFRN, CMTE

INDICATIONS

1. It is appropriate to consider extubation (removal of the endotracheal tube) when the indications for intubation are no longer present. Extubation should not be considered a procedure without risk. It is critical that the appropriate equipment and skilled personnel are present and able to intervene as indicated (Rosenblatt, 2006).
2. Extubation is also appropriate when ventilatory support is being withdrawn in anticipation of a patient's death.

CONTRAINDICATIONS AND CAUTIONS

1. Except when ventilatory support is being withdrawn pending death, extubation is contraindicated when the patient is deemed unable to protect his or her own airway or is unable to effectively ventilate without the assistance of mechanical ventilation. It is critical that a careful patient assessment is completed before removal of the endotracheal tube. Assessment findings must include the following:
   a. Level of consciousness: awake and following simple commands
   b. Objective ventilatory criteria (Rosenblatt, 2006):
      - Vital capacity of 10 ml/kg or greater
      - Tidal volume of greater than 6 ml/kg
      - Peak voluntary negative inspiratory pressure of greater than 20 cm H_2O
   c. Ability to protect airway, positive gag and swallow reflexes
   d. Hemodynamically stable
   e. Effective respiratory muscle strength
2. Difficulty encountered when originally placing the endotracheal tube. If intubation was difficult, the health care team should develop a contingency plan for airway access should extubation fail.
3. Many sources recommend extubation be accomplished early in the day to ensure adequate skilled staff available if complications present (Green et al., 2004).

EQUIPMENT

Suction set-up
Suction catheter/tonsil tip suction
30-ml syringe
Bag-mask
Oxygen delivery system

Oxygen face mask humidifier (recommended)
Pulse oximeter
Equipment to reintubate the patient if indicated (see Procedure 8)

PATIENT PREPARATION

1. To prevent aspiration, ensure that stomach contents have been evacuated.
2. Assess heart rate, respiratory rate, and breath sounds before the procedure.
3. Suction endotracheal tube, mouth, and oropharynx (see Procedure 29 and 31).
4. Elevate the head of the bed.
5. Instruct the patient that she or he will be asked to cough as soon as the tube is removed.

PROCEDURAL STEPS (Nettina, 2006)

1. Instruct the patient to take a deep breath.
2. Deflate the endotracheal tube cuff.
3. Remove the endotracheal tube at maximum inspiration (DHMC, 2006).
4. Instruct the patient to cough.
5. Suction the oropharynx as needed (see Procedure 29).
6. Apply supplemental oxygen as indicated (see Procedure 25).
7. Listen for stridor and auscultate bilateral breath sounds.
8. Monitor respirations and pulse oximetry (see Procedure 21).

AGE-SPECIFIC CONSIDERATIONS

1. Evaluation of the ratio of dead space (V_D) to tidal volume (V_T) has been found to be predictive of successful extubation in pediatric patients. Hubble and colleagues (2000) described a V_D/V_T of less than or equal to 0.5 to be reliably predictive of successful extubation. These authors suggested that routine V_D/V_T monitoring of pediatric patients may permit earlier extubation and reduce unexpected extubation failures.
2. To prevent post-extubation stridor, many sources recommend the administration of one dose of corticosteroids 24 hours before extubation and three or four subsequent doses, every 6 hours, after extubation in pediatric and neonatal patients (Markowitz & Randolph, 2002; Stein & Karam, 2006).

COMPLICATIONS

1. Extubation may fail, and the patient may require reintubation. Extubation may fail for many reasons, including airway obstruction/acute laryngeal edema, aspiration. respiratory muscle fatigue, and exacerbation of heart failure or pulmonary edema (Rosenblatt, 2006).
2. Airway obstruction, acute laryngeal edema
3. Aspiration
4. Rare: unilateral or bilateral vocal cord paralysis (Kaur & Heard, 2003).

REFERENCES

Dartmouth-Hitchcock Medical Center (DHMC), Department of Respiratory Care. (2006). *Extubation protocol*. Lebanon, NH: Author.

Green, G. B., Harris, I., Lin, G. A. & Moylan, K. C. (2004). Critical care-mechanical ventilation. In G. B. Green, I. S. Harris, & G. A. Lin (Eds.), *Washington manual of medical therapeutics* (31st ed., pp. 186-194). Philadelphia: Lippincott Williams & Wilkins.

Hubble, C. L., Gentile, M. A., Tripp, D. S., Craig, D. M., Meliones, J. N. & Cheifet, I. M. (2000). Deadspace to tidal volume ratio predicts successful extubation in infants and children. *Critical care medicine, 28*, 2034-2040.

Kaur, S. & Heard, S. O. (2003). Airway management and endotracheal intubation. In R. S. Irwin, & J. M. Rippe (Eds.), *Irwin and Rippe's intensive care medicine* (5th ed., pp. 4-16). Philadelphia: Lippincott Williams & Wilkins.

Markovitz, M. P. & Randolph, A. G. (2002). Corticosteroids for the prevention of reintubation and postextubation stridor in pediatric patients: A meta-analysis. *Journal of the Society of Critical Care Medicine, the World Federation of Pediatric Societies, the Paediatric Intensive Care Society UK and the Latin American Society, 3*(3), 223-226.

Nettina, S. M. (2006). Respiratory function and therapy. In E. J. Mills (Ed.), *Lippincott manual of nursing practice* (8th ed., pp. 201-280). Philadelphia: Lippincott Williams & Wilkins.

Rosenblatt, W. H. (2006). Airway management. In P. G. Barash, B. F. Cullen, & R. K. Stoelting (Eds.), *Clinical anesthesia* (5th ed., pp. 596-642). Philadelphia: Lippincott Williams and Wilkins.

Stein, F. & Karam, J. M. (2006). Extubation. In J. A. McMillan, R. D. Feigin, C. D. DeAngelis, & M. D. Jones (Eds.), *Oski's Pediatrics: Principles and practice* (4th ed., pp. 2573-2574). Philadelphia: Lippincott Williams & Wilkins.

PROCEDURE 14

Combitube Airway

Andrew J. Bowman, RN, MSN, CEN, CTRN, CCRN-CMC, BC, CVN-I, FAACN, NREMT-P

The Combitube and the Combitube SA (small adult) are manufactured by Nellcor Puritan Bennett, Inc. (Pleasanton, CA). The Combitube esophageal-tracheal double-lumen airway is an adjunct to emergency airway management that combines the functions of an endotracheal tube and an esophageal obturator. It has two lumens that permit ventilation whether the distal tip is positioned in the esophagus (98% of the time [Frass, 2001]) or in the trachea (Nellcor Puritan Bennett Inc, 2005).

INDICATION

The Combitube is indicated whenever emergency airway management is required but endotracheal intubation is not possible or is not permitted by the level of training of the care provider. In many emergency care scenarios, particularly in the prehospital environment, emergency personnel who are trained in tracheal intubation may not be available. Placing a Combitube does not normally require the use of a laryngoscope (Agro et al., 2001; Birnbaumer & Pollack, 2002; Frass, 2001).

CONTRAINDICATIONS AND CAUTIONS
(Nellcor Puritan Bennett, Inc., 2005)

1. The Combitube airway is contraindicated in the following situations:
   a. Responsive patient with an intact gag reflex
   b. Patient with known esophageal disease or patient who has ingested caustic substances
   c. Patient with laryngeal foreign body or pathology that has resulted in upper airway obstruction (Rich et al., 2004b)
   d. Combitube: Patient less than 5 feet (152 cm) tall. (Use Combitube SA.)
   e. Combitube SA: Patient less than 4 feet (122 cm) tall
2. The Combitube is only effective in alleviating supraglottic airway obstruction. An esophageally placed Combitube cannot alleviate a glottic or subglottic airway obstruction (Rich et al., 2004b).
3. The Combitube cannot be placed in a patient with a clenched jaw (Rich et al., 2004b).
4. It may be difficult to place a Combitube in a patient with a rigid cervical collar in place (Rich et al., 2004b).

EQUIPMENT
Oxygen delivery source
Combitube airway
Suction set-up and 12-French suction catheter (10-French for Combitube SA)
140-ml syringe (included in airway kit)
20-ml syringe (included in airway kit)
Bag-mask
Water-soluble lubricant
End-tidal CO_2 (ETCO$_2$) detection device (Rich et al., 2004a)
Esophageal detector device (optional) (Rich et al., 2004a)

PATIENT PREPARATION
1. Ensure a patent airway and ventilate the patient with bag-valve-mask and supplemental oxygen.
2. Determine Combitube cuff integrity by inflating each cuff with air with the provided syringes; the pharyngeal (proximal) cuff (blue pilot balloon) is inflated with 100 ml of air, and the esophageal/tracheal (distal) cuff (white pilot balloon) is filled with 15 ml of air (Nellcor Puritan Bennett, Inc., 2005).
3. *To avoid distal tube tip contact with the posterior pharyngeal wall during insertion and to reduce pharyngeal trauma during insertion, bend the Combitube airway following its natural curve and hold in

---

*Indicates portions of the procedure usually performed by a physician or an advanced practice nurse.

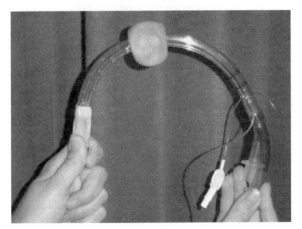

FIGURE 14-1 The Lipp maneuver to facilitate placement of the Combitube and avoid pharyngeal trauma during insertion. (Photograph courtesy of Andrew Bowman.)

this bent position until ready to insert (Lipp maneuver) (Figure 14-1) (Rich et al., 2004a).

4. Remove any sharp objects from the mouth and oropharynx (as might be found in the trauma patient) and ensure that the cuffs are not torn or damaged on insertion. Sharp teeth may also damage the cuffs (Rich et al., 2004b).

5. Suction the oropharynx if needed (see Procedure 29).

PROCEDURAL STEPS (Nellcor Puritan Bennett, Inc., 2005)
Placing the Combitube

1. Ensure that both cuffs of the Combitube are fully deflated.
2. Lubricate the distal tip with water-soluble lubricant.
3. Place the patient in a supine position, and then lift the tongue and jaw upward with one hand. Avoid the sniffing position because the Combitube is more easily placed with the head and neck in the neutral, midline position (Frass, 2001).
4. *With the other hand, hold the Combitube airway with the curve in the same direction as the anatomic curve of the pharynx. Insert the tip into the patient's mouth and guide it gently, not forcibly, behind the tongue until the two black (alveolar) rings are aligned with the teeth (or gums in the edentulous patient). If difficulty is encountered while advancing the tube, either redirect it or withdraw it completely and reattempt insertion. **Do not use force.**

---

*Indicates portions of the procedure usually performed by a physician or an advanced practice nurse.

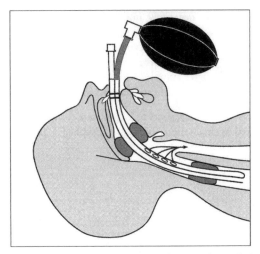

FIGURE 14-2 Combitube airway, distal tip in the esophagus with ventilation through long tube. (From Levitan, R. [2004]. *The AirwayCam^{TM} guide to intubation and practical emergency airway management* [p. 60]. Wayne, PA: Airway Cam Technologies, Inc.)

5. Inflate the proximal or pharyngeal (blue pilot balloon) first with 100 ml of air (85 ml for Combitube SA).
   a. During inflation, the pharyngeal cuff adjusts to fill and seal the pharynx by pressing against the back of the tongue and closing the soft palate in an upward fashion.
   b. Slight movement of the Combitube may be noted during proximal cuff inflation.
   c. Complete inflation with recommended volume is recommended in emergency situations. In elective cases, a minimal leak technique may be used to avoid any stress or injury to the pharyngeal mucosa (Frass, 2001).
6. Inflate the distal (white pilot balloon) cuff with 15 ml of air (12 ml for the Combitube SA).
7. Immediately attempt ventilation through the longer blue ventilation tube with a bag-valve device while observing for rise and fall of the chest. Additionally verify correct placement by auscultating for breath sounds, assessing for the presence of $ETCO_2$ and/or rapid inflation of an esophageal detector device (EDD) (Rich et al., 2004a).
   a. Rise and fall of the chest and presence of breath sounds indicate placement of the distal tip in the esophagus (Figure 14-2).
   b. The presence of $ETCO_2$ is dependent on pulmonary perfusion, and colorimetric detectors may not quickly change color during times of reduced perfusion (see Procedure 24).
8. If the chest does not rise and fall with attempted ventilation through the longer blue ventilation tube, the distal portion may have entered the trachea (Figure 14-3). Immediately switch the bag-valve device to the shorter clear

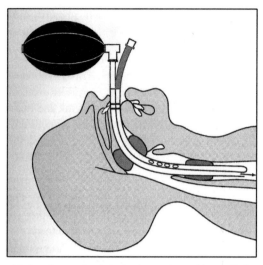

FIGURE 14-3 Combitube airway, distal tip in the trachea with ventilation through short tube. (From Levitan, R. [2004]. *The AirwayCam^TM guide to intubation and practical emergency airway management* [p. 61]. Wayne, PA: Airway Cam Technologies, Inc.)

ventilation tube. Assess for rise and fall of the chest, presence of breath sounds, as well as $ETCO_2$ and/or rapid inflation of an EDD. Positioning the distal tip in the trachea is rare (Frass, 2001).

9. If the distal portion of the Combitube is confirmed to be in the esophagus, decompress the stomach by placing a suction catheter or a nasogastric tube through the shorter, clear tube. See Procedure 98.

Replacing the Combitube With an Endotracheal Tube

1. *To replace the Combitube when ventilating through the long, blue tube:
   a. Decompress the stomach by placing a suction catheter or a nasogastric tube through the shorter, clear tube.
   b. Preoxygenate the patient.
   c. Remove all air from the proximal, pharyngeal (blue) cuff using the 140-ml syringe (Lutes & Hopson, 2004).
   d. Position the Combitube to the left side of the mouth. Insert the laryngoscope and intubate the trachea with the Combitube still in place with the distal, esophageal (white) cuff still inflated.
   e. Deflate the distal, esophageal (white) cuff by removing all of the air with the 20-ml syringe.
   f. Remove the Combitube.
   g. An alternative approach is to deflate both cuffs, remove the Combitube, and then proceed with tracheal intubation (Lutes and Hopson, 2004).

---

*Indicates portions of the procedure usually performed by a physician or an advanced practice nurse.

2. *To replace the Combitube when ventilating through the short, clear ventilation tube:
   a. Preoxygenate the patient.
   b. Pass a tube-changing stylet through the short, clear tube.
   c. Deflate both cuffs of the Combitube airway and remove the Combitube.
   d. Place an appropriately sized endotracheal tube over the stylet and intubate the patient.
3. *To remove a Combitube airway in the patient who has regained consciousness or has had return of airway protective or gag reflexes:
   a. Roll the patient to one side (if possible) and remove all air from both cuffs of the Combitube airway.
   b. Remove the Combitube and discard.
   c. Be prepared to suction as needed.

AGE-SPECIFIC CONSIDERATIONS

1. No pediatric-size Combitube is available.
2. The Combitube should not be used in a patient less than 5 feet (152 cm) tall.
3. The Combitube SA should not be used in patients less than 4 feet (122 cm) tall (Kendall Company, 1998).

COMPLICATIONS (Rich et al., 2004b; Vezina et al., 2005)

1. Bleeding from oropharynx
2. Bronchial aspiration (especially if the esophagus is not sealed adequately)
3. Vocal cord injury
4. Esophageal perforation and mediastinitis
5. Subcutaneous emphysema
6. Inadequate ventilation
7. Pneumonia
8. Bronchitis
9. Malposition with inability to ventilate through either tube
10. Upper airway obstruction from overinflation of distal esophageal cuff (Portereiko, et al., 2006)
11. Pneumothorax
12. Esophageal laceration
13. Aspiration pneumonitis

---

*Indicates portions of the procedure usually performed by a physician or an advanced practice nurse.

REFERENCES

Agro, F., Frass, M., Benumof, J., Kraft, P., Urtubia, R., Gaitini, L., & Giuliano, I. (2001). The esophageal tracheal Combitube as a non-invasive alternative to endotracheal intubation: A review. *Minerva Anestesiologica, 67*, 863-874.

Birnbaumer, D. & Pollack, C. (2002). Troubleshooting and managing the difficult airway. *Seminars in Respiratory and Critical Care Medicine, 23*(1), 3-9.

Frass, M. (2001). Combitube. *Internet Journal of Anesthesiology, 5*(2). Retrieved March 9, 2006, from http://www.ispub.com/ostia/index.php?xmlFilePath=journals/ijeicm/vol5n2/combi.xml

Kendall Company. (1998). *Combitube and Combitube SA product literature.* Mansfield, MA: Author.

Lutes, M. & Hopson, L. R. (2004). Tracheal intubation. In J. R. Roberts., & J. R. Hedges (Eds.), *Clinical procedures in emergency medicine* (4th ed). Philadelphia: Saunders.

Nellcor Puritan Bennett, Inc. (2005). *Combitube product literature.* Pleasonton, CA: Author.

Portereiko, J. V., Perez, M. M., Hojman, H., Frankel, H. L. & Rabinovici, R. (2006). Acute upper airway obstruction by an over-inflated Combitube esophageal obturator balloon. *Journal of Trauma, Injury, Infection and Critical Care, 60,* 426-427.

Rich, J. M., Mason, A. M., Bey, T. A., Krafft, P. & Frass, M. (2004a). The critical airway, rescue ventilation and the Combitube: Part 1. *American Association of Nurse Anesthetists Journal, 72,* 17-25.

Rich, J. M., Mason, A. M., Bey, T. A., Krafft, P. & Frass, M. (2004b). The critical airway, rescue ventilation and the Combitube: Part 2. *American Association of Nurse Anesthetists Journal, 72,* 115-125.

Vezina, M-C., Nicole, P. C., Trepanier, C. A. & Lessard, M. R. (2005). Retrospective study of complications associated with the Combitube. *Canadian Journal of Anesthesia, 52,* 76.

PROCEDURE 15

Cricothyrotomy

Andrew J. Bowman, RN, MSN, CEN, CTRN, CCRN-CMC, BC, CVN-I, FACCN, NREMT-P

Cricothyrotomy, also referred to as *cricothyroidotomy*, is an emergency surgical procedure that creates an opening through the cricothyroid membrane through which a cuffed endotracheal tube, tracheostomy tube, or specially created commercial cricothyrotomy tube is placed to secure an airway and, if necessary, to ventilate the patient.

INDICATIONS

To establish an airway when attempts at tracheal intubation have failed, when intubation should not be attempted due to the nature of the patient's injuries or previous condition or emergently when complete upper airway obstruction is present (Walls et al., 2004). Examples include, but may not be limited to, the following:

1. Massive midfacial trauma
2. Anatomic variants

3. Ongoing severe oral or glottic area hemorrhage
4. Upper airway obstruction
   a. Oral or pharyngeal edema from infection or space-occupying lesions
   b. Anaphylaxis
   c. Chemical inhalation or ingestion injuries
   d. Burns
   e. Foreign objects

CONTRAINDICATIONS AND CAUTIONS

1. There are no absolute contraindications according to most experts other than the ability to otherwise orally or nasally intubate the patient. However, there are some relative contraindications to the procedure. These include the following:
   a. Blunt trauma to the larynx with possible fracture
   b. Preexisting laryngeal tumor or stricture or other disease
   c. Tracheal transection
   d. Anterior neck hematoma
   e. Anterior neck infection
   f. Coagulopathies
2. Surgical cricothyrotomy is usually not recommended for children younger than 10 years. Reasons include:
   a. Poor landmarks
   b. Small size of cricothyroid membrane/space
3. Needle cricothyrotomy (see Procedure 16) may be considered in the child younger than 10 years of age but the practitioner must acknowledge that this technique does not provide optimum ventilation for prolonged periods.
4. Studies have shown that the percutaneous or Seldinger technique may be performed significantly more quickly than the standard technique of surgical cricothyrotomy (Schaumann, 2005).

EQUIPMENT

Sterile gloves
Masks
Antiseptic solution
Local anesthetic with epinephrine
Syringes and needles for infiltrating local anesthesia
Bag-mask device with supplemental oxygen source

Surgical Cricothyrotomy

Gauze dressings and sponges
Sterile drapes
No. 11 scalpel
Hemostat or tracheal spreader (Trousseau dilator)
Mayo scissors
Tracheal hook
Tape or ties to secure tube
Tracheostomy tube (No. 4 Shiley) or cuffed endotracheal tube (5–6 mm)

Melker Technique (Also Known as Seldinger Technique or Percutaneous Cricothyrotomy)

Melker tray containing:
  Syringe
  Needles
  Guidewire
  Dilator
  6-mm uncuffed or cuffed tube (depending on which kit is used)
  No. 11 blade

PATIENT PREPARATION

1. Place patient in a supine position with neck in a neutral position.
2. Cleanse the anterior neck with antiseptic solution.

PROCEDURAL STEPS
Surgical Technique (Walls, 2004)

1. Drape neck with sterile towels.
2. *Anesthetize the area with a local anesthetic, especially if the patient is conscious.
3. *Manually stabilize the thyroid cartilage and incise vertically, in the midline anterior neck, over the cricothyroid membrane (Figure 15-1).
4. *Dilate the incision with the hemostat or tracheal spreader through the cricothyroid membrane.
5. *Insert a cuffed endotracheal tube or tracheostomy tube into the cricothyroid membrane incision, directing the tube caudally into the trachea.
6. Inflate the tube cuff and ventilate the patient with bag-mask device.
7. Observe for chest rise and fall, presence of exhaled carbon dioxide ($ETCO_2$) on either a colorimetric device or capnograph (see Procedure 24) and auscultate for bilateral breath sounds.
8. Secure the tube with tape or ties. If using an endotracheal tube, note and document the centimeter marking at the skin incision line.
9. Place a sterile dressing around the incision area.

Melker Technique (Cook Critical Care, 2000)

The Melker emergency cricothyrotomy catheter set is designed to establish emergency airway access by using a percutaneous entry via Seldinger technique through the cricothyroid membrane with subsequent dilation of the tracheal entrance tract and passage of either a cuffed or uncuffed airway catheter.

1–3. Follow steps 1–3 as outlined above under "Surgical Technique."
   4. *Place a 6-ml syringe containing saline solution on the 18-G catheter and needle introducer.
   5. *Advance the 18-G catheter and needle introducer through the incision and through the cricothyroid membrane at a 45-degree angle caudally. Proper

---

*Indicates portions of procedure usually performed by a physician or an advanced practice nurse.

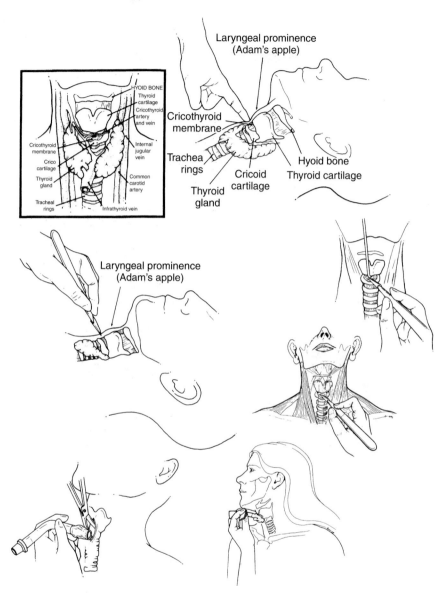

FIGURE 15-1 Surgical cricothyroidotomy. (From Mace, S. E. & Hedges, J. [2004]. Cricothyrotomy and translaryngeal jet ventilation [p.120]. In J. R. Roberts & J. R. Hedges (Eds.), *Clinical procedures in emergency medicine* (4th ed.). Philadelphia: Saunders.)

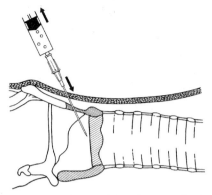

FIGURE 15-2 Advance the 18-G catheter and introducer needle through the incision into the cricothyroid membrane at a 45-degree angle in the caudad direction. Proper placement is confirmed by the aspiration on the syringe with free air return. (From Cook Critical Care. [2000]. *Melker emergency cricothyroidotomy catheter sets* [p. 6]. Bloomington, IN: Author.)

placement within the trachea is confirmed by aspiration of air bubbles into the saline-filled syringe (Figure 15-2).

6. *Remove the syringe and needle while leaving the catheter in place. Advance the guide wire through the catheter several centimeters into the airway; **do not lose control of the wire** (Figure 15-3).

7. *Remove the catheter over the guide wire, leaving the guide wire in place; **do not lose control of the wire** (Figure 15-4).

8. *Advance the dilator and airway catheter combination over the guide wire and through the cricothyroid membrane (Figure 15-5).

9. *Once the airway catheter is in place, remove the guide wire and dilator together. Inflate the cuff if using the cuffed version of the Melker tray (Figure 15-6).

10. Ventilate the patient and follow steps 7–9 as outlined earlier under "Surgical Technique" to confirm placement.

AGE-SPECIFIC CONSIDERATIONS

In children younger than 10 years, the small larynx lies much higher, at the C2–3 level, rather than at the C5–6 level as in an adult. A 12- or 14-G catheter-over-needle cricothyrotomy (see Procedure 16) is safer than a surgical cricothyrotomy in this age group (Walls, 2004).

COMPLICATIONS

1. Creation of a false passage into subcutaneous tissue with incorrect tube placement
2. Asphyxia
3. Aspiration

---

*Indicates portions of procedure usually performed by a physician or an advanced practice nurse.

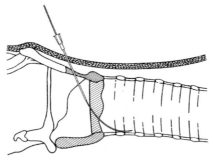

FIGURE 15-3 Remove the syringe and needle leaving the catheter. Advance the guide wire through the catheter into the airway several centimeters. (From Cook Critical Care. [2000]. *Melker emergency cricothyroidotomy catheter sets* [p. 7]. Bloomington, IN: Author.)

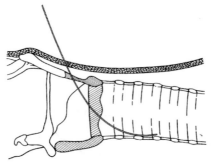

FIGURE 15-4 Remove the catheter, leaving the guide wire in place. (From Cook Critical Care. [2000]. *Melker emergency cricothyroidotomy catheter sets* [p. 8]. Bloomington, IN: Author.)

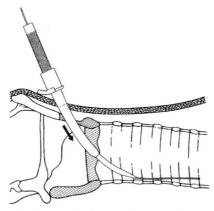

FIGURE 15-5 Advance the dilator and airway catheter over the wire through the cricothyroid membrane. (From Cook Critical Care. [2000]. *Melker emergency cricothyroidotomy catheter sets* [p. 10]. Bloomington, IN: Author.)

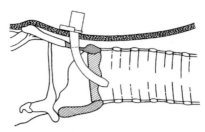

FIGURE 15-6 Once airway catheter is in place, remove guide wire and dilator simultaneously. (From Cook Critical Care. [2000]. *Melker emergency cricothyroidotomy catheter sets* [p. 11]. Bloomington, IN: Author.)

4. Hemorrhage or hematoma formation with compression of neck structures
5. Laceration or trauma to trachea, esophagus or vascular structures in the neck
6. Mediastinal emphysema
7. Pneumothorax or hemothorax
8. Vocal cord paralysis, voice changes, or dysphonia
9. Persistent stoma
10. Subglottic stenosis
11. Tracheoesophageal fistula
12. Tracheomalacia

PATIENT TEACHING
1. You will not be able to speak while the tracheal tube is in place.
2. Report any sounds of air leak or any difficulty breathing.
3. Do not touch the tracheal tube, incision site, or tapes or ties.

REFERENCES

Cook Critical Care. (2000). *Melker emergency cricothyroidotomy catheter sets*. Bloomington, IN: Author.

Schaumann N., Lorenz V., Schellongowski P., Staudinger, T., Locker, G. & Burgmann, H., et al.. (2005). Evaluation of Seldinger technique emergency cricothyroidotomy versus standard surgical cricothyroidotomy in 200 cadavers. *Anesthesiology, 102*(1), 7-11.

Walls, R., Murphy, M., Luten, R. & Schneider, R (2004). *Manual of emergency airway management* (2nd ed). Philadelphia: Lippincott Williams & Wilkins.

Percutaneous Transtracheal Ventilation

Garrett K. Chan, APRN,BC, PhD, CEN

Percutaneous transtracheal ventilation (PTV) is also known as *needle cricothyrotomy, jet insufflation, percutaneous translaryngeal ventilation,* and *percutaneous transtracheal jet ventilation* (PTJV).

INDICATION

PVT is an emergency technique that provides a temporary avenue for gas exchange until a definitive airway can be secured (Henderson, et al., 2004). PTV is an appropriate intervention for emergency nonsurgical ventilation control when intubation has been unsuccessful and mask ventilation is inadequate. PTV is considered a temporary airway to allow effective gas delivery until a more stable airway can be placed (Henderson et al., 2004). Needle cricothyrotomy is the emergent surgical airway of choice for patients younger than 12 years (Rubin & Sadovnikoff, 2004).

CONTRAINDICATIONS AND CAUTIONS

1. PTV does not provide complete control of the airway, and aspiration may occur (Danzl & Vissers, 2004).
2. Because carbon dioxide accumulates, this technique is recommended only until a definitive airway can be secured (Henderson et al., 2004).
3. The catheter may kink easily or dislodge after placement into the trachea. Constant monitoring is necessary (Higgs & Vijayanand, 2005).
4. Tracheal suctioning cannot be performed through the catheter (Bledsoe et al., 2007).
5. The patient must be able to exhale passively through the nose or mouth.

EQUIPMENT

Antiseptic solution
14-G or larger over-the-needle catheter or commercially available needle cricothyrotomy device
3-ml syringe
2-ml saline for injection (optional)
Regulating valve connected to a high-pressure oxygen source
Suction equipment (pharyngeal)
Oral and nasal airways
Endotracheal tube adaptor for a size 3 tube (optional, for use with a bag-valve-mask)

PATIENT PREPARATION

1. Place the patient in a supine position with the neck in neutral alignment.
2. Cleanse the anterior neck with an antiseptic solution.
3. Prepare the suction equipment and maintain immediate availability.
4. Restrain or sedate the patient, or do both as indicated to prevent inadvertent dislodgment of the catheter.
5. If possible, the patient should have nasal and oral airways placed to facilitate exhalation (see Procedures 5 and 6) (Walls & Vissers, 2000).
6. If possible, establish intravenous access and place the patient on standard monitoring devices including electrocardiography, pulse oxymetry, and noninvasive blood pressure (Gerig et al., 2005).

PROCEDURAL STEPS

1. *Locate the cricothyroid membrane (Figure 16-1).
2. *Pass the over-the-needle catheter (with syringe attached) at a 45-degree angle caudally, and cannulate the trachea through the cricothyroid membrane. Air will be aspirated into the syringe when the entrance to the trachea has been attained. Saline in the syringe makes it easier to see air bubbles when aspirating (Figure 16-2).
3. *Remove the syringe and needle while manually stabilizing the catheter. Advance the catheter caudally into the trachea (Figure 16-3).
4. *Reconfirm the endotracheal placement by aspirating air.
5. *Optional step—if the commercially available kit includes a J-shaped wire, a Seldenger technique may be used to ensure a caudal insertion of the transtracheal catheter.
   a. Insert the J-shaped wire through the needle or catheter, ensuring a caudal direction.
   b. Remove the needle or catheter over the guide wire while maintaining control of the guide wire.

---

*Indicates portions of the procedure usually performed by a physician or an advanced practice nurse.

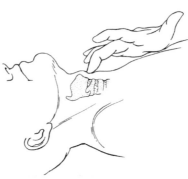

FIGURE 16-1 Locating the cricothyroid membrane. (Courtesy of P. Rosen, MD.)

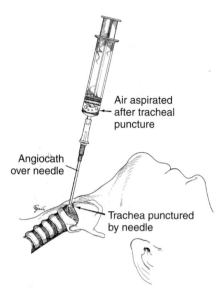

FIGURE 16-2 Tracheal cannulation. (From Wilkins, Jr., E. W. [Ed.] [1989]. *Emergency medicine: Scientific foundations and current practice* [3rd ed.] [p. 999]. Baltimore: Williams & Wilkins.)

    c. The second catheter is then railroaded into the airway over the guidewire and so follows the course of the wire caudally (Higgs & Vijayanand, 2005).

6. For most adults, attach the catheter hub to the jet ventilator device. Insufflation pressures should be between 40 and 50 psi (Gens, 2004).

7. There is no standard ventilatory device for PTV. The method described here can be accomplished with commonly available equipment. Other options include the use of intermittent high-pressure oxygen delivery by attaching

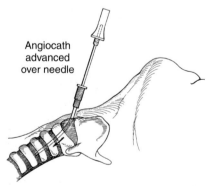

FIGURE 16-3 Catheter placement in trachea. (From Wilkins, Jr., E.W. [Ed.] [1989]. *Emergency medicine: Scientific foundations and current practice* [3rd ed.] [p. 1000]. Baltimore: Williams & Wilkins.)

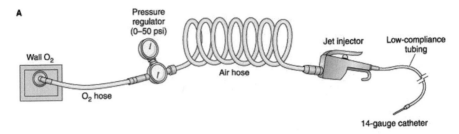

FIGURE 16-4 Jet insufflator. (From Morgan, G. E., Mikhail, M. S., & Murray, M. J. [Eds.] [2006]. *Clinical anesthesiology* [4th ed.]. New York: McGraw-Hill.)

noncollapsible tubing to an oxygen source at one end and to the catheter at the other. A regulating valve or a commercially available system (e.g., the Shrader blow gun) is attached to a high-pressure oxygen supply and placed within the system to allow for intermittent oxygen delivery (Figure 16-4). The customary frequency of inflation for is once every 5 seconds (12 breaths per minute). The inflation should occur over 1 second and the exhalation should occur over the next 4 seconds (Rubin & Sadovnikoff, 2004).

8. The chest rise is a good indicator of adequate inflation. If a high-pressure oxygen source is not available, ventilation may be attempted with a bag-valve-mask via the adaptor from a 3.0-mm endotracheal tube. Remove the adaptor from the endotracheal tube, insert it into the catheter, attach a bag-valve-mask, and ventilate (Figure 16-5). This method is less effective than a high-pressure oxygen source, and ventilation may be very difficult, if not impossible.

9. Secure the catheter by holding it manually at all times, being careful not to bend or kink it.

10. Auscultate the patient's chest to assess ventilation. Visualize the chest for rise and fall as oxygen is delivered.

11. Prepare the patient for a secondary technique to secure a more definitive airway. Needle cricothyrotomy should only be used for 10 to 20 minutes (Gens, 2004). This may require emergent transfer to the operating room for a tracheostomy.

AGE-SPECIFIC CONSIDERATION

In children aged 12 or younger, PTV is the procedure of choice for surgical airway management (Rubin & Sadovnikoff, 2004).

COMPLICATIONS

1. Subcutaneous or mediastinal emphysema, or both
2. Hemorrhage at the site of the needle puncture
3. Posterior tracheal wall or esophageal puncture
4. Pneumothorax
5. Inadequate ventilation, which may lead to hypoxia, hypotension, and cardiac collapse
6. Carbon dioxide retention

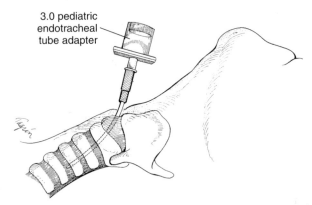

3.0 pediatric
endotracheal
tube adapter

FIGURE 16-5 Catheter attached to endotracheal tube adaptor for ventilation via bag-valve-mask. This technique is less effective than a high-pressure oxygen delivery system. (From Wilkins, Jr., E.W. [Ed.] [1989]. *Emergency medicine: Scientific foundations and current practice* [3rd ed.] [p. 1001]. Baltimore: Williams & Wilkins.)

7. Obstruction, kinking, or cephalad placement of the catheter (Higgs and Vijayanand, 2005)

REFERENCES

Bledsoe, B. E., Porter, R. S. & Cherry, R. A. (2007). *Essentials of paramedic care* (2nd ed.). Upper Saddle River, NJ: Pearson Prentice Hall.

Danzl, D. F. & Vissers, R. J. (2004). Tracheal intubation and mechanical ventilation. In J. E. Tintinalli, G. D. Kelen, S. Stapczynski, O. J. Ma, & D. M. Cline (Eds.), *Tintinalli's emergency medicine: A comprehensive study guide* (6). McGraw-Hill. Accessed December 18, 2006 at http://www.accessmedicine.com/content.aspx?aID=586639

Henderson, J. J., Popat, M. T., Latto, I. P. & Pearce, A. C. (2004). Difficult airway society guidelines for management of the unanticipated difficult intubation. *Anaesthesia, 59,* 675-694.

Higgs, A. & Vijayand, P. (2005). Prophylactic percutaneous transtracheal catheterisation. *Anaesthesia, 60,* 1245-1246.

Gens, D. R. (2004). Surgical airway management. In J. E. Tintinalli, G. D. Kelen, S. Stapczynski, O. J. Ma, & D. M. Cline (Eds.), *Tintinalli's emergency medicine: A comprehensive study guide* (6th ed., pp. 119-124). New York, NY: McGraw-Hill.

Gerig, H. J., Schnider, T. & Heidegger, T. (2005). Prophylactic percutaneous transtracheal catheterisation in the management of patients with anticipated difficult airways: A case series. *Anaesthesia, 60,* 801-805.

Rubin, M. & Sadovnikoff, N. (2004). Pediatric airway management. In J. E. Tintinalli, G. D. Kelen, S. Stapczynski, O. J. Ma, & D. M Cline (Eds.), *Tintinalli's emergency medicine: A comprehensive study guide* (6). McGraw-Hill. Accessed December 18, 2006 at http://www.accessmedicine.com/content.aspx?aID=586313

Walls, R. & Vissers, R. (2000). Surgical airway techniques. In R. Walls, R. Luten, M. Murphy, & R. Schneider (Eds.), *Manual of emergency airway management* (pp. 89-104). Philadelphia: Lippincott Williams & Wilkins.

Tracheostomy

Garrett K. Chan, APRN,BC, PhD, CEN

A tracheostomy is also known as a *trach* or a *surgical airway*. A tracheostomy may be placed surgically (also known as an *open tracheostomy*) or percutaneously. Because the percutaneous tracheostomy technique has not been well studied in emergent situations, the procedure described here focuses on the surgical/open tracheostomy technique.

INDICATIONS

To establish a definitive airway under the following emergent conditions:
1. Inability to perform endotracheal intubation or cricothyrotomy
2. Severe laryngotracheal trauma or laryngeal fracture
3. Epiglottitis, neoplasm, space abscess, or foreign body in the pharynx that prevents endotracheal intubation
4. Need for a definitive airway after a cricothyrotomy (surgical or needle) has been performed. Usually, tracheostomy is performed in the operating room in this circumstance.

CONTRAINDICATIONS AND CAUTIONS

1. Complications in the emergency setting are usually due to haste, inadequate lighting, equipment problems, and management of a patient who is struggling to breathe.
2. The complexity of this procedure mandates that it be performed by an appropriately trained professional.
3. Patients with suspected neck injuries require spinal stabilization. This precludes optimal positioning for a tracheostomy.
4. Universal precautions need to be used by all involved personnel because blood is likely to splatter during the procedure.

EQUIPMENT

Sterile gloves
Masks
Protective goggles
Antiseptic solution
Scalpel blades, Nos. 15 and 11
Local anesthetic
5-ml syringe with an 18-G needle and a 27-G needle for anesthesia
Tracheostomy tube with an obturator (appropriate pediatric or adult sizes should be available)
Metzenbaum scissors
Scissors (sharp and blunt)
Tissue forceps (with and without teeth)

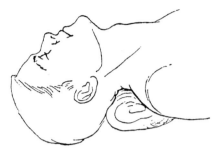

FIGURE 17-1 Patient positioning for tracheostomy. (Courtesy of P. Rosen, MD.)

Mosquito forceps
Tracheal dilator and hook
Kelly clamps
Retractors
Adhesive tape
Gauze dressings
Suction equipment, pharyngeal and tracheal
Bag-mask
High-flow oxygen source
3-0, 4-0 silk suture

PATIENT PREPARATION

1. When possible, the patient should be ventilated through an endotracheal tube, a cricothyrotomy, or another method until the tracheostomy is completed.
2. Unless there may be cervical spine injury, place the patient in a supine position with the neck in extension, and provide support under the shoulders using a blanket or small pillow (Figure 17-1). Provide manual stabilization of the head if spinal movement is contraindicated.
3. Inflate the tracheal tube cuff and check for leaks.
4. Cleanse the skin from the mandible to below the clavicles with antiseptic solution.
5. *Drape the chest and the neck.
6. *Infiltrate the skin with a local anesthetic (optional).
7. Provide analgesia. Restrain or sedate the patient as indicated.
8. Bleeding may be significant during exposure of the trachea. Prepare the tracheal and pharyngeal suction equipment and ensure immediate availability.

PROCEDURAL STEPS

1. *Make a midline skin incision vertically to expose the strap muscles (Figure 17-2).
2. *Retract the strap muscles laterally to expose the pretracheal fascia and thyroid isthmus (Figure 17-3).

---

*Indicates portion of the procedure usually performed by a physician or an advanced practice nurse.

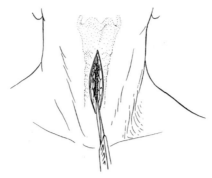

FIGURE 17-2 Midline incision. (Courtesy of P. Rosen, MD.)

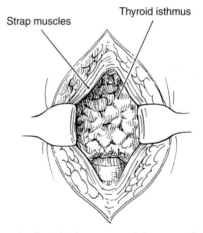

FIGURE 17-3 The thyroid isthmus exposed. (Courtesy of P. Rosen, MD.)

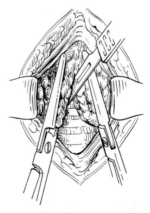

FIGURE 17-4 The trachea exposed. (Courtesy of P. Rosen, MD.)

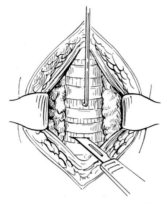

FIGURE 17-5 Tracheal entry. (Courtesy of P. Rosen, MD.)

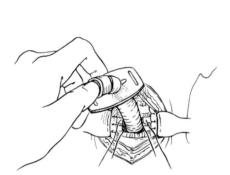

FIGURE 17-6 Insertion of tracheal tube and obturator. (Courtesy of P. Rosen, MD.)

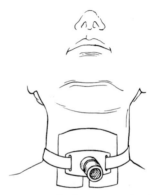

FIGURE 17-7 Tracheostomy tube tied in place. (Courtesy of P. Rosen, MD.)

3. *Clamp the thyroid isthmus and bluntly dissect to divide the isthmus and expose the trachea. Transect the thyroid isthmus and ligate it by means of sutures (Figure 17-4) (Davidson & Magit, 1996). Bleeding may be significant, so be prepared to suction.

4. *Incise through the tracheal rings to enter the trachea through the second to fourth tracheal rings (Figure 17-5) (Epstein, 2005a). Take care to control the depth of penetration to minimize the risk of injury to the posterior trachea and the esophagus (Davidson & Magit, 1996).

---

*Indicates portion of the procedure usually performed by a physician or an advanced practice nurse.

5. Suction the tracheal secretions.
6. *Insert the tracheal tube and the obturator (Figure 17-6). Remove the obturator, inflate the cuff with 5 to 8 ml of air, and ventilate the patient with a bag-mask. Auscultate the lungs to assess tube placement, and verify tube position with a chest radiograph.
7. Tie the tracheostomy tube in place around the neck with tracheostomy tape (Figure 17-7).
8. Clean and dress the insertion site.
9. Deliver humidified oxygen as soon as possible (Epstein, 2005a).

AGE-SPECIFIC CONSIDERATIONS

1. The tracheostomy procedure does not differ for the pediatric patient; however, careful attention to nearby vascular structures is necessary.
2. The smaller-diameter tracheostomy tube sizes used in infants and children require diligent pulmonary hygiene and the delivery of humidified gas to prevent the formation of mucus plugs.
3. Pulmonary edema is an additional potential complication in the pediatric population (Derkay & Buescher, 1996).

COMPLICATIONS

1. Cardiopulmonary arrest secondary to hypoxia
2. Hemorrhage and injury to the thyroid gland, esophagus, laryngeal nerve, great vessels, or trachea
3. Pneumothorax, pneumomediastinum
4. False passage of the tube into the pleura, esophagus, or surrounding vessels
5. Bradycardia or hypotension secondary to hypoxia
6. Inadvertant decannulation of the tracheostomy
7. Late complications include subglottic stenosis, granulation, tracheal stenosis, tracheomalacia, tracheoinnominate artery erosion, tracheoesophageal fistula, pneumonia, aspiration (Epstein, 2005b)

PATIENT TEACHING

1. Report any respiratory difficulty or tubing disconnections immediately.
2. Do not touch or move the tube.
3. You will not be able to speak with the tube in place.

---

*Indicates portion of the procedure usually performed by a physician or an advanced practice nurse.

REFERENCES

Davidson, T. E., & Magit, A. E. (1996). Surgical airway. In J. L. Benumof (Ed.), *Airway management: Principles and practice* (pp. 513–530). St. Louis: Mosby.

Derkay, C. S., & Buescher, S. (1996). Pediatric ear, nose and throat procedures. In H. W. Taeusch, R. O. Christiansen, & E. S. Buescher (Eds.), *Pediatric and neonatal tests and procedures* (pp. 427–445). Philadelphia: Saunders.

Epstein, S. K. (2005a). Anatomy and physiology of tracheostomy. *Respiratory Care, 50*(4), 476-482.

Epstein, S. K. (2005b). Late complications of tracheostomy. *Respiratory Care, 50*(4), 542-549.

Breathing Procedures

Positioning the Dyspneic Patient

Teresa L. Will, MSN, RN, CEN

INDICATION

To facilitate spontaneous respirations and maintain optimal oxygenation in patients with moderate to severe respiratory distress

CONTRAINDICATIONS AND CAUTIONS

These positions can only be used if the patient is responsive and has an unobstructed airway.

PROCEDURAL STEPS

1. Raise the head of the bed to an upright position at a 90-degree angle.
2. Support the patient's feet with a footboard if available.
   a. Consider using the knee gatch on the stretcher to maintain the patient's position.
   b. The knee gatch should be used for only a limited time because of pressure created on the popliteal vessels.
3. This position is known as high Fowler's position (Figure 18-1).
4. An alternative to the high Fowler's position is the orthopneic position.
   a. The patient is seated on the edge of the bed with the feet dangling, or the patient is seated in bed with an overbed table placed across the lap.
   b. The table is raised to a comfortable level and padded with a pillow or blankets. This is of particular benefit for patients with respiratory distress related to chronic obstructive pulmonary disease (COPD).
   c. This position is also known as the tripod position. In addition, this position may help relieve dyspnea related to pulmonary edema (Figure 18-2).

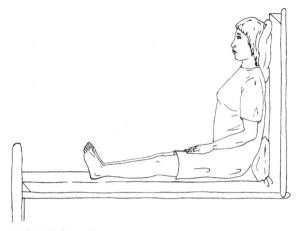

FIGURE 18-1 High Fowler's position.

AGE-SPECIFIC CONSIDERATIONS

1. It is particularly important to allow the pediatric patient to assume a position of comfort, for example, sitting on the caregiver's lap. This will decrease anxiety and facilitate spontaneous respirations. Even if it is not possible for the child to sit on the caregiver's lap, it is extremely important to allow the caregiver to be present to help alleviate the child's anxiety.

2. Infants and children will often assume a tripod position on their own to facilitate breathing when in respiratory distress.

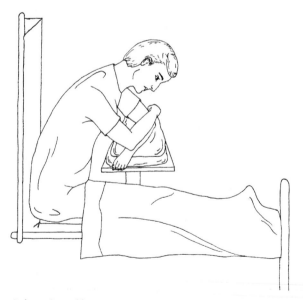

FIGURE 18-2 Orthopneic position.

3. Avoid the use of pillows in small infants as this can cause flexion of the airway and further compromise their respiratory status.
4. Before about age 6 months, infants will need to be treated in a supine position or while being held by a caregiver, because their ability to hold up the head and maintain a patent airway is compromised by their limited neck strength and relatively heavy head (ENA, 2004).

PATIENT TEACHING

1. Notify the nurse immediately if your respirations become more difficult.
2. Instruct parents to allow the patient to assume the position of choice. Ease of respiration is of the utmost importance, and the child will assume a position of comfort naturally.

REFERENCE

Emergency Nurses Association (ENA). (2004). *Emergency nursing pediatric course: Provider manual* (3rd ed.). Des Plaines, IL: Author.

PROCEDURE 19

Drawing Arterial Blood Gases

Teresa L. Will, MSN, RN, CEN, and
Jean A. Proehl, RN, MN, CEN, CCRN, FAEN

Arterial blood gases are also known as *ABGs*.

INDICATIONS

1. To evaluate acute respiratory distress and assist in determining therapeutic interventions
2. To document the existence and severity of a problem with oxygenation or carbon dioxide exchange
3. To analyze acid-base balance
4. To evaluate the effectiveness of respiratory interventions, for example, continuous ventilatory assistance or oxygen therapy

CONTRAINDICATIONS AND CAUTIONS
Proceed with caution and avoid arterial sticks in the following circumstances:
1. Previous surgery in the area (e.g., cutdown, femoral artery surgery, fistula, shunt for dialysis graft, or if artery was used in a coronary artery bypass graft)
2. Patients on anticoagulants or with known coagulopathy
3. Skin infection or other damage to the skin (e.g., burns) at the puncture site
4. Decreased collateral circulation
5. Severe atherosclerosis
6. Serious injury to the extremity
7. Fibrinolytic therapy or a candidate for it
8. Patients with femoral grafts or cellulitis (femoral punctures are contraindicated)
9. Patients who have had a cardiac catheterization via the brachial route or who have sclerotic vessels (brachial punctures are contraindicated)

EQUIPMENT
Syringe (1- to 3-ml size)

20- to 25-G needle with a clear hub (smaller gauge should be used for a radial puncture)

23- or 25-G butterfly needle (for pediatric patients)

Syringe cap

Antiseptic pledgets

Heparin 1:1000 (if the syringe is not preheparinized)

Gauze dressings

Ice

Local anesthetic (optional)

Most of the above equipment is usually available in a prepackaged kit (Figure 19-1).

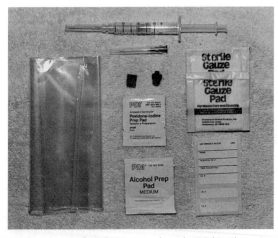

FIGURE 19-1 Typical equipment found in a prepackaged ABG kit. The syringe is preheparinized.

PATIENT PREPARATION

1. Select the puncture site on the basis of the clinical situation, how rapidly the sample must be obtained, and the circulatory status of the patient. The preferred site in most patients is the radial artery. The femoral artery is commonly used in critically ill or injured adult patients. However, hematoma or hemorrhage from a failed puncture may be more difficult to control from the femoral site.

2. If the radial artery is chosen as the puncture site, it is optional to check for the patency of the collateral circulation to the hand by performing a modified version of Allen's test. Some sources dispute the reliability and accuracy of Allen's test (McGregor, 1987; Stead & Stirt, 1985; Williams & Schenken, 1987). Interrater reliability with the Allen's test is poor, and radial artery puncture has been performed on patients with an abnormal Allen's test without subsequent hand ischemia so it should not be considered a standard of care (Barone & Madlinger, 2006).

   If used, the modified Allen's test is performed as follows:

   a. Elevate the patient's hand and arm for several seconds. Have the patient open and close the fist several times. Occlude both the radial and the ulnar arteries simultaneously until blanching occurs (Figure 19-2). If the patient is unconscious or uncooperative, elevate the hand above the level of the heart and squeeze it until blanching occurs.

   b. While maintaining pressure over the arteries, ask the patient to open the fist and relax the hand.

   c. Release pressure from the ulnar artery while maintaining pressure on the radial artery. Observe the palm closely for immediate flushing, which indicates the patency of the ulnar artery. Flushing within 7 seconds is considered normal, 8 to 14 seconds is an equivocal finding, and greater than 14 seconds is abnormal (Stroud & Rodriguez, 2004).

   d. If the modified Allen's test is abnormal, Doppler ultrasound may be performed to verify flow in the ulnar artery (Barone & Madlinger, 2006).

3. Position the extremity.

   a. *Radial:* Stabilize the wrist over a small rolled towel or washcloth. The wrist should be dorsiflexed about 30 degrees.

   b. *Brachial:* Place a rolled towel under the patient's elbow while hyperextending the elbow. Rotate the patient's wrist outward.

   c. *Femoral:* Rotate the leg slightly outward. Choose a site near the inguinal fold, approximately 2 cm below the inguinal ligament.

PROCEDURAL STEPS

1. Prepare the syringe (if not preheparinized). Draw up 1 to 2 ml of heparin and rotate the syringe to coat the barrel. Holding the syringe upright, expel the heparin and air bubbles from the syringe, leaving heparin only in the dead space of the syringe and needle.

2. Palpate the pulse and determine the point of maximal impulse. Do not insert the needle if a pulsation cannot be felt (Stroud & Rodriguez, 2004).

3. Local anesthesia may be useful in particularly anxious patients. Inject approximately 0.2 to 0.3 ml of anesthetic subcutaneously on either side and above the artery. Aspirate before injecting the anesthetic to avoid injecting

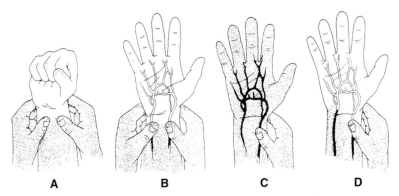

FIGURE 19-2 Allen's test. **A,** Elevate the patient's hand and arm for several seconds. Ask the patient to make a fist. Using your thumbs (or index and middle fingers), apply direct pressure over the radial and ulnar arteries simultaneously. **B,** While maintaining pressure over the arteries, ask the patient to open the fist and relax the hand. Note the blanched appearance of the palm. **C,** Release pressure from the ulnar artery while maintaining pressure on the radial artery. Observe the hand or palm closely for flushing, indicating patency of the ulnar artery. **D,** If the hand remains blanched for longer than 14 seconds, the test is abnormal. (From May, H. L. [Ed.]. [1984]. *Emergency medical procedures* [p. 84]. New York: John Wiley & Sons.)

it into the vessel. Wait 3 to 4 minutes to allow for effective anesthesia to be in place.

4. Cleanse the overlying skin with an antiseptic solution.
5. Use the index finger of your free hand to palpate the arterial pulse just proximal to the puncture site (Figure 19-3). An alternative technique is to bracket above and below the arterial pulsation with two fingers of one hand and perform the puncture between the two fingers (Figure 19-4).
6. Grasp the syringe as if holding a pencil. Direct the needle with the bevel up, and puncture the skin slowly at approximately a 30- to 45-degree angle to the radial or brachial artery (90 degrees to the femoral artery). Watch the needle hub constantly for the appearance of blood.
7. When blood appears, stop advancing the needle, and allow the blood to flow freely into the syringe. The blood should fill the syringe without aspiration, except in patients with severe hypotension. In these patients, red arterial blood should appear spontaneously in the needle hub. At this time, gentle aspiration may be used to obtain the sample. Some ABG syringes have a vented plunger that must be occluded if aspiration is necessary.
8. If the syringe fails to fill after an initial flash of blood, both walls of the artery may have been pierced. Withdraw the needle slightly until the tip reenters the artery and blood flows into the syringe. If the needle fails to enter the artery and a good pulse is still present, withdraw the needle to just above the bevel and redirect it to the point of maximal impulse.
9. The disappearance of a pulse usually indicates an arterial spasm or hematoma formation. If this occurs, withdraw the needle immediately, apply direct pressure, and select another site.

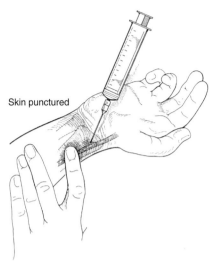

Skin punctured

FIGURE 19-3 Radial artery puncture. The index finger of one hand is used to palpate the arterial pulse just proximal to the puncture site. (From McCabe, C. J. Radial arterial puncture. In Wilkins E. W., Jr. [Ed.] [1989], *Emergency medicine: Scientific foundations and current practice* [3rd ed., p. 1013]. Baltimore: Williams & Wilkins.)

10. Obtain a sample of 1 to 2 ml. Remove the needle from the artery. Immediately apply direct pressure to the puncture site with dry gauze for 3 to 5 minutes; apply pressure for at least 10 minutes with patients receiving anticoagulants or with clotting disorders (Stroud & Rodriguez, 2004). The following steps *a* through *c* should be performed by an assistant:
    a. Prepare the blood sample for the laboratory by immediately expelling all air bubbles. With the syringe upright, finger tap the air bubbles to the

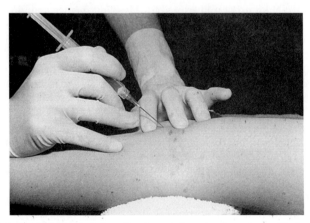

FIGURE 19-4 Brachial artery puncture. Two fingers of one hand may be used to bracket the artery and stabilize it.

top of the syringe and expel them into a gauze dressing or alcohol pledget to catch the drops of blood.

b. Activate the needlestick safety device (if present) and remove the needle. Alternately, stick the needle into a rubber stopper and remove the needle with forceps. Cap the syringe. Gently rotate the syringe between your hands to mix the heparin and the blood.

c. Label the syringe. Indicate the concentration of oxygen the patient is receiving and the patient's temperature. An elevated temperature can significantly increase the partial pressure of oxygen (PO_2). Place the syringe on ice and immediately dispatch it to the laboratory for analysis.

11. Place a dry, sterile gauze dressing over the puncture site and secure it firmly with tape. Reassess the site in 15 minutes for bleeding or hematoma formation (Stroud & Rodriguez, 2004).

AGE-SPECIFIC CONSIDERATIONS

1. Sites in children include the radial, brachial, temporal, dorsalis pedis, and posterior tibial arteries. The risk of complications is higher when the brachial artery is used so it is usually avoided. The femoral site should not be routinely used in infants and children (Lozon, 2004). The radial artery is the most frequently used site in children.

2. EMLA or ELA-Max, topical anesthetics, may be used for children, see Procedure 135 for complete information.

3. For a child, a 23- or 25-G butterfly needle attached to a syringe can be used. Both the needle and the syringe must be heparinized and the heparin must be fully expelled (Lozon, 2004).

4. In infants, continuous gentle aspiration is necessary during puncture and blood collection (Lozon, 2004).

5. Draw approximately 0.5 to 1 ml of blood for blood gas analysis in a pediatric patient; verify the minimum acceptable amount with your laboratory.

COMPLICATIONS

1. The most common complications are bleeding, hematoma, and thrombosis formation. Compression neuropathies may occur secondary to hematomas caused by arterial punctures (Stroud & Rodriguez, 2004).

2. Nerve injury may occur with inadvertent puncture of the nerve.

3. Avoiding arterial puncture in patients who take or have had heparin, warfarin, fibrinolytics, or glycoprotein IIb/IIIa inhibitors within 12 hours may assist in preventing large hematomas. If the patient is taking any of these medications, carefully consider the necessity for the arterial puncture and apply pressure for 10 minutes or longer after the artery is punctured.

4. If air bubbles are not removed from the sample, the PO_2 can increase and yield inaccurate test results.

5. The blood sample may clot if the heparin and blood are not mixed adequately.

PATIENT TEACHING

1. Do not rub the puncture site.

2. Report any bleeding, pain, numbness, or tingling following the arterial puncture.

REFERENCES

Barone, J. A., & Madlinger, R. V. (2006). Should Allen's test be performed before radial artery cannulation? *Journal of Trauma-Injury Infection & Critical Care, 61,* 468-470.

Lozon, M. M. (2004). Pediatric vascular access and blood sampling techniques. In J. R. Roberts, & J. R. Hedges (Eds.), *Clinical procedures in emergency medicine* (4th ed., pp. 357-383). Philadelphia: Saunders.

McGregor, A. D. (1987). The Allen test: An investigation of its accuracy by fluorescein angiography. *Journal of Hand Surgery (British), 12,* 82-85.

Stead, S. W., & Stirt, J. A. (1985). Assessment of digital blood flow and palmar collateral circulation. *International Journal of Clinical Monitoring and Computing, 2,* 29-34.

Stroud, S., & Rodriguez, R. (2004). Arterial puncture and cannulation. In E. F. Reichman, & R. R. Simon (Eds.), *Emergency medicine procedures* (pp. 398-410). New York: McGraw-Hill.

Williams, T., & Schenken, J. R. (1987). Radial artery puncture and the Allen test. *Annals of Internal Medicine, 106*(1), 164-165.

PROCEDURE 20

Capillary Blood Gases

Garrett K. Chan, APRN,BC, PhD, CEN

Capillary blood gases are also known as *cap gases*, *CBGs*, or *mixed venous gases*.

INDICATION

To obtain a capillary blood specimen for blood gas analysis when arterial access is unavailable or frequent sampling is indicated. Capillary blood gas values do not vary from arterial blood gas values to a degree of clinical significance when the samples are properly collected from normotensive patients (Yang et al., 2002; Yildizdas et al., 2004).

CONTRAINDICATIONS AND CAUTIONS

1. Collection and analysis may be adversely affected in the presence of poor peripheral perfusion secondary to peripheral vasoconstriction, hypothermia, or hypoperfusion (Escalante-Kanashiro & Tataleán-Da-Fieno, 2000).
2. Use a proper size of lancet (3 mm) to avoid too deep a puncture.
3. Avoid bruised or inflamed sites for sampling. Repetitive sampling from the same site may cause inflammation or scarring and should be avoided.

EQUIPMENT

Antiseptic solution or pledgets
2 × 2 gauze pad
Adhesive strip
3-mm lancet or skin-puncturing device used for blood glucose determination
1 Blood-collecting pipette
Seal for pipette (cap or clay)
Heparin solution (1:1,000), approximately 0.05 ml
2 Metal fleas
Magnet
Label
Plastic bag
Ice

PATIENT PREPARATION

1. Warm the area to be punctured for approximately 5 to 7 minutes before drawing the blood. This "arterializes" the capillary and increases the accuracy of the analysis. Warming can be accomplished with a chemical pack specifically manufactured for this purpose or a warm moist towel. If a towel is used, be sure it is not hot enough to burn the patient.

PROCEDURAL STEPS

1. Instill heparin into the pipette to coat the walls. Be careful not to leave extra heparin in the pipette; a coating of the inner wall is all that is necessary.
2. Cleanse the site with antiseptic solution and perform the puncture.
3. Wipe away the first drop of blood with gauze and then completely fill the heparinized pipette with blood, making sure that no air bubbles enter the tube. Place the tip of the capillary tube as close to the puncture site as possible to decrease exposure to environmental oxygen.
4. Seal one end of the pipette with the cap or with clay.
5. Insert two metal fleas into the open end. Run the magnet up and down along the length of the pipette to move the fleas through the blood sample and mix with the heparin.
6. Seal the open end of the pipette with a cap or with clay.
7. Label the pipette, place it in a bag on ice, and send it to the laboratory immediately. Document the FiO_2 and temperature.

AGE-SPECIFIC CONSIDERATIONS

1. For infants, punctures to the lateral or medial aspect of the heel are used to obtain capillary gas samples. The preferred sites for older children and adults are the finger or the earlobe.

2. When warming the heel of an infant, take special care so as not to burn the patient. Chemical hot packs made for adult use are too hot to be used on an infant.
3. Capillary blood gas samples should not be drawn from the heel of a patient who has begun walking and has callus development, nor should they be drawn from the fingers of neonates, to avoid nerve damage.

COMPLICATIONS
1. Inability to obtain enough blood
2. Obtaining a contaminated blood sample. Usually a blood sample becomes contaminated with interstitial fluid when the area is "milked" for blood or if not all air bubbles are removed.
3. Clotted sample from improper mixing
4. Infection or scarring at the puncture site
5. Inaccurate results if analysis of the specimen is delayed. Consult your laboratory for specimen handling and transport requirements.
6. Nerve damage

REFERENCES
Escalante-Kanashiro, R., & Tataleán-Da-Fieno, J. (2000). Capillary blood gases in a pediatric intensive care unit. *Critical Care Medicine, 28*(1)224-226.
Yang, K. C., Su, B. H., Tsai, F. J., & Peng, C. T. (2002). The comparison between capillary blood sampling and arterial blood sampling in an NICU. *Acta Paediatrica Taiwanica, 43*(3), 124-126.
Yildizdas, D., Yapicioglu, H., Yilmaz, H. L., & Sertdemir, Y. (2004). Correlation of simultaneously obtained capillary, venous, and arterial blood gases of patients in a paediatric intensive care unit. *Archives of Disease in Childhood, 89*, 176-180.

PROCEDURE 21

Pulse Oximetry and Carbon Monoxide Oximetry

Mike D. McMahon, RN, BSN

Pulse oximetry is also known as *pulse ox*, *O_2 sat*, and *SpO_2*. Carbon monoxide (CO) oximetry is also known as *pulse CO-oximetry*.

INDICATIONS
1. To monitor oxygen saturation (SpO_2) quickly and noninvasively in patients who are at risk for hypoxemia. The SpO_2 notation indicates the arterial oxygen saturation was determined by pulse oximetry rather than by arterial

blood gas analysis. This abbreviation is used because blood analysis and oximetry readings may give different readings owing to machine capabilities and patient status. The waveform that accompanies the reading is called a *plethysmograph* or *pleth*.

2. To measure CO quickly and noninvasively when occult CO poisoning is suspected. Measurements of CO saturation are available using monitor devices equipped with Masimo CO technology. The new monitors require the use of a sensor designed for both SpO_2 and CO detection. CO poisoning presents with vague symptoms such as flu-like illness, headaches, or chest pain (Kao & Nanagas, 2005). A history of a new or problematic gas appliance or using gas appliances or other methods, such as charcoal or gas generators, for heating or cooking may assist in the diagnosis. Normal CO-oximetry values are below 5% in nonsmokers and below 8% in smokers. In the setting of acute inhalation, values greater than 12% indicate moderate CO inhalation and levels greater than 25% indicate severe CO inhalation (Augustine, 2007).

CONTRAINDICATIONS AND CAUTIONS

There is no absolute contraindication for pulse oximetry; however, in some situations, data may be misinterpreted:

1. SpO_2 is a measurement of oxygen saturation, not a measurement of ventilation or acid-base status (Keogh, 2002).
2. Patient motion may interfere by mimicking a vascular waveform. Newer devices (Masimo SET, Nellcor, Oxismart) have reduced errors as a result of movement through the use of improved software algorithms.
3. At about 90% saturation level, small changes in SpO_2 can represent a large change in the patient's partial pressure of arterial oxygen (PaO_2). Readings below 70% should be considered unreliable (Scanlan & Wilkins, 2003).
4. Anemia.
5. Elevated carboxyhemoglobin levels (secondary to carbon monoxide exposure or heavy cigarette smoking) and methemoglobinemia result in falsely elevated SpO_2 readings. Pulse oximetry measures the percentage of occupied binding sites on the hemoglobin molecule without differentiating oxygen from other substances. Carbon monoxide and methemoglobin have a higher binding affinity with hemoglobin than with oxygen, so they displace oxygen from the binding sites.
6. Administration of intravenous dyes (methylene blue, indigo, carmine) results in a falsely low SpO_2 because these dyes also absorb light at a wavelength similar to that of hemoglobin.
7. Shock, cardiac arrest, excessive vasoconstriction due to hypothermia or vasopressors, peripheral vascular disease, sickle cell vaso-occlusive crisis, and low-flow states result in poor tissue perfusion, and the oximeter cannot detect hemoglobin binding accurately in this situation.
8. An arterial line or direct arterial compression of an extremity to which a sensor is applied (e.g., a blood pressure cuff, tourniquet, pneumatic antishock garment [PASG]) may result in blood flow that cannot be detected.
9. Exposure of the oximeter's photo detector to bright external light can result in false data.

10. When unsuspected CO poisoning is found, other unaware victims may be at the scene. These potential victims need to be advised of the situation and evaluated for CO poisoning (Kao & Nanagas, 2005).

EQUIPMENT

Pulse oximeter
Appropriate sensor (probe) (Figure 21-1)

PATIENT PREPARATION

Remove nail polish if possible, because some colors, especially blue (Grogan & Pronovost, 2004), interfere with pulse oximetry. If the nail polish cannot be removed rapidly and the oximeter cannot detect SpO_2 accurately, try to mount the probe side by side on a finger. This technique may also be useful for patients with extremely long fingernails.

PROCEDURAL STEPS

1. Select an appropriate sensor for patient size and placement site (see Figure 21-1).
2. Apply the sensor to the site. Accurate readings depend on the proper placement of the sensor. Sensors contain both red and infrared light sources and a photo detector. The saturation is determined by the ratio of red to infrared as sensed by the photo detector. To ensure the accuracy of the readings, it is important to place the two light sources directly opposite the photo detector.
3. If you are unable to obtain readings, assess the following:
   a. Circulation in the extremity, capillary refill, color, and temperature
   b. Sensor position in which both light sources pass through the pulsating arterial bed and reach the photo sensor
   c. Ambient light sources in the room (e.g., surgical lamps, fiberoptic lights, fluorescent lights, infrared heating lamps, direct sunlight), because the photo detector cannot differentiate bright external lights from those transmitted from the sensor light source
   d. Dirt or blood on the sensor at the light source or at the photo detector site
   e. Patient movement
4. Troubleshooting options:
   a. Change the site, the type of sensor, or both. In low-flow states, move the pulse oximeter probe to a better-perfused area, such as the nose or the earlobe, to help yield better readings.
   b. Reposition the sensor to ensure that the light sources are opposite the photo detector.
   c. Decrease the ambient light by turning off the external light sources, shutting the blinds, or covering the sensor with a dry washcloth or a blanket.
   d. Replace the probe with a new one (disposable) or clean the probe (nondisposable).
5. If the oximetry reading does not correlate with the patient's clinical presentation, assess the pulse rate apically or radially and compare it with the pulse reading on the oximeter. If the readings differ, repeat steps. 4a through 4d or obtain an arterial blood gas reading.

QUICK SENSOR APPLICATION REFERENCE

DURASENSOR® DS-100A adult digit oxygen transducer

- For patients who weigh over 40 kg (88 lbs).
- Short-term monitoring only.
- Preferred site is index finger.
- Alternate sites are smaller fingers. *No thumbs or toes!*
- For low-motion environments.
- Accuracy specifications: ± 3 digits (70–100% SaO_2) ± 1 S.D.
- Reusable durable sensor.
- Change sensor site every 4 hours.
- Never tape sensor shut.

OXISENSOR™ R-15 adult nasal oxygen transducer

- For patients who weigh over 50 kg (110 lbs).
- Only site for application is across nasal bridge.
- For no-motion environments.
- Accuracy specifications: ± 3.5 digits (80–100% SaO_2) ± 1 S.D.
- For one time use only—may *not* be reapplied.
- Requires skin preparation prior to sensor application. (Preparation solution enclosed.)

OXISENSOR D-25 adult digit oxygen transducer

- For patients who weigh over 30 kg (66 lbs).
- Preferred application site is index finger.
- Alternate sites include thumb, great toe or smaller finger.
- Accuracy specifications: ± 2 digits (70–100% SaO_2) ± 1 S.D.; ± 3 digits (50–69% SaO_2) ± 1 S.D.
- May be reused as long as adhesive quality is adequate to maintain proper placement without slippage.
- Site must be inspected every 8 hours.

OXISENSOR D-20 pediatric digit oxygen transducer

- For patients who weigh 10–50 kg (22–110 lbs).
- Preferred application site is index finger.
- Alternate sites include thumb, great toe or smaller digit.
- Accuracy specifications: ± 2 digits (70–100% SaO_2) ± 1 S.D.; ± 3 digits (50–69% SaO_2) ± 1 S.D.
- May be reused as long as adhesive is adequate to maintain proper placement without slippage.
- Site must be inspected every 8 hours.

OXISENSOR I-20 infant digit oxygen transducer

- For patients who weigh 1–20 kg (2.2–44 lbs).
- Preferred application site is great toe.
- Alternate sites include thumb or other digits.
- Use supplied additional tape to secure the I-20 to the patient's foot or hand.
- Accuracy specifications: ± 2 digits (70–100% SaO_2) ± 1 S.D. (in neonatal population); ± 3 digits (70–95% SaO_2) ± 1 S.D.
- Limited reuse with adhesive dots supplied with I-20.
- Site must be inspected every 8 hours.

OXISENSOR N-25 neonatal oxygen transducer

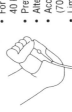

- For patients who weigh under 3 kg (6.6 lbs) or over 40 kg (88 lbs).
- Preferred application site for neonates is around ball of foot.
- Alternate site for neonates is across palm of hand.
- Accuracy specifications in neonatal population: ± 3 digits (70–95% SaO_2) ± 1 S.D.
- Limited reuse with adhesive dots supplied with N-25.
- Site must be inspected every 8 hours.

Warning: Carefully read the Directions for Use provided with each *NELLCOR* sensor for descriptions, complete instructions, warnings, cautions, and specifications.

FIGURE 21-1 Appropriate placement of various types of pulse oximeter probes. (Courtesy of Nellcor Puritan Bennett Inc., Pleasanton, CA.)

6. Vasoconstriction may alter the SpO2 waveform and numerical number (Murphy & Graham, 2006). Consider shock as a cause of decreasing values or dampened waveform.

AGE-SPECIFIC CONSIDERATIONS

1. Pulse oximetry probes may be placed around the entire foot or hand of a small infant (see Figure 21-1).
2. Pulse oximetry is accurate in the presence of fetal hemoglobin (which is normally present in neonatal patients) (Hedges, Baker, Lanoix, & Field, 2004).
3. Pediatric patients are more likely to cause false alarms due to inadvertent movement (Miyasaka, 2002).
4. Specific problems related to a newborn in the delivery room are as follows (Kopotic & Lindner, 2002):
   a. Low perfusion secondary to transitional circulation
   b. High ambient lighting, which may be found in the delivery room

COMPLICATIONS

1. False high or false low readings (see Contraindications and Cautions)
2. Reaction to the latex in some adhesive probes
3. Skin breakdown (Check the site every 8 hours and change it as indicated.)

PATIENT TEACHING

1. Hold the extremity where the sensor is placed as still as possible to obtain an accurate reading.

REFERENCES

Augustine, J. (2007). Pulse CO-oximeter utilization in the emergency scene rehab area. Retrieved February 2, 2007, from http://www.firerescue1.com/Columnists/Augustine/articles/274496/ (Page Last Updated: Wednesday, January 31, 2007 00:16 AM Pacific.)

Grogan, K. L., & Pronovost, P. J. (2004). Blood gases: Pathophysiology and interpretation. In J. E. Tintinalli, G. D. Kelen, & J. S. Stapczynski (Eds.), *Emergency medicine* (6th ed., pp. 159-167). New York: McGraw-Hill.

Hedges, J. R., Baker, W. E., Lanoix, R., & Field, D. L. (2004). Use of monitoring devices for assessing ventilation and oxygenation. In J. R. Roberts, & J. R. Hedges (Eds.), *Clinical procedures in emergency medicine* (4th ed., pp. 82-107). Philadelphia: Saunders.

Kao, L. W., & Nanagas, K. A. (2005). Carbon monoxide poisoning. *Medical Clinics of North America, 89,* 1161-1194.

Keogh, B. F. (2002). When pulse oximetry monitoring of the critically ill is not enough. *Anesthesia and Analgesia, 94,* S96-99.

Kopotic, R. J., & Lindner, W. (2002). Assessing high-risk infants in the delivery room with pulse oximetry. *Anesthesia and Analgesia, 94,* S31-36.

Miyasaka, K. (2002). Pulse oximetry in the management of children in the PICU. *Anesthesia and Analgesia, 94,* S44-46.

Murphy, M. F., & Graham, T. A. D. (2006). Monitoring the emergency patient. In J. A. Marx, R. S. Hockberger, & R. M. Walls, et al. (Eds.), *Rosen's emergency medicine: Concepts and clinical practice* (6th ed., pp. 35-41). St. Louis: Mosby.

Scanlan, C. L., & Wilkins, R. L. (2003). Analysis and monitoring of gas exchange. In R. L. Wilkins, J. K. Stoller, & C. L. Scanlan (Eds.), *Egan's fundamentals of respiratory care* (8th ed., pp. 337-369). St. Louis: Mosby.

Assessing Pulsus Paradoxus

Teresa L. Will, MSN, RN, CEN

Pulsus paradoxus is also known as *paradoxical pulse.*

INDICATION

To assess hemodynamic status in conditions that may cause a greater-than-normal decline in left ventricular outflow during inspiration. Pulsus paradoxus is an exaggeration of the normal drop in systolic blood pressure that occurs during inspiration. Conditions that result in pulsus paradoxus include cardiac tamponade, pericarditis, asthma, chronic obstructive pulmonary disease (COPD), severe congestive heart failure, tension pneumothorax, patients ventilated mechanically with large tidal volume, severe ascites, extreme obesity, and superior vena cava syndrome (Barach, 2000). Pulsus paradoxus is a quantifiable indicator of airway obstruction and will document a response to therapy over time in asthma patients (Clark et al., 2004). Pulsus paradoxus has also been studied as an objective measure of severity in croup.

CONTRAINDICATIONS AND CAUTIONS

1. Surgical procedures or disease processes that prevent blood pressure readings in both of the upper extremities (e.g., amputation, mastectomy, extraanatomic bypass, and dialysis fistula).
2. Severe arrhythmias, severe hypotension, and irregular respirations prevent accurate measurement of pulsus paradoxus.
3. A patient must be removed from a ventilator before this procedure is performed.
4. Pulses paradoxus may be absent in patients with atrial septal defect, severe aortic stenosis, and left ventricular dysfunction (Hawley & Dreher, 2002).
5. Pulsus paradoxus may be difficult to auscultate in children who are severely tachypneic, tachycardic or uncooperative.

EQUIPMENT

Blood pressure cuff (manual) and stethoscope

PROCEDURAL STEPS
Auscultory Method

1. Assess the patient for any irregular cardiac rhythms.
2. Allow the patient to assume a position of comfort and observe the patient for normal respirations. Do not ask the patient to breathe normally, because you may make the patient aware that respirations are being monitored and cause alteration of the respiratory pattern.
3. Obtain a baseline blood pressure and note the systolic finding.

4. Reinflate the blood pressure cuff slightly higher than the previous systolic reading.
5. Deflate the cuff slowly while observing the respiratory pattern. Listen for the first systolic Korotkoff sound, which can be heard during expiration. Note the systolic reading.
6. Continue to deflate the cuff slowly while listening for sounds as you continue to monitor the respiratory pattern. Note the systolic reading again when you hear the first sound during inspiration. Repeat step. 4 through 6 to validate accuracy.
7. Wait 60 seconds with cuff fully deflated between blood pressure measurements to avoid venous congestion.
8. The difference in mm Hg between the first Korotkoff sound during expiration and the first Korotkoff sound during inspiration is the measurement of the paradoxical pulse. For example, if the first Korotkoff sound on expiration is heard at 150 mm Hg and the first Korotkoff sound during inspiration is heard at 130 mm Hg, then the paradoxical pulse is said to be 20 mm Hg.
9. A difference of 10 mm Hg or less is considered to be normal (Hawley, 2002).

Arterial (Invasive) Pressure Method (Steele et al., 1995, 1997)

Pulsus paradoxus can be measured with invasive arterial pressure monitoring (when available) more easily than by auscultation. A noninvasive finger arterial pressure (Finapres) monitor has also been used to display an arterial waveform and is documented in the literature to be an accurate measurement for pulsus paradoxus when respiratory waveform and arterial waveforms are displayed at the same time.

1. Watch for inspiration peak and expiration minimum and mark each on the arterial waveform, displayed simultaneously.
2. Subtract the inspiratory systolic pressure from the expiratory systolic pressure to calculate the pulsus paradoxus.

Plethysmographic Method (Clark et al., 2004)

This method uses pulse oximetry and a standard sphygmomanometer.

1. Obtain a clear pulse oximetry waveform (see Procedure 21) with the probe on a finger.
2. Place the blood pressure cuff on the same side as the finger probe and inflate it until the waveform disappears.
3. Release the cuff slowly. Systolic expiratory pressure is noted when the first intermittent waveform is present during expiration.
4. Continue slowly releasing the cuff. Systolic inspiratory pressure is noted when the full waveform is seen.
5. Subtract the inspiratory systolic pressure from the expiratory systolic pressure to calculate the pulsus paradoxus.

REFERENCES

Barach, P. (2000). Pulsus parodoxus. *Hospital Physician, 36*(1)49-50.
Clark, J. A., Líeh-Lai, M., Thomas, R., Raghavan, K., & Sarnaik, A. P. (2004). Comparison of traditional and plethysmographic methods of measuring pulsus paradoxus. *Archives of Pediatric & Adolescent Medicine, 158,* 49.

Hawley, J., & Dreher, H. M. (2002). Cardiac tamponade: The pressure's on. *Nursing 2002, 32*(4) 32cc1-7.

Steele, D. W., Wright, R. O., Lee, C. M., & Jay, G. D., (1995). Continuous noninvasive determination of pulsus paradoxus: A pilot study. *Academic Emergency Medicine, 2,* 894-900.

Steele, D. W., Santucci, K. A., Wright, R. O., Natarajan, R., McQuillen, K. K., & Jay, G. D. (1997). Pulsus paradoxus: An objective measure of severity in croup. *American Journal of Respiratory Critical Care Medicine, 156,* 331-334.

PROCEDURE 23

Peak Expiratory Flow Measurement

Teresa L. Will, MSN, RN, CEN

Peak expiratory flow measurement is also known as *peak flow, peak expiratory flow rate,* and *PEFR.*

INDICATION

To assess peak expiratory flow rate in obstructive airway diseases (especially asthma) and to evaluate response to bronchodilator therapy. Peak flow is the most commonly used objective value that can be assessed at the bedside or at home; a declining value indicates that the patient's condition is deteriorating or is not responding to therapy (Novak & Tokarski, 2006). The peak flow rate measures how fast the maximum amount of air can be expired during a forced expiration. Increased bronchospasm or narrowing of the airways will result in a decreased speed of air flow.

CONTRAINDICATIONS AND CAUTIONS

1. Patients who are severely short of breath or who are hemodynamically unstable should not be further stressed by attempting to perform this procedure.
2. The procedure should not be performed if the patient has had recent eye surgery after which straining is contraindicated.

EQUIPMENT

Peak flowmeter
Disposable mouthpiece (if necessary)

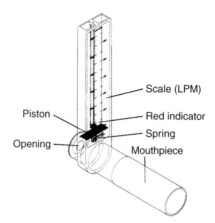

FIGURE 23-1 Peak flowmeter. (From *Assess peak flowmeter: Instructions for use.* Courtesy Health Scan Products Inc., Cedar Grove, NJ.)

PATIENT PREPARATION

1. If possible, place the patient in a sitting position with the legs dangling to maximize diaphragmatic excursion.
2. Loosen any tight or restrictive clothing.

PROCEDURAL STEPS

1. Insert the mouthpiece into the flowmeter (Figure 23-1).
2. Make sure the indicator is reset to zero.
3. Give the patient the following instructions:
   a. Stand or sit up straight, with no food or gum in your mouth.
   b. Hold the flowmeter out in front of you with the mouthpiece toward your mouth.
   c. Do not block the openings.
   d. Do not obstruct the scale.
   e. Inhale deeply until your lungs are full of air.
   f. While holding your breath, place your mouth firmly around the mouthpiece and seal the circumference with your lips.
   g. Exhale through your mouth as forcefully as possible. If exhaled air leaks through your nose, use a nose clip or pinch your nose closed.
4. Read the peak expiratory flow measurement.
5. Have the patient perform the procedure three times.
6. Document the highest value of the three.
7. The normal range for adults is 350 to 750 L/min, based on the age and height of the person (Figure 23-2). A peak flow of 40% to 69% of the patient's predicted or personal best indicates a moderate exacerbation; less than 40% is a severe exacerbation (NAEPP, 2007).

AGE-SPECIFIC CONSIDERATIONS

1. Peak flow measurements may be obtained in children as soon as they are able to understand the instructions to perform the test. This usually occurs between ages 5 and 6.

NORMAL PREDICTED AVERAGE PEAK EXPIRATORY FLOW (liters per minute)

The National Asthma Education and Prevention Program recommends that a patient's "personal best" be used as his/her baseline peak flow. "Personal best" is the maximum peak flow rate that the patient can obtain when his/her asthma is stable or under control. The following tables are intended as guidelines only.

NORMAL MALES*

Age (Years)	Height				
(in)(cm)	60" 152	65" 165	70" 178	75" 191	80" 203
20	554	575	594	611	626
25	580	603	622	640	656
30	594	617	637	655	672
35	599	622	643	661	677
40	597	620	641	659	675
45	591	613	633	651	668
50	580	602	622	640	656
55	566	588	608	625	640
60	551	572	591	607	622
65	533	554	572	588	603
70	515	535	552	568	582
75	496	515	532	547	560

NORMAL FEMALES*

Age (Years)	Height				
(in)(cm)	55" 140	60" 152	65" 165	70" 178	75" 191
20	444	460	474	486	497
25	455	471	485	497	509
30	458	475	489	502	513
35	458	474	488	501	512
40	453	469	483	496	507
45	446	462	476	488	499
50	437	453	466	478	489
55	427	442	455	467	477
60	415	430	443	454	464
65	403	417	430	441	451
70	390	404	416	427	436
75	377	391	402	413	422

NORMAL CHILDREN AND ADOLESCENTS†

Height (in) (cm)	Males & Females	Height (in) (cm)	Males & Females
43　109	147	55　140	307
44　112	160	56　142	320
45　114	173	57　145	334
46　117	187	58　147	347
47　119	200	59　150	360
48　122	214	60　152	373
49　124	227	61　155	387
50　127	240	62　157	400
51　130	254	63　160	413
52　132	267	64　163	427
53　135	280	65　165	440
54　137	293	66　168	454

* Nunn, AJH, Gregg I: Brit Med J 298:1068-70, 1989.
† Polgar G. Promadhat V: Pulmonary Function Testing in Children: Techniques and Standards. Philadelphia, W.B. Saunders Company, 1971.
NOTE: All tables are averages and are based on tests with a large number of people. The peak flow rate of an individual can vary widely. Individuals at altitudes above sea level should be aware that peak flow readings may be lower than those at sea level, which are provided in the tables.

FIGURE 23-2 Peak expiratory flow measurement chart. (From Assess peak flowmeter: Instructions for use. Courtesy Health Scan Products Inc., Cedar Grove, NJ.)

2. Children may be encouraged to stand to do their peak flow reading.
3. Pediatric normal measurements are based on the patient's height (see Figure 23-2).
4. Measurements are effort dependent. All users need to recognize the importance of taking a deep breath and exhaling forcefully. This is especially important to monitor with children.

COMPLICATIONS

1. Bronchospasm and increased dyspnea
2. Inaccurate result because of poor effort by the patient

PATIENT TEACHING

1. Keep a daily log of your peak expiratory flow when you initially start using the meter in order to establish your normal baseline. Peak expiratory flow numbers vary with gender, age, and height. Each person may have a personal best that is higher or lower than the average. When you become short of breath, use the peak flowmeter to help you decide whether you need to use your rescue inhaler or seek further medical care. If the peak expiratory flow is between 50% and 79% of your personal best, use your rescue inhaler. If the peak expiratory flow is less than 50% of your personal best, seek immediate medical care (NAEPP, 2007).
2. Often, the first sign of an "asthma attack" is a decrease in peak flow measurements, even in the absence of symptoms. Recognizing this change allows early medication intervention and can prevent severe symptoms.
3. Peak flow measurements may be used to guide medication dosages on recommendation of the primary care practitioner (NAEPP, 2002).
4. Peak flow measurements may also be taken before and after exposure to potential triggers.
5. Use the same meter for each measurement and bring your meter with you to the physician or emergency department because there can be variations between meters (NAEPP, 2007).
6. Report any increase in shortness of breath, faintness, or dizziness.
7. Keep the peak flowmeter clean because dust can affect the readings. Wash the plastic body of the meter weekly in warm soapy water, rinse, and let dry.

REFERENCES

National Asthma Education and Prevention Program (NAEPP). (2007). Retrieved September 16, 2007, from http://www.nhlbi.nih.gov/guidelines/asthma/asthgdln.pdf

Novak, R. M., & Tokarski, G. F. (2006). Asthma. In J. A. Marx, R. S. Hockberger, & R. M. Walls, et al. (Eds.), *Rosen's emergency medicine: Concepts and clinical practice* (6th ed., pp. 1078-1096). St. Louis: Mosby.

End-Tidal Carbon Dioxide Detection and Monitoring

Mike D. McMahon, RN, BSN

End-tidal carbon dioxide (ETCO$_2$) detection is also known as *capnometry* or *capnography*. Some of the devices used to measure ETCO$_2$ include Easy Cap II, Pedi-CAP, Fenem device, and STAT Cap. ETCO$_2$ monitoring allows the non-invasive measurement of exhaled CO$_2$.

DEFINITIONS

End-tidal CO$_2$ (ETCO$_2$) is the measurement of CO$_2$ at the very end of expiration. It is the maximum concentration of expired CO$_2$.
PaCO$_2$ is the partial pressure of CO$_2$ in arterial blood.
Capnometry is the measurement of expired CO$_2$ and provides a numeric display of CO$_2$ tension in mm Hg or percent CO$_2$.
Capnography is the graphic representation of expired CO$_2$ over time.
Capnograph is the measuring instrument.
Capnogram is the waveform displayed on the capnograph.

BACKGROUND INFORMATION

CO$_2$ is the byproduct waste of metabolism and used by the body to control pH level. The following formula shows the importance in the body's ability to excrete CO$_2$:

$$CO_2 + H_2O \leftrightarrow H_2CO_3 \leftrightarrow H^+ + HCO_3^-$$

The CO$_2$ and H$_2$O are excreted through the lungs and represents the body's first response to altered acid-base status (Ludy, Sole, & Ludy, 2005).

Most of the CO$_2$ produced through metabolism is expired by the lungs and can be used as a measurement of ventilatory effort. Because of the function of the lungs in the excretion of CO$_2$, detection of CO$_2$ in expired gas aids in verifying the position of an endotracheal tube (ETT) (AHA, 2005). In a patient with effective ventilatory support, the CO$_2$ levels can be used to assess pulmonary and systemic blood circulation. Additionally, capnometry may be used to determine the effectiveness of pulmonary response to treatments. High ETCO$_2$ values are almost always correlated with high PaCO$_2$ values, but low ETCO$_2$ values cannot be correlated (Sullivan, Kissoon, & Goodwin, 2005). This is due to the fact that ETCO$_2$ can be related to both pulmonary and cardiac functions.

Capnometry may be performed by means of a disposable colorimetric device that changes color in the presence of CO$_2$ or by sensors that measure the content of CO$_2$ in the flow of air from breathing. The disposable device houses a nontoxic chemical indicator that reacts to the presence of at least 4% CO$_2$ by temporarily changing color. This device attaches to the end of the endotracheal tube (ETT) and allows connection to a ventilator or a resuscitation bag. In the presence of CO_2, the device will change color with every breath. Two commonly available disposable devices turn yellow in the presence of CO_2 (Nellcor and Mercury Medical).

Capnometry may also be performed with a capnometer that measures exhaled CO_2 in intubated or nonintubated patients. There are two basic types of sensors that measure the level of CO_2 in the patient's breath: mainstream and sidestream. Mainstream CO_2 devices use a sensor that is most commonly attached to the ETT. The sensor projects infrared beams across the ETT and compares the adsorbed waveform with waveforms that have not been exposed to CO_2. Sidestream cap-nometry devices use a tube and pump to withdraw air from the patient's airway and measure the collected gas inside a separate device. Therefore, sidestream monitors can be used for the nonintubated patient. The sampling tubes can be placed inline to an ETT or may resemble an oxygen cannula and be placed in the patient's oral/nasal area. Sidestream sampling rates can be up to 100 ml/min, and low-flow technologies, such as Microstream devices, sample down to a rate of 30 ml/min. Both types can be used on the adult patient, whereas consideration should be given to using a low-flow device on the pediatric patient, who may be compromised by the additional air draw with the higher flow devices.

INDICATIONS

1. To help confirm ETT placement. The AHA (2005) lists $ETCO_2$ monitoring as a Class IIa procedure for confirmation of ETT placement in children and adults. Additionally, the American College of Emergency Physicians (ACEP) (2001) recommends "End-tidal CO_2 detection, either qualitative, quantitative, or continuous, is the most accurate and easily available method to monitor correct ETT position in patients who have adequate tissue perfusion." Unrecognized esophageal intubation has a significant impact on morbidity and mortality.

2. To help monitor the ETT position during patient transport as well as imme-diately after transferring a patient from one bed or stretcher to another.

3. To monitor continued ETT and airway patency. Secretions can build up and restrict airflow (Danzl & Vissers, 2004).

4. To monitor respiratory effectiveness during sedation (Miner, Heegaard, & Plummer, 2002).

5. To assess the effectiveness of cardiopulmonary resuscitation (CPR) and return of spontaneous circulation. $ETCO_2$ drops suddenly when cardiac cir-culation is halted and returns rapidly with the return of the patient's circula-tion. Grmec and Klemen (2001) found that patients who had $ETCO_2$ values of 10 mm Hg or less during the entire course of cardiac arrest treatment were unable to be revived.

6. In mechanically ventilated patients, the numerical value and shape of the CO_2 waveform can be used to detect hypoventilation and hyperventilation, CO_2 rebreathing, and ETT dislodgement (Murphy & Graham, 2006).

7. To guide ventilator efforts in patients with head injuries. Low CO_2 values resulting from hyperventilation can cause cerebral vasoconstriction to the point of ischemia. The goal is to keep $PaCO_2$ values in the range of 30 to 35 mm Hg (Heegaard & Biros, 2006).

8. To help confirm placement of a gastric tube. See Chapter 98 for procedural details.

9. To assist in the monitoring of patients suspected of having large pulmonary embolism (Weigand, Kurowski, Giannitsis, Katus, & Djonlagic, 2000). Low levels of $ETCO_2$ may present in the initial stage due to restricted blood flow into the lungs. As the embolism is treated, $ETCO_2$ levels should begin to return to expected normal levels.

10. Future uses may include diagnosis of obstructive and restrictive airway disease, and cardiac output on the basis of the shape of the $ETCO_2$ waveform (Murphy & Graham, 2006).

CONTRAINDICATIONS AND CAUTIONS

1. During cardiopulmonary arrest, CO_2 values may not be detectable because of the lack of circulation. With effective CPR, $ETCO_2$ levels can be in the range of 1 to 10 mm Hg during exhalation and may be detected by a CO_2 device. Other causes of low $ETCO_2$ values related to low flow include pulmonary embolism or obesity (Danzl & Vissers, 2004).

2. Use of $ETCO_2$ to detect proper placement of other airway devices (LMA, Combitube) has not been adequately studied (AHA, 2005).

3. Some colorimetric detectors (Mercury Medical) require the user to activate the device by removing a tab within the detector.

4. Colorimetric detectors have a limited life span once activated or removed from packaging. Check the manufacturer's packaging or product insert for specific time limits.

5. A false-positive detection of CO_2 may occur in esophageal intubation if the patient has recently ingested carbonated beverages or antacids; however, this CO_2 washes out in five to six breaths (Hedges, Baker, Lanoix, & Field, 2004).

6. The contamination of a colorimetric device by gastric contents, mucus, or drugs delivered endotracheally alters the reliability of the device (AHA, 2005; Nellcor, 2005).

7. Use the appropriate size of device for the patient. For both the Nellcor and Mercury Medical devices, the adult detectors have 25 ml of dead space and should be used only for patients who weigh over 15 kg (33 lb). The pediatric devices have only 3 ml of dead space and are used for patients weighing from 1 kg to 15 kg (Mercury Medical, 2004; Nellcor, 2004). A pediatric device will increase airflow resistance in a larger patient.

8. Altered end-tidal CO_2 values can be detected in the presence of mainstream bronchus intubation. Other parameters, such as equality of breath sounds and chest rise, should also be assessed.

9. Water vapor in the ETT can affect measurements by mainstream technology and cause clogging in the sidestream tube. Mainstream sensors are heated to remove moisture from the area where the infrared beam is used. Sidestream devices use a hydrophilic filter in the tubing to prevent water from entering the sensor chamber.

10. High levels of oxygen or nitrous oxide can interfere with the specific infrared wavelengths used by the sensors. Current models have become much more specific in wavelength detection, reducing the risk of error in these situations.

EQUIPMENT

End-tidal CO_2 colorimetric detector
or
Capnograph and associated tubing and cables
Bag-mask (for ETT position verification)

PROCEDURAL STEPS

Verification of Endotracheal Tube Position

Colorimetric device

1. Accomplish endotracheal intubation as outlined in Procedures 8 through 12.
2. Attach the colorimetric device between the ETT and the bag. Remove the pull tab if present (Mercury Medical device).
3. Using the ventilation bag, administer six good breaths, as evidenced by chest rise and fall and the presence of bilateral breath sounds.
4. Evaluate the exhaled CO_2 content via the color change of the device (indicated by the color yellow in the Nellcor and Mercury Medical products).
5. If CO_2 is present, continue ventilation, constantly assessing the color changes of the device. The color should change with each ventilation or expiration (purple to yellow with the Nellcor device; blue to yellow with the Mercury Medical device). If there is no indication of CO_2, or if other indicators of ETT placement are negative or questionable, remove the ETT, ventilate the patient with a bag-mask, and reattempt intubation.

Infrared-sensing devices

1. If using a mainstream device, attach the sensor to the ETT, with the sidestream device attached the connection to the end of the ETT (Figure 24-1).
2. Observe the display for $ETCO_2$ waveforms and associated numerical values (Figure 24-2).
3. Administer six breaths to wash out any gastric CO_2 content.
4. Patients who are in respiratory arrest show elevated levels of CO_2 on the monitor; those in cardiac arrest with CPR will be in the range of 2 to 10 mm Hg.
5. If there is no indication of CO_2, or if other indicators of ETT placement are negative or questionable, remove the ETT, ventilate the patient with a bag-mask, and reattempt intubation.

Ventilatory Monitoring of Nonintubated Patient During Procedural Sedation and Analgesia

Both the Emergency Nurses Association (2005) and the ACEP (2004) advise considering the use of capnometry for the patient undergoing procedural sedation and analgesia (PSA). Two studies (Burton, Harrah, Germann, & Dillon, 2006; Miner et al., 2002) found that $ETCO_2$ changes indicative of respiratory depression during PSA were commonly first detected using CO_2 measurements. Additionally, in a number of the study cases, $ETCO_2$ changes were the only indication of respiratory depression. Both studies used $ETCO_2$ criteria of an absolute change greater than 10 mm Hg, an $ETCO_2$ value greater than 50 mm Hg, or an absent waveform.

Sidestream measurements are the preferred method because specialized nasal cannulas can be used to gather exhaled CO_2. Mainstream devices can be used, but they require the patient to use a mouthpiece that may fall away as the patient becomes more sedated. Nasal cannulas are available that can be used to simultaneously administer oxygen and sample for CO_2.

1. Before sedation, establish the patient's baseline $ETCO_2$ values and waveform.
2. Follow your agency's procedures for monitoring during PSA.
3. Low values may result if the patient has hypoventilation, the collection tube (nasal cannula) falls out of the nose, or the patient mouth-breaths. If the patient is mouth-breathing and $ETCO_2$ values appear incorrect, the nasal prongs can be placed in the patient's mouth.

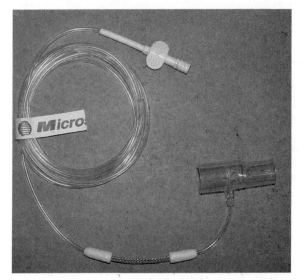

FIGURE 24-1 Microstream $ETCO_2$ sampling adapter for use with endotracheal tubes. The adapter fits between the endotracheal tube and the bag-valve or ventilator. (Photograph courtesy M. McMahon.)

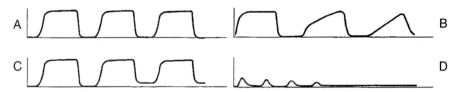

FIGURE 24-2 $ETCO_2$ waveforms (capnograms). **A,** Normal CO_2 waveform. The $ETCO_2$ measurement is taken at the end of the plateau just before the downward movement of the waveform. Normal value range is 35 to 45 mm Hg. **B,** CO_2 waveform showing obstruction. The second complex displays a "shark fin"–type appearance. This waveform can be seen in patients with obstructive lung disease (asthma) or with a mechanical obstruction in the patient's airway or ventilator circuit. **C,** CO_2 waveform showing rebreathing. The waveform is moving off the baseline, the $ETCO_2$ value may also increase. This waveform may be caused by improper mechanical ventilator setup. It also occurs in patients who are using a bag for rebreathing. **D,** CO_2 waveform showing ETT in the esophagus. The $ETCO_2$ value rapidly drops to zero. This occurs in acute esophageal intubations and if the ETT becomes dislodged. This waveform may also occur in patients who have no pulmonary circulation during CPR.

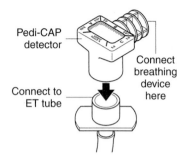

FIGURE 24-3 Connecting the Pedi-CAP to the endotracheal tube. (From *Pedi-CAP pediatric end-tidal CO₂ detector: Directions for use*. Courtesy Nellcor, Pleasanton, CA.)

4. If ETCO$_2$ decreases significantly, verbally or physically stimulate the patient to breathe.

AGE-SPECIFIC CONSIDERATIONS

1. When using a disposable detector for children who weigh less than 15 kg (33 lb), a pediatric device is indicated (Figure 24-3) because they have only 3 ml of dead space (Mercury Medical, 2004; Nellcor, 2004).
2. Keep in mind that up to 100 ml/min of air is removed by some sidestream devices, and they may not be suitable for use with infants and small children.
3. While not related specifically to ETCO$_2$ monitoring, pediatric patients are more susceptible to medications used for sedation and may have more complications during PSA (Coté & Wilson, 2006).

COMPLICATIONS

1. Increased airway resistance is encountered if the pediatric device is used on patients who weigh more than 15 kg (33 lbs). Excessive dead space is encountered if the adult device is used on patients who weigh less than 15 kg (33 lbs).
2. Attention to correct use of the technology is important because there are significant complications related to unrecognized esophageal intubation (see Procedure 8).

REFERENCES

American College of Emergency Physicians (ACEP). (2001). *Verification of endotracheal tube placement: Policy statement*. Accessed February 4, 2007, from http://www.acep.org/webportal/PracticeResources/PolicyStatements/pracmgt/VerificationofEndotrachealTubePlacement.htm

American College of Emergency Physicians (ACEP). (2004). *Clinical policy: Procedural sedation and analgesia in the emergency department*. Accessed February 4, 2007, from http://www.acep.org/NR/rdonlyres/6FF6A276-E14E-4C00-B9C7-083FDDDDDE3E/0/cpSedAnalg2Feb05.pdf

American Heart Association (AHA). (2005). American Heart Association Guidelines for cardiopulmonary resuscitation and emergency cardiovascular care. *Circulation 112*(suppl IV).

Burton, J. H., Harrah, J. D., Germann, C. A., & Dillon, D. C. (2006). Does end-tidal carbon dioxide monitoring detect respiratory events prior to current sedation monitoring practices? *Academic Emergency Medicine, 13*, 500-504.

Coté, C. J., & Wilson, S. for the American Academy of Pediatrics/American Academy of Pediatric Dentistry. (2006). Guidelines for monitoring and management of pediatric patients during and after sedation for diagnostic and therapeutic procedures: An update. *Pediatrics, 118*, 2587-2602.

Danzl, D. F., & Vissers, R. J. (2004). Tracheal intubation and mechanical ventilation. In J. E. Tintinalli, G. D. Kelen, & J. S. Stapczynski (Eds.), *Emergency medicine* (6th ed. pp. 108-119). New York: McGraw-Hill.

Emergency Nurses Association (2005). *Position statement: Procedural sedation and analgesia in the emergency department.* Accessed February 19, 2007, from http://www.ena.org/about/position/PDFs/DF08CCBA0E46430288A9EB30B835E350.pdf

Grmec, S., & Klemen, P. (2001). Does the end-tidal carbon dioxide ($ETCO_2$) concentration have prognostic value during out-of-hospital cardiac arrest? *European Journal of Emergency Medicine, 8*, 263-269.

Hedges, J. R., Baker, W. E., Lanoix, R., & Field, D. L. (2004). Use of monitoring devices for assisting ventilation and oxygenation. In J. R. Roberts, & J. R. Hedges (Eds.), *Clinical procedures in emergency medicine* (4th ed. pp. 29-50). Philadelphia: Saunders.

Heegaard, W., & Biros, M. H. (2006). Head. In J. A. Marx, R. S. Hockberger, & R. M. Walls (Eds.), *Rosen's emergency medicine: Concepts and clinical practice* (6th ed. pp. 349-382). St. Louis: Mosby.

Ludy, J. E., Sole, M. L., & Ludy, M. (2005). Ventilatory assistance. In M. L. Sole, D. G. Klein, & M. J. Moseley (Eds.), *Introduction to critical care nursing* (pp. 159-214). St. Louis: Saunders.

Mercury Medical. (2004). *StatCO$_2$®* and Mini *StatCO$_2$®* end tidal CO_2 detectors. Retrieved February 10, 2007, from http://www.66.77.149.134/index.cfm?fuseaction=act_getpagecontent&page_id=159

Miner, J. R., Heegaard, W., & Plummer, D. (2002). End-tidal carbon dioxide monitoring during procedural sedation. *Academic Emergency Medicine, 9*, 275-280.

Murphy, M. F., & Graham, T. A. D. (2006). Monitoring the emergency patient. In J. A. Marx, R. S. Hockberger, & R. M. Walls, et al. (Eds.), *Rosen's emergency medicine: Concepts and clinical practice* (6th ed. pp. 35-41). St. Louis: Mosby.

Nellcor. (2004). *CO_2 detection.* Pleasanton, CA: Author. Retrieved February 10, 2007, from http://www.nellcor.com/_Catalog/PDF/Product/CO2_Detection.pdf

Nellcor. (2005). *Easy Cap II® CO_2 detectors.* Pleasanton, CA: Author. Retrieved February 20, 2007, from http://www.nellcor.com/Serv/Manuals.aspx?ID=176

Sullivan, K. J., Kissoon, N., & Goodwin, S. R. (2005). End-tidal carbon dioxide monitoring in pediatric emergencies. *Pediatric Emergency Care, 21*, 327-332.

Weigand, U. K. H., Kurowski, V., Giannitsis, E., Katus, H. A., & Djonlagic, H. (2000). Effectiveness of end-tidal carbon dioxide tension for monitoring of thrombolytic therapy in acute pulmonary embolism. *Critical Care Medicine, 28*, 3588-3592.

Oxygen Therapy

General Principles of Oxygen Therapy and Oxygen Delivery Devices

Andrew J. Bowman, RN, MSN, CEN, CTRN, CCRN-CMC, BC, CVN-I, FACCN, NREMT-P

INDICATION

To provide supplemental oxygen (O_2) to patients with adequate and spontaneous respirations (ventilation) but inadequate oxygenation. The need for supplemental O_2 may be determined by clinical assessment of the patient, pulse oximetry, and arterial blood gas analysis. Supplemental O_2 is defined as delivery of O_2 concentration greater than room air O_2 concentration of 21% or FiO_2 (fraction of inspired O_2) of 0.21. The provision of supplemental O_2 should be treated with the same respect and caution as when administering any drug. Oxygen delivery has safe dosing ranges and may produce adverse effects, and toxic effects are possible, especially with delivery of high concentrations or with prolonged use.

CONTRAINDICATIONS AND CAUTIONS

1. In ill or injured patients, O_2 is never contraindicated. Insufficient O_2 administration may lead to hypoxia, which is a significant risk to the patient. Hypoxia may lead to cardiac arrhythmias and may damage tissues and organs. Supplemental O_2 should be delivered to maintain an O_2 saturation by pulse oximetry (SpO_2) of greater than 90%. Administering additional O_2, once the hemoglobin has fully saturated (SpO_2 99% to 100%), increases the risk of toxic effects.
2. Oxygen-induced hypoventilation, from suppression of the hypoxic respiratory drive, may occur in a small set of patients. Administration of O_2 to these patients may result in hypoventilation, further hypercapnia, and possibly hypoxia and apnea. This class of patients; often with underlying COPD, cystic fibrosis, sedation from medications for procedures, neuromuscular disease, morbid obesity, and extensive previous chest disease, requires more aggressive monitoring of their respiratory status during O_2 delivery. Oxygen therapy should be titrated to maintain an SpO_2 between 90% and 92% in these patients. If hypoxia persists, then invasive or noninvasive mechanical ventilation may be necessary.
3. A significant physical hazard of O_2 therapy is fire. Oxygen supports combustion, and smoking should not be permitted anywhere O_2 is being used.

Spark producing appliances and volatile or flammable substances should also be removed from the area. Patients may need to be searched to ensure that they do not have any matches or lighters.

4. Absorption atelectasis may occur with use of high concentrations of O_2. The usually more abundant nitrogen gas is "washed out" of the alveolus with breathing of high O_2 concentrations. When the O_2 is absorbed, the alveolus may collapse, further worsening the ability to oxygenate and ventilate the patient (Pierce, 2007).

5. Exposure of lung tissue to high O_2 concentrations can lead to pathologic changes in the tissue. After only a few hours of exposure to high O_2 levels (generally an FiO_2 greater than 0.5) mucus clearance from the lung is depressed. More prolonged exposure may lead to changes that are similar to acute respiratory distress syndrome (ARDS). The lowest FiO_2 capable of creating sufficient SpO_2 should be used in an attempt to avoid O_2 toxicity (Pierce, 2007).

6. Oxygen masks may impede care in patients with facial burns or trauma or who need frequent nursing care to the facial area. Gastric tubes may interfere with obtaining an adequate mask seal.

7. Aspiration is a potential hazard when an O_2 delivery mask is in use. Elevating the head of the bed may reduce this risk.

8. Oxygen concentration delivery is highly variable, and factors such as O_2 flow rate, ventilatory rate and depth, mask seal, and anatomic dead space all contribute to this variability (Table 25-1).

9. To deliver high O_2 concentrations, masks must have a tight seal. This tight seal may be uncomfortable and irritating to the skin.

10. Masks may interfere with patients' speech and must be removed for patients to eat meals.

11. All O_2 delivery devices must be monitored to ensure they are functioning correctly and delivering the desired concentrations of O_2.

EQUIPMENT

Appropriate O_2 delivery device (see Table 25-1)
Oxygen delivery system (extra tubing, connectors)
Flowmeter or regulator
Nut and tailpiece ("Christmas tree adapter," green nipple connector)
Oxygen source (O_2 tank or wall delivery system)
Humidification delivery adjunct (used only in select patients)

PATIENT PREPARATION

1. Explain strict no smoking instructions to the patient and all visitors.
2. When not contraindicated, allow the patient to assume a position of comfort.

PROCEDURAL STEPS

1. Attach flowmeter or regulator to O_2 source.
2. Attach the nut and tailpiece to the flowmeter. If humidified O_2 is required, attach the humidifier to the flowmeter. Humidification is not required for short-term use.
3. Attach the flared vinyl tip of the O_2 tubing to the tailpiece or humidifier.

Text continued on p. 112.

TABLE 25-1
OXYGEN DELIVERY DEVICES

O₂ Delivery Device	O₂ Flow (L/min)	FiO₂	Advantages	Disadvantages
Nasal Cannula Nasal cannula in place, attached to an O₂ flowmeter	1 2 3 4 5 6	24% 28% 32% 36% 40% 44%	Well tolerated and comfortable Patient may eat and drink without removing May be used with humidity	May cause pressure sores around nose and ears. This can be minimized by placing padding between the cannula tubing and the skin Decreased effectiveness with mouth breathing May dry and irritate nasal mucosa
Simple Mask Simple face mask attached to an O₂ flowmeter	5–6 6–7 7–8	40% 50% 60%	Simple and lightweight May be used with humidity Effective for mouth breathers or those with nasal obstruction	Insufficient O₂ flow may lead to rebreathing of CO_2; use a flow rate of at least 5-6 L/min Considered confining by some patients Limits access to face for coughing, eating, drinking, blowing nose, and delivery of oral and facial nursing care Aspiration of vomitus possible Difficulty with fitting when a gastric tube is present May cause drying of eyes

Partial Rebreather Mask

7	65%	FiO$_2$ of greater than 60% is delivered for treatment of moderate to severe hypoxia.
8–15	70%–80%	

Insufficient O$_2$ flow may lead to rebreathing of CO$_2$; reservoir bag should never completely collapse

Considered confining by some patients

Limits access to face for coughing, eating, drinking, blowing nose, and delivery of oral and facial nursing care

Aspiration of vomitus possible

Difficulty with fitting when a gastric tube is present

May cause drying of eyes

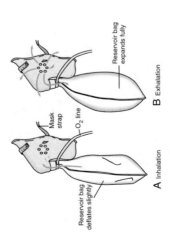

Reservoir bag deflates slightly

Mask strap

O$_2$ line

Reservoir bag expands fully

A Inhalation

B Exhalation

(Top) Partial rebreather mask in place, attached to an O$_2$ flowmeter. *(Bottom)* Arrows indicate the direction of gas movement on **(A)** inhalation and **(B)** exhalation.

Continued

TABLE 25-1
OXYGEN DELIVERY DEVICES —cont'd

O₂ Delivery Device	O₂ Flow (L/min)	FiO₂	Advantages	Disadvantages
Nonrebreather Mask (Note that masks labeled nonrebreather by some manufacturers are actually partial rebreathers.)	Set rate high enough to prevent collapse of reservoir bag. Delivers an FiO₂ of 80% or greater		Highest FiO₂ delivery for a nonintubated patient	Insufficient O₂ flow may lead to rebreathing of CO₂; reservoir bag should never completely collapse Considered confining by some patients; mask must fit snugly for optimal FiO₂ Limits access to face for coughing, eating, drinking, blowing nose, and delivery of oral and facial nursing care Aspiration of vomitus possible Difficulty with fitting when a gastric tube is present May cause drying of eyes Possible sticking of valves, limiting benefit and causing CO₂ rebreathing

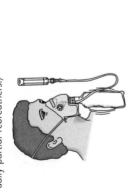

(Top) Nonrebreather mask in place, attached to an O₂ flowmeter. (Bottom) Arrows indicate the direction of gas movement on (A) inhalation and (B) exhalation.

Air Entrainment Mask
(Also known as a Venturi mask or Venti mask)

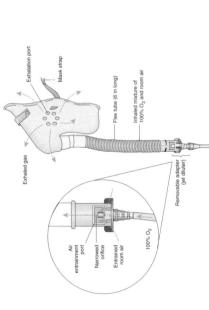

Oxygen flowing rapidly through narrowed orifice creates an area of low pressure that entrains room air through the air entrainment port.

FiO₂ changed by adjusting the air entrainment port and O₂ flow rate (per directions on each device)
Provides FiO₂ of 24% to 50%

Precise control of FiO₂
Useful in patients with COPD where excessive O₂ delivery may suppress respiratory drive

Considered confining by some patients
Limits access to face for coughing, eating, drinking, blowing nose, and delivery of oral and facial nursing care
Aspiration of vomitus possible
Difficulty with fitting when a gastric tube is present
May cause drying of eyes

Tracheal Collar
(Also known as a Puritan collar)

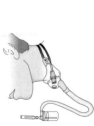

Tracheostomy collar over a tracheostomy tube attached to a flowmeter and humidification device

FiO₂ of 28% to 100%; varies with flow rate and fit of mask

High humidity prevents airway drying and maintains ciliary function
Device is lightweight and comfortable

Collar can accumulate secretions
Tubing can accumulate water, which could block delivery of O₂, could cause the collar to become dislodged, or could drain into the airway when the patient changes position

Figures from Pierce, L. (2007). *Management of the mechanically ventilated patient.* St. Louis: Saunders.

4. Adjust the O_2 to the flow rate as directed by equipment recommendations to deliver the prescribed amount of O_2. The float ball on the flowmeter should be positioned so that the flow rate line is in the middle of the ball.
5. Check to see that O_2 is flowing through the cannula or mask.
6. For nonrebreather masks, the reservoir must be filled with O_2 before it is applied to the patient. When using an O_2 mask with a reservoir bag, adjust the flow rate so that the bag does not collapse, even with a deep inspiration. These masks require a tight seal in order to deliver the highest concentration of oxygen.
7. Place the cannula prongs into the nares or apply the mask to the face. Oxygen masks have a malleable metal nose strip that can be adjusted for a better and more comfortable fit. Monitor to ensure that the mask side ports do not become blocked.
8. Padding straps with gauze or cotton may prevent irritation or discomfort.
9. If humidification is being used, periodically check and drain tubing of excess water as needed.

AGE-SPECIFIC CONSIDERATIONS

1. Allow an alert child to maintain a position of comfort.
2. Allow parents or caregivers to remain in the room with the child. Allow the parent or caregiver to hold the child if not contraindicated by patient condition.
3. Introduce O_2 delivery devices in a nonthreatening manner. A parent or caregiver may hold the O_2 delivery device to decrease the child's anxiety.
4. If a child becomes too upset by the O_2 delivery device, alternative methods may be attempted. A drinking cup decorated with colorful stickers and O_2 supply tubing inserted through the bottom of the cup is one such alternative.

COMPLICATIONS

1. Mask or cannula may be easily dislodged or removed.
2. Masks are standard size and may not fit all patients adequately and comfortably.
3. Facial irritation and skin breakdown may result if a mask is too tight.
4. Some patients may be poorly tolerant of tight fitting masks.
5. Mask must be removed for the patient to eat, drink, expectorate, or blow the nose.

PATIENT TEACHING

1. No smoking is allowed while O_2 is in the room.
2. Remove the mask only to eat, drink, blow nose, expectorate, or vomit. Replace the mask immediately.
3. Explain the proper position of mask and the importance of a snug fit. Explain that both prongs of the cannula must be in the nose.

REFERENCE

Pierce, L. (2007). *Management of the mechanically ventilated patient*. St. Louis: Saunders.

Application and Removal of Oxygen Tank Regulators

Andrew J. Bowman, RN, MSN, CEN, CTRN, CCRN-CMC, BC, CVN-I, FACCN, NREMT-P

Oxygen tanks are also known as *D-cylinder, E-cylinder, M-cylinder, H-cylinder, K-cylinder*, and so forth. Regulators are also known as *adjustable regulator, flowmeter*, or *control valve* (a regulator reduces the cylinder pressure to a working pressure before the oxygen enters the flowmeter; the flowmeter controls and measures the liter flow of oxygen to the patient). Sealing washers are also known as *O-rings* or *gaskets*. E-cylinders are the most common tanks used in the emergency department. D-cylinders are often used for prehospital transport.

INDICATIONS
Oxygen cylinders are used to provide oxygen in the following situations:
1. During the transportation of patients
2. When no piped oxygen source is available

CONTRAINDICATIONS AND CAUTIONS
1. Secure oxygen cylinders in support stand to avoid damage during transport and storage. The pressurized oxygen may turn the cylinder into a "torpedo" if damage occurs to the regulator or to the tank or valve stem (Pollack, 2005).
2. Cylinders can be heavy and cumbersome to handle. An E-cylinder weighs approximately 16 lbs. Some newer medical oxygen tanks are made of aluminum or carbon fiber. An aluminum E-cylinder weighs about 8 lbs, and a carbon fiber cylinder comparable in liter capacity to an E-cylinder weighs about 4 lbs. Do not drag, slide, or roll a cylinder. Use a portable carrier to move it to the point of use.
3. Never drop a cylinder or allow it to strike another surface.
4. To prevent fire, never permit oil, grease, or other highly flammable materials to come in contact with oxygen cylinders, valves, regulators, or fittings.
5. To prevent an accidental readjustment of oxygen flow, never drape anything over the cylinder or the regulator.
6. Use only the proper wrench or key to open or close the post valve; that is, a key that has a circular opening. *Keys that have a hexagonal opening of approximately 1 inch should be discarded. Use of an incorrectly shaped key can loosen the retaining nut on the stem of the cylinder and may result in serious injury or death.*
7. Oxygen tanks should be stored according to hospital policies and procedures based on The Joint Commission (TJC) guidelines.

8. In the United States oxygen is traditionally stored in green tanks. Each tank must also be labeled with its contents. Always read the label on the tank to confirm it contains the desired gas.

EQUIPMENT

Cylinder of oxygen (E-cylinder is the most commonly used size in the emergency department setting [Figure 26-1])

Regulator with flowmeter and cylinder pressure gauge (pin index safety system compatible with an oxygen cylinder [Figure 26-2])

Nut and tailpiece ("Christmas tree," nipple) adapter

Wrench or key (some cylinder posts may have a regulator knob, and these do not require a wrench)

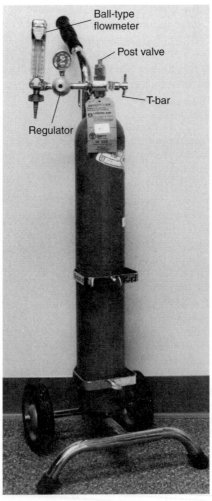

FIGURE 26-1 An E-cylinder in a portable stand with a regulator and a flowmeter attached.

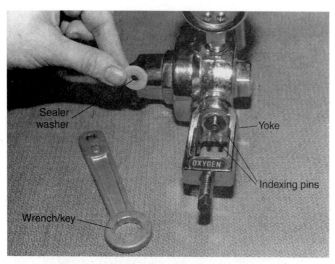

FIGURE 26-2 A sealing washer is usually provided with the dust cover. Note the two indexing pins, which indicate the appropriate regulator for an E-cylinder. Do not force regulator connectors onto cylinders or alter the indexing.

PROCEDURAL STEPS
Application of Regulator (Pollack, 2005)

1. Secure the cylinder in a support stand or assigned location on the stretcher or transport cart.
2. Remove the protective seal from the post valve. Inspect the opening to ensure that it is free of debris and dirt.
3. Turn the post-valve outlet away from any personnel. Warn anyone present that a loud noise is going to occur. Turn the post valve open (counterclockwise) and close it quickly with the key. This action produces a "whooshing" sound. That clears (cracks) the valve and eliminates any dust or foreign materials. If you have difficulty remembering which direction to turn the key, the saying "righty-tighty, lefty-loosey" may help.
4. Place the yoke on the cylinder, making sure the fittings are compatible and the gasket or sealing washers are in place (see Figure 26-2).
5. Tighten the yoke securely with an appropriate wrench or "T-bar" (Figure 26-3; also see Figure 26-2).
6. Turn off the flowmeter.
7. Slowly open the post valve until the pressure-gauge needle stops rising. Usually, one full turn is sufficient. The pressure gauge on a full E-cylinder reads about 2000 lb per square inch (psi).
8. Assess the system for any audible leaks. If a leak is heard, turn off the post valve and open the flowmeter to bleed all pressure from the regulator. Retighten the connections and open the post valve.
9. Check the pressure gauge to ascertain whether cylinder pressure is adequate for a sufficient supply of gas. Do not use the cylinder for

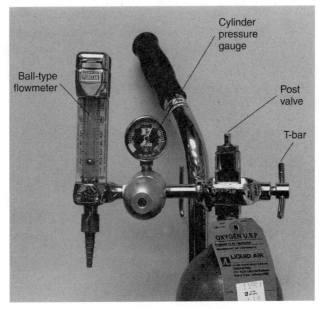

FIGURE 26-3 A close-up view of a regulator and a ball-type flowmeter on an E-cylinder.

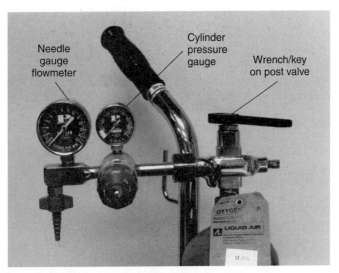

FIGURE 26-4 A close-up view of a regulator and needle-gauge flowmeter on an E-cylinder.

TABLE 26–1

TIME AT 2 L/MIN PER OXYGEN CYLINDER TYPE*

Cylinder Type	Volume (L)	Cylinder Factor	Minutes O$_2$ at 2 L/min
D	356	0.16	120 (2 hours)
E	622	0.28	210 (3.5 hours)
M	3000	1.56	1170 (19.5 hours)
H, K	6600	3.0	2250 (37.5 hours)

*Values are approximate. Volume is for a full tank.

transporting a patient if the pressure gauge reads below 500 psi. To calculate the approximate amount of oxygen left in a tank at a given flow rate, the following formula may be used (Bledsoe, Porter, & Cherry, 2006):

Tank life (in minutes) = (Tank pressure [in psi] − Safe residual pressure [500 psi]) × Cylinder factor/Flow rate (L/min)

Example: An E-cylinder O$_2$ tank has 1000 psi on the regulator. You wish to transport a patient receiving nasal cannula O$_2$ at 4 L/min. Your residual safe pressure is 500 psi.

$$(1000 - 500) \times 0.28/4 = 35 \text{ minutes of reliable tank life}$$

Table 26-1 lists the cylinder factor for the most common cylinder sizes.

10. Connect the desired form of patient oxygen delivery device (see Procedure 25).
11. Open the flowmeter to register desired flow rate. If you are using the "ball-type" flowmeter, the middle of the ball should be at the desired level (see Figure 26-3).
12. When the cylinder is not in use, turn the post valve off and bleed the system by turning the flowmeter open until the pressure gauge reads "0."

Removal of Regulator

1. Secure the cylinder in an upright position.
2. Turn the post valve off with an appropriate key or wrench.
3. Open the flowmeter to bleed the system until the pressure gauge reads "0."
4. Loosen the yoke and remove the regulator.
5. Label the tank "empty" or "in use" and store it in a rack.

COMPLICATIONS

1. Ball-type flowmeters are constructed to be used in an upright position (see Figure 26-3). Laying them on their side affects the accuracy of their reading but not the accuracy of the actual flow. An obstruction to the flow (e.g., crimped or pinched tubing) causes the ball to drop to the actual flow reaching the patient.
2. Needle-gauge flowmeters and cylinder regulators may be used in any position without affecting the accuracy of their reading (Figures 26-4 and 26-5). An obstruction to the flow causes the gauge to register higher than the actual flow being delivered to the patient.

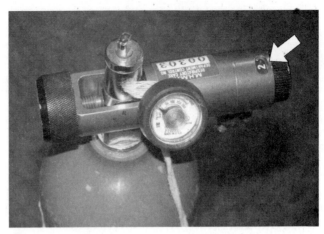

FIGURE 26-5 A cylindrical regulator set at 2 L/min (see *arrow*). (Photograph courtesy of John Markowitz.)

3. A cylinder containing less than 500 psi should not be used when transporting patients.

REFERENCES

Bledsoe, B., Porter, R., & Cherry, R. (2006). *Essentials of paramedic care* (2nd ed.). Upper Saddle River, NJ: Brady.

Pollack, A. (2005). *Emergency care and transportation of the sick and injured* (9th ed.). Boston: Jones and Bartlett Publishers.

PROCEDURE 27

Noninvasive Assisted Ventilation

Garrett K. Chan, APRN,BC, PhD, CEN

Noninvasive assisted ventilation (NIAV) or noninvasive positive pressure ventilation (NPPV) provides an alternative method to assisting an acutely ill patient's ventilations without having to place either an endotracheal tube or a tracheostomy tube into the patient's airway. The advantages of NIAV include the following (Mak, 2002):

- Allowing respiratory muscles to rest by augmenting each breath by inspiratory pressure or volume support
- Improving tidal volumes by applying pressure or increasing volume support
- Improving expiratory airflow by applying a degree of positive expiratory pressure that reduces the dynamic airway's compression and hyperinflation
- Timing breaths to compensate for the lack of central drive
- Allowing the administration of higher levels of fraction of inspired oxygen (FiO_2) without causing excessive respiratory depression

NIAV is used in chronic obstructive pulmonary disease (COPD), acute cardiogenic pulmonary edema (ACPE), and acute hypercapnic respiratory failure (AHRF). NIAV can help avoid endotracheal intubation, reduce a patient's breathlessness, decrease the complications that occur with intubation and mechanical ventilation, decrease the need for sedation and neuromuscular blockade in order to tolerate mechanical ventilation, and decrease the length of hospitalization.

There are now multiple randomized, prospective studies showing the benefit of noninvasive ventilation in respiratory failure. Not only has it been shown to be an effective therapy, but also there is evidence that it contributes to less time in the hospital, fewer complications, and decreased mortality compared with immediate intubation and ventilation (Ram, Picot, Lightowler, & Wdzicha, 2004).

INDICATIONS

1. To provide short-term (e.g., 1- to 4-day) mechanical ventilatory support to patients presenting with respiratory failure to avoid intubation and complications arising from intubation. Patients who are candidates for NIAV generally present as tachypneic, tachycardic, and possibly diaphoretic, with paradoxic respirations and increased work of breathing. The patient should be alert and able to cooperate, protect his or her airway, and understand that intubation is the probable alternative to this mode of ventilation.

2. To reduce respiratory muscle fatigue by supporting inspiratory effort, reducing the work of breathing, and providing rest to the respiratory musculature.

3. To reduce dyspnea, tachypnea, and hypercapnia associated with an exacerbation of COPD, ACPE, and AHRF (Brochard et al., 1995; Mak, 2002; Wysocki et al., 1995).

4. To correct gas exchange through the application of either positive end-expiratory pressure (PEEP) alone or with inspiratory positive airway pressure (IPAP), pressure support ventilation (PSV), or pressure control ventilation (PCV). PEEP or CPAP improves gas exchange by increasing the functional residual capacity of the lungs through alveolar recruitment. PEEP or CPAP decreases the need for intubation in patients with acute congestive heart failure (CHF) (Bersten et al., 1991).

5. To treat purely hypercapnic respiratory failure with associated respiratory muscle fatigue. NIMV is significantly less successful in avoiding intubation in patients whose mechanism of failure (other than CHF) is primarily hypoxemia (Wysocki et al., 1995). Patients presenting with an exacerbation of COPD generally have acute hypercapnia superimposed on chronic respiratory failure. Patients presenting with CHF may demonstrate either hypoxia or a combination of hypoxia and hypercapnia.

6. To facilitate the weaning of ventilator-dependent COPD patients who have failed to complete the conventional weaning process for extubation (Tebal, Marks, & Benzo, 1996).

7. To treat sleep apnea, both bilevel positive airway pressure (BiPAP) and CPAP have shown to be effective treatments.

8. To provide respiratory support to patients with progressive muscle disease, such as amyotrophic lateral sclerosis (ALS) or muscular dystrophy (MD) (Kleopa, Sherman, Neal, Romano, & Heiman-Patterson, 1999).

CONTRAINDICATIONS AND CAUTIONS

1. Immediate need for intubation to preserve life
2. Unstable cardiac status
3. Inability to protect or clear the airway of copious secretions, altered level of consciousness, or absent gag reflex
4. Facial trauma, surgery, or malformation that precludes an effective seal mask
5. Ability and willingness to cooperate are essential for an effective NIAV trial

PATIENT PREPARATION

1. Position the patient in an upright position, with the head of the bed raised at least 30 degrees. The patient's position in bed may affect the seal of the mask, and thereby the synchrony of the patient–ventilator interface.

2. Place the patient on a cardiac monitor (see Procedure 55) and a pulse oximeter (see Procedure 21).

3. The choice of either a nasal mask or a full-face mask for the delivery of NIAV rests with the caregiver. This choice depends on the caregiver's experience and comfort with the various masks and associated ventilators, and the patient's ability to adapt to the patient–ventilator interface. A properly fitting, self-sealing, clear mask is essential to the successful management of patients receiving NIAV. Most air leaks occur at the nasal bridge area (both nasal and full-face masks) or the corners of the mouth (full-face mask) and are caused by a mask that is too large. A smaller mask may solve the leakage problem. In the acute care setting, many of the caregivers in the studies cited used a full-face mask (Fernandez et al., 1993; Wysocki et al., 1993) to deliver NIAV. Nasal masks provide some advantages over full-face masks, including better comfort, ease of use, less dead space, and decreased risk of inadvertent aspiration. However, nasal ventilation may have some serious drawbacks for the critically ill patient, including the inadvertent loss of significant gas volume through the mouth and patient-ventilator dysynchrony secondary to this volume loss. Closing the mouth during nasal ventilation is mandatory. Patients in acute respiratory failure may in fact respond better to a full-face mask simply because they do not have to concentrate on breathing with a closed mouth. Synchrony with the ventilator is a key factor in reducing the work of breathing.

4. When beginning the initial trial of NIAV, the mask should be held in place rather than strapped in order to accustom the patient to the closed system. The patient should be "talked through" this initial phase to reduce the anxiety associated with NIAV. At this time the respiratory therapist or nurse should remain at the bedside for extended periods to alleviate the anxiety associated

with NIAV and to titrate the ventilator settings to best meet the patient's needs.

5. If the total system pressure (PSV, IPAP, PCV plus PEEP, or CPAP) exceeds 20 cm of water (H_2O), a gastric tube may be necessary to prevent gastric distention (see Procedure 98).

6. In most clinical settings, NIAV is delivered intermittently, with breaks of several minutes given to patients every 1 to 2 hours. Depending on the clinical scenario, the patient takes a break from the NIAV with a specific type of oxygen delivery system (e.g., a nonrebreathing mask for the CHF patient, or a precise concentration Venturi mask for the COPD patient). Most often, the first day of treatment has the greatest duration of ventilation. On subsequent days, the duration of ventilation is gradually reduced, depending on the clinical status of the patient.

7. In all types of NIAV (CPAP, BiPAP, NIAV with a ventilator), improvement in gas exchange and arterial blood gas results, and reduction in work of breathing should occur within 1 to 2 hours of initiation of treatment. Patients who do not demonstrate these improvements are at significant risk of failing the NIAV trial and may require intubation.

CONTINUOUS POSITIVE AIRWAY PRESSURE (CPAP)
Equipment
> Humidification system
> Oxygen blender, flow generator, high-flow flowmeter
> Large-bore tubing
> 500-ml to 3-L intermittent mandatory ventilation bag set-up to act as a reservoir, depending on patient size
> CPAP valve
> Low-pressure disconnect alarm with tubing
> One-way valve to prevent rebreathing
> Adaptors as necessary to assemble the unit
> Tight-fitting CPAP mask with adjustable head straps
> Many commercial CPAP systems are available. CPAP and BiPAP systems are commonly administered through ventilators. Figure 27-1 represents a schematic of a general system, but not one system in particular.

Procedural Steps
1. Attach the appropriate CPAP valve to the expiratory housing of the CPAP mask. Some valves come preset to a certain level, whereas some are adjustable. It is common to start with 5 cm H_2O of CPAP.

2. Adjust the flow of gas on the CPAP setup so the reservoir bag remains inflated throughout the respiratory cycle.

3. Adjust the disconnect alarm 2 to 3 cm H_2O below the CPAP level. Temporarily detach the system from the patient to test the alarm function.

4. Monitor the level of CPAP delivered via a pressure manometer and the delivered fraction of inspired oxygen (FiO_2) via an oxygen analyzer.

5. Assess and document the patient's response to CPAP. Monitor the patient's vital signs, work of breathing, and oxygen saturation (pulse oximetry). If CPAP does not achieve the desired response, consult the physician and

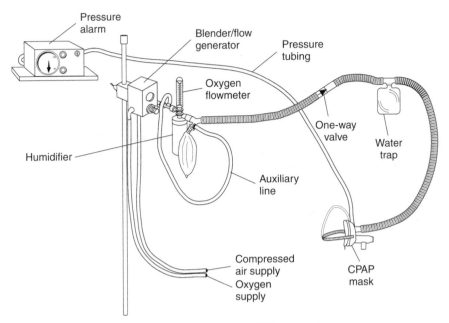

FIGURE 27–1 Continuous positive airway pressure (CPAP) mask setup.

respiratory therapist regarding an increase in the level of CPAP or a change to a system that delivers IPAP in addition to CPAP.

BILEVEL POSITIVE AIRWAY PRESSURE (BIPAP)
Equipment
The BiPAP system provides time-cycled, pressure-limited ventilation. This device is capable of delivering different pressures during inspiration (IPAP) and expiration (EPAP) (Figure 27-2).

BiPAP ventilator circuit
Humidifier
Nasal mask
Adjustable nasal mask straps
T-device for oxygen flow
Oxygen tubing

Procedural Steps
1. Set the bleed-in oxygen flow rate to achieve the desired FiO_2. Monitor FiO_2 via an in-line oxygen analyzer. A disadvantage of some BiPAP systems is inexact and varying FiO_2 delivery, particularly when high FiO_2 levels are required.
2. Initially, set the level of IPAP to accustom the patient to positive-pressure ventilation. Typical initial settings would be 5 cm H_2O of IPAP over 5 cm H_2O of PEEP (or EPAP, depending on the manufacturer's designation). Gradually increase the IPAP level as clinical needs demand. Reassess the mask seal. At higher levels of IPAP, leaks around the mask are more frequent. A leak

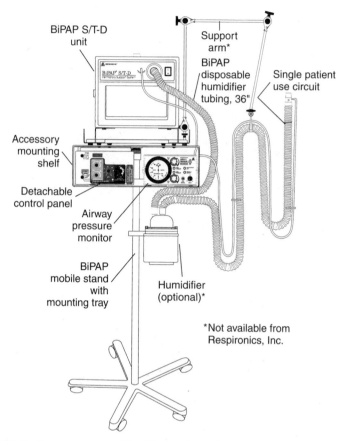

FIGURE 27-2 Commercially available bilevel positive airway pressure (BiPAP) unit. (From *The complete BiPAP S/T-D hospital system* [1992]. Courtesy Respironics Inc., Pittsburgh, PA.)

may require reseating the mask, tightening the mask straps, and repositioning the patient (Figure 27-3).

3. Assess the patient-ventilator interface for synchrony. The patient should receive IPAP on each spontaneous breath. If the patient is a mouth breather and is wearing a nasal mask, the patient's efforts may not be synchronous and fully supported by the ventilator. If the patient is unable to synchronize with the machine, consider switching to a full-face mask. If you do not have the capability to do full-face mask ventilation with the BiPAP unit, consider switching to NIMV with a mechanical ventilator with PSV and PCV modes.

NONINVASIVE VENTILATION VIA A MECHANICAL VENTILATOR
Equipment

Mechanical ventilator capable of pressure support and pressure-control modes of ventilation

Self-sealing full-face mask

Adjustable head straps

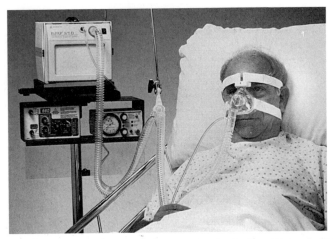

FIGURE 27–3 Correctly fitted nasal mask. (Courtesy Respironics Inc., Pittsburgh, PA.)

PROCEDURAL STEPS

1. Pressure-regulated modes of ventilation (PSV, PCV) are the most common modes of ventilation used in NIMV. Volume-targeted modes (synchronized intermittent mandatory ventilation [SIMV] assist control volume cycles) have been used successfully; however, some authors have cited better patient tolerance for pressure-regulated modes of ventilation (Foglio et al., 1994).

2. Start with low PSV levels to accustom the patient to positive-pressure breathing. Typical initial PSV levels are 5 cm H_2O. Gradually increase the PSV level until adequate tidal volume and chest excursion have been achieved.

3. Should large air leaks around the mask interfere with the synchrony of the patient-ventilator interface, you may choose to switch to the PCV mode, which is time limited, and therefore inspiration will always terminate when the inspiratory time is reached. Adjust the inspiratory time to a comfortable level for the patient.

4. Most mechanical ventilators have several types of alarms. These include high and low pressure, high and low minute volume, high respiratory rate, low tidal volume, low PEEP, and a general disconnect alarm. The alarm limits depend on the patient's status.

AGE-SPECIFIC CONSIDERATIONS

1. NIAV has been used on pediatric patient populations as young as 4 years of age (Padman, Lawless, & Von Nessen, 1994). These populations include patients with cystic fibrosis, asthma, and various neuromuscular diseases. NIAV has also been used in the pediatric setting as a treatment for atelectasis.

2. Generally, pediatric patients start at lower levels of CPAP, IPAP, and PSV than do adult patients.

3. Nasal CPAP is routinely used for infants in the neonatal intensive care unit. Indications include low gestational age, immature lungs, atelectasis, and

unresolved spells of apnea and bradycardia. Neonates are ventilated in a supine position, not upright.

COMPLICATIONS

1. Decreased cardiac output due to reduced venous return secondary to increased intrathoracic pressure. Patients may be particularly sensitive to this phenomenon if they are hypovolemic.
2. Pneumothorax secondary to increased intrathoracic pressure.
3. Gastric insufflation due to air swallowing or total inspiratory pressures greater than 20 cm H_2O.
4. Potential for aspiration due to a tight-fitting mask and gastric insufflation.
5. Conjunctivitis secondary to gas leakage around the bridge of the nose.
6. Respiratory failure secondary to the failure of NIAV to reverse respiratory muscle fatigue and correct gas exchange. In this situation, remove the patient from the ventilator and support ventilation with a bag-mask until intubation can be accomplished.

PATIENT TEACHING

1. Instruct the patient to remain in a stable, upright position to avoid creating leaks in the seal of the mask.
2. Demonstrate how to remove the mask quickly in the event of vomiting.
3. Immediately report:
   - Sudden increased difficulty in breathing
   - Nausea or vomiting
4. Hydration and mouth care are important when using NIAV. Instruct the patient to drink fluids as well as keep mouth moist.

REFERENCES

Bersten, A. D., Holt, A. W., Vedig, A. E., Skowronski, G. A., & Baggoley, C. J. (1991). Treatment of severe cardiogenic pulmonary edema with continuous positive airway pressure delivered by facemask. *New England Journal of Medicine, 325,* 1825-1830.

Brochard, L., Mancebo, J., Wysocki, M., Lofaso, F., Conti, G., & Rauss, A., et al. (1995). Noninvasive ventilation for acute exacerbations of chronic obstructive lung disease. *New England Journal of Medicine, 333,* 817-822.

Fernandez, R., Blanch, L., Valles, J., Baigorri, F., & Artigas, A. (1993). Pressure support ventilation via facemask in acute respiratory failure in hypercapnic COPD patients. *Intensive Care Medicine, 19,* 456-461.

Foglio, K., Clini, E. & Vitacca, M. (1994). Different modes of noninvasive, intermittent positive pressure ventilation (IPPV) in acute exacerbations of COLD patients. *Monaldi Archives for Chest Disease, 49,* 556-557.

Kleopa, K. A., Sherman, M., Neal, B., Romano, G. J. & Heiman-Patterson, T. (1999). BiPAP improves survival and rate of pulmonary function decline in patients with ALS. *Journal of Neurological Sciences, 164*(1), 82-88.

Mak, V. (2002). Non-invasive assisted ventilation (NIPPV/NIAV) in the management of acute hypercapnic failure secondary to COPD. *Chest medicine on-line.* Retrieved December 28, 2006, from http://www.priory.com/cmol/niav1.htm

Padman, R., Lawless, S. & Von Nessen, S. (1994). Use of BiPAP by nasal mask in the treatment of respiratory insufficiency in pediatric patients: Preliminary investigation. *Pediatric Pulmonology, 17,* 119-123.

Ram, F. S. F., Picot, J., Lightowler, J., & Wdzicha, J. A. (2004). Non-invasive positive pressure ventilation for treatment of respiratory failure due to exacerbations of chronic obstructive pulmonary disease. *Cochrane Database of Systematic Reviews 2004*, (3), CD004104.

Tebal, L., Marks, P. & Benzo, R. (1996). Non-invasive mechanical ventilation: The benefits of the BiPAP system. *West Virginia Journal of Medicine, 92*(1), 18-21.

Wysocki, M., Tric, L., Wolff, M. A, Gertner, J., Millet, H. & Herman, B. (1993). Noninvasive pressure support ventilation in patients with acute respiratory failure. *Chest, 103*, 907-913.

Wysocki, M., Tric, L., Wolff, M. A., Millet, H., & Herman, B. (1995). Noninvasive pressure support ventilation in patients with acute respiratory failure: A randomized comparison with conventional therapy. *Chest, 107*, 761-768.

PROCEDURE 28

T-Piece

Garrett K. Chan, APRN,BC, PhD, CEN

The T-piece is also known as a *T-piece aerosol nebulizer, "tee" piece, or Briggs adaptor.*

INDICATIONS

1. To provide humidification and oxygen to patients with endotracheal or tracheostomy tubes and spontaneous breathing patterns.
2. To assist with weaning from a ventilator duirng a spontaneous breathing trial (SBT) while providing humidification and oxygen to patients with endotracheal or tracheostomy tubes and spontaneous breathing patterns that generally meet the following parameters. SBTs should last approximately 30 to 120 minutes to assess the patient's readiness for extubation (MacIntyre et al., 2001). If the patient tolerates an SBT for 20 to 120 minutes, discontinuation of mechanical ventilation should be considered. It should be noted that some patients may be successfully weaned even though they do not meet all the criteria. Correlation with the clinician's physical assessment of the patient will help guide a successful extubation (MacIntyre, 2004; MacIntyre et al., 2001).

Objective Physiologic Measurements

- Adequate oxygenation (e.g., PO_2 60 mm Hg or greater on fraction of inspired oxygen [FiO_2] 0.4 or less; positive end-expiratory pressure (PEEP) 5–10 cm H_2O or less; P/F ratio (PO_2/FiO_2) 150–300 or greater)
- Stable cardiovascular system (e.g., heart rate 140 or less; stable blood pressure; no [or minimal] vasopressors)

- Afebrile (temperature less than $38°C$)
- No significant respiratory acidosis
- Adequate hemoglobin (e.g., Hgb 8–10 g/dl or greater)
- Adequate mentation (e.g., arousable, Glasgow Coma Scale score 13 or greater, no continuous sedative infusions)
- Stable metabolic status (e.g., acceptable electrolytes)

Subjective Clinical Assessments
- Resolution of disease acute phase; physician/nurse/respiratory therapist believes discontinuation is possible, adequate cough

Ventilator Measurements (selected)
- Minute ventilation (Ve) = 10–15 L/min
- Negative inspiratory force (NIF) = -20 to -30 cm H_2O
- Maximal inspiratory pressure (Pmax) = -15 to -130 cm H_2O

Measured during a Brief Period of Spontaneous Breathing
- Respiratory rate (RR) = 30 to 38 breaths per minute
- Tidal volume (VT) = 4 to 6 ml/kg
- Respiratory rate/tidal volume ratio (f/VT) = 60 to 105/L

CONTRAINDICATIONS AND CAUTIONS
1. Patients who are obtunded without spontaneous respirations or who do not meet minimum spontaneous parameters require mechanical ventilation.
2. The aerosol temperature at the patient end of the circuit should be at body temperature (optional for normothermic patients requiring short-term use).
3. Tubing must be checked and drained of excess water frequently. A water trap may be included in the circuit and is recommended if extended use is anticipated. The water trap is placed in the lowest portion of the aerosol tubing.

EQUIPMENT
Heated aerosol (optional)
Oxygen analyzer
T-piece setup (Figure 28–1)
Flowmeters (air or O_2)

PROCEDURAL STEPS
1. Assemble the aerosol nebulizer and make sure the humidifier is filled with sterile water to the appropriate mark.
2. Connect the flowmeter to the oxygen source and attach the nebulizer.
3. Set the FiO_2 of the O_2 blender or humidifier and plug in the heating element if one is being used.
4. Turn the primary flowmeter to 14 L/min of oxygen. Analyze the FiO_2 with an oxygen analyzer and label the flowmeters with the proper L/min settings. To maintain adequate flow, Table 28-1 can be used. Always run the flowmeter by powering the nebulizer at 14 L/min or greater and/or adjust the bleed until the desired FiO_2 is obtained.

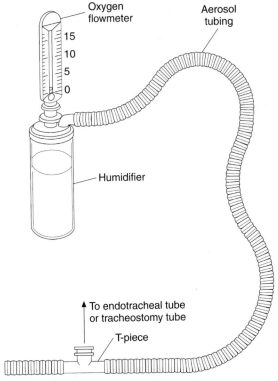

FIGURE 28-1 T-piece setup (bleed-in flowmeter, heater, and water trap not shown).

5. Check to see that mist is visible at the T-piece. If it is not visible, the unit may be faulty or the flow rate may not be high enough. Attach the T-piece to the endotracheal or tracheostomy tube.

6. It is important to maintain a high-flow system. If the patient's inspiratory flow rate exceeds the output of the nebulizer, the resultant flow deficit will result in room-air entrainment and a decreased FiO_2. To ensure a high-flow system, the Venturi should never be turned higher than the 40% setting. Any FiO_2 greater than 40% must be achieved by bleeding in additional flow to the system. This guarantees the patient at least 40 L/min

TABLE 28-1
FLOWMETER USE IN T-PIECE SETUP

FiO_2	Nebulizer Power Flow Required	Bleed-in Desired
21%	Air flowmeter	Not used
22%-27%	Air flowmeter	O_2 flowmeter
28%-45%	O_2 flowmeter	Not used
45%-80%	O_2 flowmeter	O_2 flowmeter

total flow. Be sure to analyze for proper FiO_2 after setup and equipment changes.

7. Check the heating element to ensure that it is functioning properly. The humidifier should be warm, not hot, to the touch.

COMPLICATIONS

1. FiO_2 changes can result from unsecured flowmeter controls and entrainment port handles.
2. Inadequate oxygen flow can impede the production of the mist.
3. Aspiration of water can occur if the tubing is not drained.
4. Excessive condensate can also block oxygen flow.
5. Excessive condensate can also contribute to the possibility of bacterial growth and aerosolization of bacteria into the patient's lungs.
6. Patients being weaned from a mechanical ventilator may not be able to tolerate a T-piece, especially after a prolonged period of mechanical ventilation and may require reconnection to the ventilator.

REFERENCES

MacIntyre, N. R. (2004). Evidence-based ventilator weaning and discontinuation. *Respiratory Care, 49*(7), 830-836.

MacIntyre, N. R., Cook, D. J., Ely, E. W. Jr., Epstein, S. K., Fink, J. B., Heffner, J. E., Hess, D., Hubmayer, R. D.& Scheinhorn, D. J. (2001). Evidence-based guidelines for weaning and discontinuing ventilatory support: A collective task force facilitated by the American College of Chest Physicians; the American Association for Respiratory Care; and the American College of Critical Care Medicine. *Chest, 120*(6 Suppl), 375S-395S.

Suctioning

Pharyngeal Suctioning

Teresa L. Will, MSN, RN, CEN

Pharyngeal suctioning is also known as *oropharyngeal suctioning, Yankauer suctioning, nasopharyngeal suctioning*, and *tonsillar suctioning*.

INDICATIONS

1. To clear the airway of secretions, foreign matter, or blood in patients incapable of clearing their own oropharynx or nasopharynx. Pharyngeal suctioning may be used with conscious or unconscious and intubated or nonintubated patients.
2. To stimulate coughing and deep breathing in the nonintubated patient.

CONTRAINDICATIONS AND CAUTIONS

1. Oropharyngeal secretions may be thick (e.g., blood or vomit). Use a large-bore suction catheter, a tonsillar-pharyngeal suction-tip device (Yankauer), or the suction connecting tubing alone for more effective airway clearance.
2. Excessive suctioning may traumatize the pharyngeal tissue and cause bleeding, swelling, or localized inflammation. Use a beveled tip and limit suctioning to 10 seconds per attempt to help decrease adverse effects.
3. Hypoxemia may result from prolonged suctioning.
4. Suctioning may cause coughing, gagging, or both, which increase intracranial pressure and should be avoided in patients with head injuries. If gagging leads to vomiting, aspiration and respiratory compromise may occur.
5. Suctioning may stimulate the vagal response, leading to bradycardia and hypotension, particularly in infants and younger pediatric patients.
6. If possible, use the less traumatic oropharyngeal route rather than the nasopharyngeal approach.
7. Excessive bleeding may occur in patients who have bleeding disorders or who are receiving anticoagulant therapy. Observe for bleeding and use lower suction pressures for those patients.
8. If epiglottitis is suspected, nasopharyngeal suctioning is contraindicated, because it may precipitate total occlusion of the airway.
9. Pharyngeal suctioning is considered a clean procedure. Regular examination gloves should be worn during the procedure.

EQUIPMENT

Portable or wall continuous-suction unit with regulator
Suction canister
Suction connecting tubing
Tonsillar or pharyngeal suction tip or bulb syringe
Suction catheter with an age-appropriate size of French whistle tip with a vent port or Y connector

30 to 60 ml of tap water to clear the connecting tubing and suction tip

Container to hold water (an emesis basin works well)

Water-soluble lubricant for a catheter inserted via the nasopharyngeal route

Emesis basin

Tissues

Supplemental oxygen source and oxygen delivery device

Examination gloves

PATIENT PREPARATION

1. For optimal airway alignment, place the patient in semi-Fowler's position. The sniffing position maximizes alignment of the airway for nasopharyngeal suctioning. Pharyngeal suctioning may be performed in any position.
2. The patient may feel breathless during the procedure. A high-flow oxygen mask may be set up for use between suctioning. Instruct the patient to use the oxygen mask and take deep breaths until he or she feels comfortable.
3. Warn the patient that the suctioning procedure may stimulate the gag or cough reflex. Provide an emesis basin and tissues.

PROCEDURAL STEPS

1. Assemble the suction canister and attach it to the suction unit.
2. Attach the connecting tubing to the suction canister.
3. Select an appropriate catheter or suction device. To prevent hypoxia and trauma, the suction catheter for the nasopharyngeal route should not be greater than half the diameter of the naris to be suctioned.
4. Set the suction gauge between 120 and 200 mm Hg. Full suction assists in the rapid removal of a large amount of fluid or debris from the oropharynx. Occlude the suction tubing to test the level of suction as measured by the suction gauge.

Oropharyngeal Route

1. Attach the catheter or pharyngeal suction tip to the connecting tubing.
2. Insert the catheter or pharyngeal suction tip into the back of the mouth without applying suction. If using a Yankauer tip, gently sweep the posterior pharynx while applying suction for 10 to 15 seconds.
3. If using a catheter, insert it into the area on either side of the glottis. Apply suction intermittently for 10 seconds, gently rotating as you withdraw the catheter.
4. Flush the catheter by aspirating water through the connecting tubing.

Nasopharyngeal Route

1. Nasopharyngeal suctioning is used when the oral route is not accessible (e.g., with clenched teeth or oral trauma).
2. Assess for nasal patency by inspecting each naris for any obstruction, such as polyps, structural deformity, or trauma. Occlude each naris and ask the patient to inhale to determine which side is most patent. Use the most patent naris for suctioning.
3. Attach the suction catheter to the connecting tubing. Apply a small amount of water-soluble lubricant to the catheter or lubricate with water.

4. Instruct the patient to use supplemental oxygen before the procedure and take deep breaths for 30 seconds.
5. Without applying suction, gently insert the lubricated catheter medially into the naris. As you slide the catheter to the back of the naris, instruct the conscious patient to assume the sniffing position. This position assists in passage of the catheter through the larynx and enhances access to the pharyngeal area. Slide the catheter through the naris until resistance is met or coughing is stimulated. If coughing is stimulated, pull back on the catheter slightly.
6. Apply suction intermittently for a maximum of 10 seconds and rotate the catheter slightly while withdrawing.
7. Flush the catheter by aspirating water through the connecting tubing.
8. Offer supplemental oxygen after suctioning.
9. If frequent suctioning is required, a nasopharyngeal airway may be inserted to decrease mucosal trauma and to act as a guide for the catheter. See Procedure 6.

Bulb Syringe

1. Depress the bulb syringe and gently advance into the nose or to the area of pooled secretions and debris in the oropharynx. Release the large bulb syringe to aspirate secretions and debris.
2. When suctioning an infant, insert the tip of the bulb syringe into the side pockets in the cheeks. Never put the tip of the bulb syringe in the back of the throat.
3. Depress bulb syringe into a basin to dispose of secretions and debris.
4. Flush the bulb syringe by aspirating and expelling water until clear.
5. Repeat steps 1 to 3 until the airway is clear.

AGE-SPECIFIC CONSIDERATIONS

1. Lower suction pressures may be used in children.
2. Provide supplemental oxygen as needed to prevent hypoxemia in the pediatric patient.
3. Infants and children are especially prone to vagal stimulation, so monitor heart rate and limit application of suction to 10 seconds.
4. A bulb syringe is usually used only for infants.

COMPLICATIONS

1. Infection is a potential complication of nasopharyngeal suctioning when the correct technique is not used. A new catheter must be used each time for nasopharyngeal suctioning to prevent contamination of the tracheobronchial area.
2. A catheter or pharyngeal suction tip for the oropharynx may be used repeatedly for the same patient unless it is grossly contaminated or becomes clogged with large debris.
3. Excessive suctioning may create irritation to the upper airway and result in bleeding or edema, which may further compromise the airway patency.

PATIENT TEACHING

1. Cough when possible to assist in clearing the airway.

2. Report any respiratory difficulty.
3. For a conscious patient with excessive oral secretions, a tonsil tip may be set up and the patient instructed on how to suction himself or herself.

REFERENCES

Emergency Nurses Association (ENA). (2004). *Emergency nursing pediatric course: Provider manual* (3rd ed.). Des Plaines, IL: Author.

Kattwinkel, J. (Ed.) (2006). *Textbook of neonatal resuscitation* (5th ed.). Elk Grove, IL: American Academy of Pediatrics.

PROCEDURE 30

Nasotracheal Suctioning

Teresa L. Will, MSN, RN, CEN, and
Jean A. Proehl, RN, MN, CEN, CCRN, FAEN

INDICATIONS

1. To maintain airway patency, maximize oxygenation, and reduce lower airway resistance in the nonintubated patient through removal of secretions when the patient cannot cough effectively. Evidence of secretions includes one or more of the following (AARC, 2004):
   - Visible secretions in the airway
   - Auscultation of coarse, gurgling breath sounds, rhonchi or diminished breath sounds
   - Suspected aspiration of gastric or upper airway secretions
   - Increased work of breathing
   - Hypoxemia or hypercarbia
   - Chest radiographic evidence of retained secretions resulting in atelectasis or consolidation
2. To stimulate coughing in the weak or debilitated patient who is unable to clear secretions without assistance.
3. To obtain a sputum specimen when the patient is unable to do so without assistance.

CONTRAINDICATIONS AND CAUTIONS

1. Relative contraindications for nasotracheal suctioning include the following (AARC, 2004):

- Occluded naris
- Nasal bleeding
- Acute head, facial, or neck injury
- Coagulopathy or bleeding disorder
- Laryngospasm
- Irritable airway
- Upper respiratory tract infection
- Tracheal surgery
- Gastric surgery with high anastomosis
- Myocardial infarction
- Bronchospasm

2. Do not suction patients with epiglottitis or croup (AARC, 2004).
3. To prevent hypoxia and tissue trauma, select a suction catheter no more than one half the diameter of the naris to be suctioned.
4. Suctioning may exacerbate increased intracranial pressure or severe hypertension and should be performed with caution in patients with these conditions.
5. Hypoxia may occur during suctioning, particularly in patients with a history of pulmonary or cardiac disease and in infants and small children.
6. Continuous suction may cause trauma to mucosa. Suction should be applied for no longer than 10 seconds (Chulay, 2005).
7. Nasotracheal suction should not be used for patients with severe facial or head trauma. There is risk of penetration of the cranial vault by the suction catheter.
8. Use caution in patients with narrow or obstructed nares and in those who are anticoagulated or who have bleeding disorders.

EQUIPMENT

Portable or wall continuous-suction unit with regulator
Suction canister
Suction-connecting tubing
Water-soluble lubricant
Sterile-suction catheter (14 Fr is the standard size for adults)
Sterile water or 0.9% saline solution to flush tubing
Sterile container or cup
Sterile gloves
Oxygen source with oxygen mask or nasal cannula
Towels
Emesis basin and tissues
Bag-mask (readily available)
(Commercially prepared suction catheter kits are available.)

PATIENT PREPARATION

1. For optimal airway alignment, place the patient in semi-Fowler's position. In the supine position, place the head in a neutral position. If possible, have the patient blow his or her nose to clear the nasal passages. To prevent contamination of the lower airways, suction the trachea first and then the mouth and pharynx. Alternately, suction the mouth and pharynx first and then change to a new, sterile suction catheter. (See Procedure 29.)

2. If frequent nasotracheal suctioning is necessary, a nasal airway may be placed to help prevent trauma to the naris. (See Procedure 6.)
3. Obtain baseline assessments of breath sounds, skin color, heart rate, and oxygen saturation. Monitor skin color, oxygen saturation, and heart rate during the procedure.
4. Provide an oxygen source before and after suctioning. If a nasal cannula is being used, the prongs may be adjusted so that one naris continues to receive oxygen.
5. Administer sedation or analgesia as prescribed.
6. Inform the patient that a brief feeling of breathlessness is normal during the procedure and that the procedure may stimulate the gag or cough reflex. Provide an emesis basin and tissues. Encourage the patient to expectorate any mucus produced.
7. Drape towels over the patient's chest to prevent contamination by secretions.
8. Measure from the nose to the sternal notch with the catheter. Do not contaminate the sterile catheter while measuring. This will give a rough estimate of how far to advance the catheter to reach the lower airway.

PROCEDURAL STEPS

1. Assemble the suction canister and attach it to the wall or a portable suction unit. Attach the connecting tubing to the suction canister.
2. Set the suction pressure between 100 and 150 mm Hg for an adult. Negative pressures in excess of 150 mm Hg may result in hypoxemia, trauma, and atelectasis (AARC, 2004). Occlude the suction tubing to test the level of suction, as measured by the suction gauge.
3. Examine both nares and choose a patent one. Avoid using a naris that is partially blocked by polyps, hemorrhage, or a deviated nasal septum. To prevent hypoxia and trauma, the suction catheter for the nasotracheal route should not be greater than one half of the internal diameter of the naris.
4. Preoxygenate the patient with high-flow oxygen for 2 minutes before suctioning; alternately, place the prong of a nasal cannula in the opposite naris, or have an assistant hold an oxygen mask with high-flow oxygen to the mouth. Ask patients to take slow, deep breaths through the mouth during the procedure. Preoxygenation is a key method of preventing a decrease in the patient's baseline oxygenation status.
5. Dispense a small amount of water-soluble lubricant onto a sterile field, such as the inside of the catheter package.
6. Put on sterile gloves.
7. Attach the sterile suction catheter to the connecting tubing.
8. Hold the suction catheter in your dominant hand, which must remain sterile. Your other hand, which controls the suction control vent, is considered clean.
9. Apply a water-soluble lubricant to the suction catheter.
10. Gently advance the catheter through the nasal passage in a medial, downward direction. Never apply suction upon insertion of the catheter.
11. Have the patient open his or her mouth and extend the tongue to prevent retraction of the tongue when the gag reflex is stimulated.

12. Have the patient take slow, deep breaths or cough gently. Coughing assists in opening the glottis, which permits insertion of the catheter into the trachea.
13. When the patient coughs, advance the suction catheter until resistance is met or spontaneous coughing is noted.
14. When resistance is met, withdraw the catheter 2 to 3 cm and apply suction intermittently for no more than 10 seconds. Gently rotate the catheter while withdrawing it.
15. Withdraw the suction catheter to the epiglottis area or to the point at which spontaneous coughing or gagging is absent. When secretions are excessive, necessitating repeat passes of the suction catheter, do not withdraw the catheter beyond the epiglottis. This prevents having to traverse the nasal passages again. Discontinuation of suctioning is heavily dependent on the patient's tolerance of the procedure.
16. Reoxygenate the patient with high-flow oxygen for at least 2 minutes before repeating the procedure.
17. Flush the catheter by aspirating sterile water or saline solution through the tubing.

AGE-SPECIFIC CONSIDERATIONS

1. Pediatric suction catheter sizes are 10 Fr for children and 8 Fr for infants.
2. For children, set the suction pressure as follows (AARC, 2004):
   • Neonates: 60 to 80 mm Hg
   • Infants: 80 to 100 mm Hg
   • Children: 100 to 120 mm Hg
3. To prevent hypoxia, hyperoxygenate infants and children before nasotracheal suctioning.
4. Monitor the heart rate in children during the suctioning procedure because vagal stimulation may create bradycardia. Bradycardia is usually reversed quickly with the administration of supplemental oxygen and the cessation of the suctioning procedure.

COMPLICATIONS

1. Infection of the lower respiratory tract is a potential complication because the catheter is contaminated when it is passed through the nasopharyngeal area.
2. The patient may refuse to allow the procedure to be repeated because it is very uncomfortable.
3. Prolonged suctioning may deplete the residual volume of the lung and lead to alveolar collapse, or atelectasis and hypoxia. Hypoxia can be decreased by providing adequate preoxygenation and postoxygenation and limiting suctioning to 10 seconds.
4. Suctioning may stimulate a vagal response, resulting in hypotension or bradycardia.
5. Forcing the suction catheter or inserting it repeatedly may result in mucosal damage and bleeding or local inflammation of the nasopharynx or trachea. Passing the catheter during inspiration is essential to avoid mucosal damage.
6. Laryngospasm, bronchospasm, and bronchoconstriction may occur.
7. Nasotracheal suctioning will increase intracranial pressure because of stimulation of the cough and gag reflex. Increased blood pressure may

also result. Efficient and quick suctioning will help minimize these adverse effects.

8. Aspiration is a risk especially when the gag reflex is stimulated in the presence of other factors such as decreased level of consciousness or tube feedings. Placing the patient in semi-Fowler's position helps decrease this risk.

PATIENT TEACHING

1. Cough and breathe deeply, to assist in clearing the airway.
2. Increase fluid intake to loosen and thin secretions by adequate hydration.
3. Practice good oral hygiene to decrease the risk of infection or bacterial colonization.

REFERENCES

American Association for Respiratory Care (AARC). (2004). AARC clinical practice guideline: Nasotracheal suctioning—2004 Revision & update. *Respiratory Care Journal, 49*, 1080–1089. Retrieved January 7, 2007, from http://www.rcjournal.com/contents/09.04/09.04.1080.pdf

Chulay, M. (2005). Suctioning: endotracheal or tracheostomy tube. In D. J. Lynn-McHale Wiegand, & K. K. Carlson (Eds.), *AACN procedure manual for critical care* (5th ed. pp. 9–11). Philadelphia: Saunders.

PROCEDURE 31

Endotracheal or Tracheostomy Suctioning

Teresa L. Will, MSN, RN, CEN, and
Jean A. Proehl, RN, MN, CEN, CCRN, FAEN

Endotracheal suctioning is also known as *ET suctioning*.

INDICATIONS

1. To maintain patency of an artificial airway
2. To remove secretions via an endotracheal tube (ETT) or tracheostomy tube, which may obstruct the airway and cause hypoxia, pneumonia, bronchitis, or atelectasis. The need for suctioning may be indicated by decreasing oxygen saturation, audible gurgling, adventitious breath sounds, or restlessness.

3. To obtain a sputum specimen for laboratory analysis
4. To stimulate a deep cough reflex in patients who are sedated or neurologically impaired in order to mobilize secretions to the larger airways

CONTRAINDICATIONS AND CAUTIONS

1. Suctioning may exacerbate increased intracranial pressure or severe hypertension.
2. Do not deflate the ETT or tracheostomy cuff before suctioning. The inflated cuff assists in preventing aspiration of any contents into the lungs if the gag reflex is stimulated and vomiting occurs. Positioning the patient with the head of the bed elevated 30 degrees during and after suctioning may minimize aspiration risk.
3. To prevent hypoxia, suctioning should not exceed 10 seconds per attempt (Chulay, 2005).
4. For patients receiving mechanical ventilation with positive end-expiratory pressure (PEEP), a PEEP adapter may be added to the bag-mask device to prevent interruption of pressure support.
5. Suctioning should be based on individual need and should not be a scheduled procedure. Limiting suctioning prevents excessive mucosal damage and decreases exposure to bacterial colonization.
6. Instillation of saline solution to loosen secretions is not effective and may decrease arterial oxygenation. Saline may also promote bacterial colonization of the lower airways (Chulay, 2005).

EQUIPMENT

Portable or wall continuous-suction unit with regulator
Suction canister
Suction connecting tubing
Sterile suction catheter with intermittent suction-control vent or closed-suction system device (see Alternative Technique section)
Sterile gloves
Sterile container
Sterile water or saline solution
Bag-mask or anesthesia bag connected to a high-flow oxygen source
(Commercially prepared, disposable suction catheter kits are available.)

PATIENT PREPARATION

1. Endotracheal or tracheostomy suctioning may be accomplished in any position; however, Fowler's position with neutral head alignment is optimal. If the patient is combative or uncooperative, restraints or sedation may be necessary to perform the procedure safely.
2. Obtain baseline assessments of breath sounds, skin color, heart rate, and oxygen saturation. Monitor skin color, oxygen saturation, and heart rate during the procedure.
3. Warn the patient that suctioning may stimulate uncontrolled coughing or brief periods of breathlessness.
4. To maintain airway patency in the patient who is unconscious and has an ETT inserted through the mouth, insert a bite block so that the tube is not kinked or bitten.

PROCEDURAL STEPS
Open Technique

1. If possible, obtain assistance before suctioning. To maximize oxygen delivery, one person should hyperoxygenate the patient while another person suctions. One-handed bagging usually does not achieve adequate tidal volume in an adult patient. The ventilator may also be used (Chulay, 2005).

2. Assemble the suction canister and attach it to the wall or a portable suction unit. Attach the connecting tubing to the suction canister. Be sure that all the connections are tight or the suction may not function.

3. Set the suction gauge between 100 and 120 mm Hg in adults (Chulay, 2005). Occlude the suction tubing to test the suction level, as measured by the suction gauge.

4. Select a suction catheter that is no larger than half the diameter of the ETT or tracheostomy tube to prevent interruption of ventilation during the suctioning. For example, a 14 Fr catheter will leave half the airway open in a size 7 ETT.

5. *Tracheostomy-Specific Method*: If the patient has a double-walled tracheostomy, remove the inner cannula and place it in a saline-filled basin during the procedure. The inner cannula may be cleaned with hydrogen peroxide and a pipe cleaner. Rinse it in saline and shake it dry before reinserting it (Figure 31-1).

6. Attach the suction catheter to the connecting tubing. Hold the suction catheter in your dominant hand, which must remain sterile. Use your other hand to control the suction vent. This hand is considered clean.

7. Use the ventilator to hyperoxygenate the patient or have your assistant ventilate the patient with 100% oxygen via the bag-mask for 30 seconds or at least five or six hyperinflations (Chulay, 2005).

8. Immerse the tip of the catheter into the saline and aspirate a small amount to lubricate the catheter.

9. For endotracheal suctioning, have your assistant stabilize the tube to prevent excessive movement or tube displacement.

10. Gently insert the catheter through the tube and advance the catheter until resistance is met. Pull the catheter back 1 cm. Do not apply suction during the introduction of the catheter.

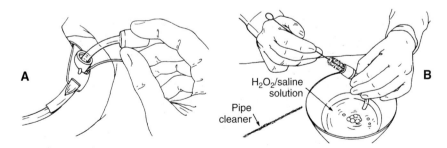

A

B

H₂O₂/saline solution

Pipe cleaner

FIGURE 31-1 A, Remove inner cannula; the cannula may need to be turned counterclockwise to release locking mechanism. **B,** Clean inner cannula. (From Kersten, L. [1989]. *Comprehensive respiratory nursing* [p. 677]. Philadelphia: Saunders.)

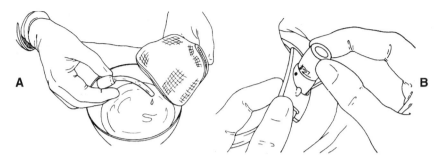

FIGURE 31-2 **A,** Rinse and shake dry. **B,** Reinsert cannula and turn clockwise to lock in place. (From Kersten, L. [1989]. *Comprehensive respiratory nursing* [p. 677]. Philadelphia: Saunders.)

11. Withdraw the catheter slowly while applying intermittent suction and rotating the catheter for no longer than 10 seconds (Chulay, 2005).
12. Use the ventilator to ventilate and hyperoxygenate the patient or have your assistant ventilate the patient with 100% oxygen via the bag-mask. Postoxygenation should be given for 30 seconds (five or six breaths) after suctioning or until the alert patient signals recovery (Chulay, 2005).
13. Reconnect the patient to the ventilator or T-piece.
14. Rinse the catheter and connecting tubing by aspirating sterile water or saline through the tubing.
15. Repeat steps 8 through 11 if excessive secretions exist. Allow the patient at least 1 minute to recover before repeating the procedure.
16. If necessary, suction the nares or the oropharynx before disposing of the catheter and gloves.
17. For a tracheostomy, dry and replace the clean inner cannula (Figure 31-2).

Closed-suction System

1. The closed-suction system device is placed between the ETT or tracheostomy tube and the ventilator or T-piece to permit suctioning without interrupting oxygenation or ventilation. The attached sheathed suction catheter passes through a seal into the tracheal tube (Figure 31-3).
2. Select a suction catheter that is no larger than half the diameter of the ETT or tracheostomy tube to prevent interruption of ventilation during the suctioning. For example, a 14 Fr catheter will leave half the airway open in a size 7 ETT. Attach the suction-connecting tubing to the open end of the closed-suction system near the lock.
3. Depress the suction-control valve and set the suction gauge per the manufacturer's recommendations. Keep the control valve depressed until the desired suction level is set.
4. Connect the T-piece of the suction system to the ventilator tubing and then attach the T-piece to the ETT or tracheostomy tube.
5. Use the ventilator to ventilate and hyperoxygenate the patient or have your assistant ventilate the patient with 100% oxygen via the bag-mask for 30 seconds or at least five or six inflations (Chulay, 2005).
6. Use your nondominant hand to stabilize the T-piece and gently advance the sleeved catheter through the tracheal tube with your dominant hand.

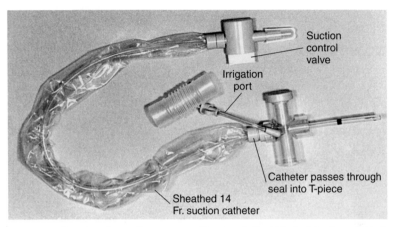

FIGURE 31-3 Closed-suction catheter system. (Courtesy Ballard Medical Products, Midvale, UT.)

7. Use your dominant hand to grasp the suction-control valve. Depress the valve intermittently while withdrawing the suction catheter in a straight motion in 10 seconds or less (Chulay, 2005). Be sure to withdraw the suction catheter completely to prevent occlusion or irritation of the airway.

8. Use the ventilator to ventilate and hyperoxygenate the patient or have your assistant ventilate the patient with 100% oxygen via the bag-mask. Postoxygenation should be given for 30 seconds (five or six breaths) after suctioning or until the alert patient signals recovery (Chulay, 2005).

9. Repeat suctioning as needed. Flush the suction catheter by instilling sterile normal saline or water through the irrigation port until the catheter and connecting tubing are clear. A self-sealing system prevents the fluid from entering the tracheal tube.

10. After flushing, lock the catheter by turning the suction control valve to the lock position or following the manufacturer's instructions on the package insert.

11. Repeat steps 5 through 8 if additional suctioning is required. To provide adequate preoxygenation, allow the patient to rest at least 1 minute before repeating the procedure.

Sputum Trap for Specimen Collection

1. Connect the suction tubing to the open port of the sputum trap. Attach the suction catheter to the port of the sputum trap by means of the soft rubber extension tubing (Figure 31-4). Use the same set-up as you would if you were preparing to suction.

2. Insert the suction catheter and use the suction technique as previously described.

3. Remove the catheter and the tubing from the sputum trap. As preparation for shipment to the laboratory, connect the rubber tubing port to the plastic port of the sputum trap.

4. Flush the suction catheter with approximately 10 ml of normal saline.

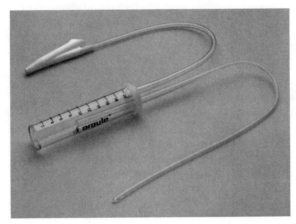

FIGURE 31-4   Sputum trap collection system. (From Argyle De Lee mucus trap with vacuum breaker [product information]. [1998]. Courtesy Sherwood Davis & Geck, St. Louis.)

AGE-SPECIFIC CONSIDERATIONS

1. Suction catheter insertion should stop short of the carina in infants and children. Using the ETT markings as a guide, insert the suction catheter only 1-2 cm beyond the tube. If resistance is met, pull the tube back 0.5-1 cm before applying suction (Curley & Thompson, 2001; Jarog, 2008).
2. For children, set the suction pressure as follows (AARC, 2004; Jarog, 2008).
   - *Neonates*: 60 to 80 mm Hg
   - *Infants*: 80 to 100 mm Hg
   - *Children younger than 8 years*: 100 to 120 mm Hg
   - *Children older than 8 years*: 120 to 150 mm Hg
3. Ventilate and oxygenate pediatric patients for at least 30 seconds before and after each passage of the suction catheter (Jarog, 2008).
4. To avoid hyperoxemia in neonates, consider using less than 100% oxygen. For preoxygenation, use 10% to 20% more oxygen than baseline and titrate to maintain the oxygen saturation at the patient's baseline.
5. Monitor the heart rate in children during suctioning because vagal stimulation may cause bradycardia. Bradycardia can usually be reversed quickly with the administration of supplemental oxygen and the cessation of suctioning.
6. Select the correct catheter size for effective suctioning. As general guidelines, use a 10 Fr to 16 Fr suction catheter for an adult, an 8 Fr to 10 Fr suction catheter for a child, and a 6 Fr to 8 Fr for a small infant. Neonatal and pediatric sizes of closed-suction catheters are available.

COMPLICATIONS

1. Prolonged suctioning may cause hypoxia or atelectasis.
2. Hypoxia, hypercarbia, or stimulation of the cough reflex during endotracheal or tracheostomy suctioning increases cerebral blood volume and intracranial pressure. Use caution when providing respiratory care to a patient with a head injury by limiting suctioning to duration and number of passes per suction event.

3. The procedure may create a feeling of suffocation in the patient and lead to excessive anxiety.
4. An improper suctioning technique may traumatize the tracheal mucosa.
5. A respiratory tract infection may result from colonization of the airway with bacteria.
6. Aspiration of vomit may occur if the tracheal cuff is faulty. Postintubation aspiration has been reduced with the advent of low-pressure, high-volume cuffs.
7. Suctioning may stimulate a vagal response that may result in hypotension or bradycardia.
8. Patients receiving anticoagulants or thrombolytics may have blood-tinged secretions. Suctioning should be limited in these patients.

PATIENT TEACHING
1. To decrease the incidence of mucosal damage at the point of entry (mouth or nose) and at the tracheal entry area, avoid touching or moving the ETT or tracheostomy tube.
2. Patient should report any respiratory distress immediately.

REFERENCES

American Association for Respiratory Care (AARC). (2004). AARC clinical practice guideline: Nasotracheal suctioning—2004 Revision & update. *Respiratory Care Journal, 49,* 1080–1089. Retrieved January 7, 2007, from http://www.rcjournal.com/contents/09.04/09.04.1080.pdf

Chulay, M. (2005). Suctioning: Endotracheal or tracheostomy tube. In D. J. Lynn-McHale Wiegand, & K. K. Carlson (Eds.), *AACN procedure manual for critical care* (5th ed. pp. 9–11). Philadelphia: Saunders.

Curley, M. A. Q. & Thompson, J. E. (2001). Oxygenation and ventilation. In M. A. Q. Curley, & P. A. Maloney-Harmon (Eds.), *Critical care nursing of infants and children* (2nd ed. pp. 233–308). Philadelphia: Saunders.

Jarog, D. L. (2008). Endotracheal tube: Suctioning and care. In J. T. Verger, & R. M. Lebet (Eds.), *AACN procedure manual for acute and critical pediatric care* (pp. 5–16). Philadelphia: Saunders.

Ventilation

Mouth-to-Mask Ventilation

Ruth L. Schaffler, PhD, ARNP, CEN

Mouth-to-mask ventilation is also known as *face-mask ventilation* and *face-shield ventilation*.

INDICATION

To ventilate a patient who has ineffective or absent spontaneous respirations while protecting the rescuer from direct contact with the patient's mouth or secretions. Mouth-to-mask ventilation may provide a greater tidal volume than ventilation with a bag-mask, especially if the rescuer is not highly skilled in the use of the bag-mask.

CONTRAINDICATIONS AND CAUTIONS

1. Clear the airway of any obstruction before ventilating the patient.
2. Masks should be made from a transparent material so that lip color, vomit, blood, or other foreign material in the airway are visible. A mask with a one-way valve is preferred.
3. Both hands of the rescuer are needed to provide an adequate seal around the mask and to maintain an open airway. If cardiopulmonary resuscitation (CPR) is indicated, two rescuers are preferred because it is difficult for one person to simultaneously open the airway and quickly reestablish the mask seal with each return to the patient's head after performing chest compressions. Use of a face shield that drapes over the patient's face facilitates CPR by one rescuer.
4. The concentration of oxygen delivered in exhaled air is approximately 16%, but delivery to the patient can be enhanced by adding supplemental oxygen via a port (present on some masks).
5. Use of a face mask may not be appropriate for patients who have severe facial trauma, trismus, excessive oral bleeding, or vomiting.
6. Face masks are not used for patients who have a postlaryngectomy stoma.
7. Low tidal volumes without supplementary oxygen may be ineffective for maintaining adequate arterial oxygen saturation, resulting in hypercarbia and acidosis.

EQUIPMENT

Face mask (Figure 32-1) or face shield (flexible plastic sheet with filter or one-way valve)
Oropharyngeal or nasopharyngeal airway (if needed)
Oxygen tubing and source (optional, but preferred)
Suction equipment (if needed)

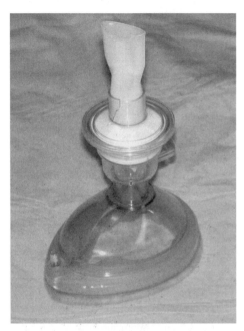

FIGURE 32-1 Example of a face mask with a one-way valve.

PATIENT PREPARATION

1. Place the patient in a supine position on a firm surface when possible. If necessary, ventilations can be delivered to patients who are seated or who are floating in water.
2. Open the airway by using the head-tilt/chin-lift maneuver if there is no evidence of head or neck trauma. If a cervical spine injury is suspected, a jaw-thrust maneuver should be used without extending the neck. If the jaw thrust does not open the airway, use the head-tilt/chin-lift method (see Procedure 3).
3. Clear the airway of any visible obstruction before ventilating the patient; blind finger sweeps are not recommended and may actually be harmful.
4. An oral airway or a nasal airway may be used to maintain airway patency (see Procedures 5 and 6).
5. The rescuer should be positioned to use either a cephalic (above the patient's head) or a lateral (beside the patient's head) technique for rescue breathing. Two rescuers are preferred to perform CPR—one to provide ventilation and maintain an adequate seal of the mask on the patient's face and the other to deliver chest compressions.

PROCEDURAL STEPS
Mouth-to-mask Ventilation

1. Place the mask over the patient's nose and mouth with the narrow end of the mask over the nose. A properly sized mask should extend from the bridge of the nose to the space between the lower lip and the chin and should provide an airtight seal on the face.

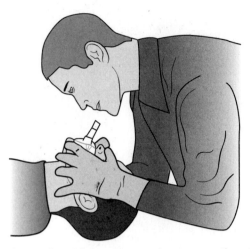

FIGURE 32-2 Mouth-to-mask ventilation. Place mask over a mouth and nose, and maintain a tight seal against the face by using both hands. Observe the rise and fall of the chest during the respiratory cycle. (Pons, P., & Cason, D. [1997]. *Paramedic field guide* [p. 270]. St. Louis: Mosby.)

2. If you are using the cephalic technique, apply pressure to both sides of the mask by using the thumbs and thenar aspects of the palms to seal the cuff of the mask tightly against the face (Figure 32-2). If you are using the lateral technique, place the thumb and index finger of your hand nearest the top of the patient's head over the upper border of the mask and the thumb of your opposite hand (closest to the patient's chin) over the lower border of the mask. Use the remaining fingers to maintain the correct jaw position.
3. Lift upward on the patient's mandible, using the index, middle, and ring fingers of your hands to maintain a head tilt.
4. If a third assistant is available, have that person apply cricoid pressure. Cricoid pressure helps prevent gastric inflation and reduces the risk of regurgitation or aspiration. It is applied by pressing down on the cricoid cartilage to compress the esophagus against the cervical vertebrae (AHA, 2006).
5. Blow into the opening of the mask and deliver a normal breath, not a deep breath, over 1 second and observe the chest rise. A rescuer is generally unable to estimate tidal volume during CPR so visible chest rise is used to determine the adequacy of ventilation.
6. For an adult, rescue breaths should be slow, at least 1 second each every 5 to 6 seconds. For a child, one breath every 3 seconds is recommended (AHA, 2006).
7. Remove your mouth from the mask opening to allow passive exhalation by the patient. This step is unnecessary if there is a one-way valve.
8. Ventilate the adult (a person older than age 8) 12 times per minute. The rate of rescue breathing for a child (aged 1 to 8 years) or an infant (younger than 1 year) is 20 times per minute. Reassess the need for continued assisted ventilation every 5 minutes.
9. Connect oxygen tubing to the mask as soon as possible (if an oxygen inlet is present) and adjust the flow rate to 10 to 12 L/min (AHA, 2006). If there is no oxygen inlet, oxygen delivery to the patient

may be enhanced if the rescuer wears a nasal cannula dispensing oxygen at a flow rate of 6 L/min.

Face Shield

1. Face shields are sheets of clear plastic or silicone to place over the victim's mouth and nose. Place the shield on the patient's face with the filter or one-way valve over the mouth.
2. Position yourself to the side of the patient's head.
3. Pinch the patient's nose by using the thumb and index finger of one hand and maintain the head tilt with the other hand.
4. Take a normal breath and blow for at least 1 second through the one-way valve on the face shield as you watch for the chest to rise.
5. Lift your mouth off the shield to allow the patient to exhale passively. Expired air will flow out under the face shield. Leave the shield on the patient's face during resuscitation.
6. Rescue breathing should be performed 12 times per minute for an adult, 20 times a minute for a child or infant.
7. Every 5 minutes, reassess the need for continued assisted ventilation.
8. Oxygen delivery to the patient may be enhanced if the rescuer wears a nasal cannula dispensing oxygen at a flow rate of 6 L/min.
9. Face shields should be replaced by mouth-to-mask or bag-mask devices as soon as possible.

AGE-SPECIFIC CONSIDERATIONS
Pediatric

1. In children, respiratory problems are a more likely cause of cardiopulmonary arrest than underlying cardiac problems (AHA, 2006). Rescue breathing should begin immediately in apneic patients. In the out-of-hospital setting, notify the emergency medical services (EMS) after the first 2 minutes of rescue efforts on a pediatric patient. Rescue efforts should begin on an adult after the EMS system is activated.
2. For pediatric patients (birth to 8 years of age), the volume of ventilations should be sufficient to cause the chest to rise without causing gastric distention. Because of a wide variation in the compliance and size of children's lungs (AHA, 2006), no prescribed volume or pressure is recommended.
3. Children's airways are small and are easily obstructed by mucus, edema, or both. Frequent suctioning may be required. The tongue is the most common cause of airway obstruction in a child (AHA, 2006).
4. Hyperextension of the neck should be avoided in an infant or a small child, because it may obstruct the narrow, pliable airway. Pushing on the soft tissues under the chin may also obstruct the airway.
5. Use appropriately sized infant and pediatric masks.
6. Rescue breaths for pediatric patients should be slow (1 second), with only enough volume to cause the chest to rise. If the chest does not rise, reposition the patient's head and reattempt ventilation.
7. Gastric distention occurs easily in infants and children, generally as a result of overly rapid delivery or excessive volume of ventilations.

Distention can be minimized by delivering rescue breaths slowly (AHA, 2006).

Geriatric

1. Geriatric patients may have decreased pulmonary function associated with aging or chronic diseases. Ventilation may be difficult because of decreased vital capacity, decreased lung compliance, and poor alveolar gas exchange.
2. Dentures may interfere with artificial ventilation efforts. If they are loose or ill fitting, they should be removed.

COMPLICATIONS

1. Loss of oxygen and tidal volume caused by an ineffective seal around the face mask
2. Insufficient airway patency as a result of improper chin-lift or head-tilt position
3. Failure to recognize an obstruction caused by vomiting, excessive secretions, or bleeding in the upper airway
4. Ineffective chest rise resulting from ventilations that are too shallow
5. Gastric distention resulting from ventilations that are excessive in volume or that are delivered too rapidly
6. Improperly assembled one-way valve that does not permit air to enter the patient's lungs

REFERENCE

American Heart Association (AHA). (2006). *Basic life support for healthcare providers.* Dallas: Author.

PROCEDURE 33

Bag-Mask Ventilation

Teresa L. Will, MSN, RN, CEN

The bag-mask is also known as a *bag-valve-mask, bag-valve device, BVM, Ambu bag, self-inflating bag,* and *manual resuscitator.*

INDICATION

To provide positive-pressure ventilatory support manually in the presence of inadequate spontaneous ventilation or apnea

CONTRAINDICATIONS AND CAUTIONS

1. Excessive airway pressure or tidal volume can cause gastric distention and pneumothorax.

2. Care should be taken to ensure a properly fitted mask and to provide a good seal. Frequently, two people are required to provide adequate ventilation to a nonintubated patient. One member of the team maintains the airway positioning and the mask seal while the other delivers the volume of air via the bag. Mouth-to-mask ventilation (see Procedure 32) may be more effective in some situations. One rescuer can provide adequate ventilation using a bag-mask device if the rescuer has some experience and practice with this device.

EQUIPMENT

Oral or nasal airway
Masks of various sizes
Pharyngeal suctioning equipment
Self-inflating bag with oxygen reservoir and attached oxygen-connecting tubing

PATIENT PREPARATION

1. Secure an open airway and position the patient's head and neck properly. See the following earlier procedures:
    Procedure 3—Airway Positioning
    Procedure 4—Airway Foreign Object Removal
    Procedure 5—Oral Airway Insertion
    Procedure 6—Nasal Airway Insertion
    Procedure 7—Laryngeal Mask Airway
    Procedures 8, 10, 11—Endotracheal Intubation
    Procedure 14—Combitube Airway
    Procedure 15—Crichothyrotomy
    Procedure 17—Tracheostomy
2. Suction any foreign matter out of the airway (see Procedure 29)

PROCEDURAL STEPS

1. Connect the oxygen tubing to the oxygen flowmeter and set at 10 to 15 L/min. Using a bag-mask with a reservoir significantly increases the oxygen concentration administered. If no oxygen is readily available, the bag-mask device can be used on room air until oxygen becomes available.
2. For the nonintubated patient, choose the appropriate size of mask and secure it to the bag. The mask should be large enough to seal around the mouth and nose without covering the eyes. Ensure that the equipment is functioning by placing the mask against your hand and noting the gas flow through the mask. Stand behind the patient's head. Seat the mask on the face by covering the nose, the mouth, and the tip of the chin. The narrow end of the mask goes over the nose. Hold the mask firmly with your thumb over the patient's nose and your fingers grasping the bony edge of the mandible (Figure 33-1). A two-person technique may be used with one team member maintaining the airway and mask seal while the other delivers the air from the bag (Figure 33-2).
3. To help minimize gastric inflation and passive regurgitation in the unconscious patient, consider the application of cricoid pressure (the Sellick maneuver) to minimize the passage of air into the esophagus. Using the fingers

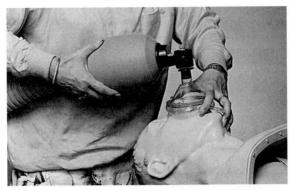

FIGURE 33-1 Application of a bag-mask by a single rescuer. (From Jesudian, M. C. et al. [1985]. Bag-mask ventilation: Two rescuers are better than one: Preliminary report. *Critical Care Medicine,* *13*[2], p. 122, with permission.)

and thumb of one hand on either side of the trachea, gently compress the cricoid ring posteriorly (toward the cervical spine). This technique occludes the esophagus (Figure 33-3).

4. For the intubated patient, attach the bag to the connector or adapter of the endotracheal tube. When one hand is needed to maintain the head position, the free hand can compress the bag and thus inflate the lungs.
5. If two hands are not available to squeeze the bag, compress the bag against your thigh or chest or the stretcher to assist in decompressing the bag and generating additional tidal volume.
6. The gentle symmetrical rise and fall of the chest signals an adequate tidal volume and mask seal or endotracheal tube to bag seal. A tidal volume of 6 to 7 ml/kg or 400 to 600 ml over 1 second is recommended for bag-mask ventilation with oxygen. When no oxygen is connected to the bag-mask

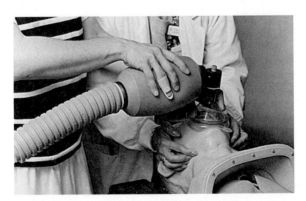

FIGURE 33-2 Application of a bag-mask by two rescuers. (From Jesudian, M. C. et al. [1985]. Bag-mask ventilation: Two rescuers are better than one: Preliminary report. *Critical Care Medicine 13*[2], p. 122, with permission.)

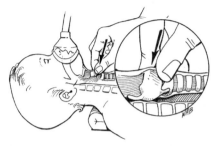

FIGURE 33-3 Gentle pressure on the cricothyroid membrane occludes the esophagus and helps prevent gastric distention during positive pressure ventilation. (From Walsh-Sukys, M. C. [1997]. Orotracheal intubation. In M. C. Walsh-Sukys & S. E. Krug [Eds.]. *Procedures in infants and children* [pp. 36–41]. Philadelphia: Saunders, with permission.)

ventilation system, a slightly larger chest rise should be seen. A tidal volume of 10 ml/kg or 700 to 1000 ml given over 1 second is recommended with room air (AHA, 2005).

7. Ventilate at the rate indicated below (AHA, 2005):
   - Adult or pediatric patient in cardiac arrest—8-10 breaths per minute
   - Adult patient with a pulse—10-12 breaths per minute
   - Pediatric patient with a pulse—12-20 breaths per minute

AGE-SPECIFIC CONSIDERATIONS

1. Children have fewer and smaller alveoli, which predisposes them to alveolar collapse owing to lower elastic recoil. To prevent barotrauma, look for a gentle rise and fall of the chest rather than an exaggerated or pronounced expansion.

2. Bag-mask devices are generally made with pop-off valves set at 30 to 35 cm H_2O pressure to prevent overinflation of the lungs. In children with poor compliance or high resistance during lung insufflation, you may not get chest rise before the valve "pops." In this instance, the pop-off valve may have to be occluded or you may have to switch to a bag without a pop-off valve for the delivery of higher pressure gradients.

3. The tidal volume to be delivered for either adults or children is 6 to 10 ml/kg of body weight. Higher tidal volumes have been associated with increased risk of barotrauma, cause regurgitation, and interfere with effective ventilation (AHA, 2005). To help minimize the risk of overinflation, inadvertent gastric inflation, or barotrauma choose the appropriate bag size. The bag size recommended for infants and children is 450 to 500 ml; and for adults, 1600 ml (AHA, 2005). Tidal volumes that are too low may result in hypoxia and hypercarbia. Supplementary oxygen will ensure the maintenance of oxygen saturation at these smaller tidal volumes

4. When applying cricoid pressure in children, gentle pressure is sufficient to occlude the esophagus effectively. You may use fewer than three fingers for compression, and a fingertip may be all that is required for the infant. In children of all ages, care should be taken to avoid excessive pressures that may produce tracheal compression and inadvertent obstruction.

5. Gastric distention commonly occurs as a result of bag-mask ventilation in children; inserting a gastric tube is a high priority to prevent complications.

COMPLICATIONS

1. Ventilation rates higher than 12 breaths per minute during cardiac arrest can cause excessive intrathoracic pressure, which results in decreased coronary blood flow and survival rates (Aufderheide et al., 2004).
2. Excessive tidal volumes cause gastric distention, leading to vomiting and aspiration or pulmonary impingement. Insert a gastric tube as soon as possible if prolonged bag-mask ventilation is necessary. Children are highly susceptible to gastric distention. See Procedure 98.
3. Excessive airway pressures can result in pneumothorax or other barotrauma.
4. An inadequate seal of the face mask can cause an air leak that may result in inadequate ventilation.
5. Ophthalmic damage can occur if the mask is too large because pressure is exerted on the eyes during ventilation.

REFERENCES

American Heart Association (AHA). (2005). American Heart Association guidelines for cardio-pulmonary resuscitation and emergency cardiovascular care. *Circulation, 112*(Suppl. IV). Available online at www.circulationaha.org

Aufderheide, T., Sigurdsson, G., & Pirrallo, R. G., et al. (2004). Hyperventilation-induced hypotension during cardiopulmonary resuscitation. *Circulation, 109*, 1960-1965.

PROCEDURE 34

Anesthesia Bag Ventilation

Teresa L. Will, MSN, RN, CEN

An anesthesia bag is also known as *flow-inflating bag, Ayre's bag, A-bag, Jackson-Rees circuit, Mapleson-F circuit, bellows, manual resuscitator,* and *balloon bag.* This type of resuscitation bag relies on a continuous source of compressed oxygen or mixed gases to deliver ventilations. No valves are in the circuit, so no additional work is imposed on the patient taking some spontaneous breaths. Occasionally, an outlet valve is present at the tail of the bag suitable for exhausting/scavenging anesthetic gases. At lower flows, some gas can be conserved; but in emergency practice, the valve is primarily used to adjust the amount of continuous positive airway pressure (CPAP) at a given flow rate.

INDICATIONS

1. To provide manual ventilation in the event of apnea or an ineffective respiratory pattern, when a continuous source of compressed gases is available. The anesthesia bag delivers the highest achievable FiO_2 to the patient with adequate flow rate if no leaks are present (Trimble, n.d.).
2. To monitor spontaneous patient breathing effort and flow.
3. To provide CPAP to maintain airway wall separation and a decrease in respiratory distress in conditions such as pulmonary edema by decreasing preload, recruiting alveoli, and enhancing oxygenation.
4. To deliver a specifically blended concentration of oxygen (up to 100%) via a compressed gas system.

CONTRAINDICATIONS AND CAUTIONS

1. Anesthesia bags are difficult to use in mask-ventilated patients. In difficult airway situations, two or three hands may be needed to manipulate the mask and airway, and an additional person may be needed to squeeze the bag. A self-filling bag-mask may be preferable in this situation (see Procedure 33).
2. Anesthesia bags cannot be operated on uncompressed room air; thus, a self-filling bag-mask device should always be available in case of failure of compressed gas sources.
3. Overinflation may result in gastric distention or pneumothorax.
4. Barotrauma can result from an inability to control gas flow. Balancing inflow, controlling leaks, and allowing sufficient outflow or exhaust are essential to prevent overinflation or underinflation.
5. A true 100% oxygen concentration is delivered (without added work imposed by valves) if the minute volume of gas is two to three times the minute tidal volume delivered (Trimble, n.d.). One must provide an outflow leak to permit exhalation either through the open tail of the bag or by lifting the mask slightly for a nonintubated patient. The tail is only occluded while assisting breathing with the incoming gas flow and/or gently squeezing the bag to direct flow into the patient. An entirely closed system must not be used on intubated patients.

EQUIPMENT

Anesthesia bag
Oxygen or air flowmeter
Oxygen-connecting tubing
Suction equipment
Mask (if patient is not intubated)
Pressure gauge or manometer (This is highly desirable if the anesthesia bag has a pressure gauge port; essential with infants and neonates. If no manometer is used, the port should be capped.)
Compressed oxygen continuous flow or compressed room air continuous flow

PATIENT PREPARATION

1. Secure an open airway and position the patient's head and neck properly. See Procedures 3 to 17 for methods of establishing an airway.
2. Suction any foreign matter out of the airway (see Procedures 29 to 31).

PROCEDURAL STEPS

1. Connect the oxygen tubing to the oxygen flowmeter and the gas inlet on the anesthesia bag. If less than 100% oxygen is indicated, an air or oxygen blender is needed.
2. Turn on the oxygen flowmeter to allow the bag to fill halfway. Adjust the flow-control valve to keep the bag approximately half full. This allows ease in compression of the bag and usually delivers adequate tidal volumes (6 to 10 L/min) (AHA/ILCOR, 2000).
3. If the patient is not intubated, choose a mask that covers the patient's nose, mouth, and the groove between the base of the lower teeth and the chin. Attach the mask or the endotracheal tube to the anesthesia bag.
4. Test the unit by placing the mask against your hand and squeezing the bag to feel the flow. Observe the cycle of inflation, gas delivery, and reinflation.
5. If there is a pressure port, attach the pressure gauge to the bag. Pressure measurement is not a primary concern in the adult patient, but the gauge must be attached for the bag to inflate properly (a small leak occurs if the port is not capped) (Figure 34-1).
6. If you are using a mask, stand behind the patient's head and seat the mask on the face by covering the nose, mouth with the lips apart, and settle the base of the mask into the ridge of the chin with the mouth open. The narrow end of the mask goes over the nose. Hold the mask firmly with your thumb over the patient's nose and your fingers grasping the bony edge of the mandible (see Procedure 33 and Figure 33-1). A two-person technique may be used with one team member maintaining the airway and mask seal while the other delivers the air from the bag (see Procedure 33 and Figure 33-2).
7. For the intubated patient, attach the bag's connector, with a slight twist, to the adaptor of the endotracheal tube.
8. With your free hand, close the tail of the bag and gently squeeze the bag to force air into the lungs. Remember, this is done gently as (unlike with a bag-mask) continuous flow coming into the bag is now also directed into the patient. If the anesthesia bag has a flow-control outlet valve, you only need to occlude the distal opening of the bag with a finger as you squeeze; the valve is intended for low-flow steady-state general anesthesia.
9. Anesthesia bags are less fatiguing to the hands in prolonged use (Trimble, n.d.). Watch for rise and fall of the chest, notice any spontaneous breathing

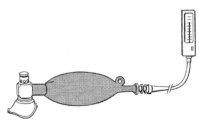

FIGURE 34-1 An anesthesia bag requires a constant gas flow to inflate. (From Walsh-Sukys, M. C. [1997]. Bag and mask ventilation [p. 29]. In M. C. Walsh-Sukys & S. E. Krug (Eds.), *Procedures in infants and children.* Philadelphia: Saunders.)

efforts, and feel for lung compliance and increasing pressure when you are squeezing the bag.

10. To help minimize gastric inflation and passive regurgitation in the unconscious, nonintubated patient, consider the application of cricoid pressure (the Sellick maneuver) to minimize the passage of air into the esophagus. Using the fingers and thumb of one hand on either side of the trachea, gently compress the cricoid ring back toward the cervical spine (see Figure 33-3). This helps occlude the esophagus.

11. Symmetrical rise and fall of the chest and good breath sounds bilaterally indicate adequate tidal volume and mask seal.

12. Ventilate at the rate indicated below (AHA, 2005):
    - Adult or pediatric patient in cardiac arrest—8-10 breaths per minute
    - Adult patient with a pulse—10-12 breaths per minute
    - Pediatric patient with a pulse—12-20 breaths per minute

AGE-SPECIFIC CONSIDERATIONS

1. Children have fewer and smaller alveoli, which are more susceptible to collapse because of lower elastic recoil; therefore, airway pressures need to be monitored carefully to prevent barotrauma.

2. The tidal volume delivered for both the child and the adult is 6 to 10 ml/kg. The size of the anesthesia bag should be chosen on the basis of volume: for neonates, 450 ml; for children, 750 ml; and for adults, 1600 ml (AHA/ILCOR, 2000).

3. When applying cricoid pressure in children, gentle pressure effectively occludes the esophagus. You may use two fingers for compression, and a fingertip may be all that is required for the infant. Care should be taken in children of all ages to avoid excessive pressures that may produce tracheal compression and inadvertent obstruction.

4. If a mask that is too large is used, pressure may be placed on the eyes. This can cause vagal stimulation, especially in children.

5. Gastric distention commonly occurs as a result of bag-mask ventilation in children, inserting a gastric tube is a high priority to prevent complications.

COMPLICATIONS
Via Bag-mask

1. Ventilation rates higher than 12 breaths per minute during cardiac arrest can cause excessive intrathoracic pressure which results in decreased coronary blood flow and survival rates (Aufderheide et al., 2004).

2. Overinflation can result in gastric distention that may lead to vomiting and aspiration or limited lung expansion. Insert a gastric tube as soon as possible to decompress the stomach (see Procedure 98).

3. Inadequate pressure on the bag leads to low delivered volume and inadequate ventilation.

4. Inadequate seal of the face mask resulting in an inadvertent air leak may cause inadequate ventilation.

5. Excessive tidal volumes, rates, or decreased inspiratory/expiratory ratios may diminish venous return, decreasing cardiac output and causing hypotension.

6. Damage to the eyes can occur if the mask is too large and pressure is exerted during the bag-mask ventilation. Gas flow onto the eyes can cause corneal drying and injury.

Via Bag-endotracheal Tube

1. Ventilation rates higher than 12 breaths per minute during cardiac arrest can cause excessive intrathoracic pressure which results in decreased coronary blood flow and survival rates (Aufderheide et al., 2004).
2. Delivery of excessive volume can result in barotrauma, such as a pneumothorax.
3. Inadequate pressure can result in inadequate ventilation.

REFERENCES

American Heart Association (AHA). (2005). American Heart Association guidelines for cardio-pulmonary resuscitation and emergency cardiovascular care. *Circulation, 112*(Suppl. IV). Available online at www.circulationaha.org

American Heart Association & International Liaison Committee on Resuscitation (AHA/ILCOR). (2000). Guidelines 2000 for cardiopulmonary resuscitation and emergency cardiovascular care: International consensus on science. *Circulation, 102*(Suppl I), I1-I384.

Aufderheide, T., Sigurdsson, G., & Pirrallo, R. G., et al. (2004). Hyperventilation induced hypotension during cardiopulmonary resuscitation. *Circulation, 109*, 1960-1965.

Trimble, T. (n.d.). Using anesthesia bags. Retrieved February 2, 2007, from http://enw.org/A-Bags.htm

PROCEDURE 35

Mechanical Ventilators

Reneé Semonin Holleran, RN, PhD, CEN, CCRN, CFRN, CTRN, FAEN, Michael Rouse, MSN, CRNA, and *Lori Carpenter, RRT*

Mechanical ventilators are also known as *ventilators, vents,* and *respirators;* they may also be known by a specific brand name.

INDICATIONS

1. The primary purpose of mechanical ventilation is to maintain alveolar ventilations or the exchange of fresh gas between the lungs and the ambient air by causing air to flow in and out of the lungs via changing airway pressures.
2. To deliver a specific and reliable concentration of oxygen to an ill or injured patient who is hypoxic or in danger of becoming hypoxic because of illness

or injury. A partial pressure of arterial oxygen (PaO_2) of less than or equal to 50 mm Hg indicates a critical level of oxygen, which requires intervention.
3. To assist or provide mechanical ventilation for the patient who is experiencing respiratory distress or impending respiratory arrest.
4. To decrease the work of breathing for the ill or injured patient and prevent respiratory muscle fatigue. Respiratory muscle fatigue results from depletion of energy stores because of an increased ventilatory workload. Disease states such as weakness, chronic obstructive pulmonary disease, and shock may lead to respiratory muscle fatigue (Burns, 2005).
5. To avoid prolonged use of a manual bag-mask device; which could cause hypocapnia or hypercapnia, during transport of patients who require ventilatory support.

CONTRAINDICATIONS AND CAUTIONS
1. There are no specific contraindications for the use of mechanical ventilation other than it must be initiated and monitored by skilled personnel who understand not only the physiologic aspects of mechanical ventilation but also how to perform a patient–ventilator systems check. However, mechanical ventilation can cause pulmonary injury as well as leave the patient at risk for respiratory infections and generalized sepsis.
2. The safety and effectiveness of positive-pressure mechanical ventilation are dependent on the proper placement of the endotracheal, tracheostomy, or cricothyrotomy tube. Assess proper tube placement before connecting the patient to the ventilator and periodically while the patient remains on the ventilator. At the first change in the patient's condition, you must confirm proper tube placement before considering other causes (see Procedure 8). If the cause of the problem cannot be determined, remove the patient from the ventilator and provide manual ventilation with a bag-mask device until the source of the alarm can be identified.
3. During positive-pressure ventilation, tidal volume for the adult patient should be determined by the patient's height. The standard is 6 to 8 ml/kg of *ideal* body weight. It is important to consult with respiratory therapy for appropriate ventilator settings for both children and adults.
4. Mechanical ventilation may cause further damage to an injured lung or may injure remaining healthy lung tissue (Burns, 2005). Patients with a chest injury or a pulmonary disease, such as asthma and emphysema, should be monitored carefully when they undergo mechanical ventilation. Increased airway pressures may lead to the development of a pneumothorax or a tension pneumothorax. In some cases, prophylactic chest tubes may be inserted to prevent the development of a tension pneumothorax.
5. Anxiety can interfere with mechanical ventilation. Sedation may be required to decrease anxiety, which in turn decreases the work of breathing and decreases oxygen consumption, allowing the patient to breathe with the ventilator. Narcotics cause respiratory depression; therefore, they may be particularly beneficial in patients who have uncontrolled tachypnea and resist or "buck" the ventilator. Some patients may require neuromuscular blocking agents (NMBAs) to facilitate mechanical ventilation. It is important to confirm that the patient is receiving adequate sedation and analgesia when NMBAs are used. A potentially fatal situation exists if a patient receiving

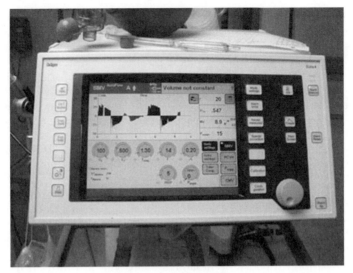

FIGURE 35-1 Example of a ventilator that may be used in an emergency department. (Courtesy Rose DeJarnette.)

NMBAs or deep sedation inadvertently becomes disconnected from the ventilator; therefore appropriate safeguards, alarms, and monitors should be in place.

6. Assess the patient–ventilator system every hour. This check should include airway pressures (inspiratory and expiratory) and fraction of inspired oxygen (FiO$_2$), tidal volume, and verification that alarms are set properly.

EQUIPMENT

Intubation equipment (see Procedure 8)
Bag-mask with oxygen reservoir connected to an oxygen source and appropriately fitting mask in case intubation fails
Suction setup
Mechanical ventilator (see following discussion) (Figure 35-1)
Oxygen source for ventilator
Compressed air source
Humidifier
Ventilator circuit to supply gas to the patient
Cardiac monitor
Pulse oximeter
End-tidal CO$_2$ monitor

Ventilators

Ventilators fall into two general categories: negative-pressure and positive-pressure ventilators.

Negative-pressure Ventilators: These ventilators work by applying subatmospheric pressure at a prescribed rate per minute to the thorax of a patient enclosed in an airtight body suit. The ventilator creates a pressure gradient that causes air to move passively into the lungs. The old iron lung is an example of a negative-pressure ventilator, although today's models in no way resemble their historic counterpart. Negative-pressure ventilation provides the advantage of not requiring an artificial airway, thus allowing the patient to communicate and eat normally. Today, negative-pressure ventilators are used in a home-care setting for patients who have normal lung function and who have neuromuscular diseases, or who require ventilatory support during sleep; they are not used in acute situations.

Positive-pressure Ventilators: These ventilators employ an artificial airway that forces air into the lungs. Expiration during positive-pressure ventilation occurs passively as a result of the elastic recoil of the lungs and the chest wall. Positive-pressure ventilators are classified according to the cycling mechanism or the method by which inspiration is terminated and expiration is initiated.

Volume-cycled Ventilators: These are the ventilators used most often in the emergency department. Inspiration ends when a preselected volume of gas has been delivered. One of the advantages of volume-cycled ventilators is that they can be programmed to overcome changes in lung compliance and airway resistance.

Pressure-cycled Ventilators: In these ventilators, inspiration ends when a preset driving pressure is attained. The pressure is constant, so that tidal volume is dependent on lung compliance and airway resistance. These ventilators are used mainly for patients who require short-term ventilation, such as those who have undergone surgery.

Flow-cycled Ventilators: In these ventilators, inspiration ends when the flow rate of gas delivered drops below a preset level. As lung volume increases and lung compliance decreases, the flow rate of gas decreases progressively and is sensed by the ventilator, which then interrupts gas flow, allowing exhalation.

Time-cycled Ventilators: These ventilators are used primarily for neonates and incorporate a timing mechanism that controls the inspiratory phase. The ventilator delivers a determined flow, for a given time, which determines tidal volume.

Ventilator Settings (Figure 35-2)

Tidal Volume: The amount of air that moves in and out of the lungs in one breath. Normally calculated at 6 to 8 ml/kg of *ideal* body weight for height.

Rate: The number of breaths delivered per minute.

FiO_2: The fraction of inspired oxygen is described as a percentage or a decimal. Room air is 21% (or 0.21) oxygen. Typically, the FiO_2 used in an emergency situation is 100% (or 1).

Peak Inspiratory Pressure (PIP): The highest pressure generated by the ventilator to deliver the preset tidal volume, PIP varies depending on airway resistance and lung compliance. In adults, PIP is optimally less than 30 cm H_2O. A pressure alarm should be set at 5 to 10 cm H_2O above the PIP. An alarm may indicate kinked ventilator tubing, the patient biting the tube or coughing, or water in the circuit. A low-pressure alarm usually signals that the patient has been disconnected from the ventilator.

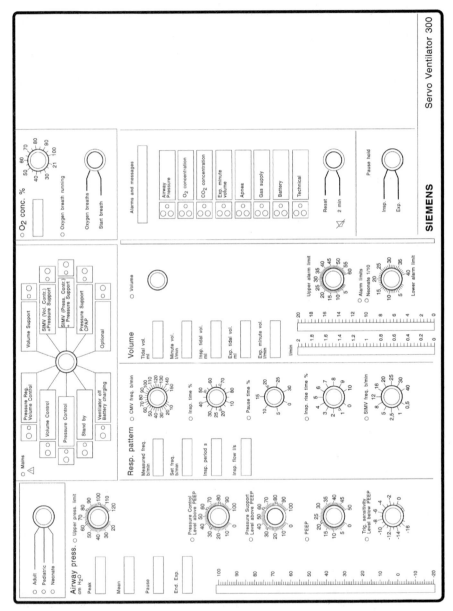

FIGURE 35-2 Ventilator control panel (Servo Ventilator 300). (Courtesy Siemens Life Support Systems, Danvers, MA.)

Positive End-expiratory Pressure (PEEP): Resistance is applied to the expiratory phase of ventilation, so that positive airway pressure is maintained throughout exhalation. The primary use of PEEP is to improve oxygenation in patients who do not respond to increases in FiO_2. PEEP also aids in preventing collapsed alveoli and in opening already collapsed alveoli to prevent atelectasis. Usually, PEEP begins at 3 to 5 cm H_2O. Low levels of PEEP may be set just to help overcome the effects of the dead space in the ventilator circuit. Severe lung disease may require a PEEP level of at least 30 cm H_2O. Patients receiving PEEP need to be monitored closely for barotrauma.

Continuous Positive Airway Pressure (CPAP): Essentially the same as PEEP, except that the patient has spontaneous respirations and is unaided by mechanical positive-pressure breaths. The positive pressure is usually delivered by mask (see Procedure 27).

Ventilation Modes

Ventilators have the capacity to operate in different ventilatory modes.

Assist Mode: When the patient begins to inhale, the ventilator senses the negative pressure created by the patient's effort and delivers a ventilator breath at the prescribed tidal-volume setting. This mode allows the patient some control over ventilation; however, if the patient becomes apneic, the machine does not deliver a breath.

Control Mode: The ventilator is not sensitive to the patient's ventilatory efforts, and it delivers a prescribed rate of ventilation per minute.

Assist/Control Mode: This mode is used most often in the setting of acute respiratory failure and is tolerated well by the awake patient. The ventilator senses the patient's effort and delivers a ventilator breath, allowing for a rate faster than the set rate on the ventilator. If the patient's inspiratory effort ceases, however, the ventilator continues to deliver mechanical breaths at the prescribed rate.

Intermittent Mandatory Ventilation (IMV): Often, this mode is used to wean patients off the ventilator. The patient on IMV breathes spontaneously between mechanical breaths delivered by the ventilator. The spontaneous breaths vary in tidal volume based on the patient's effort, but the ventilator ensures that the patient receives a prescribed number of breaths per minute.

Pressure Support Ventilation (PSV): This mode is used when the patient is spontaneously breathing. When using pressure support ventilation, inspiratory pressure, PEEP amount, and sensitivity are selected. During patient inspiration, a high flow of gas is delivered to the preselected inspiratory pressure, and this pressure is then maintained throughout inspiration.

Synchronous Intermittent Mandatory Ventilation (SIMV): The ventilator senses the patient's spontaneous breath and does not deliver a ventilator breath until the patient has completely exhaled. This avoids hyperinflation caused by the delivery of a mechanical breath during the inspiratory phase of a spontaneous, patient-initiated breath, referred to as "breath stacking."

PATIENT PREPARATION

Intubate the patient or obtain airway access surgically or percutaneously (see Procedures 8 to 12 and 14 to 17).

PROCEDURAL STEPS

1. Plug the ventilator into an oxygen source. Turn the machine on and check that the equipment is functioning properly according to the equipment manual.
2. Set the FiO_2. In the emergency department, it is usually set at 100% initially. Manipulate the oxygen setting based on the clinical and physiologic assessment of the patient, including arterial blood gases.
3. Set the tidal volume based on the patient's weight (6 to 8 ml/kg based on *ideal* body weight for height) (Byrd & Eggleston, 2007).
4. Set the respiratory rate based on the patient's age and clinical condition (adult, 10 to 12; child, 14 to 24; and infant, 20 to 40).
5. Set the ventilator mode (CMV, AC, IMV, PSV, SIMV).
6. Ensure that all of the alarms are turned on and functioning. Common alarms include disconnect alarms (low-pressure or low-volume alarms) and pressure alarms (high-pressure alarms, low-pressure alarms) minute ventilation alarms, FiO_2 alarms, silence or pause alarms.
7. Connect the endotracheal tube (or tracheostomy/cricothyrotomy tube) to the ventilator.
8. Set PEEP as indicated. Research has demonstrated that barotrauma causes serious injury and may lead to additional respiratory problems. A respiratory therapist or intensivist should be consulted when applying pressure to the airway. If respiratory care personnel are not available, PEEP should start at 5 cm H_2O or less, and the maximum airway pressure at 6 to 10 cm H_2O (Burns, 2005).
9. To evaluate the patient's clinical condition, draw arterial blood gases 15 to 30 minutes after connecting the patient to the ventilator and adjust the ventilator as indicated.
10. Monitor ECG, pulse oximetry, and end-tidal CO_2 continuously to identify early tube misplacement or problems with the ventilator or its settings.
11. Check that the humidifier has adequate distilled water and that the thermostat is adjusted to the manufacturer's recommended temperature. Drain ventilator tubing as needed to prevent condensation and aerosolization of bacteria into the patient's lungs. Alternatively, a heat-moisture exchanger (HME, or "artificial nose") that condenses exhalations to warm and moisten the next breath is commonly used. It can also act as a bacterial and viral filter.
12. Patients who remain in the emergency department for extended periods of time should be periodically repositioned. Repositioning has been shown to improve oxygenation (Vollman, 2005).

AGE-SPECIFIC CONSIDERATIONS

1. Infants' and young children's chests are more compliant, which results in a greater change in volume when there is a change in pressure.
2. The pediatric patient's alveoli fill and empty more quickly than the adult's.

3. Tidal volume for the pediatric patient is generally calculated at 6 to 8 ml/kg. However, there are times when lower tidal volumes may be used for children with acute respiratory distress syndrome (ARDS) or acute lung injury (ALI) to keep the PIP lower.
4. Infants' and young children's respiratory rates are faster than those of adults, and the ventilator rate should be set appropriately.
5. Infants are ventilated with pressure-cycled machines that leave them at risk for barotrauma, and they must be monitored closely for complications.
6. An uncuffed endotracheal tube may cause an increase in PIP without an increase in ventilation. The American Heart Association now recommends the use of cuffed endotracheal tubes in children older than 1 year when pressure is required for effective ventilation (AHA, 2005). The child should be monitored closely and an assessment includes periodic blood gas analysis and continuous pulse oximetry.
7. Owing to the short length of infant endotracheal tubes, a change of the head position may dislodge the tube. Small-diameter pediatric tubes may also become plugged and nonfunctional easily, causing deterioration in ventilation.
8. The geriatric patient who requires mechanical ventilation may have preexisting diseases that may lead to more complications with mechanical ventilation, such as emphysema or congestive heart failure. Aging leads to reduction in lung mass, decreased expansion of the rib cage, and decreased vital capacity.
9. Obesity does not increase lung size so excessive volumes and pressures should not be used. Tidal volume should be calculated on the patient's *ideal* body weight based on the patient's height (Byrd & Eggleston, 2007). However, obese patients are prone to respiratory fatigue, atelectasis, flaccidity of the airway's soft tissue, and decreased functional reserve capacity, which can lead to precipitous drops in oxygen saturation and airway compromise.

COMPLICATIONS

1. Whenever there is a complication related to mechanical ventilation that is serious enough to cause patient compromise, disconnect the patient from the ventilator and deliver manual ventilations with a bag-mask device until the problem is identified and corrected.
2. Increased intrathoracic pressure from mechanical ventilation may cause decreased venous return to the heart and hypotension. The emergency care provider should first determine whether medication or the patient's clinical condition (e.g., shock) is the cause of hypotension. This effect is exacerbated by PEEP.
3. Mechanical ventilation causes barotrauma and acute lung injury. Monitor the patient for the development of a pneumothorax or a tension pneumothorax.
4. The awake patient may "fight" the ventilator. Patients may require sedation and analgesia as well as NMBAs. Once these medications are given, spontaneous ventilatory efforts are impaired, and if the ventilator fails, the patient requires assistance with a bag-mask device until the ventilator is functioning again. Inadequate sedation and analgesia when NMBAs are used can cause

physiologic and psychological complications, such as hypertension and release of stress hormones.

5. Other complications that may occur with mechanical ventilation include cuff leak, mucus plugs in the tube, displaced tube (e.g., right main stem), tear in the ventilator tubing, malfunctioning alarms, pulmonary infections, sepsis, and lack of humidification.

PATIENT AND FAMILY TEACHING

1. When preparing the patient for respiratory support, be alert to the patient's emotional and informational needs (often overlooked in a crisis). A calm voice in the patient's ear can assure him or her of constant attendance and safety while on the ventilator.
2. Explain the need for mechanical ventilation and the importance of not touching the ventilator or any other equipment surrounding the patient.
3. Tell the patient and family to notify the nurse of system disconnections or if anything does not appear or "feel" right when the patient is being ventilated.
4. While the patient is on the ventilator, encourage family members to provide support and reassurance to the patient by means of conversation and touch.

REFERENCES

American Heart Association (AHA). (2005). American Heart Association Guidelines for cardiopulmonary resuscitation and emergency cardiovascular care. *Circulation, 112*(suppl. IV). Available on-line at www.circulationaha.org

Burns, S. (2005). Ventilatory management: Volume and pressure modes. In D. J. Lynn-McHale & K. K. Carlson (Eds.), *AACN procedure manual for critical care* (5th ed., pp. 211–225). Philadelphia: Saunders.

Byrd, R., & Eggleston, K. (2007). *Mechanical ventilation*. Retrieved January 7, 2007, from www.emedicine.com.

Vollman, K. M. (2005). Manual pronation therapy. In D. J. Lynn-McHale & K. K. Carlson (Eds.), *AACN procedure manual for critical care* (5th ed., pp. 108–124). Philadelphia: Saunders.

Inhalation Therapy

Nebulizer Therapy

Margo E. Layman, MSN, RN, RNC, CN-A, and
Jean A. Proehl, RN, MN, CEN, CCRN, FAEN

Nebulizer therapy is also known as *neb*, *updraft*, *SVN* (small-volume nebulizer), and *acorn neb*.

INDICATIONS

To deliver medications directly to the respiratory tract to treat the following:
1. Acute bronchospasm due to reactive airway disease (asthma) and other causes
2. Excessive mucus buildup
3. Croup
4. Epiglottitis

CONTRAINDICATION AND CAUTIONS

1. A metered-dose inhaler (MDI) with a spacer is preferred over a nebulizer, even for administering bronchodilators during severe asthma exacerbations (GINA & NHLBI, 2005). Nebulizers are not preferred for maintenance treatment either because they are expensive, not very portable, more difficult to use and maintain, and do not provide precise drug delivery unless equipped with a dosimeter (GINA & NHLBI, 2005).
2. Patients who are in distress, confused, or who cannot cooperate with the procedure, or whose history-taking requires talking while receiving treament will benefit from an aerosol mask fitted closely to the face with corrugated mist tubing extensions placed in the exhalation ports. Commonly referred to as *horns*, *whiskers*, or *tusks*, these act as a reservoir for aerosolized medication that would otherwise have been wasted to the atmosphere. The constant flow and the looseness of the mask prevent CO_2 rebreathing.
3. Patients with chronic obstructive pulmonary disease should generally receive nebulizer treatments with compressed air instead of oxygen. Supplemental oxygen dosing may be individualized without alteration by the rapid flow of the nebulizer. The nebulizer can be adapted to the side port of a Venturi mask providing fixed oxygen concentrations.
4. Nebulized medications are contraindicated in the presence of absent or severely diminished breath sounds unless the nebulized medication is delivered through an endotracheal tube that uses positive pressure. A patient with decreased air exchange may not be able to move the medication adequately into the respiratory tract.
5. Many bronchodilators are catecholamines and should be used with caution in patients with cardiac irritability. When inhaled, catecholamines increase the cardiac rate and may precipitate dysrhythmias.

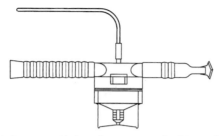

FIGURE 36-1 Nebulizer assembled to allow corrugated tubing to function as a reservoir.

EQUIPMENT

Nebulizer and connecting tubing (Figure 36-1)
Short, corrugated tubing
Oxygen cannula
Compressed gas source (oxygen or air) or air compressor
Medication to be administered by nebulizer (Table 36-1)

PATIENT PREPARATION

1. Place the patient in an upright position (40 to 90 degrees), which allows deep ventilation and maximal diaphragmatic movement.
2. Assess the breath sounds, pulse rate, respiratory status, oxygen saturation (see Procedure 21), and peak flow (see Procedure 23), if possible, before administering the medication.
3. Assess the heart rate during the treatment. If the heart rate increases by 20 beats per minute, stop the nebulizer treatment. In pregnant patients, the fetal heart rate should also be assessed (see Procedure 108).
4. Instruct the patient take slow deep breaths through the mouth and hold at end inspiration.

PROCEDURAL STEPS

1. Place the patient on supplemental oxygen (see Procedure 25), with the device and flow rate determined by the patient's condition, pulse oximetry, and/or arterial blood gases.

TABLE 36-1
MEDICATIONS COMMONLY ADMINISTERED VIA NEBULIZER

Generic Name	Type of Medication	Trade Name
Albuterol	Bronchodilator	Ventolin, Proventil
Ipratropium bromide	Anticholinergic bronchodilator	Atrovent
Albuterol + ipratropium	Combination of bronchodilators	DuoNeb
Levalbuterol HCl	Bronchodilator	Xopenex
Metaproterenol	Bronchodilator	Alupent
Racemic epinephrine	Bronchodilator	Vaponefrin
Cromolyn sodium	Mast cell stabilizer, antiasthmatic	Intal

2. Assemble the nebulizer and the tubing and instill the medication into the nebulizer.

3. Add normal saline diluent to the nebulizer if required (2.5 ml is a common amount of diluent). Most medications come prediluted with saline.

4. Attach the nebulizer to a source of compressed gas. Oxygen (6 to 8 L/min) can be used, but room air via an air compressor increases the humidity of the inhaled gas because of the water vapor content in room air. Adjust the flow rate until a light mist is created. If too forceful a stream is generated, the medication may be wasted.

5. Attach the corrugated tubing to the nebulizer. Some references place the tubing between the nebulizer and the mouthpiece to allow large droplets to "rain out" into the tubing; this decreases deposition of these droplets on the tongue and may reduce side effects. Other sources place the tubing on the opposite side of the nebulizer to serve as a reservoir.

6. Give the patient the mouthpiece or place the mask on the patient. Emphasize avoiding spillage of the medicine and avoiding wasted medicine due to talking or otherwise interrupting the treatment.

7. Coach the patient in the correct breathing technique to improve the effectiveness of the treatment. Instruct the patient to breathe slowly in and out through the mouthpiece or mask. Keep the lips sealed around the mouthpiece.

8. Tap the sides of the nebulizer occasionally to cause condensation droplets to return to the pool from which it is nebulized.

9. Continue treatment until nebulizer no longer delivers medicine mist or droplets.

10. Reassess breath sounds, pulse rate, oxygen saturation, respiratory rate, and peak flow.

11. Medications may be combined in the nebulizer.

AGE-SPECIFIC CONSIDERATIONS

1. Use of a mask guarantees better compliance for the elderly patient as well as the pediatric patient who is unable to cooperate by holding a nebulizer mouthpiece and inhaling appropriately. Never administer nebulizer treatments to a crying child; crying prevents absorption of nebulized medications (Fink, 2000).

2. If a child resists wearing a mask, the medication stream can be directed into the face in a blow-by fashion.

3. In infants and young children, a loose face mask on a nebulizer may be more acceptable than the close-fitting face mask of a spacer on an MDI. However, encourage parents to continue to attempt to use an MDI because of the advantages it has over a nebulizer (GINA & NHLBI, 2005).

COMPLICATIONS

Nausea, vomiting, tremors, bronchospasm, headache, and tachycardia are common medication-related side effects.

PATIENT TEACHING

If the nebulizer is sent home with the patient, instruct him or her to wash the nebulizer in soapy water, rinse, and air dry daily. Additional cleansing should be performed according to manufacturer's recommendations.

REFERENCES

Fink, J. B. (2000). Aerosol device selection: evidence to practice. *Respiratory Care*, 45, 874-884.

Global Initiative for Asthma (GINA) & National Heart, Lung, and Blood Institute (NHLBI). (2005). Global strategy for asthma management and prevention. Bethesda, MD: Authors. Retrieved January 11, 2007, from http://www.guidelines.gov/summary/summary.aspx?doc_id=8227 &nbr=004592&string=beta+AND+agonists+AND+asthma

PROCEDURE 37

Metered-Dose Inhaler

Margo E. Layman, MSN, RN, RNC, CN-A

Metered-dose inhalers are also known as *MDIs* or *puffers*. They disperse medication into the lungs through aerosol spray, mist, or fine powder.

INDICATIONS

To administer medications directly to pulmonary structures, to assist in relief of bronchospasm in reversible obstructive airway disease, and to prevent exercise-induced bronchospasm. Advantages of medication delivery via MDI include a decreased likelihood of systemic side effects and an immediate relief of symptoms. The types of medications used with MDIs include the following:

- Bronchodilators, which relax the muscles around the bronchial tubes
- Corticosteroids, which decrease inflammation and swelling in the airways
- Cromolyn, which reduces the reactions to antigens in the airways
- Insulin, for blood sugar management

CONTRAINDICATIONS AND CAUTIONS

1. Improper technique results in medication not reaching the bronchial tubes or air passages. Some devices, such as dry powder inhalers (DPIs) and insulin inhalers, require a different technique for optimal medication delivery. Review the manufacturer's recommendations for the specific device in use.
2. Remember to remove the mouthpiece cap and shake the canister to mix the medication properly.
3. The patient may be unable to use an MDI because of extreme shortness of breath with decreased air exchange or an altered level of consciousness.

EQUIPMENT

MDI with prescribed medication
Spacer (e.g., AeroChamber) (optional)
Facial tissues (optional)
Cup of water (for patient to rinse mouth when a steroid is used)

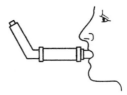

FIGURE 37-1 Metered-dose inhaler attached to a spacer. (From Proehl, J. A., & Jones, L. M. [1998]. *Mosby's emergency department patient teaching guides.* St. Louis: Mosby.)

PATIENT PREPARATION

1. Assess breath sounds, heart rate, respiratory rate, oxygen saturation (see Procedure 21), and peak flow (see Procedure 23).
2. Assist the patient to an upright sitting position.

PROCEDURAL STEPS

1. Warm inhaler canister by rolling it in your hands, and shake the canister immediately before using. Remove the protective cap and make sure the metal canister is firmly seated in the plastic case.
2. Hold the mouthpiece 2.5 to 5 cm (1 to 2 inches) from the mouth, keeping the canister in an upright position.
3. At the end of deep expiration, depress the metal canister (with two of your fingers on top of the canister and your thumb on the bottom of the plastic MDI) while the patient inhales deeply and slowly through the mouth (Fink, 2005).
4. Have the patient hold the breath as long as possible, at least 5 to 7 seconds (Fink, 2005).
5. Wait 30 to 60 seconds, and then repeat steps 2 to 4.
6. To use a spacer, insert the canister into the spacer and put the mouthpiece into the patient's mouth before activating the MDI (Figure 37-1). The spacer traps the medication mist inside the chamber, allowing the patient to inhale and exhale slowly several times without removing the mouth from the spacer. This ensures maximal medication delivery.

AGE-SPECIFIC CONSIDERATIONS

1. Hand strength diminishes with age or arthritis and may cause difficulty in ensuring enough pressure on the canister for the patient to receive a proper dose of medication.
2. Inhalers require specific inhalation techniques and children or older patients with decreased mental and/or cognitive status may not be able to use the inhaler correctly (Rau, 2005).
3. A child may need the nose plugged during inhalation.
4. Spacers can be used with a mask attachment for infants and small children; this allows the child 5 or 6 breaths to inhale medication. Children are not able to use an MDI without a spacer until they are old enough to understand and perform the technique. A mask can be used and a nurse, parent, or caretaker can depress the MDI with the child's inspiration.

COMPLICATIONS

1. Cardiac arrhythmias (tachycardia)
2. Hyperventilation with dizziness, lightheadedness, tingling, and palpitations
3. Paroxysmal bronchospasm
4. Thrush in patients receiving corticosteroid inhalations. Use of a spacer and a thorough mouth rinse after each application helps prevent thrush.

PATIENT TEACHING

1. Do not attempt to instruct the patient on using the MDI during an episode of shortness of breath.
2. Proper technique is important for drug delivery and ultimate effectiveness. Patients are frequently not adequately instructed on proper MDI use (Fink, 2005). Consider asking a respiratory care practitioner to consult and assist with patient instruction.
3. Use a placebo MDI to demonstrate the correct technique (Fink, 2005). Placebo MDIs are available from pharmaceutical companies.
4. Clean the MDI plastic canister after each use with warm water and dry it thoroughly. This prevents clogging of the valve in the mouthpiece.
5. Observe the MDI to make sure it is dispensing medication.
6. Notify a physician if shortness of breath or difficulty in breathing persists after the MDI is used as prescribed.
7. Use the short-acting "rescue" bronchodilator first when short of breath. Space doses 1 or 2 minutes apart so each inhalation penetrates deeper than the preceding one. Use "control" medicines such as steroids or long-acting combinations last.
8. Rinse the mouth with water ("swish and spit") after steroid inhalations to help prevent thrush.

REFERENCES

Fink, J. B. (2005). Inhalers in asthma management: Is demonstration the key to compliance? *Respiratory Care, 50,* 598-600.

Rau, J. L. (2005). The inhalation of drugs: Advantages and problems. *Respiratory Care, 50,* 367-382.

Pleural Decompression

Emergency Needle Thoracentesis

Deborah A. Upton, MSN, ARNP-BC, CEN

Emergency needle thoracentesis is also known as *needling a chest.*

INDICATIONS

To provide immediate decompression of a tension pneumothorax with respiratory compromise, cardiovascular compromise, or both. Tension pneumothorax is suspected in the presence of one or more the following:

- Respiratory distress
- Unilateral decreased or absent breath sounds
- Signs of hypoxemia
- Jugular venous distention (indicates elevated central venous pressure)
- Hypotension
- Unilateral hyperresonance
- Tracheal deviation
- Pulseless electrical activity, especially when preceded by trauma

Performance of needle thoracentesis converts a tension pneumothorax to a simple pneumothorax, but tension may recur if the needle is removed without prompt placement of a chest tube.

CONTRAINDICATIONS AND CAUTIONS

1. If this procedure is used in the absence of a tension pneumothorax, there is a risk of producing a pneumothorax, causing damage to the lung or blood vessels (ACS, 2004).
2. Needle thoracentesis is performed as an interim procedure until tube thoracostomy (chest tube placement) can be carried out. Anticipate thoracostomy as a follow-up procedure.
3. Initial presentation of a traumatic ruptured diaphragm with herniation of abdominal contents into a hemithorax can mimic a tension pneumothorax. Placement of a needle in this instance can result in bacterial contamination of the pleural cavity. Suspect a ruptured diaphragm in a patient with a history of sudden, compressive force to the abdomen.
4. Owing to the urgent nature of a tension pneumothorax, consideration should be given to training nursing and ancillary personnel in this procedure in areas that have no immediate access to a physician. The patient may suffer cardiac arrest without immediate intervention.

5. Research demonstrates that in some adults, the standard 3-cm, over-the-needle catheter may not reach the pleural cavity at the second intercostal space. Insufficient cannula length may contribute to the failure of the procedure. A minimum length of 4.5 cm (1.77 inches) is recommended (Britten, Palmer, & Snow, 1996).
6. Reinforced cannulae such as used for needle cricothyrotomy may be more resistant to kinking than intravenous cannulas.

EQUIPMENT

Antiseptic solution
Local anesthetic
Syringe and needles for local anesthesia
10- to 18-G over-the-needle catheter (4.5 to 6 cm in length)
3-inch collapsible tubing for flutter valve (Penrose drain or Heimlich valve)
   or sterile rubber glove
Suture ties or small rubber band

PATIENT PREPARATION

1. Chest radiography may be deferred initially, depending on the patient's presentation. If a ruptured diaphragm is suspected, consider obtaining films before performing needle thoracentesis.
2. If time allows, cleanse the chest with an antiseptic solution on the side of the tension pneumothorax. The usual site for needle insertion is the second intercostal space at the midclavicular line (Figure 38-1).
3. If cervical spine pathology is ruled out and the patient's condition permits, place the patient in an upright position.
4. Administer high-flow oxygen.

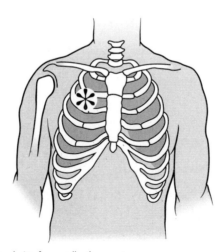

FIGURE 38-1 The usual site for needle thoracostomy.

PROCEDURAL STEPS

1. *If the patient is conscious and the patient's condition permits, infiltrate the area with local anesthetic.
2. *Insert the needle with a catheter through the skin at the second intercostal space, just superior to the third rib at the midclavicular line, 1 to 2 cm from the sternal edge, and direct it toward the top of the second rib. Hold the needle perpendicular to the chest wall when inserting over the top of the rib (intercostal nerves and arteries run inferior to the rib) and into the pleural space.
3. *Egress of air confirms the diagnosis of tension pneumothorax. If no air is released or if signs and symptoms do not improve, consider the presence of pericardial tamponade, myocardial contusion, or air embolism.
4. *Remove the needle and leave the catheter in place. The catheter may now be secured with tape and left open to the air. A simple pneumothorax now exists.
5. Assemble the equipment and prepare for subsequent chest tube placement (see Procedure 39). If there is a delay in chest tube placement (e.g., during transport), a flutter valve can be placed over the hub of the catheter. A simple form of flutter valve could be a 2-inch sterile rubber drain or a finger of a sterile glove with the tip removed. The flutter valve can then be secured to the hub of the catheter with tape or a suture (Figure 38-2). Alternately, intravenous extension tubing can be attached to the catheter with the distal end of the tubing submerged a few centimeters into sterile fluid to create a water seal.
6. Intubated patients receiving positive-pressure ventilation do not necessarily require a flutter valve or water seal to the needle as this is a short-term intervention and the positive pressure of ventilation will force out any air that does enter the chest cavity.
7. After chest tube placement is carried out, remove the catheter. Apply antibiotic ointment and a sterile dressing over the puncture site.
8. Obtain a chest radiograph after the procedure.

---

*Indicates portions of the procedure usually performed by a physician or an advanced practice nurse.

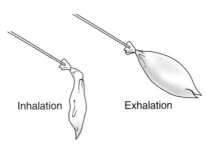

Inhalation   Exhalation

FIGURE 38-2 Flutter valve made from the finger of a rubber glove.

AGE-SPECIFIC CONSIDERATIONS

1. The use of accessory muscles and nasal flaring may also be indicators of tension pneumothorax in children.
2. Landmarks and insertion techniques are the same in children and adults. A relatively smaller needle/catheter is used for children.

COMPLICATIONS

1. Creation of a pneumothorax if a tension pneumothorax did not exist before procedure was performed.
2. Hematoma at insertion site, lung laceration (ACS, 2004).
3. Perforation of abdominal viscera if ruptured diaphragm or herniation of abdominal contents is present.
4. Placement of the needle close to the sternum may result in a laceration of the internal mammary artery with significant blood loss and resultant hemothorax.
5. Failure to decompress a tension pneumothorax with resulting patient deterioration.
6. Infection of puncture site (late).
7. Pleural infection/empyema (late).

REFERENCES

American College of Surgeons (ACS). (2004)Advanced trauma life support (7th ed). Chicago: Author.

Britten, S., Palmer, S. H., & Snow, T. M. (1996). Needle thoracocentesis in tension pneumothorax: Insufficient cannula length and potential failure. *Injury, 27*, 321–322.

PROCEDURE 39

Chest Tube Insertion

Deborah A. Upton, MSN, ARNP-BC, CEN

Chest tube insertion is also known as *tube thoracostomy.*

INDICATIONS

1. To remove air, blood, or both from the pleural cavity in the presence of a pneumothorax (free air in the pleural space), hemothorax (free blood in the pleural space), or hemopneumothorax (combination of air and blood).
2. To remove fluid from the pleural cavity in the presence of a large pleural effusion, empyema, or chylothorax. Iatrogenic pleural collections are most commonly seen after central venous access procedures.

3. To provide prophylactic chest drainage in patients with severe blunt chest trauma (flail chest or pulmonary contusions) who will require positive-pressure ventilatory support. Prophylactic chest tubes may also be inserted in patients with penetrating thoracic injuries, even in the absence of evidence of pneumothorax.

CONTRAINDICATIONS AND CAUTIONS

1. A patient's hemodynamic status may deteriorate rapidly after the evacuation of a massive hemothorax (larger than 1000 to 2000 ml). Initiate fluid resuscitation before performing chest decompression and anticipate the need for high-volume resuscitation. Autotransfusion may be indicated if available. A large left hemothorax may signal an aortic or great vessel injury.
2. The use of trocar chest tubes is controversial and is not recommended by most authors because trocar use has been associated with damage to the thoracic and abdominal structures. If a trocar is used, it should be used only to guide the tube through an opening already created by blunt dissection, rather than to enter the chest forcibly (Kirsch & Mulligan, 2004).
3. A patient with a previous thoracostomy may have scar tissue and adhesions, making chest tube placement difficult.
4. Consideration should be given to decompression of a pneumothoraces before attempting air transport, because the size of the pneumothorax may increase with altitude.
5. Chest tube insertion is not indicated if an emergency thoracotomy is imminent.

EQUIPMENT

Antiseptic solution
Local anesthetic
Syringes and needles for local anesthesia
No. 10 or 15 scalpel
Large, curved hemostat
Suture scissors
Needle holder
Sterile towels or drapes
Chest tube
36 Fr to 40 Fr for blood or viscous fluid
12 Fr to 22 Fr for air only
Large silk suture (0-0 to 2-0)
3-in tape
Occlusive dressing (gauze impregnated with petroleum jelly) (optional)
Gauze dressings (4 × 4, split drain sponges)
Chest-drainage device
Autotransfusion equipment if indicated or available
(Most institutions have preassembled trays containing most of this equipment.)

PATIENT PREPARATION

1. Provide supplemental oxygen.

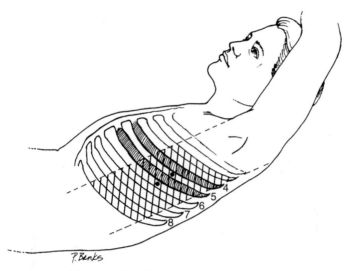

FIGURE 39-1 Acceptable and preferred locations for chest tube placement. (From Dalbec, D., & Krome, R. L. [1986]. Thoracostomy. *Emergency medical clinics of North America, 4*, 449.)

2. Obtain a chest radiograph unless the patient's condition mandates immediate chest tube placement.
3. In nonemergent circumstances, establish intravenous access, electrocardiographic monitoring, and pulse oximetry.
4. If time allows, cleanse the insertion site with antiseptic solution. The usual site for chest tube placement is the fourth or fifth intercostal space in the anterior or midaxillary line (Figure 39-1). Alternatively, the level of the nipple line can be used as a marker, especially in the unstable patient who requires immediate tube placement. In women with pendulous breasts, the lateral crease of tche breast is a more stable landmark. Insertion through a lower site risks subdiaphragmatic placement, possibly into the liver or spleen.
5. Place the patient in a supine position with the arm over the head on the involved side. If the patient's injuries permit, elevate the trunk to a 30- to 60-degree angle.
6. Administer antibiotics as prescribed to prevent empyema and pneumonia (Maxwell et al., 2004).
7. Administer sedation and analgesia as prescribed. This is an extremely uncomfortable and painful procedure.
8. Prepare the chest-drainage device (see Procedures 40 to 46).
9. Prepare autotransfusion equipment if indicated (see Procedures 77 to 80).

PROCEDURAL STEPS

1. *Cleanse the insertion site with an antiseptic solution.

---

*Indicates portions of the procedure usually performed by a physician or an advanced practice nurse.

2. *Drape the chest with sterile drapes.
3. *Infiltrate the area with a local anesthetic if the patient is conscious and if the patient's condition permits.
4. *Using the chest tube, measure the distance from the insertion site to the apex of the lung and note the distance on the tube.
5. *Make a 2- to 4-cm incision through the chest wall parallel to the ribs of the fifth intercostal space. The incision is made one interspace below the desired interspace. Making an incision below the pleural cavity entry site permits blunt dissection over the superior surface of the rib and creates a tunnel that allows later removal of the tube without an air leak.
6. *Bluntly dissect over the superior surface of the rib with the curved hemostat (nerves and arteries run inferior to the ribs). Enter the pleural cavity with the hemostat. The patient will experience pain as the pleural cavity is entered (Figure 39-2).

---

*Indicates portions of the procedure usually performed by a physician or an advanced practice nurse.

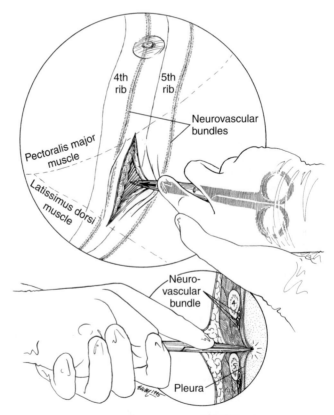

FIGURE 39-2 Enter the pleural space with a Kelly clamp. (Rosen, P., Chan, T., Vilke, G., & Sternbach, G. [2001]. *Atlas of emergency procedures* [p. 41]. St. Louis: Mosby.)

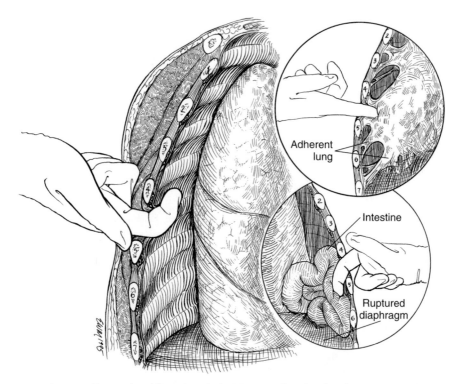

Adherent
lung

Intestine

Ruptured
diaphragm

FIGURE 39-3   Place a gloved finger into the incision to confirm the pleural penetration and assess for the presence of adhesions. (From Rosen, P., Chan, T., Vilke, G., & Sternbach, G. [2001]. *Atlas of emergency procedures* [p. 42]. St. Louis: Mosby.)

7.   *Widen the pleural opening and the skin incision by pulling the opened hemostat back out of the chest wall.

8.   *With a gloved finger, palpate through the incision to verify entry into the pleural space and to check for adhesions of the pleura and for intrathoracic or intraabdominal organs (Figure 39-3).

9.   *Direct the chest tube upward through the incision. Use a large hemostat to introduce the tube. Advance the tube to the premeasured distance (approximately 15 to 25 cm). The immediate return of blood, air, or both confirms the appropriate placement.

10.   *Connect the chest tube to the chest-drainage device.

11.   Tape all connections in the chest-drainage system. One inch of tape is placed horizontally, extending over connections. Reinforce this with tape placed vertically so that it encircles both ends of the connector (Figure 39-4).

12.   *Suture the chest tube in place with silk suture.

---

*Indicates portions of the procedure usually performed by a physician or an advanced practice nurse.

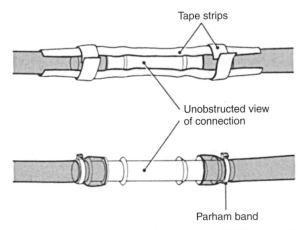

FIGURE 39-4 Securing of connection points. (Kersten, L. D. [1989]. Comprehensive respiratory nursing. *Dimensions of critical care nursing, 14,* 6–13.)

13. Apply an occlusive dressing to the insertion site. Petroleum-impregnated gauze may be wrapped around the tube close to the insertion site if the air leak is large. However, this may cause maceration of the skin and is not routinely necessary (Barefoot, 2005) (Figure 39-5).
    a. Apply split drain sponges around the chest tube, one over the top and one underneath the tube.
    b. Apply two or three gauze pads (4 × 4) on top of the split sponges.
    c. Tape the dressing to the skin.
14. Tape the chest tube to the skin.
15. Obtain a chest radiograph to confirm the correct tube placement (the last hole on the tube should be inside the pleural space) and to assess the status of the pneumothorax or hemothorax.
16. Monitor the chest-drainage device for the presence of large, continuous air leaks (may signal esophageal or large-airway damage) or excessive blood loss. Indications for surgical intervention include massive blood loss

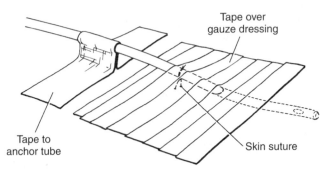

FIGURE 39-5 Occlusive chest tube dressing. (Kersten, L. D. [1989]. Comprehensive respiratory nursing. *Dimensions of critical care nursing, 14,* 6–13.)

TABLE 39–1

APROXIMATE SIZES FOR PEDIATRIC THORACOTOMY TUBES BY AGE
AND WEIGHT

Age	Approximate Weight (kg)	Tube Size (French)
Newborn to 9 months	3.5-8	12-18
10 to 17 months	10	14-20
18 months to 3 years	12-15	14-24
4 to 7 years	17-22	20-32
8 years	28	28-32
9 years and older	35 and higher	28-38

(greater than 1000 to 1500 ml initially or 300 ml in the first hour) or massive or persistent air leaks (Kirsch & Mulligan, 2004).

AGE-SPECIFIC CONSIDERATIONS

1. For newborn infants, the tube is placed in the fifth intercostal space of the anterior axillary line and directed anteriorly (Kirsch & Mulligan, 2004).
2. In a small infant, be sure that the dressing is not so large as to splint a large part of the chest wall and interfere with effective ventilation (MacDonald, 2004).
3. Approximate sizes for pediatric thoracostomy by age and weight are shown in Table 39-1.

COMPLICATIONS

1. A malpositioned, nonfunctioning tube (with the last hole in the tube outside of the pleural space or the tube malpositioned in the subcutaneous space)
2. Bleeding from the skin incision, from intercostal arteries or veins, or from a pulmonary artery or vein (risk is increased if chest tube with trocar is used)
3. Organ or structure injury (diaphragm, liver, spleen, stomach, or colon); the risk is increased if chest tube with trocar is used
4. Vasovagal response
5. Dyspnea
6. Hypovolemia secondary to rapid fluid loss with a hemothorax
7. Hemothorax
8. Reexpansion pulmonary edema
9. Occlusion or kinking of the tube (which may result in the formation of a tension pneumothorax)
10. Pain with reexpansion of the lung
11. Local hematoma
12. Local cellulitis (late)
13. Atelectasis or pneumonia due to splinting by the patient (late)
14. Reoccurrence of pathology after removal of the tube
15. Empyema (late)

PATIENT TEACHING

1. Request assistance when moving or turning in bed or when getting out of bed.
2. Immediately report any shortness of breath, chest pain, or disconnections in the system.
3. Do not lie on the tubing or allow it to be kinked.

REFERENCES

Barefoot, W. (2005). Chest tube placement (perform). In D. J. Lynn-McHale Wiegand, & K. K. Carlson (Eds.), *AACN procedure manual for critical care* (5th ed. pp. 145–149). Philadelphia: Saunders.

Kirsch, T. D., & Mulligan, J. P. (2004). Tube thoracostomy. In J. R. Roberts, & J. R. Hedges (Eds.), *Clinical procedures in emergency medicine* (4th ed., pp. 187–209). Philadelphia: Saunders.

MacDonald, M. (2004). Thoracostomy in the neonate: A blunt discussion. *NeoReviews, 5*, 301–306.

Maxwell, R. A., Campbell, D. J., & Fabian, T. C., et al. (2004). Use of presumptive antibiotics following tube thoracostomy for traumatic hemopneumothorax in the prevention of empyema and pneumonia: A multicenter trial. *Journal of Trauma, 57*, 742–749.

PROCEDURE 40

Management of Chest-Drainage Systems

Deborah A. Upton, MSN, ARNP-BC, CEN

The information contained in this procedure should be used in conjunction with that in the procedures pertaining to specific chest-drainage systems (see Procedures 42 through 46).

INDICATION

To evacuate air, fluid, or both from the pleural space and reexpand the lung by restoring negative intrapleural pressure.

CONTRAINDICATIONS AND CAUTIONS

1. Water-seal devices must be kept upright; otherwise, intrapleural negativity may be lost with air entry into the pleural space.
2. Do not clamp the tube unless it is absolutely necessary (to change the chest-drainage device or to check for air leaks), because a tension pneumothorax may develop.
3. Do not raise the device above the patient's chest level because fluid may reenter the chest and increase the probability of infection (applies to water-seal systems only).

4. Do not allow the tubing to coil below the top of the device or lie on the floor, because dependent fluid-filled loops require increased intrathoracic pressure to continue the emptying of the pleural space.

5. "Milking," or stripping, chest tubes can result in more than 400 cm H_2O of negative pressure within the pleural space (Duncan & Erickson, 1982). This negative pressure may damage the lung tissue and, therefore, stripping of chest tubes should not be performed routinely. Milking may be necessary when a visible clot is obstructing the tube, as is the case when the flow of sanguinous drainage suddenly slows or stops. To milk the tube, fold the tubing over on itself three times. Each fold should be approximately 3 inches long. Squeeze the folded tubing three or four times and release.

GENERAL INFORMATION

1. The fluid level in the water-seal tube/chamber should rise with inspiration and fall with expiration. If fluctuations are not present, the lung is either fully reexpanded or there is an obstruction. Check the tubing for kinks or occlusions. The most common cause is the patient lying on the tubing. Positive-pressure ventilation dampens these fluctuations.

2. For water-seal units, bubbles should be present in the the water in the water-seal chamber only in the presence of an air leak. Intermittent bubbling can occur when the suction is initially turned on due to air being displaced in the collection chamber, or a small leak in the pleural space, or upon exhalation and/or coughing. To determine the etiology of bubbles in the water seal chamber:

   a. Intermittently occlude, for less than 1 minute, the chest tube near the insertion site. If the bubbling stops, the leak is from either the insertion site or the patient's lung.

   b. Reinforce the occlusive dressing over the chest tube insertion site. If the bubbling continues, the air leak is coming from the patient's lung. If this is a new finding, report the observation to the physician immediately.

   c. If the bubbling continues after occluding at the insertion site, then the air leak is located either in the tubing or in the equipment. Check the integrity of the unit and all its connections. If a prefabricated, disposable unit is in use (Emerson, Pleur-Evac, Atrium, or Argyle), replace the entire unit. An extra chest-drainage unit should always be readily available for this purpose.

AGE-SPECIFIC CONSIDERATIONS

1. Adult chest-drainage units may be used for children; however, pediatric chest-drainage devices are available from most manufacturers. The pediatric collection chamber is smaller than its adult counterpart and has smaller incremental markings for accurate measurement of small volumes. Autotransfusion is not usually available on pediatric units, but adult auto-transfusion units may be used instead.

2. Negative 10 to 20 cm H_2O is the suction level usually recommended for pediatric patients.

3. Milking or stripping of chest tubes is contraindicated in children.

COMPLICATIONS

1. A tension pneumothorax may develop if there are obstructions in the system. Kinked or clamped tubing is the most likely source of obstruction.
2. If the device breaks or the system becomes disconnected, a loss of intrapleural negativity may result, and an open pneumothorax may develop. If the tubing becomes disconnected at any site, clean the connectors with alcohol and reconnect. If the device breaks, place the end of the drainage tubing (approximately 2.5 cm) in a container of sterile water until another chest-drainage device can be prepared.
3. Accidental dislodgement of the chest tube: If this happens, have the patient cough or exhale forcibly. Apply an occlusive dressing to the area and tape it on three sides. Notify the physician immediately. Check the oxygen saturation as measured by pulse oximetry (SpO$_2$) and administer oxygen. Monitor the patient closely for the development of a tension pneumothorax until another chest tube can be inserted.

PATIENT TEACHING

1. Turn and reposition yourself every 2 hours. Request assistance when moving or turning in bed or when getting out of bed.
2. Cough and deep breath every 2 hours, splinting the affected side.
3. Report any shortness of breath, chest pain, or disconnections in the system immediately.
4. Do not lie on the tubing or allow it to be kinked.

REFERENCE

Duncan, C., & Erickson, R. (1982). Pressures associated with chest tube stripping. *Heart & Lung*, *11*, 166–171.

One-Way Valve

Deborah A. Upton, MSN, ARNP-BC, CEN

A one-way valve is also known as a *Heimlich, flap,* or *flutter valve.*

INDICATION

To allow air and fluid to drain from the pleural cavity and simultaneously prevent reentry of air into the pleural space. Patients who have chronic pneumothorax or pleural effusion can benefit from a one-way valve because no other chest drainage device is required. Using the one-way valve, these patients can ambulate and, in some cases, can be discharged from the hospital. The valve can also be used during interhospital transport instead of, or in addition to, a chest-drainage unit.

CONTRAINDICATIONS AND CAUTIONS

1. If the valve is placed going in the wrong direction, air egress will be prevented and tension pneumothorax may result. Be sure the collapsed end of the valve is distal to the patient and the chest tube (see Figure 41-1).
2. If a hemothorax or pleural effusion is present, it may be necessary to replace the valve or add a regular chest-drainage unit for fluid collection.

EQUIPMENT

One-way valve
Adhesive tape
Padded hemostat
Urinary catheter drainage collection bag or sterile glove (if necessary for fluid collection)
Sutures ties or small rubber band

PATIENT PREPARATION

1. Insert a chest tube or chest-drainage catheter (see Procedure 39).
2. Instruct the patient to rest during the procedure and report pain or shortness of breath.
3. If possible, have the patient sit at a 45- to 90-degree angle.

PROCEDURAL STEPS

1. If the chest tube is connected to a chest-drainage unit, untape the connection.
2. If drainage of blood or other fluid is anticipated, attach a urinary catheter collection bag to the distal end of the valve. A sterile glove can be used if only a small amount of drainage is present.
3. Disconnect the chest tube from the chest-drainage unit and immediately connect to the blue end of the one-way valve. The "collapsed end" of the valve is the distal end, which allows the fluid or air to drain out of the pleural space but does not allow the air to reenter (see Figure 41-1). If fluid is draining

Open to atmosphere or attach to suction

To patient

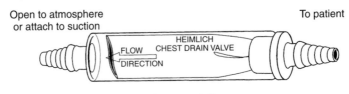

One-way air flow

FIGURE 41-1 Heimlich or one-way valve. The "collapsed end" is placed distally to allow drainage out of the chest. (From Kirsch, T. D., & Mulligan, J. P. [2004]. Tube thoracostomy. In J. R. Roberts & J. R. Hedges (Eds.), *Clinical procedures in emergency medicine* [4th ed., p. 201]. Philadelphia: Saunders.)

actively, the chest tube may be clamped briefly during this step. Do not clamp the chest tube until you are ready to place the valve, and remove the clamp as soon as the valve is in place.

4. Ask the patient to cough or exhale forcibly.
5. Tape the connections securely and anchor the chest tube and valve to the patient's chest.
6. Intubated patients receiving positive pressure ventilation do not necessarily need a flutter valve unless there is a bronchopleural fistula.
7. Obtain a chest radiograph to determine whether air has reentered the pleural cavity.

COMPLICATIONS

1. Infection resulting from a break in aseptic technique
2. Tension pneumothorax if the valve is inserted incorrectly or the chest tube is clamped, kinked, or occluded

PATIENT TEACHING

1. Report chest pain, shortness of breath, or any disconnection in the system immediately.
2. Do not attempt to reposition the chest tube or valve.

Chest-Drainage Bottles

Deborah A. Upton, RN, MSN, ARNP-BC, CEN

The information in this procedure should be used in conjunction with that in Procedure 40.

NOTE: *Chest-drainage bottle systems are no longer manufactured. They have been replaced with the disposable drainage sets. However, some institutions are still using the chest drainage bottle system. Also, study of this system clarifies understanding of the integrated devices, and improvisation may be needed in austere conditions.*

INDICATION
See Procedure 40.

CONTRAINDICATIONS AND CAUTIONS
1. See Procedure 40.
2. The one-bottle system can be used for removing fluid; however, a two- or three-bottle system is preferred because it reduces the need for frequent readjustment of the water-seal tube to maintain appropriate submersion (the same bottle is used as a water-seal and as a collection chamber). Also, suction cannot be used with a one-bottle system.
3. The bottle system is rarely used now because most facilities have replaced it with prefabricated, disposable chest-drainage systems. The prefabricated systems can be used as either gravity or suction-drainage systems. They are easier to set up and maintain, and their components are less fragile than those of glass bottles.

PATIENT PREPARATION
Insert a chest tube (see Procedure 39).

ONE-BOTTLE SYSTEM: GRAVITY DRAINAGE
Equipment
Sterile water-seal device or collection bottle (Figure 42-1)
Sterile water or saline
Holder for bottle
3 to 4 ft of sterile tubing
Tubing connectors, ¼-in internal diameter
Adhesive tape

Procedural Steps
1. Add enough sterile water or saline solution to the bottle to submerge the end of the water-seal tube 2.5 cm below the water level. The water-seal tube is

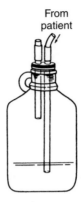

From
patient

FIGURE 42-1 One-bottle chest-drainage system.

attached to the tubing that exits the patient. This provides the water seal necessary for preventing back flow. The short, rigid tube is the vent tube (see Figure 42-1).

2. Attach the chest tube to the drainage tubing with a connector.
3. Connect the drainage tubing to the water-seal tube.
4. Secure the connection sites with adhesive tape.

TWO-BOTTLE SYSTEM: GRAVITY DRAINAGE
Equipment
Sterile collection and water-seal bottles (Figure 42-2)
Sterile water or saline solution
Holder for bottles
3 to 4 ft of sterile tubing
Tubing connectors, ¼-in internal diameter
Adhesive tape

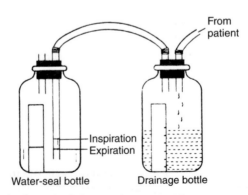

From
patient

Inspiration
Expiration

Water-seal bottle   Drainage bottle

FIGURE 42-2 Two-bottle gravity-drainage system.

Procedural Steps

1. Add enough sterile water or saline solution to the water-seal bottle to sub-merge the end of the water-seal tube 2.5 cm below the water level. This provides the water seal necessary for preventing back flow. The short, rigid tube is the vent tube.
2. Attach the drainage bottle to the water-seal bottle via the short length of sterile tubing that is attached to the water-seal tube.
3. Attach the chest tube to the drainage tubing via a connector.
4. Connect the drainage tubing to the other short, rigid tube in the drainage bottle (see Figure 42-2).
5. Secure the connections with adhesive tape.

TWO-BOTTLE SYSTEM: SUCTION DRAINAGE
Equipment

    Sterile water-seal/collection bottle and suction-control bottle (Figure 42-3)
    Sterile water or saline solution
    Holder for bottles
    3 to 4 ft of sterile tubing
    Tubing connectors, ¼-in internal diameter
    Suction setup
    Adhesive tape

Procedural Steps

1. Add enough sterile water or saline solution to the water-seal/collection bottle to submerge the end of the water-seal tube 2.5 cm below the water level. This provides a water seal necessary for preventing back flow.
2. The suction-control bottle has three openings in the cap. The long, rigid tube in the center works as the manometer tube. Fill the suction-control bottle with enough sterile water or saline to submerge the manometer tube in about

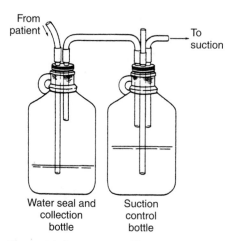

From patient → To suction

Water seal and collection bottle   Suction control bottle

FIGURE 42-3 Two-bottle chest-drainage system with suction.

10 cm of water. Connect the suction-control bottle to the water-seal/collection bottle with a short length of sterile tube. Connect the other short, rigid tube in the suction-control bottle to the continuous-suction device. The level of submersion of the manometer tube, rather than the suction regulator device, determines how much suction is applied (Brunner & Suddarth, 1988):

$$1 \text{ cm manometer of submersion} = 1 \text{ cm of negative water pressure}$$

3. Attach the chest tube to the drainage tubing with a connector.
4. Attach the drainage tube to the water-seal tube of the collection bottle (see Figure 42-3).
5. Secure the connections with adhesive tape.

THREE-BOTTLE SYSTEM
Equipment
Sterile collection, suction, and water-seal (overflow) bottles (Figure 42-4)
Sterile water or saline
Holder for bottles
4 to 5 ft of sterile tubing
Tubing connectors, ¼-in internal diameter
Adhesive tape
Suction setup

Procedural Steps
1. Add enough sterile water or saline solution to one of the bottles with two openings in the cap to submerge the end of the long, rigid tube 2.5 cm below the water level. This provides the water seal necessary for preventing back flow. This is the water-seal and collection overflow bottle.
2. The other bottle with two openings in the cap is the collection bottle. One of the short, rigid tubes is connected to the drainage tubing, and the other is connected to the water-seal tube via a short length of sterile tubing.

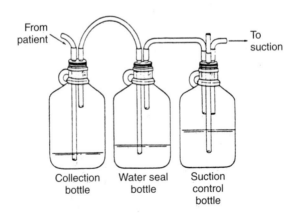

From patient   To suction

Collection bottle   Water seal bottle   Suction control bottle

FIGURE 42-4 Three-bottle chest-drainage system.

3. The suction bottle has three openings in the cap. The long, rigid tube in the center is the manometer tube. Fill the suction bottle with enough sterile water to submerge the manometer tube in about 10 cm of water. Connect one of the short, rigid tubes of the suction bottle to the water-seal bottle via a short length of sterile tubing. Connect the other short rigid tube in the suction bottle to the suction device. The depth the manometer tube submerged in the water, rather than the suction regulator device, determines the amount of suction that is applied (Brunner & Suddarth, 1988).

$$1 \text{ cm manometer of submersion} = 1 \text{ cm of negative water pressure}$$

4. Attach the chest tube to the drainage tube via a connector.
5. Attach the drainage tube to the other short, rigid tube of the collection bottle (see Figure 42-4).
6. Secure the connection sites with adhesive tape.

COMPLICATIONS

1. See Procedure 40.
2. When the suction source is functioning there is continuous bubbling from the manometer tube in the suction bottle. If the bubbling stops, check the suction source. If the suction source is malfunctioning, disconnect the manometer tube from the suction bottle to provide an air vent for gravity drainage.

PATIENT TEACHING

See Procedure 40.

REFERENCE
Brunner, L. S., & Suddarth, D. S. (1988). *Textbook of medical-surgical nursing* (6th ed). Philadelphia: J.B. Lippincott.

Chest-Drainage Devices: Emerson

Deborah A. Upton, MSN, ARNP-BC, CEN

The information in this procedure should be used in conjunction with that in Procedure 40.

NOTE: The Emerson pump bottle set is no longer manufactured but may still be in use because the bottles are reusable. Also, portable pumps might be used as disaster medical equipment.

INDICATION

See Procedure 40.

CONTRAINDICATIONS AND CAUTIONS

1. See Procedure 40.
2. The Emerson pump is a high-pressure, high-flow system capable of generating pressures of 60 cm H_2O. Bottles are used infrequently because most facilities now use low-pressure, prefabricated, disposable chest-drainage systems.

EQUIPMENT

Emerson pump-bottle set (connectors, drainage tubes, bottles, bottle cap assemblies, bottle tubes, large tubing, pump, mobile stand with a triangular tray)

or

Disposable Emerson chest-drainage unit for Emerson pump or wall-suction setup (for disposable unit with manometer only)

Sterile water or saline solution

Tape

PATIENT PREPARATION

Insert a chest tube (see Procedure 39).

PROCEDURAL STEPS

Bottle System for Emerson Pump (Figure 43-1) (Emerson, 1989c)

1. Add enough sterile water or saline solution to the water-seal collection bottle to fill it up to the water line. Write the time and date on the bottle. Attach the two, short, rigid, narrow tubes to the underside of the cap via three connectors. These tubes should be submerged in 1 to 2 cm of sterile water in the bottle. This provides the water seal necessary for preventing back flow.

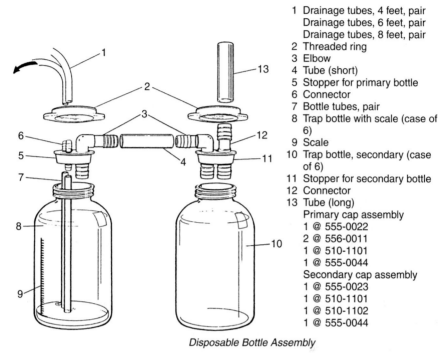

1 Drainage tubes, 4 feet, pair
  Drainage tubes, 6 feet, pair
  Drainage tubes, 8 feet, pair
2 Threaded ring
3 Elbow
4 Tube (short)
5 Stopper for primary bottle
6 Connector
7 Bottle tubes, pair
8 Trap bottle with scale (case of 6)
9 Scale
10 Trap bottle, secondary (case of 6)
11 Stopper for secondary bottle
12 Connector
13 Tube (long)
   Primary cap assembly
   1 @ 555-0022
   2 @ 556-0011
   1 @ 510-1101
   1 @ 555-0044
   Secondary cap assembly
   1 @ 555-0023
   1 @ 510-1101
   1 @ 510-1102
   1 @ 555-0044

Disposable Bottle Assembly

FIGURE 43-1 Emerson bottle setup. (Courtesy J. H. Emerson Co., Cambridge, MA.)

2. If the patient has only one chest tube, cover one of the openings in the bottle cap with the plastic adapter.
3. Attach the water-seal bottle and the fluid-trap bottle via the short, wide connection tube.
4. Attach the fluid-trap bottle to the pump via the large, wide connection tube.
5. Plug in the machine and make sure that the red indicator light goes on.
6. Plug in the two small connectors on the primary bottle cap and adjust the speed of the motor until the desired suction is attained (-20 to -30 cm H_2O).
7. Remove the cap(s) and connect the long tube(s) (if there are two chest tubes) to the cap of the water-seal collection bottle.
8. Connect the drainage tube(s) to the chest tube(s).
9. Tape all the connections and make sure the caps are tight.
10. Turn on the machine and adjust the pressure to the prescribed level.
11. To determine the negative pressure in the patient's pleural space, subtract the depth of submersion of the tube tips in the water-seal collection bottle from the pressure on the machine. For example, if the pressure on the machine is set at -30 cm of water and the tubes in the water-seal collection bottle are submerged to 20 cm of water, then the pressure in the patient's pleural space is -10 cm of water. Therefore, to maintain the desired pressure, it is necessary to increase the pressure setting on the machine as fluid accumulates in the water-seal collection bottle. Fluid should not be allowed

to fill more than one quarter of the bottle (the machine capacity is −60 cm H_2O; higher fluid levels require increased pressure settings on the machine to maintain the desired pressure level).

Disposable System for Emerson Pump (Figure 43-2) (Emerson, 1989a)

1. Add water through the suction port up to the water-seal mark.
2. Place the disposable unit in the stand (Figure 43-3) or suspend it from the bed by using ties or accessory metal hangers.
3. Connect the patient tube(s) to the patient fittings on the disposable unit.
4. Connect the flexible corrugated tube to the suction port on the disposable unit and the fitting on the bottom of the Emerson pump.
5. Turn on the pump. The level of accumulated fluid in the disposable unit does not affect the vacuum level applied to the patient, because there is no underwater seal in the primary collecting compartment.

Disposable System for Wall Suction (Figure 43-4) (Emerson, 1989b)

1. Add water through the suction port up to the water-seal mark.
2. Add water through the manometer air intake to the desired level of suction. The air intake port must be left uncapped to allow air to enter and relieve excess negativity.
3. Connect the patient tube(s) to the patient fittings on the disposable unit.
4. Connect the reducing adapter to the suction port and attach it to the wall-suction device. Adjust the wall-suction device until bubbles appear in the bottom of the manometer column.

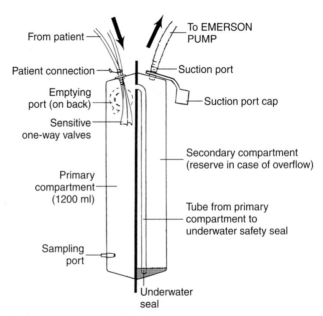

FIGURE 43-2 Emerson disposable thoracic drainage set for use with the Emerson suction regulator or the Emerson pump. (Courtesy J. H. Emerson Co., Cambridge, MA.)

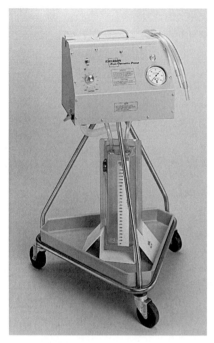

FIGURE 43-3 Emerson pump with disposable chest drainage unit. (Courtesy J. H. Emerson Co., Cambridge, MA.)

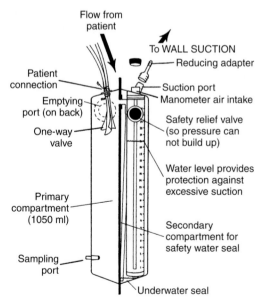

FIGURE 43-4 Emerson disposable thoracic drainage set (with manometer) for use with any regulated suction source. (Courtesy J. H. Emerson Co., Cambridge, MA.)

AGE-SPECIFIC CONSIDERATION

There are no pediatric versions of the bottle or disposable units, but the adult units can be used for infants and children.

COMPLICATIONS

1. See Procedure 40.
2. When available, the pump should be connected to a power supply with automatic emergency generator power supply back-up. If there is a loss of electrical power or if the Emerson pump malfunctions, the internal vacuum blower has an air vent to the atmosphere, so there is no danger of pressure accumulation (R. Felt, personal communication, February 1998).

PATIENT TEACHING

See Procedure 40.

REFERENCES

J. H. Emerson Co. (1989a). *Emerson disposable thoracic drainage set: Instructions for use.* Form 903-6001-2. Cambridge, MA: Author.

J. H. Emerson Co. (1989b). *Emerson disposable thoracic drainage set: Instructions for use with wall suction.* Form 902-4001. Cambridge, MA: Author.

J. H. Emerson Co. (1989c). *Emerson post-operative pumps: Operation and maintenance.* Cambridge, MA: Author.

PROCEDURE 44

Chest-Drainage Devices: Pleur-Evac

Deborah A. Upton, MSN, ARNP-BC, CEN

Pleur-Evac and Sahara chest-drainage units are products of the Deknatel Product Group, Teleflex Medical OEM (Research Triangle Park, NC).

The information in this procedure should be used in conjunction with the information in Procedure 40.

INDICATIONS

1. See Procedure 40.
2. The Sahara units are totally dry and, thus, quick and easy to set up.

3. All Sahara units have 100% latex-free pathway and tubing.
4. The Sahara and dry suction-control units can achieve greater levels of suction (as much as -40 cm H_2O) than the wet suction-control units.

CONTRAINDICATIONS AND CAUTIONS
See Procedure 40.

EQUIPMENT
Pleur-Evac (wet or dry suction control) water-seal unit or Sahara (dry) chest-drainage unit
Sterile water
Adhesive tape
Suction setup
Needle and a 30-ml syringe (to fill the air-leak chamber of the Sahara unit)

PATIENT PREPARATION
Insert a chest tube (see Procedure 39).

PROCEDURAL STEPS
Pleur-Evac: Wet Suction Control (Figure 44-1) (Deknatel, 1997b)
1. Attach a funnel to the suction-tubing connector and fill it to the 2-cm level with sterile water (approximately 70 ml). Use the "Fill to Here" mark as a guide. The water turns blue for enhanced visibility. Disconnect the funnel. If necessary, the unit can now be attached to the patient.
2. Remove the atmospheric vent cover (muffler) and fill the suction-control chamber with enough sterile water to achieve the desired level of suction; -20 cm H_2O is the standard setting. Replace the muffler, making sure that you do not occlude the atmospheric vent.
3. Attach the long tube from the collection chamber to the patient's chest tube and tape all the connections securely.
4. Attach the tubing from the suction-control chamber to a suction source. Adjust the suction until gentle, continuous bubbling occurs in the suction-control chamber. Increasing the suction from the suction source increases bubbling and air flow through the system but does not increase the suction delivered to the pleural cavity; additional water must be added to the chamber to accomplish this.
5. If gravity drainage is desired, omit step 4 and leave the suction tubing open and unclamped to prevent positive-pressure buildup.

Pleur-Evac: Dry-suction Control (Figure 44-2) (Deknatel, 1997c)
1. Attach a funnel to the suction-tube connector and fill it to the 2-cm level ("Fill to Here" mark) with sterile water (approximately 70 ml). The water turns blue for enhanced visibility. Disconnect the funnel.
2. Attach the long tube from the collection chamber to the patient's chest tube and tape all connections securely.
3. Attach the tubing from the suction-control chamber to a suction source. The suction is controlled by a dial that is preset at -20 cm H_2O. Turn on the suction and increase it until the orange float is visible in the suction-control indicator window. Increasing the suction from the source increases the

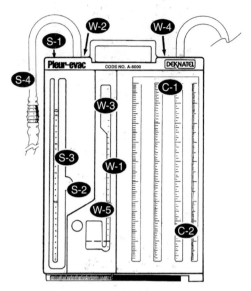

FIGURE 44-1 Pleur-Evac A-8000 chest-drainage unit.

S-1: Atmospheric vent: Fill the suction-control chamber through this opening. Do not cover the vent with anything other than the muffler provided. The muffler allows air to enter the suction-control chamber, but it decreases evaporation and noise.

S-2: Self-sealing diaphragm to inject or withdraw fluid to adjust the water level in the suction-control chamber.

S-3: Suction-control pressure scale.

S-4: Suction tubing.

W-1: Water-seal pressure scale: Oscillations (tidaling) occur in this chamber with respirations, but they may not be present when the suction is on, the lung is fully expanded, or the tubing is obstructed or kinked.

W-2: Positive-pressure relief valve: Opens to vent increased positive pressure within the system and prevent pressure accumulation (tension pneumothorax).

W-3: High-negativity float valve: Preserves the water seal in the presence of high negativity. The high-negativity relief valve may be used to reduce negativity.

W-4: Filtered high-negativity relief valve: Depress this button to relieve excess negativity within the system (i.e., after "milking" or stripping the tube to clear clots). If this button is depressed in the absence of suction, negative pressure may be lost and atmospheric pressure may be attained.

W-5: Self-sealing diaphragm: Injects or withdraws fluid to adjust the water level in the water-seal chamber.

C-1: Collection chamber: 2500-ml capacity with overflow from one compartment to the next.

C-2: Self-sealing diaphragm on the back of the collection chamber: Obtains laboratory samples of drainage. (From Deknatel. [1989]. *Pleur-Evac: Instructions for use.* Teleflex Medical OEM, Research Triangle Park, NC. Copyright 1989 by Pfizer Hospital Products Group.)

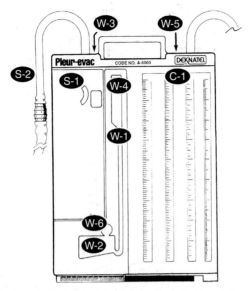

FIGURE 44-2 Pleur-Evac A-6000 dry-suction control chest-drainage unit.

S-1: Suction-control dial and indicator: When the orange float appears in this window, the suction is operating at the level indicated by the dial.

S-2: Suction tubing: Connects to the suction source.

W-1: Water-seal pressure scale: Oscillations (tidaling) occur in this chamber with respirations, but they may not be present when the suction is on, the lung is fully expanded, or the tubing is obstructed or kinked.

W-2: Patient air-leak meter: The higher the number of the column in which bubbles are seen, the larger the air leak.

W-3: Positive-pressure relief valve: Opens to vent increased positive pressure within the system and prevent pressure accumulation (tension pneumothorax).

W-4: High-negativity float valve: Preserves the water seal in the presence of high negativity. The high-negativity relief valve may be used to reduce negativity.

W-5: Filtered high-negativity relief valve: Depress this button to relieve excess negativity within the system (i.e., after "milking" or stripping the tube to clear clots). If this button is depressed in the absence of suction, negative pressure may be lost and atmospheric pressure may be attained.

W-6: Self-sealing diaphragm: Injects or withdraws fluid to adjust the water level in the water-seal chamber.

C-1: Collection chamber, 2500-ml capacity with overflow from one compartment to the next. (From Deknatel. [1989]. *Pleur-Evac: Instructions for use.* Teleflex Medical OEM, Research Triangle Park, NC. Copyright 1989 by Pfizer Hospital Products Group.)

air flow through the system without increasing the negativity delivered to the patient; if more negativity is desired, change the suction-control dial. If the suction level is decreased after the initial setup, the negativity delivered to the patient may not change unless the excess negativity is vented with the high-negativity relief valve.

4. If gravity drainage is desired, omit step 3 and leave the suction tubing open and unclamped to prevent positive-pressure buildup.

Sahara (Figure 44-3) (Deknatel, 1997a)

1. Attach the long tube from the collection chamber to the patient's chest tube and tape all connections securely (Figure 44-4). No fluid needs to be added to

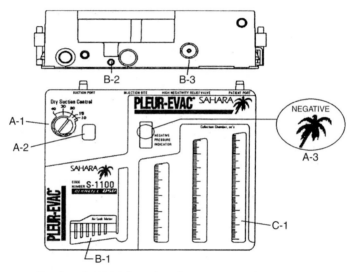

FIGURE 44-3 Pleur-Evac S-1100 Sahara chest-drainage system.

A-1: Suction dial: Preset to 20 cm H_2O.

A-2: Suction indicator: When the orange float appears in this window, the suction is operating at the level indicated by the dial.

A-3: Negative-pressure indicator: If a palm tree can be seen in this window, negative pressure exists within the collection chamber. The palm tree should be continuously visible when suction is in use. During gravity drainage, the palm tree may be visible intermittently.

B-1: Air-leak meter: When filled with fluid, this chamber indicates the degree of air leak from the chest cavity. The higher the number of the column in which bubbles are seen, the larger the air leak.

B-2: Positive-pressure relief valve: Opens to vent increased positive pressure within the system and prevent pressure accumulation (tension pneumothorax).

B-3: Filtered high-negativity relief valve: Depress this button to relieve excess negativity within the system (i.e., after "milking" or stripping the tube to clear clots). If this button is depressed in the absence of suction, negative pressure may be lost and atmospheric pressure attained. There is an automatic high-negative, pressure-relief valve that limits negative pressure to approximately 50 cm H_2O.

C-1: Collection chamber: 2000-ml capacity with overflow from one compartment to the next. (From Deknatel DSP. [1996]. Pleur-Evac Sahara (product insert). Teleflex Medical OEM, Research Triangle Park, NC. Author. Copyright 1996 by DSP Worldwide, Inc.)

the system before it is connected to the patient, because there is a one-way valve, not a water seal, which prevents air from reentering the thoracic cavity.

2. Use an 18-G or smaller needle and a 30-ml syringe to inject 30 ml of sterile water or saline through the injection port of the unit into the patient air-leak meter.

3. Connect the suction source to the suction port. The suction-control dial is preset at −20 cm H_2O; if a different level of suction is prescribed, turn the dial until it clicks into place. Increase the suction from the suction source until the orange float appears in the suction-control indicator window (Figure 44-5). Increasing the suction from the source increases the air flow through the system without increasing the negativity delivered to the patient; if more negativity is desired, change the suction-control dial. If the suction level is

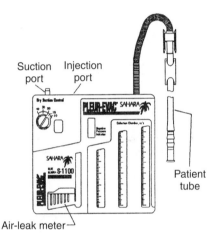

FIGURE 44-4 Pleur-Evac S-1100 Sahara chest-drainage system components for basic setup. (From Deknatel DSP. [1996]. *Pleur-Evac Sahara (product insert)*. Teleflex Medical OEM, Research Triangle Park, NC. Author. Copyright 1996 by DSP Worldwide, Inc.)

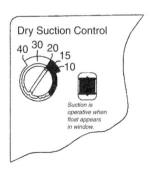

FIGURE 44-5 Pleur-Evac S-1100 Sahara chest-drainage system suction indicator window. (From Deknatel DSP. [1996]. Teleflex Medical OEM, Research Triangle Park, NC: Copyright 1996 by DSP Worldwide, Inc.)

decreased after the initial setup, the negativity delivered to the patient may not change unless the excess negativity is relieved by use of the high-negativity relief valve.

4. If gravity drainage is desired, omit step 3 and leave the suction port open to prevent positive-pressure buildup.

AGE-SPECIFIC CONSIDERATIONS

1. All these devices may be used for children. Infant versions are available for both wet and dry water-seal devices. The most significant differences in the infant versions are that the drainage chamber is smaller than its adult counterpart, with finer gradations for accurate measurement of drainage and no autotransfusion capability. There is no infant version of the Sahara drainage device.

2. See Procedure 40.

COMPLICATIONS

See Procedure 40.

PATIENT TEACHING

See Procedure 40.

REFERENCES

Deknatel Product Group, Genzyme Surgical Products. (1997a). *Pleur-Evac Sahara* (*product insert*). Teleflex Medical OEM, Research Triangle, NC: Author.

Deknatel Product Group, Genzyme Surgical Products. (1997b). *Pleur-Evac adult/pediatric single-use chest drainage unit: A-8000* (*product insert*). Teleflex Medical OEM, Research Triangle, NC: Author.

Deknatel Product Group, Teleflex Medical OEM, Research Triangle Park, NC. (1997c). *Pleur-Evac adult/pediatric single-use chest drainage unit: Dry suction control A-6000* (*product insert*). Teleflex Medical OEM, Research Triangle Park, NC: Author.

Chest-Drainage Devices: Argyle

Deborah A. Upton, MSN, ARNP-BC, CEN

The information in the procedure should be used in conjunction with the information in Procedure 40.

INDICATION
See Procedure 40.

CONTRAINDICATIONS AND CAUTIONS
See Procedure 40.

EQUIPMENT
Chest-drainage unit (Aqua-Seal, Thora-Seal III, or Sentinel Seal)
Sterile water
1- or 2-in tape
Suction setup

PATIENT PREPARATION
Insert a chest tube (see Procedure 39).

PROCEDURAL STEPS
Aqua-Seal **(Figure 45-1)** (Tyco, 2002a)
1. Fill the water-seal chamber. Lower the preattached syringe and fill it to the top with approximately 45 ml of sterile fluid (Figure 45-2). Raise the syringe and allow the fluid to flow into the water-seal chamber up to the 2-cm line. The water turns blue for enhanced visibility. Remove the tubing and the syringe from the water-seal chamber and discard them. If necessary, the unit can be connected to the patient now. If the water-seal level needs to be adjusted later, use the needleless access port on the back of the water-seal chamber.
2. Fill the suction-control chamber. Pour sterile fluid directly into the "suction-control fill opening" to the prescribed level; -20 cm H_2O is the usual setting for patients who are older than 6 months. Close the suction-control chamber with the attached cap; make sure that the cap snaps into place (suction greater than -25 cm H_2O can be achieved with the suction-control bypass adaptor on the back of the unit; see the package insert for more information).
3. Attach the chest tube to the thoracic catheter connector (if not done in step 1). Tape the connection securely.

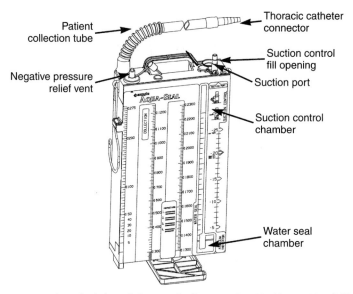

FIGURE 45-1 Aqua-Seal chest-drainage unit. (Courtesy Tyco Healthcare, Mansfield, MA.)

4. Turn the black valve on the suction port clockwise to the closed position (Figure 45-3). Connect a regulated suction source to the suction port. Turn the vacuum on and open the black suction valve until a gentle bubbling is achieved in the suction-control chamber.

5. Excess negative pressure can be relieved with the negative-pressure relief vent on the top of the unit. Excess positive pressure is automatically relieved by a valve on top of the unit.

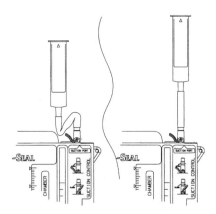

FIGURE 45-2 Filling the water-seal chamber of the Aqua-Seal. (Courtesy Tyco Healthcare, Mansfield, MA.)

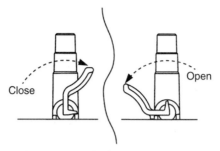

FIGURE 45-3 Aqua-Seal suction-control valve. (Courtesy Tyco Healthcare, Mansfield, MA.)

Thora-Seal III (Figure 45-4) (Tyco, 2002b)

1. Fill the water-seal bottle. Remove the water-seal cap from the top of the unit (middle bottle). Pour approximately 110 ml of sterile fluid directly into the opening to the line indicated on the water-seal bottle. Replace the cap. If necessary, the unit can be connected to the patient now.
2. Fill the suction-control bottle. Pour sterile fluid into the opening on the top of the suction-control bottle to the prescribed level: −20 cm H_2O is the usual setting for patients who are older than 6 months.
3. Attach the chest tube to the thoracic catheter connector (if this did not occur in step 1). Tape the connection securely.

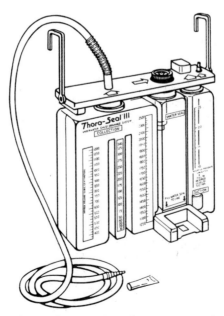

FIGURE 45-4 Thora-Seal III underwater chest drainage system. (Courtesy Tyco Healthcare, Mansfield, MA.)

4. Attach the suction tubing to the connection port on top of the suction bottle, turn on the vacuum, and adjust until a gentle bubbling is achieved in the suction-control bottle.
5. To change the collection bottle, remove the floor stand. With the physician's approval, clamp the patient's connecting tubing for a brief time. Rotate the collection bottle clockwise and pull it down. Insert a new bottle into the manifold and rotate until the bottle neck snaps into a locked position. Remove the clamp from the patient's connecting tubing. Replace the floor stand.

Sentinel Seal (Figure 45-5) (Tyco, 2002c)

1. Fill the underwater-seal chamber. Remove the "suction regulator" from the top of the unit by twisting it at the base. Pour approximately 90 ml of sterile fluid through the opening and fill to the red "2" line on the suction control chamber. Replace the suction regulator and twist it into place. Remove the red protector ring from the suction regulator and discard it.
2. Fill the patient assessment chamber. Remove the instruction tape from the top of the unit and fill the chamber to the red line with approximately 35 ml of sterile fluid. The fluid turns blue for enhanced visibility.
3. Attach the chest tube to the thoracic catheter connector. Tape the connection securely.

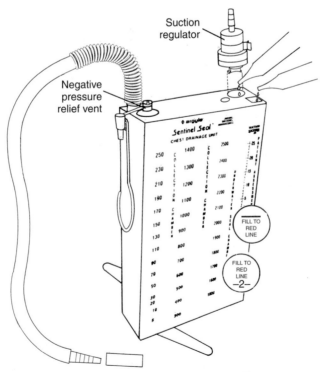

FIGURE 45-5 Sentinel-Seal chest drainage unit. (Courtesy Tyco Healthcare, Mansfield, MA.)

4. Connect the suction source to the suction regulator. Set the wall suction source to at least 160 mm Hg (set a portable suction source to at least 50 cm H_2O). Watch the patient assessment chamber while turning the suction regulator until the fluid reaches the prescribed suction level; −20 cm H_2O is the usual setting for patients who are older than 6 months. To increase the vacuum level, clamp the tubing connected to the chest tube briefly and turn the regulator clockwise until the fluid in the manometer rises to the required level, remove the clamp from the chest tube. To decrease the vacuum level, clamp the tubing connected to the chest tube then depress the negative pressure release valve and simultaneously turn the suction regulator counterclockwise while observing the drop in the left column in the patient manometer. Remove the clamp from the tubing. Do not depress the negative-pressure relief vent unless the unit is connected to the suction source or the intrapleural negativity may be lost.

5. For gravity drainage, disconnect the suction tubing from the suction regulator.

AGE-SPECIFIC CONSIDERATION

Argyle does not make a pediatric chest-drainage unit, but all units can be used for pediatric patients.

COMPLICATIONS

1. See Procedure 40.
2. Tipping the units may result in mixing of fluid from some chambers or loss of the water seal.

PATIENT TEACHING

See Procedure 40.

REFERENCES

Tyco Healthcare. (2002a). *Aqua-Seal three chamber thoracic drainage system.* Retrieved February 3, 2007, from http://www.tycohealth-ece.com/files/d0000/ty_ajvbbw.pdf

Tyco Healthcare. (2002b). *Thora-Seal III four chamber thoracic drainage system.* Retrieved February 3, 2007, from http://www.tycohealth-ece.com/files/d0000/ty_uyxcd3.pdf

Tyco Healthcare. (2002c). *Sentinel Seal four chamber thoracic drainage system.* Retrieved February 3, 2007, from http://www.tycohealth-ece.com/files/d0000/ty_sprz6j.pdf

Chest-Drainage Devices: Atrium

Deborah A. Upton, MSN, ARNP-BC, CEN

The information in this procedure should be used in conjunction with the information in Procedure 40.

INDICATIONS

1. See Procedure 40.
2. The dry-suction system has the advantages of quick setup, quiet operation, and the ability to use high levels of controlled suction.

CONTRAINDICATIONS AND CAUTIONS

See Procedure 40.

EQUIPMENT

    Atrium chest-drainage unit (wet- or dry-suction control)
    Sterile water or saline
    Tape
    Suction setup

PATIENT PREPARATION

Insert a chest tube (see Procedure 39).

PROCEDURAL STEPS

Wet-suction Control (Figure 46-1) (Atrium, 2006a)

1. Turn the suction-control stopcock to the on position. Fill the water-seal chamber with sterile water by holding the preattached funnel level with the unit. Add water to the top of the funnel. Raise the funnel and empty the water into the water-seal chamber up to the 2-cm line. The water turns blue to assist in air-leak detection. If too much water is added, the excess can be removed by inserting a needle and syringe through the face grommet. When the water has passed to the chamber, the suction-control stopcock must be returned to the off position before it is connected to the unregulated suction device. Discard the funnel after use or use it to fill the suction-control chamber.
2. To fill the suction-control chamber, remove the suction-control vent plug and pour into the chamber the amount of sterile water or saline needed to achieve the desired suction pressure in the suction-control chamber (Table 46-1). The water turns blue when the chamber is filled. The usual setting for adults is -20 cm H_2O.
3. Replace the suction-control vent plug.

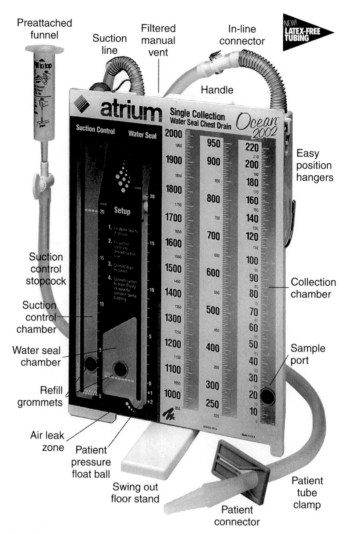

FIGURE 46-1 Atrium water seal chest-drainage unit with wet-suction control. (Courtesy Atrium Medical Corporation, Hudson, NH.)

TABLE 46-1
WATER NEEDED FOR VARIOUS SUCTION LEVELS

Suction Pressure	Water/Saline Volume Needed
-20 cm H_2O	320 ml
-15 cm H_2O	190 ml
-10 cm H_2O	80 ml

From Weimer, C. (2006) Personal communication. Atrium.

4. Remove the cap from the patient-tube connector and attach it to the chest tube.
5. Position the unit below the patient's chest level and keep it upright by using either the bed attachment hooks or the floor stand.
6. Connect the suction source to the suction-control stopcock. Tape all the connections to prevent accidental disconnections.
7. Turn on the suction-control stopcock and increase the suction pressure slowly until constant gentle bubbling occurs in the suction-control chamber. To increase or decrease the suction pressure delivered to the patient, adjust the fluid level in the suction-control chamber by injecting or withdrawing water via the face grommet.
8. Observe the water seal for air leaks and changes in pressure in the water seal chamber. Absence of bubbling with minimal float-ball oscillation indicates that there is no air leak. Constant or intermittent bubbling, with air bubbles going from right to left in the air-leak zone, indicates a leak in either the chest-drainage system or the thoracic cavity (Figure 46-2).
9. Changes in patient pressure are detected by observing the float ball in the calibrated water-seal column. When the chest tube is connected to the suction chamber, the suction pressure delivered to the patient is equal to the suction-control setting plus the float-ball level. Accumulated positive pressure is automatically released by the in-line positive-pressure valve in the calibrated water-seal column.

Dry-Suction Control (Figure 46-3) (Atrium, 2006b)

1. Turn the suction-control stopcock to the on position. Fill the water-seal chamber with sterile water by holding the preattached funnel level with the unit. Add water to the top of the funnel. Raise the funnel and empty the water into the water-seal chamber up to the 2-cm line. The water turns blue to assist in air-leak detection. If too much water is added, the excess can be removed by inserting a needle and syringe through the face grommet.
2. Remove the cap from the patient-tube connector and attach it to the chest tube.

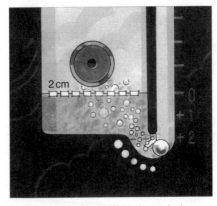

FIGURE 46-2 Atrium water seal with float ball in the air-leak zone. (Courtesy Atrium Medical Corporation, Hudson, NH.)

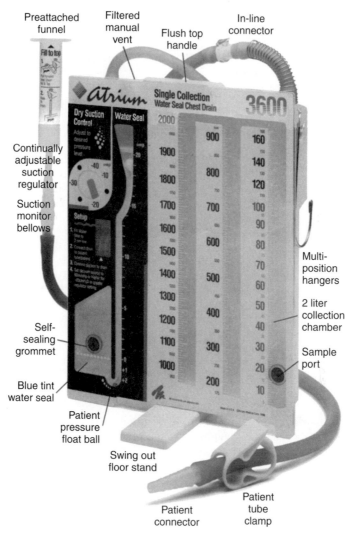

FIGURE 46-3 Atrium dry-suction collection unit. (Courtesy Atrium Medical Corporation, Hudson, NH.)

3. Connect the chest-drain suction line to the suction source. The suction-control regulator is preset to −20 cm H$_2$O. Increase the suction source to −80 mm Hg or higher. The suction-monitor bellows must be expanded to the mark or beyond it for a −20 cm H$_2$O or higher setting. The monitor bellows does not expand when suction is not operating or is disconnected. The regulator-control dial on the side of the drain can be set at −10 to −40 cm H$_2$O (Figure 46-4). To change the suction pressure, dial down to lower the suction pressure and up to increase it.

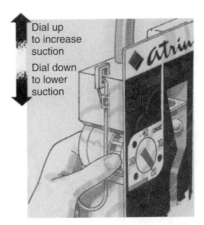

Dial up to increase suction

Dial down to lower suction

FIGURE 46-4 Dry-suction control regulator. (Courtesy Atrium Medical Corporation, Hudson, NH.)

4. Observe the calibrated water-seal column for changes in patient pressure. When the suction is operating, the patient pressure equals the suction-control setting plus the water-seal column level. For gravity drainage, the patient pressure equals the calibrated water-seal column level only.
5. Observe the water seal chamber for air leaks. Absence of bubbling with minimal float-ball oscillation indicates that there is no air leak. Constant or intermittent bubbling indicates a leak in either the chest-drainage system or the thoracic cavity (see Figure 46-2).

AGE-SPECIFIC CONSIDERATION

Infant or pediatric collection units are available in either a wet- or dry-suction control model. The drainage chamber is smaller than the adult counterpart, and it has large, easy-to-read drainage gradations. The pediatric units do not have autotransfusion capability.

COMPLICATIONS

See Procedure 40.

PATIENT TEACHING

See Procedure 40.

REFERENCES

Atrium Medical Corporation. (2006a). *Atrium 2002 single collection water seal drainage unit instruction sheet.* Hudson, NH: Author.
Atrium Medical Corporation. (2006b). *Atrium 3600 single collection dry suction chest drainage manual.* Hudson, NH: Author.

Thoracentesis

Deborah A. Upton, MSN, ARNP-BC, CEN

INDICATION

To remove fluid (pleural effusion) from the pleural cavity for diagnostic or therapeutic purposes. Air or fluid in the pleural space may affect ventilatory mechanisms. Emergency needle thoracentesis for tension pneumothorax is discussed in Procedure 38.

CONTRAINDICATIONS AND CAUTIONS

1. An absolute contraindication for thoracentesis is needle insertion into an area of infection.
2. Relative contraindications include bleeding dyscrasias and anticoagulant therapy. In this situation, emergent correction of coagulopathy may be indicated prior to thoracentesis for patients who are not in distress.
3. Caution should be used in the presence of a compromised respiratory status (e.g., ventilator dependency, ruptured diaphragm, emphysema) or pleural adhesions, because of a higher incidence of pneumothorax secondary to lung perforation.
4. Uncooperative patient
5. Cardiac hemodynamic or rhythm instability

EQUIPMENT

Antiseptic solution
Sterile towels
Local anesthetic
Gauze dressings
Tape
Syringes and needles for local anesthesia
For aspiration:
- 18- to 22-G needle, 3.75 to 5 cm long or
- 16- to 20-G over-the-needle catheter or
- 14- to 16-G through-the-needle catheter with plastic sleeve or
- 50- to 60-ml syringe

Three-way stopcock
Two curved hemostats
Intravenous (IV) extension tubing
18-G needle
Sterile basin (if vacuum bottle is not used)
500- to 1000-ml vacuum bottle(s) (optional)
(Preassembled kits containing some of this equipment are available.)

PATIENT PREPARATION

1. Place the patient in a sitting position, leaning forward on a bedside table with arms crossed. If the patient cannot tolerate a sitting position, place him or her in a supine position.
2. Cleanse the site with an antiseptic solution. For the patient in a supine position, drape the area with a sterile towel. For the removal of pleural fluid, the insertion site is the posterior axillary line one intercostal space below the top of the fluid (Barefoot, 2005) (Figure 47-1).
3. Administer atropine, if prescribed, to prevent a vasovagal response.
4. Instruct the patient to refrain from coughing during the procedure to prevent trauma to the lung.

PROCEDURAL STEPS

1. *Infiltrate the area with a local anesthetic directly inferior to the selected site. The needle-insertion site is directly over the top of the rib. Change to the 22-G needle and continue the anesthetic infiltration to the periosteum. If a rigid needle is used to withdraw fluid, advance the anesthetic needle until the pleural space is entered and fluid can be withdrawn. Note the depth of penetration at which fluid is aspirated by clamping a hemostat at the skin line of the anesthetic needle.

---

*Indicates portions of the procedure usually performed by a physician or an advanced practice nurse.

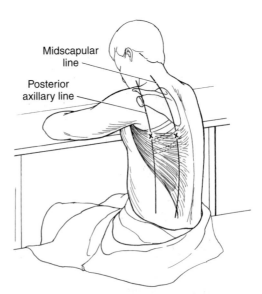

Midscapular line

Posterior axillary line

FIGURE 47-1 Anatomic landmarks for thoracentesis. (From Rosen, P., Chan, T. C., Vilke, G. M., & Sternbach, G. [2001]. *Atlas of emergency procedures* [p. 37]. St. Louis: Mosby.)

2. *Insert the needle or catheter into the pleural space. The needle should be inserted directly over the top of a rib. A pop may be felt as the pleural space is entered.

   a. *Rigid needle:* Attach a 50- to 60-ml syringe to the needle via a three-way stopcock. Place a hemostat on the needle at the same depth as the hemostat on the anesthetic needle. Insert the needle to the depth of the hemostat.

   b. *Over-the-needle catheter:* Attach a 14- to 18-G over-the-needle catheter to a 50- to 60-ml syringe. Aspirate as the needle is advanced. After entering the pleural space, advance the catheter off the needle and withdraw the needle. Cover the open end of the catheter with a sterile, gloved finger when the needle is withdrawn.

   c. *Through-the-needle catheter:* Attach a three-way stopcock to the catheter and turn it to the off position. Insert the needle into the pleural space. Guide the catheter, within the plastic sleeve, through the needle. Discard the plastic sleeve. Withdraw the needle, leaving the catheter in the pleural space (Figure 47-2). Cover the needle with the plastic needle guard.

3. *Withdraw fluid via a syringe and stopcock or a vacuum bottle.

   a. *Syringe and stopcock:* Attach the 50- to 60-ml syringe to the needle or catheter via a three-way stopcock. Withdraw the fluid and then turn the stopcock off to the patient to empty the syringe into a basin. Repeat until the desired amount of fluid is withdrawn.

   b. *Vacuum bottle:* Attach one end of the IV extension tubing to the catheter via a three-way stopcock, and the other end to an 18-G needle. Insert the needle into the top of the vacuum bottle and open the stopcock between the bottle and the patient (see Figure 47-2).

---

*Indicates portions of the procedure usually performed by a physician or an advanced practice nurse.

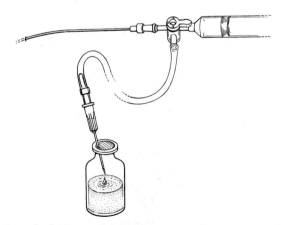

FIGURE 47-2 Set-up for fluid removal during thoracentesis. (From Rosen, P., Chan, T. C., Vilke, G. M., & Sternbach, G. [2001]. *Atlas of emergency procedures* [p. 37]. St. Louis: Mosby.)

4. *Withdraw the desired amount of fluid; 50 to 100 ml of fluid is required for laboratory diagnosis. For therapeutic drainage, fluid is removed in 50-ml increments until respiratory distress is relieved. It is recommended that no more than 1000 to 1500 ml of fluid be removed at a time owing to the risk of postprocedure pulmonary edema, hypovolemia, or hypoxemia (Barefoot, 2005). Turn the stopcock off to the tubing and withdraw the needle from the patient.

5. Apply a sterile dressing and obtain a chest radiograph.

6. Fluid from the syringe or the bottle may be sent to the laboratory for analysis. Analyses that are performed frequently include Gram stain, culture and sensitivity, acid-fast staining and culture, differential cell count, cytology, pH, specific gravity, total protein, glucose, and lactate dehydrogenase.

AGE-SPECIFIC CONSIDERATION

Landmarks and insertion techniques are the same for both pediatric and adult patients. A smaller needle or catheter is used for pediatric patients.

COMPLICATIONS

1. Reexpansion pulmonary edema can result from removal of a large quantity of fluid. Do not remove more than 1000 to 1500 ml of fluid at one time.

2. Shearing of the plastic catheter may occur if a through-the-catheter is withdrawn through the needle.

3. Hypoxia may develop in patients with underlying respiratory pathology.

4. A hemothorax can result from laceration of the lung, diaphragm, or intercostal vessels.

5. Lung perforation can create a pneumothorax. Other internal organs, such as the spleen and liver, may also be perforated.

6. A hematoma may appear at the insertion site.

7. Vasovagal response

8. Syncope

9. Air embolism

PATIENT TEACHING

1. Immediately report any shortness of breath, faintness, bloody sputum, or chest pain.

2. Rest in a position of comfort for 1 hour after the procedure.

---

*Indicates portions of the procedure usually performed by a physician or an advanced practice nurse.

REFERENCE

Barefoot, W. (2005). Performing thoracentesis. In L. McHale-Wiegand, & K. K. Carlson (Eds.), *AACN procedure manual for critical care* (5th ed. pp. 174–185). Philadelphia: Saunders.

Circulation Procedures

Positioning the Hypotensive Patient

Maureen T. Quigley, MS, ARNP

Also known as modified *Trendelenburg position*.

INDICATION

To temporarily treat symptomatic hypotension caused by hypovolemia, vasovagal reaction, or medication.

CONTRAINDICATIONS AND CAUTIONS

1. Ensure the adequacy of airway, breathing, and circulation before initiating treatment.
2. Because of the many potential adverse consequences of the traditional Trendelenburg position (i.e., head lower than body), it is no longer recommended for treatment of hypotension.
   - Reflex vasodilation and congestion of vessels in lung apices occur when the head of the body is placed lower than the feet (Warner, 2006).
   - Central venous pressure, intracranial and intraocular pressure, myocardial work, and pulmonary venous pressure are all increased in the Trendelenburg position.
   - Pulmonary compliance and functional residual capacity are decreased (Faust, 2004).
   - The Trendelenburg position should be avoided in the presence of potential head or spinal cord injuries.
   - Use of Trendelenburg position is contraindicated in patients with lower extremity ischemia (Bridges & Jarquin-Valdiviva, 2005).
3. In the obese patient, supine positioning can cause ventilatory impairment, with compression on the aorta and inferior vena cava (Babatunde & Whitten, 2006).
4. Patients who are in cardiogenic or anaphylactic shock may not be able to tolerate a supine or modified Trendelenburg position.

PROCEDURAL STEPS

1. Place the patient in a supine position.
2. Raise the lower extremities to a maximum elevation of 45 degrees. This is known as the modified Trendelenburg position (Figure 48-1).
3. Do not lower the patient's head below the level of the body, because this places pressure on the diaphragm that may result in respiratory distress. See the Contraindications and Cautions for the traditional Trendelenburg position listed earlier.

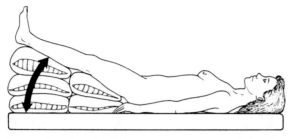

Lower extremities elevated   Patient flat

FIGURE 48-1 Modified Trendelenburg position. (From Finis, N. M. [1995]. Abdominal trauma. In S. Kitt, J. Selfridge-Thomas, J. A. Proehl, & J. Kaiser [Eds.], *Emergency nursing: A physiologic and clinical perspective* [2nd ed., p. 241]. Philadelphia: Saunders.)

PATIENT TEACHING

1. Explain that the position is temporary.

2. Immediately report any difficulty in breathing.

REFERENCES

Babatunde, O., & Whitten, C. (2006). Anesthesia and obesity. In P. G. Barash, B. F. Cullen, & R. K. Stoelting (Eds.), *Clinical anesthesia* (5th ed., pp. 1040–1051). Philadelphia: Lippincott Williams & Wilkins.

Bridges, N., & Jarquin-Valdiviva, A. (2005). Use of the Trendelenburg position as the resuscitation position: To T or not to T? *American Journal of Critical Care, 14,* 364–368.

Faust, R. J. (2004). Patient positioning. In R. D. Miller (Ed.), *Miller's anesthesia* (6th ed., pp. 1151–1167). Philadelphia: Churchill Livingstone.

Warner, M. (2006). Patient positioning. In P. G. Barash, B. F. Cullen, & R. K. Stoelting (Eds.), *Clinical anesthesia* (5th. pp. 643–667). Philadelphia: Lippincott Williams & Wilkins.

Doppler Ultrasound for Assessment of Blood Pressure and Peripheral Pulses

Maureen T. Quigley, MS, ARNP

INDICATIONS

1. To measure the blood pressure, pulse, or both, when auscultation by stethoscope is unsuccessful (i.e., in the presence of hypotension, hypothermia, or shock; when the pulse is faint or weak; extremity edema; faint Korotkoff sounds; or in a noisy environment). Fetal heart tones can also be assessed by Doppler; see Procedure 108.
2. To assess peripheral blood flow when circulatory impairment or vascular trauma is suspected.

CONTRAINDICATIONS AND CAUTIONS

1. Use of an ultrasonic transmission gel recommended by the vendor assists in optimal sound transmission and protects the crystals, which are found in the probe. The crystals transmit and receive ultrasonic waves. In emergency situations, any surgical jelly or lubricant may be substituted for a conductive gel but ECG paste or cream should never be used as it may damage the probe (Parks Medical Electronics, 2005).
2. The probe should be checked regularly for damage to the electrode and integrity of the crystals.
3. Improper probe placement may lead to erroneous interpretations. Care should be taken to verify that the signal is coming from the intended vessel and not from a collateral vessel. This can be determined by assessing the quality of the sound, as described in the Complications section of this procedure.
4. Excess pressure on the probe may compress the artery and abolish the signal.
5. Verify sensitivity when signals are absent from a position where they would normally be expected. Sensitivity may be verified by checking one's own pulses with the Doppler device.
6. The presence of a signal does not always indicate that circulation and perfusion are adequate to maintain viable tissue, just as absence of a signal does not always indicate that there is no blood flow through the vessel.

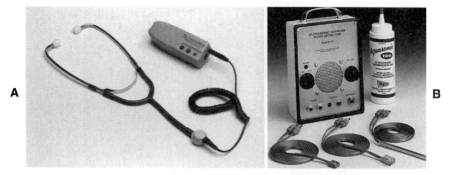

FIGURE 49-1 Examples of two commercially available Doppler devices. (Courtesy Medasonics, Newark, CA, and Parks Medical Electronics, Aloha, OR.)

7. Tissue penetration varies, depending on which Doppler probe is used. A high-frequency (8 to 10 Hz) probe is usually used on the surface vessel sites; this probe is typically long and narrow. A low-frequency probe is usually used for deeper tissue sites, such as fetal heart tones; this probe is typically short and wide.

8. Falsely elevated pressures may be observed in patients with diabetes, obesity, or calcified vessels (Gorgas, 2004).

EQUIPMENT

Doppler probe with a frequency of 5 to 10 MHz (for limb arteries and veins) and an amplifier (Figure 49-1)

Ultrasonic transmission gel

Blood pressure cuff

Wet towel or tissue

PROCEDURAL STEPS
Blood Pressure Measurement

1. Place the blood pressure cuff on the upper arm, the thigh, or the ankle and apply a transmission gel to the skin over the brachial-popliteal artery or the posterior-tibial artery. Be sure the cuff is high enough on the limb that the Doppler probe can access the area with the strongest pulse.

2. Turn on the Doppler instrument and turn down the volume. Insert the stethoscope earpieces, if applicable.

3. Adjust the volume control as necessary.

4. Identify the brachial-popliteal pulse or the posterior-tibial pulse with the Doppler instrument.

5. Position the probe over the artery and tilt it so that it is at a 45-degree angle along the length of the vessel to optimize frequency shifts and signal amplitude (Figure 49-2).

6. Inflate the blood pressure cuff until the arterial sounds are no longer audible.

7. Deflate the cuff slowly, listening for the first sound, which reflects the systolic pressure. Diastolic pressure is recorded at the point at which there is a decrease in arterial wall motion (Pickering, 2002).

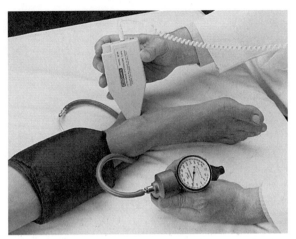

FIGURE 49-2 Measurement of systolic blood pressure in the ankle. (Courtesy Medasonics, Newark, CA.)

8. Clean the gel from the patient's skin with a wet towel or tissue.
9. Clean the face of the Doppler probe with a soft tissue. Do not use alcohol or other organic solvents to clean the probe. If the gel has dried on the probe, clean the probe with warm (not hot) running tap water but do not immerse the probe. The probe may be gas (ethylene oxide) sterilized at the lowest temperature consistent with good sterilization not to exceed 60° C [140° F]). A sterile water wash after sterilization is recommended (Parks Medical Electronics, 2005).

Assessment of Peripheral Blood Flow

1. Apply a transmission gel to the skin over the vessel.
2. Turn on the Doppler instrument and turn down the volume. Insert the stethoscope earpieces, if applicable.
3. Place the probe over the vessel to be assessed and tilt the probe so that it is at a 45-degree angle to the vessel. Standard arterial locations include the brachial, radial, femoral, popliteal, dorsalis pedis, and posterior tibial pulses.
4. Adjust the volume control as necessary.
5. Mark the pulse location with a waterproof marker. Compare the blood flow bilaterally. Begin assessment of the extremity at its most distal aspect. If you do not find a pulse with the Doppler instrument, move to a more proximal site. Continue to move more proximally until you are able to identify the blood flow. The findings may then be recorded by describing the pulses at each location as absent, present, or diminished.

AGE-SPECIFIC CONSIDERATION

In infants, auscultation or Korotkoff sound techniques may underestimate true systolic pressure, and ultrasonic flow detectors are recommended (Pickering, 2002).

COMPLICATIONS

1. Absence of a Doppler signal may be due to any of the following:
   a. Blood flow at a speed less than the Doppler instrument can detect
   b. Excess pressure on the probe, causing occlusion of the vessel
   c. Volume setting that is too low
   d. Insufficient transmission gel
   e. Dead battery
   f. Damaged equipment
2. The signal may be misinterpreted. Arterial sounds are loud, pulsatile, pumping sounds that are repeated with each cardiac cycle. Venous sounds are normally cyclic. They occur with respirations, and on expiration, they produce a high-pitched sound that resembles a rushing wind.
3. Static may occur. Possible causes are hair movement on the body, air bubbles in the gel popping, and radio interference.
4. The output of ultrasonic signals from diagnostic Doppler applications is very low; nevertheless, prolonged, unnecessary exposure to ultrasonic signals should be avoided to prevent tissue damage.

REFERENCES

Gorgas, D. L. (2004). Vital sign measurement. In J. R. Roberts, & J. R. Hedges (Eds.), *Clinical procedures in emergency medicine* (4th ed., pp. 3–28). Philadelphia: Saunders.
Parks Medical Electronics, Inc. (2005). *Parks Flo-Lab operating manual.* Aloha, OR: Author.
Pickering, T. G. (2002). Principles and techniques of blood pressure measurement. *Cardiology Clinics, 20*(2), 207–223.

PROCEDURE 50

Measuring Postural Vital Signs

Margo E. Layman, MSN, RN, RNC, CN-A

Postural vital signs are also known as *orthostatic vital signs* and *tilt test*.

INDICATIONS

1. To noninvasively evaluate a patient's symptoms of cerebral hypoperfusion or disease associated with orthostatic hypotension (hemorrhage or profound volume loss) (Bradley & Davis, 2003).
2. To assess response to a change in position in the elderly or ill.

3. To evaluate a patient with a history of known or suspected fluid loss secondary to vomiting, diarrhea, diaphoresis, bleeding, blunt abdominal or chest trauma, abdominal pain, unexplained syncope, weakness or dizziness, or autonomic dysfunction.

CONTRAINDICATIONS AND CAUTIONS

1. The value of orthostatic vital signs is disputed as there is no universal definition of how to perform them or what blood pressure and heart rate changes constitute "positive orthostatics." Euvolemic patients may have orthostatic changes, whereas hypovolemic patients may not. Therefore, the vital signs should be interpreted in the context of the patient's other signs and symptoms such as dizziness and visual dimming.
2. An assistant may be necessary because a patient with orthostatic hypotension may experience dizziness, lightheadedness, or syncope when moving from a lying to a standing position for postural vital sign measurement. Do not leave the patient alone during this procedure.
3. Orthostatic vital signs are contraindicated in patients with supine hypotension, shock, or a severe alteration in mental status, as well as in those who may have spinal, pelvic, or lower-extremity injuries (Gorgas, 2004).
4. Certain medications, such as sympatholytic drugs, diuretics, nitrates, narcotics, antihistamines, psychotropic agents, barbiturates, antihypertensives, and anticholergenics, can predispose a patient to orthostatic hypotension in the absence of hypovolemia. Studies have demonstrated a significant incidence of orthostatic hypotension, even in euvolemic patients (Irvin & White, 2004).
5. Paradoxical bradycardia may be observed in hypovolemic patients who have rapid and massive bleeding; this may be interpreted as orthostasis (Gorgas, 2004).
6. Prevent unreliable results by avoiding invasive or painful procedures during the measurement of postural vital signs.

PATIENT PREPARATION

Have the patient lie in a supine position for 2 to 3 minutes before taking the initial measurements.

PROCEDURAL STEPS

1. Measure the blood pressure and heart rate measurements after the patient has been in supine position for 2 to 3 minutes. Taking two sets of measurements and using the second set as baseline helps prevent false-positive results that are based on patient's sympathetic response (Bradley & Davis, 2003).
2. Have the patient move from the supine to the sitting position (if three measurements are taken) or from supine to standing. If the patient is unable to stand for blood pressure measurement, try the high Fowler's position, although the results may be less credible. A supine-to-standing measurement is more accurate than a supine-to-sitting measurement (Gorgas, 2004).
3. Question the patient about weakness, dizziness, or visual dimming associated with a change of position. Note any pallor or diaphoresis. These symptoms are as important as the measurement of vital signs. If the patient becomes

extremely dizzy and needs to lie down or becomes syncopal, the measurement should be terminated.

4. Take the standing or sitting blood pressure (in the same arm as the initial readings) and the heart rate measurement within 1 minute. Support the patient's forearm at heart level when taking the blood pressure to prevent an inaccurate measurement.

5. If an intermediate sitting measurement was taken, have the patient move into the standing position and repeat steps 3 and 4.

6. Return patient to supine or sitting position.

7. Note all measurements on the patient record, including the position in which they were taken (i.e., with the patient lying, sitting, or standing). Positive findings in adults are usually considered to be a heart rate increase of 30 beats/min, a decrease in systolic blood pressure of 20 mm Hg, a diastolic blood pressure decrease of 10 mm Hg, or symptoms of cerebral hypofusion, such as dizziness and syncope (Bradley & Davis, 2003). Other authors state that changes in blood pressure are too variable to be considered a reliable indicator of blood loss (Gorgas, 2004). The results of one study indicate that the two most valuable predictors for hypovolemia are a pulse increase of 30 beats/min or severe dizziness on standing (McGee, Abernethy, & Simel, 1999).

AGE-SPECIFIC CONSIDERATIONS

1. The usefulness of orthostatic vital signs in children is not clear. Postural near-syncope or an increase in heart rate of 25 beats/min or more may be a predictor of dehydration in children (Gorgas, 2004). Assessment of dehydration in children should be based on preillness and postillness weight, capillary refill, and clinical assessment (Gorelick, Shaw, & Murphy, 1997).

2. Patients with nondemand pacemakers or those taking beta-blocking medications may not have significant changes in heart rate.

COMPLICATIONS

Weakness, dizziness, syncope, and falls

PATIENT TEACHING

Educate elderly patients and other patients with postural symptoms about the importance of sitting for 5 minutes before getting out of bed or of standing slowly after sitting for an extended length of time.

REFERENCES

Bradley, J. G., & Davis, K. A. (2003). Orthostatic hypotension. *American Family Physician, 68,* 2393–2398.

Gorelick, M. H, Shaw, K. N., & Murphy, K. O. (1997). Validity and reliability of clinical signs in the diagnosis of dehydration in children. *Pediatrics, 99,* 6–18.

Gorgas, D. L. (2004). Vital-sign measurement procedures. In J. R. Roberts, & J. R. Hedges (Eds.), *Clinical procedures in emergency medicine* (4th ed. pp. 3–28). Philadelphia: Saunders.

Irvin, D. J., & White, M. (2004). The importance of accurately assessing orthostatic hypotension. *Geriatric Nursing, 25,* 100–101.

McGee, S., Abernethy, W. B., & Simel, D. L. (1999). Is this patient hypovolemic? *Journal of the American Medical Association, 281,* 1022–1029.

Pneumatic Antishock Garment

Reneé Semonin Holleran, RN, PhD, CEN, CCRN, CFRN, CTRN, FAEN

Pneumatic antishock garment is also known as *PASG, military antishock garment (MAST)*, or *shock pants*.

INDICATIONS

Indications, contraindications, and cautions remain controversial and depend on local protocols. PASGs are no longer used in many areas. If used, PASG should be considered a short-term intervention until definitive care can be initiated. Indications for the use of PASG may include the following:

1. Decompensated shock
2. Stabilization of pelvic fractures with hypotension (ACS, 2004; McSwain Frame, & Salomone 2003)
3. Significant trauma (see 1 and 2 above) with a transport time of 20 to 40 minutes (Salomone, Ustin, McSwain, & Feliciano, 2005)

CONTRAINDICATIONS AND CAUTIONS

1. Absolute contraindications to the application of a PASG include the following:
   - Pulmonary edema
   - Congestive heart failure
   - Penetrating thoracic injuries
2. Relative contraindications to the use of a PASG include the following:
   - Cautious use during pregnancy (attempt to stabilize the patient by using the proper position [left lateral recumbent, tilted 15 degrees to the left] and inflation of the leg compartments only)
   - Abdominal evisceration
   - Impaled foreign body
3. The application of PASG for isolated lower-extremity fractures is not recommended because of the risk of the development of compartment syndrome (McSwain, Frame, & Salomone, 2003). A traction splint provides a better method of stabilizing femur fractures.
4. In conditions that require long inflation times (20 to 40 minutes or greater), significant alterations in fluid and electrolyte balance may occur and may complicate management and recovery. The patient is also at greater risk of developing pressure sores as well as compartment syndrome the longer the pants remain inflated.
5. PASG application should always be used in combination with oxygen administration and intravenous (IV) fluid resuscitation.

6. If the patient is transported to a higher altitude (air transport or over mountain passes), the air in the PASG expands and the pressure inside the garment increases. Monitor the PASG pressures carefully in these situations.

EQUIPMENT

Pneumatic antishock garment (Figure 51-1)
Long spine board or scoop stretcher
Foot pump or inflation device that comes with the pants
Board straps or cravats

PATIENT PREPARATION

1. If the mechanism of injury warrants immobilization, place the patient on a long spine board or a scoop stretcher (see Procedure 111). Position the garment on the board or the scoop stretcher before the patient. The patient may be log rolled onto the garment and the garment slid up under the patient (technique A), or, alternatively, the garment may be placed on the patient like trousers (technique B).
2. Remove all clothing and anything else below the waist to prevent compression injuries from objects such as belts when the pants are inflated.

PROCEDURAL STEPS
Inflation

1. Place the garment on the patient by using one of the following techniques:

Technique A (see Figure 51-1)

   a. Release the leg and abdominal Velcro closures. Lay the garment out flat. Maintain in-line spinal immobilization if indicated.
   b. One or more persons may then slide the garment underneath the patient. Raise the feet and slide the PASG under the buttocks. Elevate the buttocks slightly to place the pants properly.
   c. Match the Velcro straps on the leg compartments and secure them (some models color code the Velcro closures). Fasten the Velcro straps on the abdominal compartment.

Technique B

(This method is contraindicated in persons with suspected or confirmed spinal fractures.)

   a. Lay the garment out flat near the patient. Match the Velcro closures. Close the Velcro straps loosely on all three compartments.
   b. Maintain in-line spinal immobilization, if appropriate. Position at least one person on each side of the patient near the patient's hips. If additional people are available, they may help elevate the hips or feet. Simultaneously, elevate the feet carefully while sliding the trousers over the feet and up the legs. Elevate the hips to allow the proper placement of the garment.
   c. Readjust the Velcro straps to ensure a snug fit.
2. The abdominal compartment should be placed just below the rib cage so as not to reduce vital capacity and impair respiration.

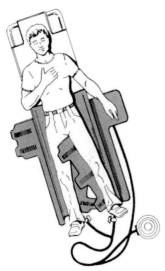

Put the patient on the MAST face up (supine) so that the top of the garment will be just below the lowest rib. Align patient with spine line label.

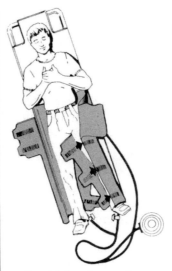

Wrap left leg of garment around the patient's left leg and secure it with fastener strips.

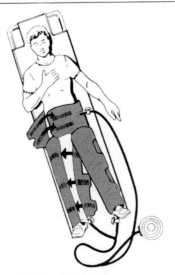

Wrap the right leg of garment around the patient's right leg and secure it with fastener strips.

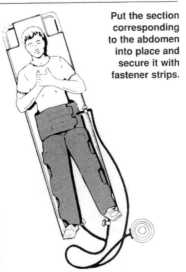

Put the section corresponding to the abdomen into place and secure it with fastener strips.

Using the foot pump, inflate the trousers until air exhausts through the relief valves and/or the patient's vital signs become stable. Close the inflation/deflation valves.

FIGURE 51-1 Application of pneumatic antishock garment. (From *Medical anti-shock trouser*, Boston: David Clark Company, page 9, 1997.)

3. Close the stopcock to the abdominal compartment and open the stopcocks to the leg compartments.
4. Attach the tubing from the foot pump to the three compartments. Some models have color-coded tubing for the different compartments.
5. Inflate the leg compartments with the pump until the pressure gauge (if present) indicates the appropriate amount of pressure. Some pants have a pop-off valve that limits the inflation pressure to 104 mm Hg. Crackling of the Velcro closures also indicates sufficient inflation. The goal is to achieve a systolic pressure of 100 mm Hg while using the lowest inflation pressure possible (less than 40 mm Hg). Patients in extremis may need rapid, simultaneous inflation of all three compartments to 100 mm Hg immediately on application of the garment. If the foot pump is not available, sufficient pressures may be obtained by manually inflating the compartments.
6. Recheck the patient's vital signs. Inflation should be stopped when the systolic pressure reaches 100 mm Hg.
7. If the systolic pressure has not increased to more than 100 mm Hg, inflate the abdominal compartment. (Note: Pregnancy is a relative contraindication for inflation of the abdominal compartment.)
8. Assess vital signs and respiratory effort frequently.
9. Secure the patient to the long board or scoop stretcher as necessary.

Monitoring Chamber Pressure

1. The pressure monitoring assembly consists of interconnecting tubing, pressure gauge, hand bulb, air flow control valve, and inflation/deflation valve (Figure 51-2).
2. Connect the monitor between the foot pump and the PASG as shown in Figure 51-2.

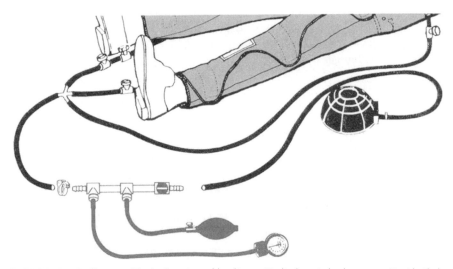

FIGURE 51-2 Pressure Monitoring Assembly. (From *Medical anti-shock trouser,* David Clark Company, page 12, 1997.)

3. Increase or decrease the pressure in the leg or abdominal chambers based on the patient's response to resuscitation and comfort.

Deflation

1. Any patient who has had the PASG applied and inflated must be stabilized before the garment is deflated. Stabilization may be accomplished via intravenous fluids, hemorrhagic control, vasopressors, or surgical intervention. Deflation of the garment must be done slowly. *Remind all providers that this device should never be cut off!*
2. Assess vital signs while the garment is inflated.
3. Gradually release air from the abdominal compartment and recheck the vital signs. If the blood pressure has dropped more than 5 mm Hg, deflation should be stopped and more fluids administered (if necessary) to restore pressure. In addition to the drop in pressure, some protocols suggest stopping deflation if the heart rate increases by 10 beats/min after deflation. If pressure is not restored, reinflate the abdominal compartment.
4. Continue to release air from the abdomen, assessing the patient's vital signs each time. Some protocols suggest waiting 5 minutes between each step of deflation, although this has not been fully researched or documented.
5. Release air from one leg of the PASG at a time, following the same procedure as above. If one leg is injured, release the pressure from the uninjured leg first.
6. Reassess the patient's condition frequently after deflation.
7. Do not remove the deflated garment from the patient, in the event that rapid reapplication is necessary.

AGE-SPECIFIC CONSIDERATIONS

1. Use of the PASG for children is not recommended in the prehospital setting (NHTSA, 1998).
2. Pediatric and toddler-sized PASGs are available.
3. If an adult-sized PASG must be used for a child, inflate the leg compartments only (Eichelberger et al., 1998).

COMPLICATIONS

1. Sudden and severe hypotension may ensue after sudden removal of the garment.
2. Metabolic acidosis may develop after prolonged use of the garment as a result of a release of lactic acid from peripheral tissues.
3. Respiratory compromise may occur as a result of decreased vital capacity or pulmonary congestion (see Contraindications and Cautions).
4. Decreases in renal blood flow may result in a decline in renal perfusion, glomerular filtration rate, and urine output.
5. Inflation of the abdominal compartment may aggravate lumbar instability because of the circumferential compartment expansion.
6. Bleeding from extremity wounds may increase with increased blood pressure.
7. Skin breakdown and decubitus ulcer formation may occur.
8. Compartmental syndrome may develop in the lower extremities.

PATIENT TEACHING

1. The PASG is a temporary measure to help increase blood pressure or splint pelvic fractures.
2. Report any increases in pain in areas under the PASG.

REFERENCES

American College of Surgeons (ACS), Committee on Trauma (2004). *Advanced trauma life support manual* (7th ed.). Chicago: Author.

Eichelberger, M. R., Partsch, G. S., Ball, J. W., & Clark, J. R., et al. (1998). *Pediatric emergencies: A manual for prehospital care providers* (2nd ed). Upper Saddle River NJ: Brady Communications, Prentice-Hall.

McSwain, N., Frame, S., & Salomone, J (2003). *Basic and advanced prehospital trauma life support*. St. Louis: Mosby.

National Highway Transportation and Safety Administration (NHTSA) (1998). *Emergency medical technician: National standard curriculum*. Washington, DC: Author.

Salomone, J. P., Ustin, J. S., McSwain, N. E., & Feliciano, D. V. (2005). Opinions of trauma practitioners regarding prehospital interventions for critically injured patients. *Journal of Trauma, 58*, 509–515.

PROCEDURE 52

Therapeutic Phlebotomy

Maureen T. Quigley, MS, ARNP

Therapeutic phlebotomy is also known as *blood letting*.

INDICATIONS

1. To decrease iron stores in iron overload syndromes, such as hemochromatosis, porphyria cutanea tarda, and African dietary iron overload (previously known as African siderosis). For every 500 ml of blood withdrawn, 200 to 250 mg of iron is removed (Heaney & Andrews, 2004). Iron is then mobilized from tissue stores by the bone marrow as it replaces the lost hemoglobin.
2. To decrease red blood cell mass in the presence of high blood viscosity (e.g., polycythemia vera). In patients with severe polycythemia (hematocrit greater than 55%), phlebotomy provides a means to reduce mean pulmonary artery pressure and pulmonary vascular resistance and enhance exercise performance (Wiedemann, 2004).
3. Rarely, therapeutic phlebotomy is advised in the patient with acute decompensation of cor pulmonale with marked polycythemia or for the rare patient who continues to have significant polycythemia despite appropriate long-term oxygen therapy (Wiedemann, 2004).

CONTRAINDICATIONS AND CAUTIONS

1. A physician from transfusion medicine should be involved in the decision to perform therapeutic phlebotomy (AABB, 2006).
2. Monitor patients who have bleeding disorders and those who are taking anticoagulant medications closely.
3. Generally, less than 500 ml of blood is removed slowly; the volume can be replaced with normal saline (Hamilton & Janz, 2006).
4. For patients with known cardiovascular disease, take care to prevent a large reduction in blood volume at one time (Means, 2004).
5. Prompt initiation of phlebotomy is critical following the diagnosis of iron overload because accumulation of iron can lead to cardiac arrhythmias, cardiomyopathy, and sudden death (Tavill, 2001).

EQUIPMENT

500-ml vacuum bottle or blood collection bag if available
Phlebotomy tubing with needles on both ends
or
Saf-T donor set (36-inch tubing with a 17-G needle on one end and a 15-G stopper-piercing needle on the other end) (anticoagulant is not required)
Blood pressure cuff or tourniquet
Antiseptic solution
Local anesthesia (optional)
Occlusive dressing
Gauze dressing
Hemostat

PROCEDURAL STEPS

1. Obtain an order including the diagnosis, most recent hemoglobin or hematocrit value, and the amount of blood to be removed.
2. Apply the tourniquet or blood pressure cuff and locate the most suitable antecubital vein. Remove the tourniquet or deflate the blood pressure cuff.
3. Cleanse the site with antiseptic solution.
4. Clamp the tubing with the hemostat at the patient's end and insert the other end into the vacuum bottle. If using the Saf-T donor set, clamp the tubing to maintain the vacuum in the bottle and connect the 15-G stopper-piercing needle to the bottle.
5. Reapply the tourniquet or inflate the blood pressure cuff to a pressure between the patient's systolic and diastolic readings.
6. Inject 1 to 2 ml of local anesthetic intradermally at the venipuncture site (optional).
7. Perform the venipuncture with the needle on the proximal end of the tubing.
8. Tape the needle in place and cover the site with an occlusive dressing.
9. Unclamp the hemostat and collect the desired amount of blood, usually 250 to 500 ml, in the collection bottle or bag.
   a. If the blood return is slow, have the patient pump his or her hand. Reapply the tourniquet or blood pressure cuff. Increase the distance between the patient and the collection bottle. Check the position of the needle.

    b. When the blood collection takes longer than 10 to 15 minutes, a blood pressure cuff is more comfortable than a tourniquet. Release the cuff every 10 to 15 minutes.

10. Reclamp the tubing with the hemostat.

11. Release the tourniquet or deflate the cuff.

12. Withdraw the needle and apply pressure with a gauze dressing until the bleeding stops.

13. Assess and document the patient's vital signs.

AGE-SPECIFIC CONSIDERATION

Removal of smaller volumes of blood during therapeutic phlebotomy is recommended in the elderly.

COMPLICATIONS

1. Adverse effects include fainting, weakness, chills, nausea, vomiting, and muscular twitching. If adverse effects occur, clamp the tubing and notify the physician.

2. Hematoma, bruising, and tenderness at the IV insertion site may occur.

PATIENT TEACHING

1. Rest for 15 minutes before moving to a sitting or standing position.

2. Eat and drink before the procedure, and drink after the procedure if not contraindicated.

3. Avoid vigorous exercise within 24 hours of therapeutic phlebotomy.

4. Do not take iron supplements if you have iron overload problems. Vitamin C supplements, which increase the absorption of iron, should also be avoided.

5. Avoid alcohol if you have iron overload problems; alcohol is toxic to the liver.

6. Patients with porphyria can contact the American Porphyria Foundation (http://www.porphyriafoundation.com/) for additional information. For patients with hemochromatosis, information on treatment with therapeutic phlebotomy is available at:http://www.cdc.gov/ncbddd/hemochromatosis/training/pdf/phlebotomy_info.pdf

REFERENCES

American Association of Blood Banks (AABB) (2006). *Standards for blood banks and transfusion services: Technical manual* (24th ed). Bethesda MD: Author.

Hamilton, G. G., & Janz, T. G. (2006). Anemia, polycythemia and white blood cell disorders. In J. A. Marx, R. S. Hockberger, & R. M. Walls, et al. (Eds.), *Rosen's emergency medicine: Concepts and clinical practice* (6th ed. pp. 1867–1884). St. Louis: Mosby.

Heaney, M. M., & Andrews, N. C. (2004). Iron homeostasis and inherited iron overload disorders: An overview. *Hematology Oncology Clinics of North America, 18,* 1379–1403.

Means, R. (2004). Polycythemia vera. In J. P. Greer, J. Foerster, J. N. Lukens, G. M. Rodgers, F. Paraskevas, & B. Glader (Eds.), *Wintrobe's clinical hematology* (11th ed. pp. 2259–2272). Philadelphia: Lippincott Williams & Williams.

Tavill, A. S. (2001). American Association for the Study of Liver Diseases guidelines: Diagnosis and management of hemochromatosis. *Hepatology, 33,* 1321–1328.

Wiedemann, H. L. (2004). Cor pulmonale. *UpToDate, version 14.3.* Uptodate.com.

Pericardiocentesis

Andrew A. Galvin, APRN,BC, CEN

Pericardiocentesis is also known as *pericardial tap*.

INDICATIONS

1. To assist in the diagnosis of pericardial tamponade in patients with decreased cardiac output, elevated central venous pressure with jugular vein distention, muffled heart tones, and hypotension (also known as Beck's triad) who have sustained blunt or penetrating trauma to the chest. Ultrasound is the preferred diagnostic technique as it is noninvasive and easily performed at the bedside.
2. To relieve pericardial tamponade secondary to infection, tumor, bleeding diathesis, or recent intracardiac instrumentation, such as pacemaker insertion.
3. To assist in the diagnosis and treatment of patients in pulseless electrical activity.
4. Placement of an indwelling "pigtail catheter" may be considered for serial drainage if effusion is likely to recur.

CONTRAINDICATIONS AND CAUTIONS

1. Ideally, pericardiocentesis is performed in the cardiac catheterization laboratory using fluoroscopic or echocardiac guidance. In the emergency department, ultrasound or echocardiography may be useful adjunctive techniques for this procedure (Ciccone, 2004; Tang, 2005; Tibbles & Porcaro, 2004). The electrocardiogram (ECG)-assisted "blind" technique for pericardiocentesis is associated with significant morbidity, and therefore, it is only recommended when there may be a considerable delay in obtaining an ultrasound or a fluoroscope (Harper, 2004). If the patient is stable and ultrasound is not available, a computed tomography (CT) scan can provide definitive diagnosis of pericardial effusion (Harper, 2004).
2. Extreme caution is necessary when performing pericardiocentesis on patients who are taking anticoagulant medication.
3. All equipment must be secured and properly grounded to prevent small current leaks, which may result in arrhythmias.
4. Pericardiocentesis may be inadequate for traumatic pericardial tamponade; a pericardial window or other operative intervention may be necessary to remove clots in the pericardium.

EQUIPMENT

16- or 18-G cardiac or spinal needle or 6-inch over-the-needle catheter
60-ml syringe
Three-way stopcock

Alligator clamps/cable
Kelly clamp
Tape
12-lead ECG machine or 5-lead ECG monitor
Antiseptic solution
Gauze dressings
Local anesthetic (optional)
Syringe and needles for local anesthetic (optional)
Sterile gloves
Gown and mask
Cardiac resuscitation equipment at the bedside
Specimen containers for requested diagnostic tests (e.g., culture, cytology)
Resuscitation equipment (defibrillator, suction, etc.) should be readily available

PATIENT PREPARATION

1. If possible, obtain a chest x-ray film and a 12-lead ECG before starting the procedure (see Procedure 56). Initiate pulse oximetry and ECG monitoring (Procedures 21 and 55).
2. If the patient is stable and able to tolerate sitting, place the patient in the semi-Fowler's position to facilitate the pooling of blood in the apex of the heart, bring the heart closer to the anterior wall and lower the diaphragm and abdominal organs.
3. Insert a nasogastric tube to decompress the stomach (see Procedure 98).
4. Connect the ECG limb leads to the patient if not done previously.

PROCEDURAL STEPS
Standard Pericardiocentesis

1. Cleanse the chest from the left costal margin to the xiphoid process with an antiseptic solution.
2. *Infiltrate the area with a local anesthetic (if indicated).
3. *Nick the skin with the No. 11 blade (optional).
4. Attach the alligator clamp to the metal hub of the needle and to any anterior chest V lead or the chest lead of a five-lead system. The rhythm of the V lead will be observed for contact with the ventricle. If the patient does not have an organized electrical rhythm with an obvious ST segment, ECG monitoring via the alligator clamp is not indicated.
5. *Palpate the junction of the xiphoid process and the left costal arch. To minimize the risk of myocardial puncture and assess for the completeness of fluid removal, the subxiphoid approach is most commonly used (LeWinter & Kabbani, 2005). Insert the needle with obturator below the xiphoid process at a 30- to 45-degree angle and direct it toward the left shoulder (Figure 53-1). As soon as the needle punctures the skin, remove the obturator and attach a 60-ml syringe with a three-way stopcock.

---

*Indicates portions of the procedure usually performed by a physician or an advanced practice nurse.

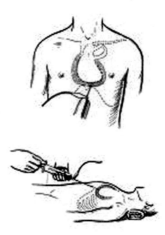

FIGURE 53-1 Pericardiocentesis with alligator cables to ECG machine. (From Dunmire, S. M., & Paris, P. M. [1994]. *Atlas of emergency procedures* [p. 64]. Philadelphia: Saunders.)

6. *Aspirate the plunger of the syringe gently as the needle is advanced. If the needle is inserted under electrocardiographic guidance, observe the V lead for a significant elevation of the ST segment or premature ventricular contractions (see Procedure 86: Temporary Transvenous Pacemaker Insertion, Figure 86-2, for an illustration of ST-segment elevation).

7. *After a blood flash is seen, the following may occur:
   a. If blood is obtained and the monitor does not show ST-segment or T-wave changes; large, widened QRS complexes; or premature ventricular contractions; then as much blood or fluid as possible is withdrawn.
   b. Should any of the above ECG changes occur (indicating that the needle is in the epicardium or the myocardium), the needle is withdrawn slowly until the patient's baseline rhythm returns. It is important to note that myocardial scarring due to an infarction or disease may prevent an injury pattern from occurring (Harper, 2004).

8. *If the syringe becomes full during the aspiration of blood, use the stopcock to expel the blood from the syringe into an emesis basin instead of disconnecting the needle. After as much blood as possible is aspirated (anywhere from 10 to 150 ml), the syringe is removed, the three-way stopcock closed, and the needle is taped securely to the chest or sutured in place, or the Kelly clamp is attached at the level of the skin and secured to prevent advancement or displacement of the needle. Blood removed from the pericardial sac generally does not clot; however, brisk bleeding may result in blood being withdrawn from the ventricle before defibrination occurs and, therefore, the blood may clot (Harper, 2004).

9. Monitor the patient closely for recurring symptoms of cardiac tamponade.

---

*Indicates portions of the procedure usually performed by a physician or an advanced practice nurse.

CT-guided Pericardiocentesis

1. Place the patient in a supine position on the movable CT tabletop.
2. *Determine the entry site based on contiguous slices of the heart and the pericardium.
3. The base of the guidance device is placed under the patient at the level of the entry site.
4. *Disinfect the skin site and place a sterile, radiopaque grid over the entry area.
5. *The needle path, direction, and depth is determined by the radiologist, and the puncture is performed when the needle tip reaches the determined site.
6. *The needle placement is confirmed and the fluid is drained.
7. The patient is monitored as noted earlier.

Echocardiographic-guided Pericardiocentesis

1. *The skin is anesthetized and the probe is positioned on the skin. The subxiphoid approach utilizing echocardiographic guidance is most commonly used (LeWinter & Kabbani, 2005).
2. *The puncture is made, and after the tip of the needle enters the pericardial space, as seen on the monitor, a J wire is inserted through the needle until its tip enters the pericardial space.
3. *The needle is removed and an angiographic catheter is inserted. This may be replaced with a pigtail catheter.
4. *The effusion is drained and the catheter is connected to the extension tubing for continuous drainage.
5. The patient is monitored as noted above.

COMPLICATIONS

1. Laceration of the ventricle or a coronary vessel, which may result in tamponade or myocardial infarction
2. Puncture of the lung resulting in a pneumothorax
3. Cardiac arrhythmia, including cardiac arrest
4. Puncture of the aorta, inferior vena cava, esophagus, stomach, liver, or peritoneum
5. Decreased cardiac output caused by continued leakage into the pericardial sac
6. Venous air embolism
7. Pericarditis (late)

---

*Indicates portions of the procedure usually performed by a physician or an advanced practice nurse.

REFERENCES

Ciccone, T. J. (2004). Cardiac ultrasound. *Emergency Medicine Clinics of North America, 22,* 621–640.

Harper, R. J. (2004). Pericardiocentesis. In J. R. Roberts, & J. R. Hedges (Eds.), *Clinical procedures in emergency medicine* (4th ed. pp. 305–322). Philadelphia: Saunders.

LeWinter, M. M., & Kabbani, S. (2005). Pericardial diseases. In D. P. Zipes (Ed.), *Braunwauld's heart disease: A textbook of cardiovascular medicine* (7th ed. pp. 1768–1769). Philadelphia: Saunders.

Tang, A. (2005). Emergency department ultrasound and echocardiography. *Emergency Medicine Clinics of North America, 23,* 1179–1194.

Tibbles, C. D., & Porcaro, W. (2004). Procedural applications of ultrasound. *Emergency Medicine Clinics of North America, 22,* 797–815.

PROCEDURE 54

Emergency Thoracotomy and Internal Defibrillation

Andrew A. Galvin, APRN,BC, CEN, and
Jean A. Proehl, RN, MN, CEN, CCRN, FAEN

Emergency thoracotomy is also known as *open* or *resuscitative thoracotomy* and *cracking the chest.*

INDICATIONS

To maximize resuscitative efforts for penetrating trauma patients in the face of actual or impending cardiac arrest. The specific goals of emergency thoracotomy are the following (Boczar & Rivers, 2004):

1. To relieve cardiac tamponade
2. To support cardiac function via direct cardiac compression, cross-clamping of the aorta, and internal defibrillation
3. To control hemorrhage from the heart or great vessels

CONTRAINDICATIONS AND CAUTIONS

1. The health care team is at significant risk for exposure to blood or body fluids due to the emergent nature of the procedure and the potential for injury from sharp instruments or fractured patient ribs (Phelan, 2006).
2. Emergency thoracotomy is not indicated for patients who have massive central nervous system injuries, blunt trauma, or other injuries that are incompatible with life. If the patient is presumed or known to have been in cardiac arrest for a prolonged period of time, the chance for survival after emergency thoracotomy is small. Asystole following blunt trauma should be considered an absolute contraindication to thoracotomy in the emergency department

(Boczar & Rivers, 2004). Indicators of poor prognosis include multiple major injuries; blunt trauma to the thorax, abdomen, or both; absent pupillary reflexes; no respiratory effort; and no palpable pulse.

3. The ideal location for a thoracotomy is the operating room. A thoracotomy should be performed in the emergency department only when the patient is too unstable to be transported to the operating room. If no operating room or surgeon is available to assume the patient's care after initial management in the emergency department, this procedure should not be performed.

4. In the patient who has intraabdominal bleeding, a major risk associated with thoracotomy is release of abdominal tamponade before aortic control can be achieved. This results in rapid exsanguination and death.

5. Patients with the best prognosis for survival after an emergency thoracotomy are those who have sustained an isolated, penetrating injury to the chest and who have lost vital signs within 10 minutes of arrival to the emergency department (Meredith & Hoth, 2007; Powell, 2004).

6. On rare occasions, patients regain consciousness during thoracotomy. In this event, chemical and physical restraint are required immediately to prevent the patient from causing further injury by pulling on clamps, tubes, and so forth. Analgesics and sedatives should also be provided.

EQUIPMENT

Antiseptic solution
Gown, gloves, mask, and protective eyewear for all team members
Suction setup with long extension tubing and a Yankauer tip
Sterile thoracotomy tray consisting minimally of the following:
    Knife handles (two long and two short)
    No. 11 and 20 blades
    Rib cutter
    Rib spreaders
    Long scissors (Mayo), curved and straight
    Vascular clamps (Mixter), extra long, medium long, and regular Satinsky clamp
    Needle holders, regular and 9-in vascular
    Tissue forceps (Russian, DeBakey, and thoracic DeBakey)
    Toothed forceps (Brown, 8-in Peons)
    Noncrushing clamps (bronchial)
    Lebsche knife and mallet (optional)
    Lap pads (sterile gauze sponges in packages of five, each marked with a blue tab for ease in counting, which are used to absorb blood)
    Gigli saw handles and blade (for clamshell technique)
    Heavy duty (trauma) scissors (for clamshell technique)
Cardiac monitor and defibrillator
Internal defibrillator paddles and cable
Pledgets
Nonabsorbable suture (e.g., 3-0 silk)
Skin stapler with 6-mm staples (optional)
Sterile saline solution
Gauze dressings

PATIENT PREPARATION

1. If time allows, prepare the patient's chest by scrubbing it with an antiseptic solution, wiping it with a sterile towel, and applying antiseptic as a paint solution. In most situations, time does not permit thorough skin cleansing, and pouring full-strength antiseptic solution on the patient's chest before making the incision is acceptable (Wise et al., 2005).
2. Mechanical ventilation via an endotracheal tube must be in progress.
3. Establish large-bore intravenous (IV) access and request blood for transfusion immediately.
4. For patients in cardiac arrest, continue external cardiac massage until the thoracic incision is made.
5. Attach the electrocardiograph leads to the patient's limbs (see Procedure 55).

PROCEDURAL STEPS

1. Turn on full-strength suction and attach it to a sterile Yankauer tip via the extension tubing. Assemble the internal paddles.
2. *Assemble the rib spreaders (if they are not preassembled).
3. *Enter the chest via a left anterolateral incision or bilateral anterior incisions ("clamshell").
    a. Left anterolateral incision. A left-sided anterolateral incision is made in the fourth or fifth intercostal space (Figure 54-1) to expose the intercostal muscles. The pleural space is entered by pushing the index finger through the intercostal space near the sternal border, and then, posteriorly, running along the superior border of the rib (Figure 54-2). Ventilations should be interrupted until the incision is complete.
    b. Bilateral anterior incisions or "clamshell" (Wise et al., 2005). Bilateral anterior incisions through the intercostal muscles and the parietal pleura are made in the fifth intercostal spaces and connected with a deep skin incision across the sternum. The heavy-duty scissors are then

---

*Indicates portions of the procedure performed by a physician.

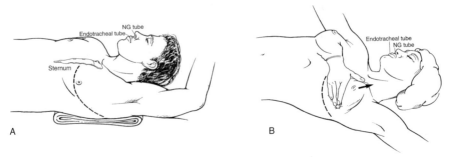

FIGURE 54-1 Left anterolateral incision sites for thoracotomy for **(A)** male or **(B)** female patients. (From Boczar, M. E., & Rivers, E. [2004]. Resuscitative thoracotomy. In J. R. Roberts & J. R. Hedges [Eds.], *Clinical Procedures in Emergency Medicine* [4th ed., p. 343]. Philadelphia: Saunders.)

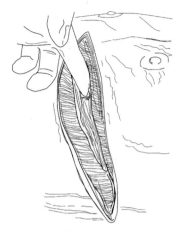

FIGURE 54-2 The fastest way to enter the pleural space without risking injury to the underlying lung is to push the index finger through the intercostal space near the sternal border and then forcefully push it posteriorly, running it along the superior border of the rib. (From Wahlstrom, H. E., Carroll, B. J., & Phillips, E. H. [1986]. Emergency thoracotomy: Indications and technique. *Surgical Rounds*, 9, p. 25.)

used to cut through all muscle and pleura while the lung is pushed back with two fingers inserted into the incisions. The remaining sternal bridge is cut with the scissors or Gigli saw. To use a Gigli saw, one end of the wire blade is pulled under the sternum with a large clamp, the handles are attached to each end, and the sternum is cut from the inside out with long smooth strokes.

4. *The rib spreaders are inserted in order to expose the pleural cavity. The pericardium is opened with scissors taking care to avoid severing the phrenic nerve (Figure 54-3).

5. *The heart is inspected for penetrating injury, which can be occluded temporarily with direct pressure by placing a finger or gauze into the hole. Alternatively, a large Foley catheter (e.g., 28 Fr) can be inserted, and the inflated balloon can be used to occlude the hole. Inflate the balloon with 10 ml or less of sterile fluid (a larger balloon may decrease stroke volume excessively) and clamp the catheter to prevent blood egress (Wise et al., 2005). Alternately, blood and IV fluid can be infused directly into the heart via the catheter. The defect is then sutured with a nonabsorbable suture and pledgets. Pledgets are used to help hold the sutures in the friable myocardial muscle (Figure 54-4). The defect may also be stapled shut with a skin stapler for temporary control of hemorrhage (Boczar & Rivers, 2004).

*Indicates portions of the procedure performed by a physician.

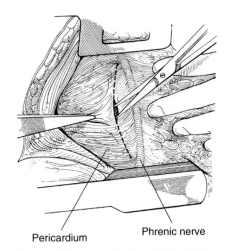

Pericardium   Phrenic nerve

FIGURE 54-3 Release of pericardial tamponade. (From Wilkins, E. W., Jr. [Ed.]. [1989]. *Emergency medicine: Scientific foundations and current practice* [3rd ed., p. 1019]. Baltimore: Williams & Wilkins.)

6. *Cardiac massage may be performed with either one or two hands by compressing the heart against the sternum. Compress in a superior-to-inferior direction to mimic the normal blood flow from the atria to the ventricles.
7. *The lung is then retracted and the descending aorta is inspected. The descending aorta may be occluded until the intravascular volume is restored and the blood pressure returns to normal. This is accomplished by compressing the aorta against the spine or by cross-clamping.

---

*Indicates portions of the procedure performed by a physician.

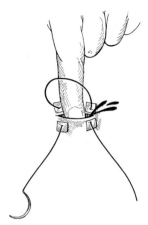

FIGURE 54-4 Use of Teflon pledgets to close a myocardial defect. (From Wilkins, E. W., Jr. [Ed.]. [1989]. *Emergency medicine: Scientific foundations and current practice* [3rd ed., p. 1020]. Baltimore: Williams & Wilkins.)

8. Document the time that the aorta is clamped.
9. *Pulmonary injuries may be controlled by clamping across the parenchyma proximal to the injury or across the hilum of the lung, or by wrapping the hilum with a Penrose drain and then providing traction to occlude the vessels and control hemorrhage.
10. To perform internal defibrillation:
    a. Open the paddles and maintain the packaging as a sterile field. Pick up the end of the cable without contaminating the field or have the physician hand off the connector end of the cable. Plug it into the defibrillator.
    b. Pour saline on gauze dressings to use between the paddles and the myocardium. This improves conduction of electricity and decreases myocardial injury.
    c. Turn on the defibrillator and charge the paddles (usually 30 to 50 Joules [J] for adults). Internal paddles are programmed to deliver no more than 50 J.
    d. *Place the paddles on opposite sides of the myocardium (Figure 54-5). Make sure all personnel clear the stretcher; state, "All clear," and discharge the current into the paddles. (NOTE: Some monitors or defibrillators require a second person to discharge the paddles from the defibrillator. In either instance, the physician holding the paddles should say "All clear" before the paddles are discharged.)
    e. Monitor the electrocardiograph for improvement in rhythm and repeat these steps as necessary.
11. If the patient appears to be salvageable, prepare for immediate transport to the operating room. In anticipation of the transfer, notify the operating room and prepare the patient (e.g., move all IV fluids, the portable oxygen tank, the cardiac monitor, and so forth, to the stretcher). If necessary, have the security personnel or other staff members clear the corridors and secure an elevator to expedite the transfer.

---

*Indicates portions of the procedure performed by a physician.

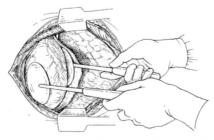

FIGURE 54-5 Internal defibrillation. (From Rosen, P., & Sternbach, G. L. [1983]. *Atlas of emergency medicine* [2nd ed., p. 55]. Baltimore: Williams & Wilkins.)

AGE-SPECIFIC CONSIDERATIONS

1. Small-scale equipment is needed for pediatric patients, including rib spreaders, vascular clamps, and internal paddles for defibrillation. Four-centimeter paddles are used for large children, whereas 2-cm paddles are used for infants and toddlers (Clemence, 2000).
2. Only 5 to 20 J are used for internal defibrillation in pediatric patients, compared with 30 to 50 J for adults (Clemence, 2000).
3. Emergent thoracotomy should be reserved for those pediatric patients who present with penetrating chest injury with detectable vital signs that worsen despite conventional therapy (Pitetti & Walker, 2005).

COMPLICATIONS

1. Lung injury during incision into the pleural space
2. Phrenic nerve transection causing diaphragmatic paralysis
3. Injury to coronary arteries while suturing lacerations or attempting to relieve a pericardial tamponade
4. Injury to the heart while performing compressions against a fractured sternum or rib
5. Hemorrhage from internal mammary arteries
6. Organ and tissue ischemia from aortic clamping. If the systolic blood pressure cannot be raised above 70 mm Hg after 30 minutes of cross-clamping the aorta, resuscitative efforts should be discontinued (Boczar & Rivers, 2004).

REFERENCES

Boczar, M. E., & Rivers, E. (2004). Resuscitative thoracotomy. In J. R. Roberts, & J. R. Hedges (Eds.), *Clinical procedures in emergency medicine* (4th ed. pp. 336–353). Philadelphia: Saunders.

Clemence, B. (2000). Emergency department thoracotomy: Nursing implications for pediatric cases. *International Journal of Trauma Nursing, 6*(4) 123–127.

Meredith, J. W., & Hoth, J. J. (2007). Thoracic trauma: When and how to intervene. *Surgical Clinics of North America, 87*(1), 95–118.

Phelan, H. A. (2006). Thoracic damage-control operation: Principles, techniques, and definitive repair. *Journal of the American College of Surgeons, 203*, 933–941.

Pitetti, R. D., & Walker, S. (2005). Life-threatening chest injuries in children. *Clinical Pediatric Medicine, 6*(1) 16–22.

Powell, D. W. (2004). Is emergency department resuscitative thoracotomy futile care for the critically injured patient requiring prehospital cardiopulmonary resuscitation? *Journal of the American College of Surgeons, 199*, 211–215.

Wise, D., Davies, G., & Coats, T., et al. (2005). Emergency thoracotomy: "How to do it." *Emergency Medicine Journal, 22*, 22–24.

Electrocardiographic Monitoring

Mike D. McMahon, RN, BSN

Electrocardiographic monitoring is also known as *ECG* or *EKG monitoring* or *cardiac monitoring*. The abbreviation EKG is derived from the term "Elektrokardiogramme," used by Einthoven over 100 years ago.

INDICATION
To continuously monitor cardiac rate and rhythm.

CONTRAINDICATIONS AND CAUTIONS
1. All equipment should be grounded to prevent electrical shock and electrical interference on the ECG tracing.
2. Always remember to treat the patient and not the monitor, because the patient's clinical condition is more important than the rhythm.
3. Monitors and printers may be capable of displaying heart rhythms at different frequency ranges. Diagnostic frequency (0.05 to 150 Hz) should be used for interpreting such points as waveform duration and ST-segment changes. If the monitor and the printer are at different frequencies, subtle changes may be seen in the ECG between the two sources. Twelve-lead ECGs are interpreted at the frequency range of 0.05 to 150 Hz.
4. Standard calibration is 1 mV = 10 mm, and standard speed is 25 mm/sec. Changes in either parameter should be documented in the patient's record.
5. Changes in body position may cause changes in the patient's rhythm, the same as changing electrode positions.

EQUIPMENT
Cardiac monitor
ECG cable (three- or five-lead system)
Pregelled disposable electrodes (three to five)
Razor (optional)
Alcohol wipes (optional)
Dry gauze dressings (optional)

PROCEDURAL STEPS
1. Turn on the monitor.
2. Select the desired lead (Figures 55-1 through 55-4). Lead II is the most commonly used monitoring lead. Marriott's modified chest lead 1 (MCL[1]) aids in QRS morphology differentiation and atrial activity (Wagner, 2001).

3. Connect the electrodes to the lead wires and place electrodes on clean, dry skin at the appropriate sites, per Figures 55-1 to 55-4. Avoid placing the electrodes over large muscle masses and bony structures. Attempt to place the electrodes where they will not be in the way if defibrillation pads need to be applied emergently.

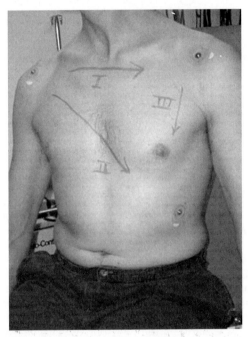

FIGURE 55-1 Electrode placement for leads I, II, and III. The *arrows* point to the positive electrode. (Courtesy Mike D. McMahon.)

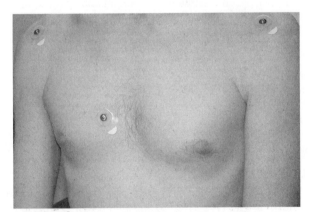

FIGURE 55-2 Marriott's MCL$_1$ using a three-wire cable. The right and left arm leads remain in the standard position. The left leg lead is placed at the V$_1$ position, and the monitor is set to display lead III. (Courtesy Mike D. McMahon.)

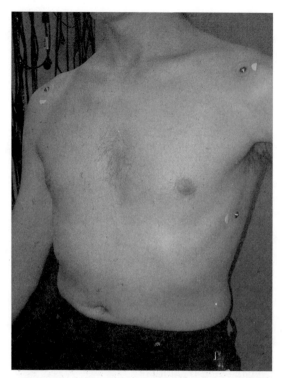

FIGURE 55-3 Marriott's MCL$_6$ using a three-wire cable. The right and left arm leads remain in the standard position. The left leg lead is placed at the V$_6$ position, and the monitor is set to display lead III. (Courtesy Mike D. McMahon.)

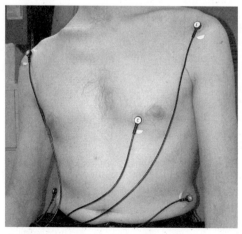

FIGURE 55-4 Five-wire placement. The limb leads are placed in the standard positions, and the chest lead can be placed across the chest. V$_3$ lead placement is shown here. (Courtesy Mike D. McMahon.)

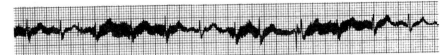

FIGURE 55-5 Common ECG problem patterns: alternating-current electrical interference (60 cycles per second).

4. Observe the ECG tracing. Ideally, the tracing should be free of excessive artifact and should have an R wave that is adequate to allow for accurate heart rate determinations.
5. Set the heart rate alarm limits (based on institutional or unit policy and standards) and turn on the alarms.

TROUBLESHOOTING ECG TECHNICAL PROBLEMS

1. Alternating current interference (also known as 60-cycle interference) (Figure 55-5)
   a. Possible causes
      - Nearby electrical equipment, power cords, electrical wiring in room walls and floors
      - Improper grounding of electrical equipment in the area
      - Unshielded lead wires or patient cable
      - Loose connections in the system (e.g., electrodes, lead wires, cable)
      - Inadequate skin preparation
      - Dry electrodes
      - Stress on patient cables
   b. Solutions
      - Ground equipment in patient area properly.
      - Verify connections of electrodes, leads, and cable.
      - Prepare the skin by performing the following procedure:
         - Clip hair as necessary
         - Cleanse the skin with an alcohol wipe
         - Abrade the skin with a dry gauze pad
         - Apply new electrodes
2. Low voltage (Figure 55-6)
   a. Possible causes
      - Low-gain setting on the ECG monitor
      - Poor electrode contact or disconnected electrode
      - Broken or disconnected lead wire
      - Loose cable connection
      - Low amplitude of QRS signal due to changing the patient's position

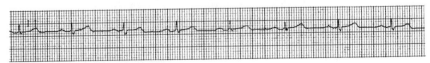

FIGURE 55-6 Common ECG problem patterns: low voltage.

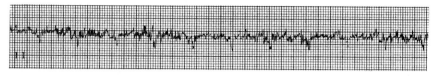

FIGURE 55-7 Common ECG problem patterns: excessive artifact.

    b. Solutions
- Increase the gain on the monitor.
- Verify that all the connections are intact.
- Change the electrodes.
- Select another lead to monitor.

3. Excessive artifact (Figure 55-7)
    a. Possible causes
- Patient movement
- Loose electrode, lead, or cable connections
- Intermittent electrical interference

    b. Solutions
- Verify the placement of the electrodes, or move the electrodes to new locations, where there is less skeletal muscle.
- Replace any loose electrodes.
- Check the connections.
- Support the lead wires and the cable to prevent tension on the cable-lead system caused by patient movement.

4. Wandering baseline (Figure 55-8)
    a. Possible causes
- Cable movement with respirations or patient movement
- Poor electrode contact or location
- Excess tension on the cable-lead system

    b. Solutions
- Reposition the cable to a place where there is less movement.
- If necessary, change the electrodes and select a new location.
- Secure the cable-lead system to reduce tension.

5. Frequency response (Figure 55-9)
    a. Problem. ST-segment changes and QRS complex morphology can be altered by frequency response filtering. Diagnostic 12-lead ECG acquire and print/display waveforms at 0.05 to 150 Hz. Many ECG monitors display waveforms at a reduced range (1 to 40 Hz). The narrower monitor frequency response may hide or, in some cases create false, ST-segment changes.

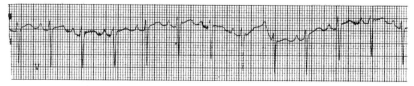

FIGURE 55-8 Common ECG problem patterns: wandering baseline.

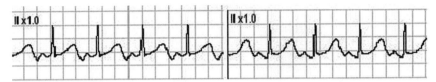

FIGURE 55-9 The same waveform viewed with two different frequency response settings. The first waveform is seen at 1 to 40 Hz and demonstrates no ST-segment elevation; the second waveform is at 0.05 to 40 Hz with 1 to 2 mm of ST-segment elevation.

   b. Solution. Do not rely on monitors to determine the presence of ST changes.

PATIENT TEACHING

1. Report any chest discomfort, palpitations, shortness of breath, or related symptoms immediately.
2. Report any disconnections in the system.

REFERENCE

Wagner, G. S. (2001). *Marriott's practical electrocardiography* (10th ed.). Philadelphia: Lippincott.

PROCEDURE 56

12-, 15-, and 18-Lead Electrocardiograms

Mike D. McMahon, RN, BSN

The 12-lead electrocardiogram (ECG) is also known as a *12-lead ECG* or *EKG*. The 15-lead ECG, also known as a *right-side ECG*, involves adding using right-sided chest wall lead placements of leads V_{4R}, V_{5R}, and V_{6R} in the ECG. The 18-lead ECG, also known as a *posterior ECG*, includes the left posterior leads, V_7, V_8, and V_9.

INDICATIONS

1. To aid in the diagnosis of acute myocardial ischemia, injury, or infarction (MI):
   a. Implementation of a 12-lead ECG program in urban and suburban emergency medical services (EMS) systems is an American Heart Association Class I recommendation (AHA, 2005).

b. AHA (2005) recommends a time limit of 10 minutes between emergency department (ED) admission and acquisition of a 12-lead ECG for patients presenting with symptoms of acute coronary syndrome (ACS).

c. A 15-lead ECG is used to determine right ventricular MI. A 15-lead ECG is indicated when an inferior wall MI, or right ventricular infarction, is suspected (Green & Hill, 2004). Patients who present with a right ventricular infarction associated with an inferior wall MI have a worse in-hospital mortality rate compared with patients without a right-sided infarct (Antman et al., 2004).

d. An 18-lead ECG is used to determine posterior wall MI. An 18-lead ECG is indicated when there is isolated ST-segment depression in the precordial leads (V_1 through V_3) of the 12-lead ECG (Wung & Drew, 2005).

e. The AHA (2005) recommends classifying patients who present with signs of ACS (chest discomfort suggestive of ischemia) into one of three groups:

- *ST-elevation MI (STEMI)*: ST-segment elevation greater than 1 mm in two or more contiguous precordial leads, or two or more adjacent limb leads, or presumed new left bundle-branch block (LBBB).
- *High-risk unstable angina/non–ST elevation MI, or right ventricular infarction, (UA/NSTEMI)*: ST-segment depression 0.5 mm or greater or dynamic T-wave inversion with pain or discomfort. Also included is nonpersistent or transient ST-segment elevation of 0.5 mm or greater or less than 20 minutes duration.
- *Intermediate/low-risk unstable angina:* Normal ECG, or ST-segment deviation of less than 0.5 mm, or T-wave inversion of 2 mm or less.

2. To diagnose and differentiate cardiac arrhythmias and conduction defects.

CONTRAINDICATIONS AND CAUTIONS

1. The sensitivity of a 12-lead ECG in the diagnosis of acute STEMI is approximately 50% on initial presentation to the ED. Another 20% to 30% of patients will have changes suggestive of myocardial ischemia (Green & Hill, 2004).

2. All electrical equipment, including the ECG machine, should be grounded to prevent electrical shock and electrical interference on the ECG tracing.

3. Do not touch the ECG machine, the patient cable, or the patient during cardioversion or defibrillation.

4. When recording ECGs with placements other than the standard lead placements, the lead placements that were used should be labeled on the printout.

5. There can be significant differences in ST-segment measurements between 12-lead ECG printouts and ECG monitoring devices. This is due to the frequency response of the devices. Diagnostic 12-leads require a frequency range of 0.05 to 150 Hz (ANSI/AAMI, 2001), whereas ECG monitoring devices may have a much narrower range of 1 to 40 Hz. See Procedure 55 (Electrocardiographic Monitoring) for more information and examples.

EQUIPMENT

Multiple-lead ECG machine, including cable and leads

Electrodes (pregelled disposable electrodes, suction cups, or plates)

Electrical conductive gel (if suction cups or plates are used)

PATIENT PREPARATION

1. Center the patient on the bed so that no part of the body touches the side rails, the head, or the foot of the bed.
2. To obtain a good tracing, place the head of the bed as flat as the patient can tolerate. Position the patient in a comfortable position and support with pillows as necessary to promote relaxation.

PROCEDURAL STEPS

1. Connect the power cord to a grounded electrical outlet and turn on the ECG machine.
2. Enter the patient demographic information necessary for your equipment.
3. Apply limb leads. If plates or suction cups are used, a conductive gel must be used. Limb leads are placed on the medial aspect of each lower leg. Plates and suction cups are placed on the medial aspect of each forearm or pre-gelled electrodes are placed on the outer aspect of each upper arm.
4. Apply the precordial leads.
   a. Standard lead placement. Lead V_1 is located in the fourth intercostal space (ICS) along the right sternal border. Lead V_2 is located in the fourth ICS along the left sternal border. Lead V_4 is located in the fifth ICS at the midclavicular line. Lead V_3 is located midway between V_2 and V_4 in the fifth ICS. Lead V_6 is located at the midaxillary line. Lead V_5 is at the fifth intercostal space, anterior axillary line. Leads V_4 through V_6 share the horizontal axis (Figure 56-1).
   b. Alternative lead placement (EASI). EASI is a 12-lead ECG system that uses five electrodes—four chest and one reference. The signals from this system are converted into 12 leads through the use of specific monitoring equipment manufactured by Philips (EASI; Philips Medical Systems). Multiple studies (Chantad et al., 2006; Sejersten et al., 2006; Wehr et al., 2006) have looked at the use of the EASI system in both hospital and field environments and found that while the waveforms may differ between the EASI system and standard 12-lead devices, the changes are not clinically significant. The leads are placed at the lower sternum (E) at the level of the fifth intercostal space, at the right and left midaxillary lines (I and A) at the same level as the E electrode, and on the upper sternum (S), and the fifth electrode (reference) can be placed anywhere on the patient's torso (see Figure 56-2).
5. Connect the electrodes to the appropriate lead wires. Lead wires are labeled for each location.
6. Instruct the patient to relax and lie as still as possible. Assure the patient that this procedure takes only 10 to 15 seconds.
7. Press the appropriate button to record the ECG.
8. Precordial lead placement for the 15-lead ECG (right-sided) is as follows (Figure 56-3). V_{1R} is at the fourth ICS along the left sternal border (same as V_2). V_{2R} is at the fourth ICS along the right sternal border (same as V_1). V_{4R} is at the fifth ICS at the right midclavicular line. V_{3R} is placed between leads V_{2R} and V_{4R}. V_{6R} is at the right midaxillary line, and V_{5R} is placed between V_{4R} and V_{6R}. V_4 through V_{6R} share the same horizontal axis.
9. For the 18-lead ECG (posterior) placement, lead V_7 is placed on the posterior axillary line, lead V_8 is placed on the posterior midclavicular line, and lead V_9

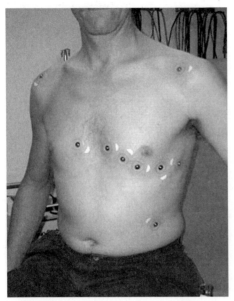

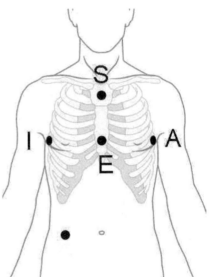

FIGURE 56-1 Standard precordial chest lead placement for a 12-lead ECG. Limb leads shown on chest and abdomen in this example. (Courtesy Mike D. McMahon.)

FIGURE 56-2 EASI lead placement. (Courtesy Philips Medical Systems).

is placed on the left paraspinal border. Leads V_7 through V_9 share the same horizontal axis as leads V_{4-6} (Figure 56-4).

10. Repeat step. 5 through 7 to record the additional leads, and mark the printed ECG to show the changed lead positions.
11. Remove the cables from the electrodes. If the patient is likely to undergo a repeat ECG, you may leave the pregelled electrodes in place; otherwise, remove the electrodes and cleanse the skin as needed.

AGE-SPECIFIC CONSIDERATIONS

1. Pediatric patients should have an ECG that includes leads V_{3R} through V_{4R} to evaluate the possibility of right ventricular hypertrophy.
2. Leads V_{1R} through V_{4R} display a prominent R wave up to age 8.
3. Flat or inverted T waves may be a sign of hypothyroidism.
4. T waves in lead V_1 should never be positive before age 6; this may continue into adolescence (Bernstein, 2004).

COMPLICATIONS

1. Equipment malfunction
2. Electric microshock

TROUBLESHOOTING ECG TECHNICAL PROBLEMS

1. Alternating current interference (see Procedure 55)
2. Wandering baseline (see Procedure 55)

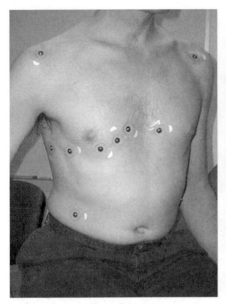

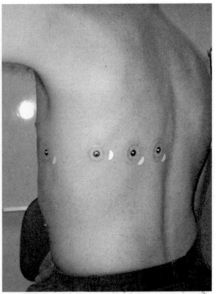

FIGURE 56-3 Precordial leads for right-sided ECG. (Courtesy Mike D. McMahon.)

FIGURE 56-4 Precordial lead positions for posterior-view ECG. (Courtesy Mike D. McMahon.)

3. Tremor
   a. Possible causes
      • Patient is tense or uncomfortable.
      • If electrode plates are used, the straps may be too tight.
   b. Solutions
      • Help the patient to find a comfortable position and encourage the patient to relax.
      • Loosen the electrode straps.
4. Intermittent or jittery waveforms
   a. Possible causes
      • Loose connections
      • Broken lead wires
      • Poor skin preparation
      • Contaminated conductive gel
      • Patient movement and tension
   b. Solutions
      • Check all the connections.
      • Test the lead wires for breaks by wiggling them and watching for the effect on the recording.
      • Reapply the electrodes with proper skin-preparation technique and with fresh electrode-conductive gel.

PATIENT TEACHING

1. Lie as still as possible with your muscles relaxed.
2. Do not talk during the recording.

REFERENCES

American Heart Association (AHA). (2005). American Heart Association guidelines for cardiopulmonary resuscitation and emergency cardiovascular care. *Circulation*, *112*(suppl. IV).

American National Standards Institute and Association for the Advancement of Medical Instrumentation (ANSI/AAMI). (2001). *Diagnostic electrocardiographic devices* (2nd ed.), ANSI/AAMI EC11:1991/(R)2001. Washington, DC/Arlington, VA: Authors.

Antman, E. M., Anbe, D. T., Armstrong, P. W., Bates, E. R., Green, L. A., & Hand, M., et al. (2004). ACC/AHA guidelines for the management of patients with ST-elevation myocardial infarction: Executive summary: A report of the ACC/AHA Task Force on Practice Guidelines (Committee to Revise the 1999 Guidelines on the Management of Patients With Acute Myocardial Infarction). *Circulation*, *110*, Available at www.acc.org/clinical/guidelines/stemi/index.pdf.

Bernstein, D. (2004). Electrocardiography. In R. E. Behrman, R. M. Kliegman, & H. B. Jenson (Eds.), *Textbook of pediatrics* (17th ed. pp. 1489–1492). Philadelphia: Saunders.

Chantad, D., et al. (2006). Derived 12-lead electrocardiogram in the assessment of ST-segment deviation and cardiac rhythm. *Journal of Electrocardiology, 39*, 7–12.

Green, B. B., & Hill, P. M. (2004). Approach to chest pain and possible myocardial ischemia. In J. E. Tintinalli, G. D. Kelen, & J. S. Stapszynski (Eds.), *Emergency medicine* (pp. 333–343). New York: McGraw-Hill.

Sejersten, M., et al. (2006). Comparison of EASI-derived 12-lead electrocardiograms versus paramedic-acquired 12-lead electrocardiograms using Mason-Likar limb lead configuration in patients with chest pain. *Journal of Electrocardiology, 39*, 13–21.

Wehr, G., et al. (2006). A vector-based, 5-electrode, 12-lead monitoring ECG (EASI) is equivalent to conventional 12-lead ECG for diagnosis of acute coronary syndromes. *Journal of Electrocardiology, 39*, 22–28.

Wung, S., & Drew, B. (2005). Extra electrocardiographic leads: Right precordial and left posterior leads. In D. J. Lynn-McHale Wiegand, & K. K. Carlson (Eds.), *AACN procedure manual for critical care* (5th ed. pp. 421–429). St. Louis: Saunders.

PROCEDURE 57

Continuous ST-Segment Monitoring

Mike D. McMahon, RN, BSN

INDICATIONS

1. To assist with the early detection and identification of myocardial ischemia or myocardial infarction (MI) in patients who present with acute coronary syndromes, especially ST-segment elevation MI (STEMI). Patients should be monitored for at least 12 to 24 hours after resolution of symptoms (Antman, Anbe, Armstrong, Bates, Green, & Hand, 2004).

2. To assist with the early detection and identification of myocardial ischemia or MI in situations, such as general anesthesia, in which the patient is unable to communicate with the staff (Landesberg, Mosseri, Wolf, Vesselow, & Weissman, 2002).
3. To facilitate the ruling out of myocardial infarction in low- to moderate-risk outpatients who do not have active chest pain, laboratory changes, or ischemic electrocardiogram (ECG) changes.
4. To monitor patients with asymptomatic forms of ischemia and unstable angina.
5. To monitor patients for reocclusion following thrombolytic therapy or percutaneous coronary intervention (PCI) (Antman et al., 2004; Kucia & Zeitz, 2002).
6. To follow the clinical progress of an MI (Schröder et al., 2001).

CONTRAINDICATIONS AND CAUTIONS
The following are clinical conditions that may alter ST-segment findings:
1. Acute pericarditis (Wagner, 2001)
2. Acute cor pulmonale
3. Pulmonary emphysema
4. Hyperkalemia
5. Digitalis
6. Balloon inflation during percutaneous transluminal coronary angioplasty
7. Pericardial tamponade
8. Intracranial hemorrhage (related to T-wave changes)
9. Hypothermia
10. Bundle-branch blocks
11. Body position changes (Adams & Pelter, 2005)
12. Paced beats
13. Changes in cardiac rhythm
14. Noisy signals
15. Misplacement of leads
16. Elevation just before reperfusion (Kucia & Zeitz, 2002)
17. Left ventricular hypertrophy (Brady, 2006)
18. Benign early repolarization
19. Ventricular aneurysm
20. ST-segment changes have been documented during exercise ECG testing. Rapid up-sloping of the ST segment is a normal finding during exercise (Chaitman, 2005). ST-segment changes in three or more consecutive leads may be considered abnormal.
21. Myocarditis (Mirvis & Goldberger, 2005)
22. Left ventricular tumor
23. Hypercalcemia
24. Hyperventilation
25. Drinking cold water
Situations that may invalidate ST-segment findings include the following:
1. Low-frequency filters on the cardiac monitors. Some new monitors have software that is activated to adjust to ST-segment monitoring automatically.
2. Poor electrode contact. Reduce the resistance across the skin to allow for a clean ECG tracing.

3. Poor patient positioning. The precordial leads are especially susceptible to shifts.
4. Improper electrode placement

EQUIPMENT
ST-segment ECG monitor
ECG cable: 3-, 5-, or 12-lead
Electrodes
Alcohol sponges
Gauze sponges
Razor (optional)
Scissors

PATIENT PREPARATION
1. If possible, choose flat, nonmuscular areas for electrode placement (see Procedure 55).
2. Good skin preparation and electrode placement are essential to perform the sensitive analysis of an ECG signal, to detect ST-segment changes, and to reduce artifact and false alarms (Antman et al., 2004). Clip or shave the chest hair as necessary. Cleanse the electrode placement sites with a mild soap and water to remove all oily residue and dead skin.
3. Allow the skin to dry and then apply the electrodes.

PROCEDURAL STEPS
1. Follow the manufacturer's instructions for setting up your monitoring system. Equipment that is currently available can analyze 2, 3, 4, and 12 leads, depending on the model. Some systems have stand-alone ST-segment trending and can trend ST segment, T waves, QRS fractionation, and QRS difference in all leads.
2. If the patient's condition allows, obtain 12-lead ECGs while the patient is lying on both right and left sides (Procedure 56). This may help determine if ST-segment changes occur as a result of patient movement (Adams & Pelter, 2005).
3. Choose the appropriate grouping of leads for ST-segment monitoring. Determine the patient's ischemic "fingerprint" from a 12-lead ECG, noting which leads show the most ST-segment displacement. Use the lead or leads with the most ST-segment displacement as the bedside ST-segment monitoring leads. If no ischemic fingerprint is available, consider the following recommendations (Table 57-1). Landesberg et al. (2002) found that V_4 is the most sensitive precordial lead for ischemia and infarction while the patient is undergoing surgery. If you are unsure about where the occlusion is located or if the patient has no ECG changes, leads II, III, and V_1 usually provide good data regarding all three vessels.
4. A dominant rhythm is identified, from which the monitor creates a template. The template develops a median beat from each monitored lead. The ST segment is isoelectric (a flat line). The amplitude of the ST segment is determined from the J point (junction point, at the end of the S wave) to the beginning of the T wave (Figure 57-1).

TABLE 57-1

MONITORING LEADS FOR DIFFERENT AREAS OF THE MYOCARDIUM

Infarct Location	Primary Leads	Reciprocal Leads	Artery Involved
Anterior wall	V_2, V_3, V_4	II, III, aV_F	Left coronary artery
Lateral wall	I, aV_L, V_5, V_6	II, III, aV_F	Circumflex branch of left anterior descending coronary artery (LAD)
Posterior wall	V_1, V_2, V_3		Right coronary artery (RCA), circumflex branch of LAD
Inferior wall	II, III, aV_F	I, aV_L	RCA

(Marquette Electronics, Inc. [1995]. From *The golden minutes and ST segment monitoring*. Milwaukee, WI: Author.)

5. When the ST-segment baseline analysis is complete, the monitor continuously updates changes in specific time intervals. A change of the ST segment off the baseline represents myocardial ischemia.
6. If changes in ST-segment amplitude exceed the alarm parameters for more than the set duration, an alarm sounds. A 12-lead ECG should verify these changes in case the alarm has been triggered by artifact. Assess the patient to determine the cause of the changes (e.g., hypothermia, hyperventilation, or suctioning versus myocardial ischemia).
7. After detecting a change in the ST segment, the system automatically resets the template based on the new ST-segment level. After treating the patient

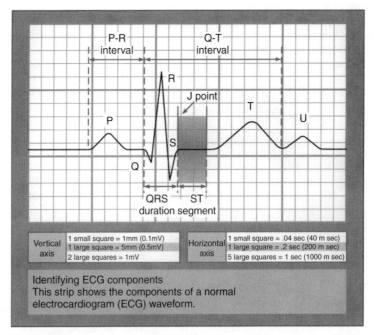

FIGURE 57-1 ECG wave form with J point. (From *12 lead ECG monitoring*. [1996]. (poster). Milwaukee, WI: Author. Courtesy Marquette Medical Systems Worldwide, Milwaukee, WI.)

(for a non–MI-related cause of the alarm), you may need to reset the parameters of the monitor to create a new template.

TROUBLESHOOTING

See Procedure 55.

PATIENT TEACHING

1. Report any chest pain, palpitations, shortness of breath, or related symptoms immediately. Any unusual signs and symptoms should also be reported, taking into account that women are at a higher risk for unrecognized ischemia compared with men (de Torbal et al., 2006; Sweitzer & Douglas, 2005).
2. Report any disconnections in the system.
3. If the patient is discharged to home, aftercare instructions should include the following:
   a. Signs and symptoms that indicate myocardial ischemia (pain in the chest, jaw, epigastrium, or shoulder; sweating; shortness of breath; a feeling of impending doom; nausea; palpitations)
   b. How to access the emergency medical services system; stress the importance of accessing emergency care quickly if symptoms of myocardial ischemia occur
   c. Risk factors for coronary artery disease and follow-up with a primary care provider to develop a plan to decrease risks (e.g., smoking cessation, diet modification, exercise, medications)
   d. A copy of the resting 12-lead ECG, which the patient can bring to future visits in the emergency department or to the primary care provider

REFERENCES

Adams, M. G., & Pelter, M. M. (2005). ST segment monitoring. In D. J. Lynn-McHale Wiegand, & K. K. Carlson (Eds.), *AACN procedure manual for critical care* (5th ed., pp. 430–437). Philadelphia: Saunders.

Antman, E. M., Anbe, D. T., Armstrong, P. W., Bates, E. R., Green, L. A., & Hand, M., et al. (2004). ACC/AHA guidelines for the management of patients with ST-elevation myocardial infarction: Executive summary: A report of the ACC/AHA Task Force on Practice Guidelines (Committee to Revise the 1999 Guidelines on the Management of Patients With Acute Myocardial Infarction). *Circulation, 110,* Available at www.acc.org/clinical/guidelines/stemi/index.pdf.

Brady, W. J. (2006). ST segment and T wave abnormalities not caused by acute coronary syndromes. *Emergency Medicine Clinics of North America, 24,* 91–111.

Chaitman, B. R. (2005). Exercise stress testing. In D. P. Zipes, P. Libby, R. O. Bonow, & W. Braunwald (Eds.), *Braunwald's heart disease: A textbook of cardiovascular medicine* (7th ed., pp. 153–185). Philadelphia: Saunders.

de Torbal, A., Boersma, E., Kors, J. A., van Herpen, G., Deckers, J. W., & van der Kuip, D. A. M., et al. (2006). Incidence of recognized and unrecognized myocardial infarction in men and women aged 55 and older: The Rotterdam Study. *European Heart Journal, 27,* 729–736.

Kucia, A. M., & Zeitz, C. J. (2002). Failed reperfusion after thrombolytic therapy: Recognition and management. *Heart & Lung, 31,* 113–121.

Landesberg, G., Mosseri, M., Wolf, Y., Vesselov, Y., & Weissman, C. (2002). Perioperative myocardial ischemia and infarction. *Anesthesiology, 96,* 264–270.

Mirvis, D. M., & Goldberger, A. L. (2005). Electrocardiography. In D. P. Zipes, P. Libby, R. O. Bonow, & W. Braunwald (Eds.), *Braunwald's heart disease: A textbook of cardiovascular medicine* (7th ed., pp. 107–151). Philadelphia: Saunders.

Schröder, K., Wegscheider, K., & Zeymer, U., et al. (2001). Extent of ST-segment deviation in the single ECG lead of maximum deviation present 90 or 180 minutes after start of thrombolytic therapy best predicts outcome in acute myocardial infarction. *Z Kardiol, 90*, 557–567.

Sweitzer, N. K., & Douglas, P. S. (2005). Cardiovascular disease in women. In D. P. Zipes, P. Libby, R. O. Bonow, & W. Braunwald (Eds.), *Braunwald's heart disease: A textbook of cardiovascular medicine* (7th ed., pp. 1951–1964). Philadelphia: Saunders.

Wagner, G. S. (2001). *Marriott's practical electrocardiography* (10th ed.). Philadelphia: Lippincott Williams & Wilkins.

PROCEDURE 58

Phlebotomy for Laboratory Specimens

June F. Stacey, RN, BSN, CEN

Phlebotomy for laboratory specimens is also known as *blood draw, blood collection, blood tests,* and *venipuncture.*

INDICATION
To obtain blood for laboratory studies.

CONTRAINDICATIONS AND CAUTIONS
1. Patients undergoing thrombolytic therapy should have as few punctures as possible. If venipuncture is absolutely necessary, use the smallest possible needle (i.e., a 23-G needle).
2. Whenever possible, patients should have blood specimens drawn when the intravenous (IV) line is started; this limits the number of punctures. This does increase the likelihood of hemolysis (Grant, 2003). However, in the author's emergency department, it results in only 4% to 8% incidence of hemolysis, and thus 92% to 96% of patients can benefit from this technique by only having one puncture (Proehl, 2006).
3. Blood should never be drawn close to a running IV line. It is preferable to draw from the other arm, but if this is not possible, turn off the fluids before drawing blood. Withdrawing and discarding 5 ml of blood before withdrawing the laboratory samples will minimize the chance of inaccurate results from dilution.

4. Because of the risk of syncope, never perform a venipuncture on a standing patient.

5. Avoid venipuncture in an arm that has an arteriovenous shunt or fistula or on the same side as a radical mastectomy.

6. Label all tubes immediately after blood collection while at the bedside. Do not allow unlabeled tubes to leave the patient's bedside or the phlebotomist's possession.

7. Neonatal or pediatric blood-sample tubes may be necessary for patients from whom it is very difficult to draw blood or those who should not have large volumes of blood drawn, such as patients who are receiving hemodialysis or who have blood dyscrasias.

8. Informed consent may be required before you perform testing for the human immunodeficiency virus. Refer to your institution's policy for more information.

9. Vacuum collection may cause veins to collapse in the very young or the very old patient.

EQUIPMENT

Tourniquet or blood pressure cuff

Antiseptic solution or preparation pads

Blood-sampling options:

- Needles (21- or 23-G) and syringe
- 21- or 23-G butterfly needle and syringe or vacuum-tube adapter
- Tube holder and needle or vacuum-tube adapter (Figure 58-1)

Cotton balls or 2 × 2-in gauze dressings

Tape

Patient labels

Evacuated tubes (Check with your laboratory for specific requirements. Common color codes include a purple top for hematology; a red, gold, green, or speckled top for chemistry; a blue top for coagulation; and a yellow top [sterile] for blood cultures.)

PATIENT PREPARATION

1. Make a positive identification of the patient.

2. Check for restrictions, such as IV, shunts, thrombolytic therapy, or an uncooperative patient.

3. Place the patient in a sitting position with the arm extended and supported comfortably or in a supine position with the arm extended at the side.

4. To prevent aspiration in the event of syncope, be sure the patient does not have gum, candy, or any other substance in his or her mouth.

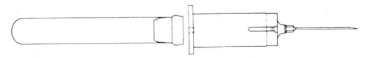

FIGURE 58-1 Vacutainer blood collection set. (Courtesy Becton Dickinson Vacutainer Systems, Franklin Lakes, NJ.)

PROCEDURAL STEPS

1. Assemble equipment (with extra tubes, needles, and syringes) within easy reach.
2. Select a site. The most common sites are the veins in the antecubital fossa—the cephalic, basilic, and median cubital (also known as the median basilic) veins—but any vein may be used. The median cubital is a good choice because it is fairly stationary and close to the surface, and nerves and tendons are farther away than they are from some other veins.
3. Apply the tourniquet or cuff within 3 to 4 inches above the intended puncture site. Note that some specimens, such as those for lactate levels, must be drawn without a tourniquet.
4. Have the patient make a fist and hold it.
5. Palpate to locate the vein. Even if the vein is visible, palpation is necessary to confirm location, direction, and suitability. A vessel that pulsates is an artery, whereas a vein feels like an elastic tube. Thrombosed veins roll and feel hard or rigid. Tendons may feel like veins. If in doubt, release the tourniquet while palpating; fullness should disappear if the structure is a vein.
6. Find the best vein, but do not leave the tourniquet on for more than 2 minutes because it may alter some laboratory values. It may be necessary to release the tourniquet, wait a few minutes, and reapply before performing the venipuncture (Miller & Lunde, 2003).
7. If you are having difficulty finding a vein, try the following:
   a. Be sure the arm is in a dependent position.
   b. Switch to the other arm.
   c. Gently massage the arm from wrist to elbow.
   d. Flick over the vein site with your finger.
   e. Apply a warm compress.
   f. Use a blood pressure cuff instead of a tourniquet.
8. Cleanse the site according to institutional policy and anchor the selected vein by placing your nondominant thumb 1 to 2 inches below the intended venipuncture site. If blood is being drawn for blood alcohol determination, use a nonalcohol cleaning solution, such as povidone-iodine or saline.
9. Perform the venipuncture with the bevel of the needle up and inserted at approximately a 15-degree angle in line with the vein. The needle may be inserted directly over the vein or off to the side and then directed into the vein.
10. If no blood is obtained, try the following:
    a. Reposition the needle by withdrawing, advancing, or rotating it slightly. Do not probe, because it is painful to the patient.
    b. Loosen the tourniquet; if it is too tight, it may be obstructing blood flow.
    c. Select a different tube, because some tubes lack an adequate vacuum.
    d. Choose another venipuncture site.
11. Withdraw the blood.
    a. *Using a syringe:* With one hand, pull the plunger gently while stabilizing the syringe and needle with the other hand. Aspirating too forcefully may collapse the vein or hemolyze the specimen. The syringe method is

often used when the veins are small, such as those in the hand or those in elderly or chronically ill patients, because a vacuum tube may provide too much suction. After the blood is drawn, remove the stopper from the tube and the needle from the syringe and expel the blood gently into the tube. Blood that is injected through the stopper with a needle has a higher risk of hemolysis and this method also increases the risk of a dirty needle stick. Replace the stopper and vent with a needle puncture. Devices to transfer blood from syringe to evacuated tube are also available.

b. *Vacuum-tube method:* The first tube may be placed in the holder and pushed to the line without loss of vacuum before you perform the venipuncture. One hand stabilizes the holder while the other presses the tube onto the needle. The tube fills and automatically stops when the vacuum is exhausted. If multiple samples are drawn, keep the holder and the needle stable as the tubes are exchanged. Be sure to use a multiple-sample needle to prevent blood from leaking as the tubes are changed. If no blood enters the tube and the needle is thought to be in the vein, change the tube before withdrawing the needle to ensure that the tube does have a vacuum.

c. *Butterfly method:* A butterfly (winged collection set) may be used with either a syringe or a tube holder and an adapter for difficult veins. This method allows you to withdraw blood with very little manipulation of the needle within the vein.

d. *Intravenous catheter:* Adapters are available to facilitate drawing directly from IV catheters into vacuum tubes during the placement of an IV line, although this method increases the likelihood of hemolysis (Grant, 2003).

12. To prevent contamination of samples with bacteria (in the case of cultures) or tube additives, blood samples should be collected (or specimen tubes filled) in the following order described in Table 58-1 (NCCLS, 2003) or as specified by your institution. Special considerations include:

a. Blood cultures (see the special procedural steps that follow)

b. Blue-top tubes. There are two common sizes of blue-top tubes for coagulation studies. The half-draw tube requires 2.7 ml, and for accurate test results, it must be allowed to fill completely to the line indicated on the label. If there is no line on the label, the tube is a full-draw tube and should be filled to the top of the label (4.5 ml). When using a butterfly for venipuncture for a citrate (blue top) tube, first draw a discard tube (use a nonadditive or a citrate tube) to fill the tubing's dead space with blood. The discard tube does not need to be completely filled, it is only used to remove the air from the tubing. Then draw the blue top tube; this ensures the proper blood-to-additive ratio (Becton, Dickinson & Company, 2004).

13. Have the patient open the hand as soon as the blood flow is established.

14. To properly mix samples, invert the collection tubes gently as indicated in Table 58-1 as soon as they are filled. Do not shake the tubes.

15. The tourniquet may be released as soon as blood enters the collection system, or it may be left on throughout the procedure.

TABLE 58-1
CORRECT ORDER OF DRAW AND ADDITIVES FOR BLOOD SPECIMEN TUBES

Order of Draw	Stopper Color	Purpose/Common Uses	Additive	Mix by Inverting
1	Varies	Blood cultures	—	8-10 times
2	Blue	Coagulation studies	Sodium citrate	3-4 times
3	Red, red-black speckled, gold, gold-black speckled	Serum samples	No anticoagulant May contain gel separator and/or clot activator, or no additive	5 times
4	Green, green-black speckled	Plasma sample Chemistry studies	Heparin	8-10 times
5	Purple, lavender	Whole blood or plasma samples Hematology	EDTA	8-10 times
6	Gray	Plasma sample Glucose, ethanol	Fluoride	8-10 times

EDTA, Ethylenediaminetetraacetic acid, an anticoagulant. From NCCLS, 2003; Becton, Dickinson, and Company, 2004.

16. On completion of the blood collection, release the tourniquet (if not previously released). Activate needle blunting device (if used).
17. Apply a gauze dressing over the site and gently withdraw the needle. Activate the needle shielding device (if used). Apply pressure until the bleeding has stopped.
18. Tape the gauze dressing firmly in place.
19. Label the blood samples according to institutional policy.
20. Place specimens on ice if necessary. Specimens that commonly require cooling include ammonia, lactic acid, gastrin, catecholamines, and parathyroid hormone. Check with your laboratory for specific requirements.

Blood Cultures

Cultures are performed in an effort to evaluate bacteremia, which may be intermittent, transient, or continuous. The ideal time to obtain cultures is before the onset of fever or chills because there is usually a delay between the influx of bacteria and a fever spike or chill. However, this is rarely possible in the emergency department setting and generally the patient is sick enough to warrant antibioctic treatment before even preliminary results are available. There is controversy and debate about how useful blood cultures are in the outpatient setting, but they are still routinely ordered (Dean & Lee, 2004). Two blood cultures from two separate sites may be obtained before antimicrobial therapy is initiated. Multiple bottles from the same site should be considered a single sample. For confirmation of bacteremia and to rule out contamination or a lapse in skin-cleaning technique, both cultures must be positive.

1. Remove the covers from the blood culture bottles and cleanse the bottle tops with 70 percent isopropyl alcohol, povidone-iodine, chlorhexidine, or other antiseptic soulution indicated by institutional policy. Allow them to air dry.
2. Cleanse the venipuncture site per institutional requirements. Two common methods are:
   a. Clean the site vigorously with 70% isopropyl alcohol and allow it to air dry for 1 to 2 minutes. Next, apply povidone-iodine to the site, starting in the center and moving outward in a circular pattern. Allow the site to air dry for 1 to 2 minutes. A double application of alcohol may be used for patients who are allergic to iodine.
   b. Scrub the site vigorously back and forth with chlorhexidine for 30 seconds and allow to air dry.
3. Apply the tourniquet and perform the venipuncture. Obtain 20 to 30 ml of blood by following procedural steps 13 through 19 above. Sterile gloves may be worn to avoid contaminating the prepared skin. Holders that allow direct collection into the blood-culture bottle are available; however, they are bulky and should be used in conjunction with a butterfly needle to minimize difficulty in positioning during the venipuncture.
4. If a syringe is used, it is preferable to draw two syringes in order to inoculate each bottle with a different syringe and reduce the risk of aerosolization of blood during inoculation. Change to a sterile needle before inoculating the culture bottle. Inject at least 10 ml of blood into each culture bottle.
5. Swab the bottle tops with 70% isopropyl alcohol and allow them to air dry.

6. Care should be taken to prevent contamination at all steps of the collection process (Dean & Lee, 2004).
7. On the laboratory slip, note the time, site, and any previous administration of antibiotics.

AGE-SPECIFIC CONSIDERATIONS

1. Consult your laboratory regarding the minimal sample volume and the appropriate collection tubes for blood studies in infants, small children, and the elderly.
2. Small blood-collection tubes, which allow the collection of capillary blood from a heel stick, are available. See Procedure 20 for capillary blood collection technique.
3. A butterfly needle facilitates venipuncture in small children because it is easier to obtain samples without moving the needle.
4. Additional personnel may be necessary to stabilize the extremity or restrain young children.
5. Use of a tight tourniquet on elderly patients with friable veins may cause the vein to rupture if it is punctured. Use a loose tourniquet or no tourniquet at all.
6. Evacuated tubes may cause vein collapse in children and the elderly.

COMPLICATIONS

1. Vasovagal syncope
2. Failure to obtain blood, usually due to incorrect needle positioning or a tube without a vacuum
3. Hematoma formation at the puncture site
4. Hemolysis of the sample. Hemolysis is more likely to occur when blood is drawn through IV catheters, especially when an adaptor is used to draw directly into vacuum tubes (Grant, 2003). Tips to help prevent hemolysis include:
   a. Allow the site to air dry before venipuncture.
   b. Make sure the needle is tight on the syringe to prevent frothing during collection.
   c. Angle the tube so that the blood runs down the side during collection.
   d. Aspirate gently when using a syringe. Hemolysis can be associated with either large- or small-gauge needles if excessive force is applied via syringe or evacuated tube.
   e. Gently invert the tube to mix additives; do not shake.
   f. Fill tubes completely. Partially filled tubes are more prone to hemolysis when they are transported via a pneumatic tube system.
   g. Avoid injecting blood from a syringe through a needle via the stopper of the tube. Use a blood transfer device or remove the needle from the syringe and the stopper from the tube and gently fill the tube.
5. Clotted sample that was not mixed properly when drawn. Gently invert each tube several times to ensure mixing.
6. Local reaction to skin-cleansing agent. Remove any residual iodine solutions after venipuncture and before dressing application.

PATIENT TEACHING

Report ongoing bleeding or pain at the venipuncture site.

REFERENCES

Becton, Dickinson & Company (2004). *BD* Vacutainer® order of draw for multiple tube collections. Franklin Lakes, NJ: Author. Retrieved January 13, 2007, from http://www.bd.com/vacutainer/pdfs/plus_plastic_tubes_wallchart_orderofdraw_VS5729.pdf.

Dean, A. J., & Lee, D. C. (2004). Bedside laboratory and microbiologic procedures. In J. R. Roberts, & J. R. Hedges (Eds.), *Clinical procedures in emergency medicine* (4th ed., pp. 1403–1405). Philadelphia: Saunders.

Grant, M. S. (2003). The effect of blood drawing techniques and equipment on hemolysis of ED laboratory blood samples. *Journal of Emergency Nursing, 29*, 116–121.

Miller, D. T., & Lunde, J. R. (2003). Laboratory specimen collection. In L. Newberry (Ed.), *Sheehy's emergency nursing: Principles and practice* (5th ed., pp. 130–132). St Louis: Mosby.

National Committee for Clinical Laboratory Standards (NCCLS). (2003). *Procedures for the collection of diagnostic blood specimens by venipuncture; approved standard* (5th ed.), *23*(32). Wayne, PA: Author.

Proehl, J. A., (2006). Emergency department hemolysis rates in laboratory specimens. Unpublished data, Dartmouth-Hitchcock Medical Center, Lebanon, NH.

PROCEDURE 59

Blood Glucose Monitoring

Daun A. Smith, RN, MS

Blood glucose monitoring is also known as *finger stick glucose*.

INDICATION
To measure whole-blood glucose levels at the bedside.

CONTRAINDICATIONS AND CAUTIONS
1. Do not obtain blood from a site that is vascularly compromised (cold, mottled, cyanotic); the sample may not produce an accurate result.
2. Severely decreased peripheral blood flow, such as occurs in the presence of hypotension, shock, peripheral vascular disease, or the severe dehydration of diabetic ketoacidosis or hyperglycemic hyperosmolar nonketotic syndrome, may lead to inaccurate results. An initial serum glucose determination performed simultaneously with a bedside blood glucose test determines concordance (Blake & Nathan, 2004).
3. There are many types of blood glucose meters, and each has specific test strips. The user must be familiar with the test strips that must be used for the

model that he or she operates. Some meters test only capillary whole blood. Others can also accommodate venous, arterial, neonatal, or capillary blood (Blake & Nathan, 2004). Some strips require blood to be placed on top of the test area; others pull the blood onto the test area from the side of the strip.

4. An accurate result depends on a competent operator, properly stored supplies, and clean, functional equipment that is calibrated correctly and tested routinely for quality control.

5. If the results are inconsistent with the patient's clinical picture or otherwise appear inaccurate, validate the result with a serum glucose test, recheck the blood glucose meter manufacturer's instructions, review the test procedure, verify that the quality control results are in the desired range, check the expiration date of the test strips, and repeat the test (Fain, 2004).

6. For results that are critically high or low (hospital policy may dictate these values) or for other questionable results, validate the result with a serum glucose test.

7. Limitations of the procedure may include a very high or low hematocrit or elevated uric acid, oxygen, or ascorbic acid levels (Blake & Nathan, 2004). Falsely high glucose results may occur in patients who use EXTRANEAL (icodextrin) peritoneal dialysis solution (Baxter Healthcare Corporation, 2001). See the blood glucose test strip package insert for specific limitations.

EQUIPMENT

Lancet or lancet device
Alcohol swab
Cotton balls or gauze pad
Blood glucose meter
Blood glucose test strip

PATIENT PREPARATION

1. Select a puncture site. The fingertip or earlobe is acceptable for adults.
2. Cleanse the site with alcohol. Allow to dry. If the site is cold, warm it with a hot pack to increase vasodilatation.

PROCEDURAL STEPS

NOTE: Each blood glucose meter or system has specific procedural steps. Consult the meter manual for the specific system to be used.

1. Prepare the meter by turning it on and making sure that the calibration code on the meter matches the code on the package of test strips. If indicated, enter operator and patient identification.

2. Ensure that the meter and strip are ready to accept the drop of blood.

3. Cleanse the intended puncture site with alcohol. Prepare the lancet or lancet device.

4. Hold the lancet firmly to the site and perform the puncture.

5. Gently squeeze the finger and release to allow blood to flow. Obtain a drop of blood that is adequate to fill the test area of the strip.

6. Lightly touch the reagent area of the strip to the drop of blood, filling the entire area. Avoid smearing the blood. (Some meters allow the addition of a second drop if the first is insufficient. Check the meter manual.) When applying blood to the test strip from a syringe, obtain

a drop at the tip of the syringe and allow the capillary action of the strip to draw the blood.

7. Read the value at the conclusion of the test.

AGE-SPECIFIC CONSIDERATION

The heel may be used as a puncture site in neonates; toes should not be used.

COMPLICATIONS

1. Discomfort at the puncture site
2. Infection (rare)
3. Inaccurate blood glucose result

PATIENT TEACHING

1. Review home blood glucose monitoring procedure and interpretation of the results.
2. Watch for signs and symptoms of infection.
3. Alternate sites, such as the forearm, should not be used if hypoglycemia is suspected or within 1 hour of a meal or insulin injection (Jungheim & Koschinsky, 2002).

REFERENCES

American Diabetes Association (ADA). (2003). Position statement: Bedside blood glucose monitoring in hospitals. *Diabetes Care, 26*(Suppl. 1), S119.

Baxter Healthcare Corporation. (2001). *EXTRANEAL product insert.* McGaw Park, IL: Author.

Blake, D. R., & Nathan, D. M. (2001). Point-of-care testing for diabetes. *Critical Care Nursing Quarterly, 2*(2), 150–161.

Fain, J. A. (2004). Blood glucose meters. *Nursing, 34*(11), 48–51.

Jungheim, K., & Koschinsky, T. (2002). Glucose monitoring at the arm: Risky delays of hypoglycemia and hyperglycemia detection. *Diabetes Care, 25,* 956–960.

Vascular Access

Peripheral Intravenous Cannulation

Margo E. Layman, MSN, RN, RNC, CN-A, and
Jean A. Proehl, RN, MN, CEN, CCRN, FAEN

INDICATION

To establish venous access for the administration of fluids, electrolytes, intravenous (IV) medications, blood components, or total parenteral nutrition.

CONTRAINDICATIONS AND CAUTIONS

If the patient has a coagulation disorder, care should be taken to prevent bleeding from unsuccessful venipuncture sites.

1. Avoid veins in limb on side of radical mastectomy with lymph node stripping, limbs that have sustained third-degree burns, or limbs with dialysis shunts (Josephson, 2004).
2. A hematoma may form if the needle punctures both the anterior and the posterior walls of the vein.
3. Attempt to draw any necessary blood specimens through the IV catheter to decrease the number of venipunctures the patient has to undergo (see Procedure 58).
4. Avoid placing IV lines over joints, because the movement of the joint may cause infiltration.
5. Rotate IV sites in adult patients every 72 to 96 hours to help prevent the development of phlebitis and infection (O'Grady et al., 2002).
6. Remove IV catheters inserted under emergency conditions and restart at a new site within 48 hours (O'Grady et al., 2002).
7. Remove IV catheters promptly on evidence of edema, redness, phlebitis, pain, or subcutaneous infiltration.
8. Do not apply antibiotic ointment or creams to insertion sites, because they may promote fungal infections and antibiotic resistance (O'Grady et al., 2002).
9. Shaving the site for intravenous cannulation may promote bacterial growth; if hair removal is necessary, clipping is preferred.
10. Never withdraw the catheter over the needle; this could shear off the catheter inside the vein.
11. Although rare, IV sites may generate emboli in patients with poor venous return. In adults, the feet and ankles are poor sites for IV cannulation because venous return may be sluggish.

EQUIPMENT

IV solution and tubing *or* IV lock and saline flush

Over-the-needle IV catheter

T-piece or short extension set

Tourniquet

Antiseptic swabs (Acceptable skin cleansing solutions include 2% chlorhexidine, tincture of iodine, an iodophor, or 70% alcohol [O'Grady et al., 2002].)

Gauze dressings

Transparent dressing (optional)

Tape

Vacuum tubes, syringe, or adapter for blood sampling (optional)

Local anesthetic or saline, tuberculin syringe with needle (optional)

Arm board (optional)

PREPARATION

Assemble IV fluid and tubing or a saline lock. A T-piece or short extension set is recommended on all IV sites to facilitate tubing changes with minimal catheter hub manipulation and dressing changes.

PROCEDURAL STEPS

1. Apply a tourniquet 5 to 6 inches above the intended site of cannulation. Tuck the tail of the tourniquet under the tourniquet to permit one-handed release as soon as the vein is cannulated.

2. Identify a vein. If the vein is not distended and is easily palpable, lightly pat the area. Have the patient open and close the fist and lower the extremity below the level of the heart. An alternative is to apply a warm pack to help distend a vein. Make the initial venipuncture in the distal extremity to preserve proximal sites for potential later use. If possible, use the nondominant arm so the patient retains use of the dominant hand. Bifurcations are good sites for venipuncture because they are stable and are not prone to roll. Applying multiple tourniquets distally from the most proximal joint or transilluminator may be necessary to visualize a vein in obese or edematous patients (Rosenthal, 2005).

3. Cleanse the skin with an antiseptic solution by using a firm, circular swabbing motion outward from the center of the site. Allow the skin to air dry for 30 seconds (povidone-iodine should be allowed to dry for at least 2 minutes).

4. Inject an intradermal wheal of local anesthetic or saline solution at the intended puncture site (optional). This is not recommended when the vein is difficult to see, because the skin wheal may obscure the site.

5. Using the thumb of your nondominant hand, apply slight traction to the distal vein to help stabilize the vein during venipuncture. Insert the needle through the skin at a 10- to 30-degree angle with the bevel up, in line with and alongside the vein. Alternatively, you may insert the needle directly over the vein, but there is an increased risk of posterior wall puncture with this technique (Figure 60-1).

6. When the vein is punctured, a flash of blood appears in the hub of the catheter. Advance the needle and stylet another ⅛ inch into the vein (adult patient).

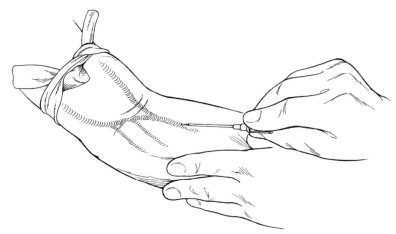

FIGURE 60-1 Insert the intravenous catheter along the vein while stabilizing the vein with your other thumb. (From Rosen, P., Chan, T., Vilke, G., & Sternbach, G. [2001] *Atlas of emergency procedures* [p. 69]. St. Louis: Mosby.)

7. Advance the catheter over the needle and into the vein. If any resistance is met on advancement of the catheter, stop immediately, remove the needle and catheter, and apply pressure to the site. Activate any needle shield or safety device as indicated.

8. To prevent blood leakage when connecting and disconnecting tubing and syringes, use your non-dominant hand and compress the vein just proximal to the tip of the catheter with the ring or middle finger while holding the catheter hub with the thumb and index finger.

9. If blood specimens are to be drawn through the IV catheter, attach the syringe or vacuum-tube adapter to the needle hub and withdraw the required samples (see Procedure 58).

10. Release the tourniquet.

11. Connect the IV tubing and open the roller clamp or attach the saline lock.

12. Apply ¼-in tape across the hub of the catheter to secure it. Do not place the tape over the insertion site or at the junction of the needle and tubing. Place a small sterile dressing over the insertion site. Alternatively, apply a transparent dressing over the site and needle hub.

13. Tape the IV tubing or saline lock securely.

14. Tape a label to the IV site with the date, the time, the size of the catheter, and your initials.

15. Adjust the drip rate as ordered or flush the saline lock. Assess the site for infiltration.

16. Before injecting medication through an injection port, clean the port with 70% alcohol or an iodophor (O'Grady et al., 2002).

AGE-SPECIFIC CONSIDERATIONS
Pediatric

1. Pediatric patients should not have routine rotation of IV sites; replace peripheral catheters only when clinically indicated (O'Grady et al., 2002).

2. Pediatric or elderly patients may require an arm board to protect the IV site. Wrapping the extremity with gauze can help prevent the patient from manipulating the catheter.
3. It may be helpful to secure the hand of a small child to an IV board before the venipuncture.
4. In infants and small children, advance the catheter off of the needle as soon as you see the blood flashback. This helps avoid puncture of the posterior wall of the vein. In adults with large, rope-like veins, advance the needle and stylet together approximately ¼ inch to prevent the catheter tip from catching on the thick wall of the vein.
5. In pediatric patients not yet walking, a foot vein may be appropriate. Avoid the child's dominant hand or the favored hand for thumb/finger sucking (Rosenthal, 2005).
6. Scalp veins can be used for IV access in infants, although they are inadequate for large volumes of fluids or medications that must be administered quickly. A rubber band can be used as a tourniquet to distend the veins (Figure 60-2). Determine which direction the blood is flowing by occluding the vein with your finger and "milking" it. The IV catheter should be inserted in the same direction the blood is flowing. The rubber band has to be cut away carefully after the IV catheter is in place. A plastic medicine cup can be used to protect the IV line (Figure 60-3). Place padding between the cup and the scalp before taping it in place.
7. Use a T-piece or a short extension set on all pediatric IV lines to facilitate the injection of medications near the site and to avoid flushing long lengths of tubing to ensure that the medication has been infused.
8. An intradermal local anesthetic may not be the best option in children who approach any puncture with fear. An topical anesthetic cream (eutectic mixture of local anesthetics [EMLA] or lidocain) may be used to anesthetize the site, but this takes 20 to 60 minutes to be effective. School-aged children may

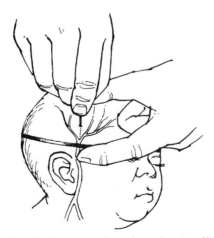

FIGURE 60-2 Use a rubber band as a tourniquet for scalp veins. (From Lozon, M. M. [2004]. Pediatric vascular access and blood sampling techniques. In J. R. Roberts & J. R. Hedges [Eds.], *Clinical procedures in emergency medicine* [4th ed., p. 367]. Philadelphia: Saunders.)

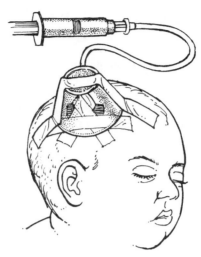

FIGURE 60-3 A plastic medicine cup can be used to protect a scalp intravenous line. (From Lozon, M. M. [2004]. Pediatric vascular access and blood sampling techniques. In J. R. Roberts & J. R. Hedges [Eds.], *Clinical procedures in emergency medicine* [4th ed., p. 367]. Philadelphia: Saunders.)

be able to decide whether they want intradermal local anesthesia, which can be described as "a sting that makes the skin go to sleep so the needle doesn't hurt so much."

Geriatric

1. Avoid using a tourniquet in elderly patients who have fragile veins to decrease the risk of blowing the vein. Using a blood pressure cuff upside down instead of a tourniquet will prevent skin tears in elderly patients. Inflate the cuff to just below diastolic pressure for effective compression (Rosenthal, 2005).
2. Using vacuum tubes to draw blood directly from the IV catheter increases the risk of blowing the vein in elderly patients.

COMPLICATIONS

1. Hematomas may form at unsuccessfully cannulated sites.
2. Inadequate cleansing of the skin at the cannulation site may result in the introduction of bacteria into the vein, which can lead to local infection or bacteremia.
3. Phlebitis may develop.
4. Catheter embolism may occur if the catheter shears off as it is withdrawn over the stylet.
5. Infiltration of the surrounding tissue can occur because of a displaced catheter. Some medications can cause serious tissue damage if they infiltrate into the tissue.

PATIENT TEACHING

1. Do not bend, pinch, or adjust the flow rate of the tubing.

2. Report any sensations of swelling, heat, pain, or drainage at the puncture site.

REFERENCES

Josephson, D. (2004). Patient preparation and site selection for peripheral intravenous infusion therapy. In D. Josephson (Ed.), *Intravenous infusion therapy for nurses: Principles & practices* (2nd ed., p. 153). New York: Thomson Learning.

O'Grady, N. P., Alexander, M., & Dellinger, E. P., et al. (2002). Guidelines for prevention of intravascular catheter–related infections. *Morbidity and Mortality Weekly Report, 51*, 1-28.

Rosenthal, K. (2005). Tailor your IV insertion techniques for special populations. *Nursing, 35*, 37-41.

PROCEDURE 61

Rapid-Infusion Catheter Exchange

Reneé Semonin Holleran, RN, PhD, CEN, CCRN, CFRN, CTRN, FAEN

Rapid-infusion catheter exchange is also known as *RIC*.

INDICATIONS

1. To increase the size of a functioning peripheral intravenous (IV) line.
2. To provide access for volume resuscitation of the patient in shock.
3. To provide percutaneous access for the introduction of invasive monitoring lines, diagnostic catheters, or temporary pacing wires.

CONTRAINDICATIONS AND CAUTIONS

1. These catheters are for peripheral IV use only.
2. A 20-G or larger catheter must be established before this device can be used.
3. Patency of the established catheter must be ensured through an adequate blood return.

EQUIPMENT

Antiseptic solution
Local anesthetic

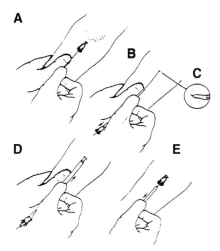

FIGURE 61-1 Percutaneous insertion of a 7- to 8.5-Fr introducer (see text for explanation). (Reproduced from Herron, H., Falcone, R., Dean, B., & Werman, H. [1997]. 8.5 French peripheral intravenous access during air medical transport of the injured patient. *Air Medical Journal, 16*[1], 8).

Rapid-infusion catheter exchange set (guide wire, sheath or dilator combination, No. 11 scalpel, 7- or 8.5-Fr catheter)
IV dressing supplies

PATIENT PREPARATION

1. Place the patient in a supine position.
2. Remove the IV dressing over the established catheter.
3. Ensure that the existing peripheral IV catheter is 20-G or larger and looks for signs of infiltration such as edema, erythema, or pain.

PROCEDURAL STEPS

1. *Infiltrate the area around the catheter with a local anesthetic.
2. Cleanse the entire area, including the puncture site and indwelling catheter, with an antiseptic solution.
3. *Disconnect the IV tubing from the catheter and insert the guide wire through the indwelling catheter and into the vein (Figure 61-1, *A*). If resistance is met, withdraw the guide wire and reinsert. If resistance persists, the procedure must be stopped.
4. *When the guide wire has been inserted into the indwelling catheter, remove the existing catheter.
5. *Pass the sheath or dilator over the guide wire (Figure 61-1, *B*).
6. *Nick the skin with the scalpel blade at the insertion site (approximately 5 mm) (Figure 61-1, *C*).

---

*Indicates portions of the procedure usually performed by a physician or an advanced practice nurse.

7. *Thread the tapered tip of the dilator over the guide wire and advance the dilator and sheath into the vessel, using a slight twisting motion (Figure 61-1, *D*).
8. *Advance the sheath over the dilator by grasping the skin and using a slight twisting motion.
9. *Make sure the sheath is held in place and then remove the dilator and guide wire. The free flow of blood demonstrates that the catheter is in place (Figure 61-1, *E*).
10. Connect the catheter to the IV tubing. Blood tubing or large-bore tubing should be used if fluid resuscitation is indicated.
11. Secure the catheter with tape or a suture. Apply a dressing.

AGE-SPECIFIC CONSIDERATION

This procedure is not recommended for infants and small children because of the size of the peripheral catheter. All patients receiving fluids through this catheter must be closely monitored because excessive amounts of fluid may be delivered, which can be deleterious to the patient (Clark, 2002).

COMPLICATIONS

1. Rupture of the vein and hematoma formation may occur when the catheter being inserted is larger than the vessel.
2. Leaving the vessel dilator in place after catheter insertion may lead to limited function as well as the potential for the dilator to dislodge from the vessel and enter the systemic circulation.
3. Infiltration and infusion of fluids, blood, or medications into surrounding tissues may occur with this procedure.

PATIENT TEACHING

1. Keep the limb where the catheter is inserted immobilized to prevent dislodgement of the catheter.
2. Report immediately dampness, pain, or swelling at the IV site, or any disconnection in the equipment.

---

*Indicates portions of the procedure usually performed by a physician or an advanced practice nurse.

REFERENCE

Clark, D. Y. (2002). Prehospital care of the trauma patient. In K. McQuillan, K. Von Rueden, R. Hartsock, M. Flynn, & E. Whalen (Eds.), *Trauma nursing: From resuscitation through rehabilitation* (3rd ed., pp. 94-106). Philadelphia: Saunders.

External Jugular Venous Access

Reneé Semonin Holleran, RN, PhD, CEN, CCRN, CFRN, CTRN, FAEN

Although the external jugular vein is usually considered a peripheral intravenous (IV) site, some institutions consider the external jugular site to be central line access instead of peripheral line access. Consult your institution's policies and procedures for clarification on whether registered nurses may insert external jugular catheters.

INDICATIONS

1. To obtain peripheral venous access for fluid resuscitation, blood products, or medication administration.
2. To obtain peripheral venous access when no sites are available on the extremities.
3. To obtain peripheral venous access to draw blood for laboratory evaluation.

CONTRAINDICATIONS AND CAUTIONS

1. External venous access may be contraindicated if the patient has a suspected cervical spine injury and the patient's head must be moved to gain vascular access (Campbell, 2004).
2. Use of the external jugular vein is contraindicated in a patient who has a penetrating injury to the neck, and it should be avoided when there is significant blunt trauma and soft tissue injury to the face, neck, or upper chest.
3. External jugular venous access should be used with caution in patients who cannot tolerate a supine or head-down position.
4. External jugular venous access should be used with caution when the anatomy of the external jugular vein is not clearly discernible.
5. Securing an external jugular venous line can be difficult, and this increases the potential for accidental dislodgement.
6. Patients taking anticoagulants are at increased risk of bleeding around the catheter. This could result in the development of an expanding hematoma and airway compromise.

EQUIPMENT

Antiseptic solution
Caps, masks, and sterile gloves
IV solution and tubing
IV needle and catheter (size and length are dependent on the need for the line)
Dressing supplies

5-ml syringe; 18-, 25-, or 27-G needles for local anesthesia
Local anesthetic
20- to 30-ml syringes to obtain blood samples
Assorted blood collection tubes

PATIENT PREPARATION

1. Place the patient in a supine, head-down position, with the head turned away from the side where the catheter is to be inserted. Please note that external jugular vein access may be obtained in the trauma patient, but the patient's head cannot be moved or lowered.
2. If this procedure is to be performed on a patient with a suspected cervical spine injury, the cervical collar must be opened or the front portion removed and someone assigned to ensure cervical spine protection (Campbell, 2004).
3. Cleanse the area overlying the external jugular vein with antiseptic solution. The external jugular vein runs downward and backward obliquely behind the angle of the mandible and across the sternomastoid muscle. It then courses deeply into the neck just above the midclavicular area. The external jugular vein enters the subclavian vein (Figure 62-1).

PROCEDURAL STEPS

1. *If the patient is conscious, anesthetize the insertion site with a local anesthetic.
2. *Attach the IV catheter to a syringe and align the needle with the external jugular vein, directing the needle tip toward the ipsilateral shoulder.
3. *Lightly "tourniquet" the distal end of the external jugular vein (just above the clavicle) with the opposite index finger. The opposite thumb can also be used on the proximal portion of the vein to assist in anchoring it for puncture (Figure 62-2).

---

*Indicates portions of the procedure usually performed by a physician or an advanced practice nurse.

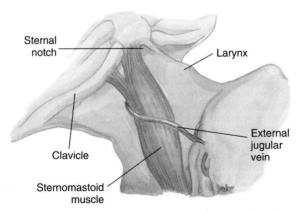

FIGURE 62-1 Anatomy of the external jugular vein. (From Sanders, M. [2001]. *Mosby's paramedic textbook* [2nd ed., p. 326]. St. Louis: Mosby).

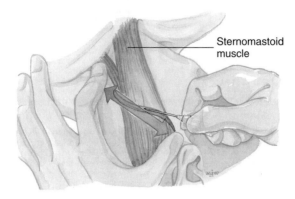

Sternomastoid muscle

FIGURE 62-2 External jugular venipuncture. (From Sanders, M. [2001]. *Mosby's paramedic textbook* [2nd ed., p. 326]. St. Louis: Mosby).

4. *Perform the venipuncture midway between the angle of the jaw and the clavicle.
5. *When a blood return is noted in the syringe, advance the catheter off the needle to the hub. If you are using another type of device (i.e., a triple-lumen catheter), advance it according to the manufacturer's instructions.
6. *If blood is to be obtained, withdraw the desired amount. Detach the syringe and place a gloved finger over the hub to prevent the introduction of air.
7. Connect the IV tubing and initiate the flow of the fluid. Monitor for signs of infiltration.
8. *Secure the catheter with sutures, tape, or surgical tape closures. Skin adhesive will help secure tape or surgical tape closures. Looping the IV tubing around the ear may add additional security. Apply a dressing over the area. Sedation may be required to help keep the patient from moving and dislodging the catheter (Fleck, 2005).

AGE-SPECIFIC CONSIDERATIONS

1. For the pediatric patient, the external jugular vein is a relatively safe place to gain venous access, because it is superficial and visible (Markenson, 2002).
2. The pediatric airway may be compromised when the child's head is turned for placement.

COMPLICATIONS

1. Infection and phlebitis. Risk factors associated with the development of infection and phlebitis include type of catheter, frequency of catheter manipulation, and patient-related factors (O'Grady et al., 2002).
2. Turning a patient's head for better visualization of the external jugular vein may cause airway compromise.

---

*Indicates portions of the procedure usually performed by a physician or an advanced practice nurse.

3. Hematoma formation at the site of the insertion may cause airway compromise.
4. Inadvertent puncture of the carotid artery may occur.
5. The catheter may shear and an embolus may form.
6. An air embolus can result from the insertion.

PATIENT TEACHING

1. Avoid excessive head movement.
2. Report any pain, shortness of breath, bleeding, or dampness at the site immediately.

REFERENCES

Campbell, J. E. (Ed.). (2004). *Basic trauma life support* (5th ed.). Upper Saddle River, NJ: Pearson Prentice Hall.

Fleck, D. (2005). Central line insertion (perform). In D. J. Lynn-McHale, & K. K. Carlson (Eds.), *AACN procedure manual for critical care* (5th ed., pp. 638-650). Philadelphia: Saunders.

Markenson, D. S. (2002). *Pediatric prehospital care*. Upper Saddle River, NJ: Prentice Hall.

O'Grady, N. P., Alexander, M., & Dellinger, E. P., et al. (2002). Guidelines for prevention of intravascular catheter-related infections. *Morbidity and Mortality Weekly Report, 51*, 1-28.

PROCEDURE 63

Subclavian Venous Access

Reneé Semonin Holleran, RN, PhD, CEN, CCRN, CFRN, CTRN, FAEN

INDICATIONS

1. To obtain central venous access through the subclavian vein when peripheral access is unobtainable, such as occurs in a patient who is in profound shock or cardiac arrest, or in a patient with peripheral vascular access limitations, such as an intravenous substance abuser or one with severe peripheral vascular disease.
2. To monitor the patient's central venous pressure (CVP).
3. To administer intravenous fluids, blood products, or medications, especially those likely to cause complications if administered via a smaller peripheral vein.
4. To administer long-term parenteral nutrition.
5. To provide a site for the insertion of a transvenous pacemaker or a pulmonary-artery catheter.

CONTRAINDICATIONS AND CAUTIONS

1. Insertion of a subclavian line should only be performed by a skilled physician, advanced practice nurse, or other appropriately trained practitioner (ACS, 2004).
2. A patient who has a coagulopathy from either a disease process or a medication must be monitored carefully for bleeding. A femoral site is preferred because the vessel can be compressed if bleeding should occur.
3. Fibrinolytic therapy must be administered with extreme caution when any central line is in place.
4. A patient who is agitated or uncooperative is at risk for injury during the procedure.
5. Subclavian access should be avoided in a patient who has had surgery or trauma to the clavicle, first rib, or subclavian vessels; has undergone radiation therapy to the clavicular area; has significant chest wall deformities; or is cachexic or obese (Mickiewicz, Dronen, & Younger, 2004).
6. Cannulization of the subclavian vein should be avoided in patients receiving positive end-expiratory pressure or continuous positive-airway pressure or in patients with pulmonary emphysema because of the increased risk of causing a pneumothorax.

EQUIPMENT

Antiseptic solution
Local anesthetic
5-ml syringe; 18-, 25-, or 27-G needles for local anesthesia
Central venous access kit (Most kits contain an 8.5-Fr introducer, which can be used for large fluid-volume resuscitation or for the introduction of a transvenous pacemaker or a pulmonary artery catheter.)
or
Multiple-lumen catheter (used for fluid administration and allows insertion of invasive lines, transvenous pacemakers as well as ports for medication administration and obtaining blood)
or
16-G, 8-inch, single-lumen catheter
No. 11 scalpel
IV solution and tubing
Flush solution (heparinized solution or 0.9% saline solution per institutional policy)
Silk suture (2-0 or 3-0) with a needle holder
Sterile towels
Masks, caps, goggles, sterile gloves, and gowns
Dressing supplies (gauze or a transparent dressing) (NOTE: When the patient is diaphoretic or the site is oozing, it should be covered with gauze instead of a transparent dressing [O'Grady et al, 2002].)

PATIENT PREPARATION

1. Place the patient on a cardiac monitor and pulse oximeter (see Procedures 21 and 55).
2. Place the patient in a supine, 20-degree Trendelenburg position with a small, rolled towel placed between the shoulder blades to improve access. If the

patient cannot tolerate the Trendelenburg position, elevate the legs for a modified Trendelenburg position (see Procedure 48). Turn the patient's head to the side opposite the insertion site.

3. *Cleanse the chest with an antiseptic solution. The subclavian vein rises as a continuation of the axillary vein, with its origin near the lateral portion of the first rib. The vein runs medially, passing under the middle third of the clavicle, and unites with the internal jugular vein near the sternum to form the brachiocephalic (innominate) vein.

4. *Drape the patient, using a sterile technique. In addition to gloves, masks and goggles should be worn for this procedure.

5. If a multiple-lumen catheter is being used, be sure that the ports have been flushed using the solution recommended by the hospital's policies and procedures.

6. The right subclavian is the preferred site because the vein is shorter and provides a more direct route (Fleck, 2005).

PROCEDURAL STEPS

1. *Locate the landmarks for the subclavian vein and anesthetize the insertion site.

2. *Place the middle finger of your nondominant hand in the suprasternal notch.

3. *Locate the tubercle, which is approximately one third of the distance along the clavicle from the sternum.

4. *With the middle finger still in the suprasternal notch and the thumb on the inferior tubercle of the clavicle, insert the needle attached to the syringe under the tubercle along the undersurface of the clavicle, directing it toward the suprasternal notch (Figure 63-1). If the patient is awake and cooperative, have him or her take a deep breath and hold it during needle insertion.

5. *While aspirating, advance the needle approximately 3 to 5 cm.

6. *When the vein has been located, detach the needle from the syringe and place a gloved finger over the hub to prevent the introduction of air.

7. *Gently insert the guide wire through the needle hub (see Figure 63-1).

8. *After the guide wire is in place, remove the needle and allow the wire to remain in the vein.

9. *Use the No. 11 blade to make a small nick in the skin where the wire enters (see Figure 63-1).

10. *Some kits contain a separate dilator, whereas others have the catheter and dilator joined together. If the dilator is separate, insert it into the hub and leave the wire in place.

11. *Insert the catheter over the wire, making sure to maintain control of the wire at all times.

12. *Once the catheter has been inserted, remove the wire and the dilator (if it is joined to the catheter).

13. *Aspirate and ascertain that there is good blood flow.

14. Draw the blood as needed for the laboratory evaluation.

---

*Indicates portions of the procedure usually performed by a physician or an advanced practice nurse.

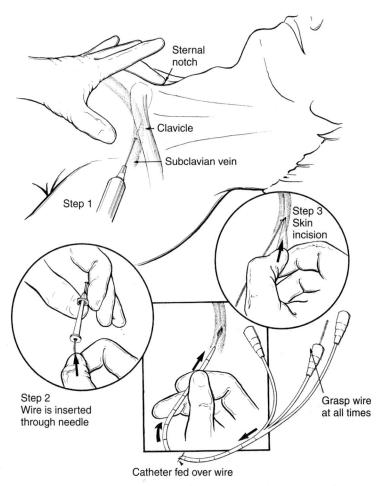

Sternal
notch

Clavicle

Subclavian vein

Step 1

Step 2
Wire is inserted
through needle

Step 3
Skin
incision

Catheter fed over wire

Grasp wire
at all times

FIGURE 63-1 Subclavian vein cannulation. (From Dunmire, S., & Paris, P. [1994]. *Atlas of emergency procedures* [p. 199]. Philadelphia: Saunders.)

15. Attach the catheter to the IV solution.
16. *Suture the catheter in place.
17. Apply a sterile gauze or transparent dressing and tape it to secure the catheter and the tubing (O'Grady et al., 2002).
18. Obtain a chest radiograph to verify the catheter placement and to rule out any postprocedural complications, such as a pneumothorax.
19. Attach the catheter to the monitoring device, that is, the CVP monitor (if indicated).

---

*Indicates portions of the procedure usually performed by a physician or an advanced practice nurse.

AGE-SPECIFIC CONSIDERATIONS

1. For a young child, an infraclavicular approach may be a good route because it allows the catheter to be secured comfortably to the chest wall (Buntain, 1995; Fernandez et al., 1997, Lozon, 2004). The landmarks for the infraclavicular approach are the bend of the clavicle and the suprasternal notch. The needle is inserted a few millimeters caudally and a few millimeters medially to the bend of the clavicle. The needle should be "walked" along the clavicle and kept parallel to the chest. The needle is advanced toward the suprasternal notch. When a blood return has been obtained, the procedure should be continued as previously described (Buntain, 1995; Lozon, 2004).
2. Complications related to central venous cannulation are more common in children than in adults; therefore, it is recommended that the procedure be performed or supervised by an experienced practitioner.
3. The femoral vein is the area of choice for placement of a central line in the pediatric patient (Fernandez et al., 1997; Lozon, 2004).
4. The size of the catheter is based on the child's age and weight (Evans & Bishop-Kurylo, 1996; Lozon, 2004):
   - Younger than 1 year and weight less than 10 kg: 3-Fr catheter
   - Aged 1 to 12 and weight 10 to 40 kg: 4-Fr catheter
   - Older than age 12 and weight more than 40 kg: 5- to 6-Fr catheter

COMPLICATIONS

1. Pneumothorax resulting from an overly acute angle of insertion
2. Insertion in the subclavian artery. In this event, remove the needle immediately and apply direct pressure.
3. Ventricular dysrhythmia as the result of insertion of the guide wire into the right ventricle
4. Air embolism as the result of not keeping the hub of the needle covered at all times (unless connected to the IV solution)
5. Guide wire embolism if the guide wire is not controlled during insertion
6. Hematoma formation from multiple attempts that may cause tracheal obstruction
7. Infection and phlebitis. Risk factors associated with the development of phlebitis include type of catheter, frequency of catheter manipulation, and patient-related factors (O'Grady et al., 2002).
8. Tracheal perforation and/or endotracheal cuff from needle insertion
9. Nerve injury to the phrenic or brachial nerves
10. Cerebral infarct from a clot related to insertion or an air embolism

PATIENT TEACHING

1. Report any chest pain or shortness of breath, as well as any disconnections or dampness around the dressing site.
2. Do not touch the area where the catheter has been inserted.

REFERENCES

American College of Surgeons (ACS). (2004). *Advanced trauma life support course for doctors* (7th ed.). Chicago: Author.

Buntain, W. (1995). *Management of pediatric trauma*. Philadelphia: Saunders.

Evans, T., & Bishop-Kurylo, D. (1996). Pediatric procedures. *Topics in Emergency Medicine, 18,* 30-45.

Fernandez, E., Sweeney, M., & Green, T. (1997). Central venous catheters. In R. Dieckmann, D. Fiser, & S. Selbst (Eds.), *Pediatric emergency and critical care procedures* (pp. 196-202). St. Louis: Mosby.

Fleck, D. (2005). Central venous catheter insertion (perform). In D. J. Lynn-McHale, & K. K. Carlson (Eds.), *AACN procedure manual for critical care* (5th ed., pp. 638-650). Philadelphia: Saunders.

Lozon, M. M. (2004). Pediatric vascular access and blood sampling techniques. In J. R. Roberts, & J. R. Hedges (Eds.), *Clinical procedures for emergency medicine* (4th ed., pp. 357-383). Philadelphia: Saunders.

Mickiewicz, M., Dronen, S., & Younger, J. (2004). Central venous catheterization and central venous pressure monitoring. In J. R. Roberts, & J. R. Hedges (Eds.), *Clinical procedures for emergency medicine* (4th ed., pp. 413-446). Philadelphia: Saunders.

O'Grady, N. P., Alexander, N. P., & Dellinger, E. P., et al. (2002). Guidelines for prevention of intravascular catheter-related infections. *Morbidity and Mortality Weekly Report, 51,* 1-28.

PROCEDURE 64

Internal Jugular Venous Access

Reneé Semonin Holleran, RN, PhD, CEN, CCRN, CFRN, CTRN, FAEN

INDICATIONS

1. To obtain central venous access when peripheral access is unattainable, such as occurs in a patient who is in profound shock or cardiac arrest or in a patient who is an intravenous (IV) drug abuser. There is a lower risk of pleural puncture when using the internal jugular (IJ) vein than when using the subclavian vein. In the obese or elderly patient, the IJ vein may afford easier access than the subclavian vein (Feldman, 2004).

2. To place a catheter to monitor central venous pressure.

3. To provide a site for insertion of a transvenous pacemaker or a pulmonary artery catheter.

4. To administer large amounts of fluid, blood products, or medications, especially those likely to cause complications if they are administered via a smaller peripheral vein.

5. Emergency venous access during CPR because the insertion location is out of the way and does not interfere with chest compressions (Mickiewicz, Dronen, & Younger, 2004).

CONTRAINDICATIONS AND CAUTIONS

1. This procedure is contraindicated in any patient with a potential cervical spine injury because positioning the patient for this procedure requires movement of the head.
2. Proceed with caution in the presence of an anatomic distortion (e.g., massive soft tissue injury) or patient habitus (obese, short neck) that interferes with the location of the anatomic landmarks.
3. A patient with a coagulopathy or at risk for coagulopathy, either from a disease process or from medication, must be monitored carefully for bleeding at the insertion site.
4. An infection in the area of the insertion precludes the use of that site.
5. If a hematoma develops on one side of the neck, insertion on the other side should be avoided or should be accomplished with extreme caution because of the potential for airway compromise if hematomas form bilaterally.
6. When selecting a site to insert a central line, several things should be considered, including selecting a site with the lowest risk of complications, anticipated duration of catheter placement, and type of fluids or medications that are to be administered through the device (McGee & Gould, 2003; O'Grady et al., 2002).

EQUIPMENT

Ultrasound equipment (optional)
Antiseptic solution
Local anesthetic
5-ml syringe; 18-, 25-, or 27-G needles for local anesthesia administration
Central venous kit (Most kits contain an 8.5-Fr introducer, which can be used for fluid-volume resuscitation or for the introduction of a transvenous pacemaker or a pulmonary-artery catheter.)
or
Multilumen catheter (used for fluid administration and allows insertion of invasive lines, transvenous pacemakers, as well as ports for administering medication and obtaining blood)
or
16-G, 8-in single-lumen catheter
No. 11 scalpel
Intravenous solution and tubing
Normal saline flush
Silk suture (2-0 or 3-0) with a needle holder
Masks, caps, goggles, sterile gloves, and gowns
Dressing supplies (gauze or a transparent dressing). (NOTE: When the patient is diaphoretic or the site is oozing, it should be covered with gauze instead of a transparent dressing [O'Grady et al, 2002].)

PATIENT PREPARATION

1. Place the patient on a cardiac monitor (Procedure 55) and pulse oximeter (Procedure 21).
2. Place the patient in a Trendelenburg position and turn the head away from the site of insertion. Placing a pillow or towel roll under the patient's shoulder can facilitate patient positioning. If the patient cannot tolerate the

Trendelenburg position, elevate the legs for a modified Trendelenburg position (Procedure 48). Turn the patient's head to the side opposite the insertion site.

3. *Cleanse the area of insertion with an antiseptic solution. The IJ vein runs posteriorly and laterally to the internal and common carotid artery. As the vein nears the thoracic area, it becomes more lateral and more anterior to the common carotid artery. Another landmark used for accessing the IJ vein is the sternocleidomastoid muscle. The IJ vein runs medially to this muscle in its upper part and then passes posteriorly to the inferior heads of the muscle in its midportion. Landmarks for the IJ vein are the angle of the mandible, the clavicle, the suprasternal notch, the external jugular vein and the carotid pulsation, the two heads of the sternocleidomastoid muscle, and the triangle formed by the two heads and the clavicle (Figure 64-1).

4. *Drape the patient's head with sterile towels.

PROCEDURAL STEPS

1. *Locate the landmarks of the IJ vein and infiltrate the area of insertion with a local anesthetic. Some research has demonstrated that the use of ultrasound guided IJ vein catheterization in the emergency department setting has been associated with a higher success rate and fewer complications (Leung, Duffy, & Finckh, 2006).

---

*Indicates portions of the procedure usually performed by a physician or an advanced practice nurse.

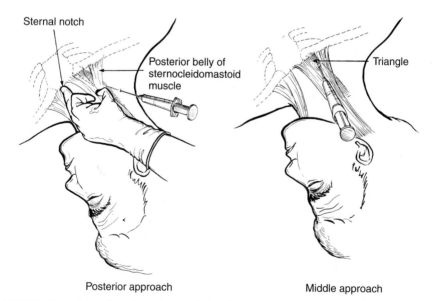

Sternal notch

Posterior belly of sternocleidomastoid muscle

Triangle

Posterior approach

Middle approach

FIGURE 64-1 Internal jugular vein cannulation. (From Dunmire, S., & Paris, P. [1994]. *Atlas of emergency procedures* [p. 201]. Philadelphia: Saunders.)

2. The three approaches to accessing the IJ vein are the middle, the anterior, and the posterior approaches. The posterior and middle approaches are the most commonly used and are described as follows (see Figure 64-1):
   a. *Middle approach:* Locate the triangle formed by the bifurcation of the sternocleidomastoid muscle and the clavicle. Attach the needle to a syringe and insert it at the apex of the triangle at a 30- to 45-degree angle to the skin. During insertion, the needle should be directed at the ipsilateral nipple. The needle should not be inserted farther than 5 cm. If the vein cannot be located immediately, the needle should be withdrawn and redirected just lateral to the ipsilateral nipple.
   b. *Posterior approach:* Locate the posterior border of the sternocleidomastoid muscle and insert the needle attached to a syringe under the posterior border, directing the needle toward the sternal notch. If the vein is not located after 4 to 6 cm of insertion, remove the needle and redirect it toward the contralateral nipple.
3. *Once the vein has been located, detach the syringe and place a gloved finger over the hub. Gently thread the guide wire through the hub of the needle. When the wire has been inserted 8 to 20 cm, remove the needle and leave the guide wire in place. Using the No. 11 blade, make a nick in the skin where the wire enters the skin. If there is a vein dilator, thread it over the wire to the hub and then remove the dilator, leaving the wire in place. Sometimes, the catheter and the dilator are inserted together over the wire. During insertion, always maintain control of the wire to prevent embolization into the circulation. Once the catheter is inserted, remove the wire and the dilator, if it is present. When the catheter is in place, confirm its location again by withdrawing some blood. Blood may also be drawn for a laboratory evaluation. If catheter patency is confirmed, connect it to the intravenous solution.
4. *Suture the catheter in place.
5. Apply a dressing and secure the catheter and the tubing with tape.
6. Obtain a chest radiograph to check the line placement and to rule out complications, such as a pneumothorax.

AGE-SPECIFIC CONSIDERATIONS

1. Only skilled personnel (or less-experienced providers under the direct supervision of a skilled clinician) can safely access the IJ vein in an infant or a young child (Lozon, 2004).
2. The right IJ vein is the preferred site for the pediatric patient because it has a lower risk of causing a pneumothorax or possible damage to the thoracic duct than does the left IJ vein. Accessing the right IJ vein in the pediatric patient increases the likelihood that the catheter may pass into the superior vena cava instead of the right subclavian vein (Lozon, 2004).

COMPLICATIONS

1. Pneumothorax

---

*Indicates portions of the procedure usually performed by a physician or an advanced practice nurse.

2. Hematoma formation from either a venous or an arterial bleed. If the carotid artery is nicked, apply direct pressure to control bleeding.
3. Air embolism resulting from the introduction of air into the catheter or guide-wire embolism if control of the wire is not maintained
4. Thoracic duct injury because of a perforation of the thoracic duct
5. Infection and phlebitis. Risk factors associated with the development of infection and phlebitis include type of catheter, frequency of catheter manipulation, and patient-related factors such diabetes and medication use (steroids) (McGee & Gould, 2003; O'Grady et al., 2002).

PATIENT TEACHING

1. Report any chest pain or shortness of breath or any disconnections or dampness around the dressing site immediately.
2. Do not touch the area where the catheter is inserted.
3. Report any signs of infection such as redness, swelling, or tenderness in the area where the catheter is inserted.

REFERENCES

Feldman, R. (2004). Central venous access. In E. F. Reichman, & R. R. Simon (Eds.), *Emergency medicine procedures* (pp. 314-337). New York: McGraw-Hill.

Leung, J., Duffy, M., & Finckh, A. (2006). Real-time ultrasonographically-guided internal jugular vein catheterization in the emergency department increases success rates and reduces complications: A randomized, prospective study. *Annals of Emergency Medicine, 48,* 540-547.

Lozon, M. M. (2004). Pediatric vascular access. In J. R. Roberts, & J. R. Hedges (Eds.), *Clinical procedures in emergency medicine* (4th ed., pp. 357-383). Philadelphia: Saunders.

McGee, D., & Gould, M. K. (2003). Preventing complications of central venous catheters. *New England Journal of Medicine, 348,* 1123-1133.

Mickiewicz, M., Dronen, S., & Younger, J. (2004). Central venous catheterization and central venous pressure monitoring. In J. R. Roberts, & J. R. Hedges (Eds.), *Clinical procedures in emergency medicine* (4th ed. pp. 413-446). Philadelphia: Saunders.

O'Grady, N. P., Alexander, M., & Dellinger, E. P., et al. (2002). Guidelines for prevention of intravascular catheter–related infections. *Morbidity and Mortality Weekly Report, 51,* 1-28.

Femoral Venous Access

Reneé Semonin Holleran, RN, PhD, CEN, CCRN, CFRN, CTRN, FAEN

INDICATIONS

1. To obtain vascular access for the administration of medications, intravenous (IV) fluids, and blood products.
2. To gain central-venous access during cardiopulmonary resuscitation (CPR) for rapid distribution of medications and/or fluids.
   NOTE: During CPR, venous return from below the diaphragm is diminished. For this reason, if the femoral site is used for access, the catheter should be long enough to pass above the level of the diaphragm, and large quantities of flush solution are recommended after IV medication.
3. To provide access for insertion of invasive devices, such as pulmonary artery catheters, transvenous pacemakers, hemodialysis catheters, and cardiac catheters.

CONTRAINDICATIONS AND CAUTIONS

1. Relative contraindications for femoral-access devices include an abnormal vascular anatomy of the lower extremities, congenital malformation of the lower extremity, femoral hernia, abdominal or pelvic tumor or trauma, abdominal ascites, and infection of the tissue overlying the puncture site (Lavelle & Costarino, 1997).
2. Caution should be exercised if a patient is receiving an anticoagulant or fibrinolytic therapy. In such a patient, femoral vein cannulation should be performed by using the single-wall puncture technique (Bodhey, Gupta, Sreedhar, & Manohar, 2006). The patient should be monitored continuously for excessive bleeding.

EQUIPMENT

Commercially available central line kit or assemble the following:
Polyurethane, radiopaque, indwelling catheter
   6- to 9-Fr catheter or a 10-cm-long catheter with or without side ports for infusions while monitoring central venous pressure
   14- to 18-G or 20-cm, single- or multiple-lumen catheters
Vessel dilator
J-tip spring-wire guide
Percutaneous entry needle (18 G, 7 cm)
10-ml syringe
Local anesthetic (e.g., lidocaine 1%)
Syringe and needles for local administration of anesthesia
Scalpel (No. 11 blade)
Needle holder

Suture scissors
Suture (2-0 silk or nylon)
Sterile gloves
Antiseptic solution
Saline flush
Dressing supplies (gauze or a transparent dressing) (NOTE: When the patient is diaphoretic or the site is oozing, it should be covered with gauze instead of a transparent dressing [O'Grady et al., 2002].)
Tape
IV solution and tubing
Blood-collection tubes

PATIENT PREPARATION

1. Place the patient in a flat, supine position with the legs fully extended.
2. Clip the hair around the insertion site as needed and cleanse the area with an antiseptic solution.

PROCEDURAL STEPS

1. *Locate the femoral artery (Figure 65-1, A) by palpating the pulsation 1 to 3 cm below the inguinal ligament, which runs from the anterosuperior iliac spine to the pubic tubercle. The femoral vein lies approximately 1 to 2 cm medial to the artery, along a parallel course. Easy location of the vein depends on the presence of a pulse in the femoral artery. During CPR, the arterial pulse may be weak or absent, but it may also be present in the femoral vein because of venous backflow during CPR. Therefore, unsuccessful attempts to cannulate the vein medial to the pulsations should lead to a more lateral approach.
2. *Infiltrate the insertion site with a local anesthetic by creating a linear intradermal wheal with a short needle. Once the dermal layer is anesthetized, make a small transverse skin puncture with a No. 11 scalpel. Replace the needle with a longer needle and continue to infiltrate the tissue with lidocaine to the periosteum.
3. *Attach a 10-ml syringe to the 18-G, 7-cm percutaneous entry needle and enter the insertion site at the transverse skin puncture. Approach the femoral vein at a 45- to 90-degree angle cephalad, and aspirate gently with the syringe while advancing. Once the wall of the vein is penetrated, blood should be aspirated freely.
   NOTE: After any unsuccessful attempts at venous wall puncture, apply pressure at the site for 5 minutes.
4. *If only blood samples are desired, aspirate the quantity needed and withdraw the needle. Apply pressure to the site for 5 minutes. Monitor the site frequently for continued bleeding.
5. *As soon as the blood is aspirated freely from the femoral vein, remove the syringe and place the J-tip spring wire through the needle into the vein. (Figure 65-1, *B*).

---

*Indicates portions of the procedure usually performed by a physician or an advanced practice nurse.

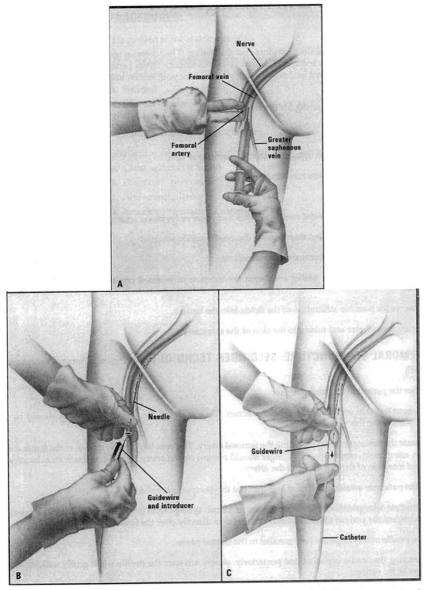

FIGURE 65-1 Cannulation of the femoral vein using a guidewire technique. See text for further information. (From American College of Surgeons. [2004]. *Advanced trauma life support* [7th ed., p. 90]. Chicago: Author.)

6. *Withdraw the needle while holding the J-wire firmly with the left hand to ensure that it remains in the vein. After the needle is removed, wipe the protruding wire with a moistened gauze pad to remove clotted blood and facilitate the advancement of the dilator or catheter.
7. *Thread the catheter or the dilator-catheter over the J-wire into the vein (Figure 65-1, C). Advance the dilator-catheter until it is seated at the hub. Remove the J-wire and then the dilator, if used. Aspirate the blood via the catheter to remove any air bubbles. Attach the primed IV tubing and the solution to the catheter.
8. The IV fluid should flow freely. The catheter position in the vein can be verified by withdrawing the blood or lowering the IV bag below the level of the entrance site and noting the blood reflux into the IV tubing.
9. *Secure the catheter to the skin. This is generally accomplished by suturing the catheter hub to the patient's skin.
10. Apply a dressing to the site.

AGE-SPECIFIC CONSIDERATIONS
1. For pediatric patients, slightly rotate the leg externally (Lozon, 2004).
2. For children, the femoral site is the first choice for emergency placement of a central venous catheter because the anatomic landmarks are easily identifiable, hemostatic pressure can be applied easily in the event of bleeding at the site, and there is no interference with airway management or chest compressions (Lavelle & Costarino, 1997).

COMPLICATIONS
1. Hematoma at the puncture site of the vein or femoral artery
2. Arteriovenous fistula
3. Inadvertent cannulation of the femoral artery
4. Infection and phlebitis. Risk factors associated with the development of infection and phlebitis include type of catheter, frequency of catheter manipulation, and patient-related factors (O'Grady et al., 2002).
5. Thrombosis
6. Injury to the femoral nerve

PATIENT TEACHING
1. Avoid flexion of the affected leg.
2. Report any wetness felt at the site or any blood on the dressing.
3. Report any pain, numbness, or tingling in the leg.

---

*Indicates portions of the procedure usually performed by a physician or an advanced practice nurse.

REFERENCES
Bodhey, N. K., Gupta, A. K., Sreedhar, R., & Manohar, S. R. (2006). Retroperitoneal hematoma: An unusual complication after femoral vein cannulation. *Journal of Cardiothoracic and Vascular Anesthesia, 20,* 859-861.
Lavelle, J., & Costarino, A. Jr. (1997). Central venous access. In F. M. Henretig, & C. King (Eds.), *Textbook of pediatric emergency procedures* (pp. 251-277). Baltimore: Williams & Wilkins.

Lozon, M. M. (2004). Pediatric vascular access and blood sampling techniques. In J. R. Roberts, & J. R. Hedges (Eds.), *Clinical procedures in emergency medicine* (4th ed. pp. 357-383). Philadelphia: Saunders.

O'Grady, N. P., Alexander, M., & Dellinger, E. P., et al. (2002). Guidelines for prevention of intravascular catheter–related infections. *Morbidity and Mortality Weekly Report, 51*, 1-28.

PROCEDURE 66

Venous Cutdown

Reneé Semonin Holleran, RN, PhD, CEN, CCRN, CFRN, CTRN, FAEN

INDICATION

To provide venous access when other sites are either unavailable or inadequate.

CONTRAINDICATIONS AND CAUTIONS

1. Venous access via cutdown may be more time consuming than percutaneous central venous access; other types of venous access should be considered before a venous cutdown is performed.
2. This procedure is contraindicated in patients who have injury proximal to the cutdown site (ACS, 2004).
3. The presence of a coagulapthy is a contraindication (ACS, 2004).

EQUIPMENT

Intravenous (IV) setup (fluid and tubing)
T-piece or short extension set
Intravenous catheter
Antiseptic solution
Tourniquet (optional)
Local anesthetic
Syringe and needles for local anesthetic administration
Scapel with No. 11 blade
Tissue scissors (iris or Metzenbaum)
Tissue forceps
Vein retractor
Hemostats
Needle holder
Plastic catheter introducer or lifter
4-0 Silk suture

4-0 Nylon suture on cutting needle
Dressing supplies (gauze or transparent)
Antibiotic ointment
(NOTE: Most facilities have prepackaged venous cutdown trays with much of
    this equipment already assembled.)

PATIENT PREPARATION

1. Assemble the IV solution and tubing. Prime the T-piece with the saline solution and leave a syringe of saline attached.
2. Place the chosen extremity in an extended position. The sites most commonly used are the saphenous vein (just anterior and superior to the medial malleolus of the tibia or superficial and medial to the femoral artery and vein in the groin) or the basilic vein (medial aspect of antecubital fossa). The cephalic vein (lateral aspect of the antecubital fossa) can also be used, but passing a catheter through the sharp angulation where the vein enters the axillary vein makes this route difficult if central access is desired (Dronen & Lanter, 2004).
3. Place a venous tourniquet proximally if a distal extremity site is chosen (optional).

PROCEDURAL STEPS

1. Cleanse the site with an antiseptic solution and then drape it.
2. *Infiltrate the area over the vein with a local anesthetic for patient comfort.
3. *Make a transverse skin incision over the vein (Figure 66-1).

---

*Indicates portions of the procedure usually performed by a physician or an advanced practice nurse.

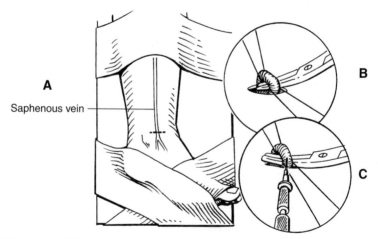

FIGURE 66-1 **A,** Make a transverse incision over the distal saphenous vein. **B,** Use silk ligatures to isolate and expose the vein. **C,** Cannulate the exposed vein. (From Krug, S. [1997]. Venous cutdown. In M. C. Walsh-Sukys & S. E. Krug, [Eds.], *Procedures in infants and children* [p. 96]. Philadelphia: Saunders.)

4. *Dissect bluntly down to the vein.
5. *Isolate the vein with silk ligatures proximally and distally.
6. *Tie the distal ligature.
7. *Make a small incision into the vein between the ligatures and insert the catheter toward the heart. A catheter introducer may facilitate this procedure. Alternatively, cannulate the vein with an over-the-needle or through-the-needle catheter (ACS, 2004)
8. Remove the tourniquet (if used).
9. Connect the primed T-piece and syringe assembly to the catheter and aspirate to confirm the placement. Flush the tubing with saline, disconnect the syringe, and connect the IV tubing to the T-piece.
10. *Tie the proximal ligature to secure the catheter in place.
11. *Suture the skin around the catheter and suture the catheter in place.
12. Apply a dressing.
13. Tape the tubing securely.
14. Observe the patient closely for signs of swelling from a hematoma formation or a fluid infiltration.

AGE-SPECIFIC CONSIDERATION

For children, the saphenous vein at the ankle is the preferred peripheral cutdown site, and the saphenous vein at the groin is the preferred central cutdown site (ACS, 2004).

COMPLICATIONS

1. Blood loss
2. Inadvertent "cannulation" of a tendon or an artery, or false passage of the catheter between layers of the vessel wall
3. Loosening of ligatures with resultant bleeding and hematoma formation
4. Embolization
5. Infiltration of IV fluid
6. Thrombophlebitis
7. Infection and sepsis
8. Injury to adjacent nerves and arteries

PATIENT TEACHING

1. Do not manipulate or move the catheter.
2. Report any disconnections or dampness at the site immediately.

---

*Indicates portions of the procedure usually performed by a physician or an advanced practice nurse.

REFERENCES

American College of Surgeons (ACS). (2004). *Advanced trauma life support for doctors* (7th ed.). Chicago: Author.
Dronen, S., & Lanter, P. (2004). Venous cutdown. In J. R. Roberts, & J. R. Hedges (Eds.), *Clinical procedures in emergency medicine* (4th ed., pp. 447-456). Philadelphia: Saunders.

Intraosseous Access

Reneé Semonin Holleran, RN, PhD, CEN, CCRN, CFRN, CTRN, FAEN

INDICATIONS

To gain rapid access to the circulation for administering fluids or medications. Intraosseous (IO) infusion should be initiated any time intravenous (IV) cannulation is either too difficult or too time consuming to accomplish. IO needles are recommended for resuscitation in any age group (AHA, 2005). Some specific indications include the following:

1. Administration of crystalloids, colloids, or blood for resuscitation of patients in shock states. However, flow rates may not be sufficient to fully treat severe hypovolemia or hemorrhagic shock.
2. Administration of medications.
3. Specimens for diagnostic studies, such as electrolytes, blood cultures, blood gases, and hemoglobin, may be obtained through the IO route, although these studies are not primary indications for this procedure.
4. Used by the military for special operations where conditions make obtaining IV access difficult.
5. May be used to deliver anesthesia, particularly for short dental procedures.

CONTRAINDICATIONS AND CAUTIONS

1. IO needle insertion is not recommended in fractured extremities because of the risk of fluid and medication infiltration into the surrounding tissue.
2. Avoid placing the IO line through burned or infected tissue to decrease the risk of infection.
3. General contraindications may include patients who have bone disorders, such as osteoporosis and osteogenesis imperfecta.
4. Avoid placing the needle in a site where there is obvious soft tissue infection.
5. Do not infuse marrow-toxic medications (e.g., certain antibiotics) via the IO route.

EQUIPMENT

Antiseptic solution

Local anesthetic (optional, but should be used if the patient is conscious)

Several large-bore (18-G or larger) IO needles (Figures 67-1 and 67-2); products that are commonly available include the following:

Jamshidi Illinois sternal (Baxter Healthcare): 15- to 18-G, adjustable plastic sleeve to control depth of penetration.

Cook IO needle (Cook Critical Care): 16- to 18-G, relatively large, round, detachable handles; various tips include bevel, pencil-point tip, and 45-degree trocar.

Sur-Fast (Cook Critical Care): Threaded shaft to assist in more secure needle placement.

B.I.G. bone injection gun (WaisMed, 2000): Available in two sizes: a blue case for the 15-G needle (adults and children older than age 12) and a red case for the 18-G needle (children up to age 12). This device is a triggered mechanism, which inserts a trocar needle into the bone.

F.A.S.T. IO infusion system (Pyng Medical Corp., 2001): An adult IO needle that is inserted in the sternum. Each kit contains a 16-G introducer with depth control, an infusion tube, a protector dome, target/strain-relief patch, and a remover.

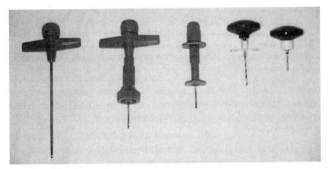

FIGURE 67-1 Types of intraosseous needles. (From Stanley, R. [2004]. Intraosseous infusion. In J. R. Roberts & J. R. Hedges [Eds.], *Clinical procedures in emergency medicine* (4th ed., p. 478]. Philadelphia: Saunders.)

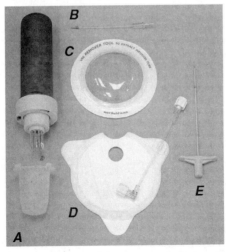

FIGURE 67-2 The F.A.S.T. intraosseous infusion system. **A,** Introducer with depth control. **B,** Infusion tube. **C,** Protector dome. **D,** Target/strain-relief patch. **E,** Remover. (Courtesy the Pyng Medical Corp., Richmond, BC.)

EZ-IO (*Vidacare, 2007*): A battery-powered device that penetrates the bone with a beveled, hollow drill tipped needle. Available for adult (over 40 kg) and pediatric patients (3-39 kg).

Syringe for aspiration

Normal saline solution for irrigation

Tape, an arm or leg board, or hemostats, for stabilization of the needle

Dressing supplies

IV tubing and a fluid bag or bottle

Pressure infusion bag

PROCEDURAL STEPS
Insertion

1. Select the potential site for the infusion. Consider the patient's age, size, site accessibility, and any other procedures that may be needed. The tibial plateau (approximately 1 cm below the tibial tuberosity and medially on the tibial plateau) is the most popular and common site for insertion of the needle (AHA, 2006) (Figure 67-3). This location is preferred because it is a relatively flat surface and there is very little overlying soft tissue, which facilitates stabilizing the needle. The medial malleolus site (approximately 2 cm proximal to the tip of the medial malleolus) may also be used, although it may be more difficult to stabilize the needle over the rounded bony prominences. The distal femur and the iliac crest are occasionally used, but they may be more difficult to access because of greater amounts of overlying tissue and rounded bone. The needle should be inserted 2 to 3 cm above the femoral condyles at an angle of 10 to 15 degrees from the vertical position (Stanley, 2004). In the adult patient, the manubrium on the midline and 1.5 cm (⅝ inch) below the sternal notch can be accessed for IO insertion with a specifically designed device. Two additional access sites include the posterior-distal metaphysis of the radius opposite the radial pulse and the anterior head of the humerus.
2. Position the patient (depending on the site of the insertion) and stabilize the area for insertion.
3. Cleanse the area with an antiseptic solution.
4. Anesthetize the area (this is not necessary in moribund or obtunded patients).

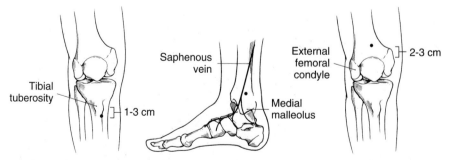

FIGURE 67-3 Examples of insertion sites for intraosseous needles. (From Stanley, R. [2004]. Intraosseous infusion. In J. R. Roberts & J. R. Hedges [Eds.], *Clinical procedures in emergency medicine* (4th ed., p. 479]. Philadelphia: Saunders.)

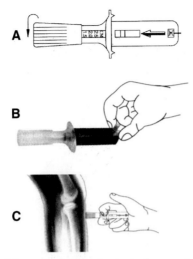

FIGURE 67-4 Insertion of the B.I.G. **A,** Adjust the depth of penetration. **B,** Pull out the safety latch. **C,** Trigger the device by pressing the rear part against the shoulder of the housing. (Courtesy WaisMed Ltd., Kress USA Corp., Overland Park, KS.)

5. Insert the needle.
   a. *Manual insertion:* With the needle pointed slightly away from the joint or at a 90-degree angle (Stanley, 2004), puncture the skin, and use a rotary motion to push the needle into the bony cortex. Feel for a "pop." The needle should feel firm in the bone but not stable.
   b. *Bone injection gun (B.I.G.)* (WaisMed, 2000) (Figure 67-4): Adjust the depth of penetration by unscrewing the sleeve from the cylindrical housing. Squeeze the sides of the safety latch together and remove it. Place the device against the insertion site and hold it firmly against the extremity while triggering it. The kickback of the device can push your hand back and prevent the needle from entering the bone if you do not hold it firmly enough. Trigger the device by pushing the rear part against the two shoulders of the housing. Remove the B.I.G. and separate the trocar needle from its housing.
   c. *F.A.S.T.* (Pyng Medical Corp., 2001) (Figure 67-5): Locate the patient's manubrium and place the target patch (Figure 67-5, *A*). Place the introducer in the target zone on the patch, perpendicular to the skin (Figure 67-5, *B*). Push on the introducer and then pull it straight back. This will expose the infusion tube and a two-part support sleeve (Figure 67-5, *C*), which will fall away. Correct placement is verified by observation of marrow entering the infusion tube. Connect the IV to the infusion tube. Place the protective dome over the site and press down firmly over the target patch to engage the Velcro fastening. This prevents the needle from moving. A remover must be used must be disengage the infusion tube from the bone.

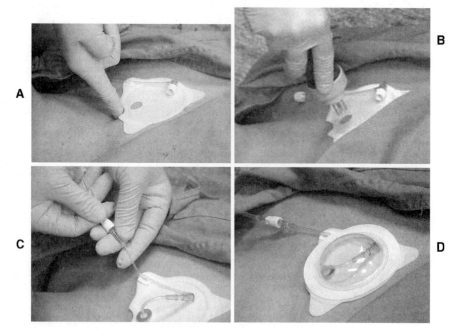

FIGURE 67-5 Insertion of the F.A.S.T. intraosseous infusion system. (Courtesy Pyng Medical Corp., Richmond, BC.)

  d. *EZ-IO* (Vidacare, Inc., 2007) (Figure 67-6): Locate the anatomical landmarks. Clean the insertion site and administer anesthesia if needed. Prepare the EZ-IO Driver and Needle Set (Figures 67-6). Begin insertion of the EZ-IO. Position the driver at the insertion site with the needle at a 90-degree angle to the surface of the bone. Power the needle through the skin until the bone is felt. Apply steady and firm pressure on the driver until into the bone. Stop when the needle flange touches the skin or a sudden decrease in resistance. Remove the driver from the needle set. If the patient is conscious, administer 10 ml of 1% lidocaine directly into the IO needle over 30-45 seconds while supporting the hub. Then, carefully remove the syringe while supporting the hub and attach the EZ-Connect tubing. Allow the lidocaine to remain in the medullary space for about 30 seconds and then administer a 10 ml saline bolus through the EZ-Connect tubing to open up the medullary space (M. Moss, personal communication, 9/28/2007). Note that because of the risk of dislodging the needle, the lidocaine bolus just described is the only time the manufacturer recommends attaching a syringe directly to the needle.

6. Remove the stylet and confirm the placement by aspirating the blood or the marrow contents (except for the EZ-IO) or irrigating with a normal saline solution. In addition, the IV fluid should run steadily. Remember that laboratory tests can be obtained from the bone marrow, if needed. Radiographic films may also be used to confirm placement.

To Insert Needle Set:

1. Protect yourself (BSI)
2. Identify indication
3. Check for contraindication
4. Locate landmarks **A***
5. Clean site **B**
6. Prepare driver and needle set
7. Stabilize leg
8. Insert EZ-I0® needle set **C**
* multiple sites available

9. Remove driver from needle set
10. Remove stylet from catheter **D**
11. Confirm placement
12. Attach EZ-Connect™
13. Inject I0 20-40 mg of 2% Lidocaine in alert patients
14. Syringe bolus (flush) I0 with 10 mL NS **E**
15. Start infusion under pressure **F**
16. Secure tubing and catheter

Do Not Leave the EZ-I0 catheter in for more than 24 hours

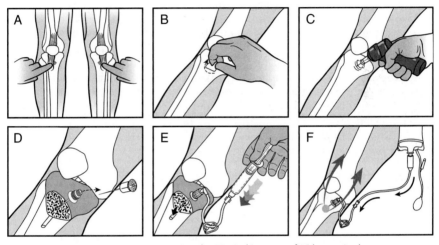

FIGURE 67-6 Insertion the EZ-I0. (Courtesy of Vidacare, Inc.)

7. Connect the syringe or the IV tubing. Administer fluids under pressure for maximum flow rate.
8. Apply a sterile dressing and stabilize the needle and the tubing. Stabilize site with tape and dressings or hemostats. If the B.I.G. is used, the safety latch can be placed around the needle to provide additional stabilization. If the F.A.S.T. is used, a protector dome is supplied for stability. A small plastic cup can be placed over the needle to provide further protection against dislodgment.
9. If the EZ-IO is used, apply a wrist band and a dressing. The wristband serves a reminder of EZ-IO placement and need for timely removal.
10. Monitor patency of the IO device.

Removal

It is important to know how to remove an IO needle once it has been inserted. The manufacturers of the needles do supply educational materials, including posters that demonstrate how to remove each of the products. The following is a summary of the removal of the F.A.S.T. Needle and the EZ-IO.

Removal of the F.A.S.T. needle

1. Obtain the remover that comes in the kit. If the remover has been lost or is not available, open another kit or contact the provider who placed the needle so that a remover can be obtained. Separately packaged removers are available and may be stocked in the event this occurs.
2. Remove the dome that covers the needle while holding the patch against the patient's skin.
3. Disconnect the infusion tube; ensure the IV flow is turned off.
4. Insert the remover in the tubing while holding the infusion tube perpendicular to the patient. *If no remover is available, make an incision next to the introducer and grasp it with a hemostat to pull it out of the bone. Do not pull on the tubing that is exiting the skin because it may separate from the introducer.
5. Advance the remover, and turn it clockwise until the remover stops; this engages the thread into the metal (proximal) tip of the infusion tube.
6. Remove the infusion tube. *Do not pull* on the luer connector or tubing. Hold the remover using the T-shaped knob, and pull straight out, perpendicular to the infusion site, while holding down the target patch.
7. Remove the target patch.
8. Dress the infusion site using aseptic technique.

Removal of the EZ-IO

1. Stabilize the patient's extremity.
2. Connect a sterile Luer-Lok syringe to the hub of the catheter.
3. Rotate the catheter clockwise while gently pulling.
4. When the catheter has been removed, place it in an appropriate container.
5. Apply a dressing to the area using aseptic technique.

AGE-SPECIFIC CONSIDERATIONS

1. IO access is widely recommended for use in the pediatric population (AHA, 2006), and it is now recommended in the management of adult patients who are critically ill (Frascone, Dries, Gisch, Kaye, & Jensen, 2001; Stanley, 2004; Waisman & Waisman, 1997).
2. The F.A.S.T. (sternal site) is contraindicated in pediatric patients.
3. The lower femur can be used safely only in small infants (Krug, 1997).
4. Adult patients with sternal trauma or chest deformities should not have a sternal IO line placed.
5. IO line placement in adult patients may be difficult because of the thickness of the bony cortex.
6. The EZ-IO can be placed in either pediatric or adult patients.

COMPLICATIONS

1. Unsuccessfully attempting to penetrate the bony cortex or bending the needle by use of excessive force delays vascular access (Figure 67-7).

---

*Indicates portions of the procedure usually performed by a physician or an advanced practice nurse.

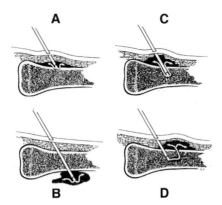

FIGURE 67-7   Placement should be carefully assessed to avoid leakage of fluid around the insertion site. **A,** Incomplete penetration of the bony cortex. **B,** Penetration of the posterior cortex. **C,** Fluid escaping around the needle through the puncture site. **D,** Fluid leaking through a nearby previous puncture site. (From Stanley, R. [2004]. Intraosseous infusion. In J. R. Roberts & J. R. Hedges [Eds.], *Clinical procedures in emergency medicine* [4th ed., p. 483]. Philadelphia: Saunders.)

2. Puncture of the posterior cortex as a result of excessive pressure during the insertion of the needle (see Figure 67-7).
3. Fluid leakage from the infusion site. Fluid extravasation may occur, especially if the insertion was difficult or both cortices were penetrated (see Figure 67-7). This fluid extravasation may lead to compartment syndrome.
4. Fat embolism resulting from use of high-pressure volume infusions (Iserson & Criss, 1986; O'Neill, 1945).
5. Potential osteomyelitis, which appears to be associated with prolonged continuous infusions (Heinild, Sondergaard, & Tudvad, 1947).
6. Clot formation within the bone marrow needle, causing slowing of the rate of infusion. The use of a pressure bag often alleviates this problem.
7. Tibial fractures

REFERENCES

American Heart Association (AHA). (2005). American Heart Association guidelines for cardiopulmonary resuscitation and emergency cardiovascular care. *Circulation, 112*(Suppl. IV). Available at www.circulationaha.org

American Heart Association (AHA). (2006). *Pediatric advanced life support.* Dallas: Author.

Frascone, R., Dries, D., Gisch, T., Kaye, K., & Jensen, J. (2001). Obtaining vascular access: Is there a place for the sternal IO? *Air Medical Journal, 20*(6), 20-22.

Heinild, S., Sondergaard, T., & Tudvad, F. (1947). Bone marrow infusion in childhood. *Journal of Pediatrics, 30,* 400-412.

Iserson, K. V., & Criss, E. (1986). Intraosseous infusions: A usable technique. *American Journal of Emergency Medicine, 4,* 540.

Krug, S. (1997). Intraosseous infusion. In M. C. Walsh-Sukys, & S. Krug (Eds.), *Procedures in infants and children* (pp. 134-139). Philadelphia: Saunders.

O'Neill, J. F. (1945). Complications of intraosseous therapy. *Annals of Surgery, 2,* 266.

Pyng Medical Corp. (2001). *F.A.S.T.*^{TM} *intraosseous infusion system with depth control (product brochure)*. Richmond, BC: Author. Available at http://www.pyng.com/.

Stanley, R. (2004). Intraosseous infusion. In J. R. Roberts, & J. R. Hedges (Eds.), *Clinical procedures in emergency medicine* (4th ed., pp. 475-485). Philadelphia: Saunders.

Waisman, M., & Waisman, D. (1997). Bone marrow infusion in adults. *Journal of Trauma, 42,* 288-293.

WaisMed, Ltd. (2007). *Bone injection gun (B.I.G.*^{TM}*) instructions*. Retrieved February 11, 2007, from http://www.waismed.com/

Vidacare, Inc. (2007). *EZ-IO instructions*. San Antonio, TX: Author. Retrieved February 11, 2007, from http://www.vidacare.com

PROCEDURE 68

Umbilical Vessel Cannulation

Tamara Bleak, RN, BSN

Umbilical lines are commonly used for vascular access in the critically ill neonate. The umbilical vein (UV) is larger and easier to access than the umbilical artery (UA) and is the first choice of access in emergency situations. If the practitioner is placing both a UA and a UV line, it is suggested that the UA line be placed first to increase the likelihood of success.

UMBILICAL ARTERY CATHETERIZATION
Indications

1. Frequent monitoring of arterial blood gases.
2. Continuous monitoring of arterial blood pressure.
3. Emergency resuscitation (UV line may be first choice).
4. Administration of fluids and medications.

Contraindications and Cautions

1. Contraindications to UA catheterization include omphalocele, necrotizing enterocolitis, omphalitis, peritonitis, acute abdominal etiology, or local vascular compromise in lower limbs or buttock area.
2. Do not force the catheter past an obstruction.
3. Do not advance the catheter once it has been placed and secured and the sterile field has been broken.

4. Obtain radiographic confirmation of catheter position before starting an infusion.

Equipment

Cap, mask, surgical gown, and gloves

Umbilical catheter with Luer-lok connection if possible. If no Luer lok catheter is available, a blunt-end needle may be used to connect catheter to stopcock. In general, catheter size guidelines are as follows (MacDonald, 2002a):

- 3.5 Fr for an infant weighing less than 1200 g
- 5 Fr for an infant weighing more than 1200 g

3-way stopcock with Luer-lok connections

10-ml syringe of either normal saline or normal saline with 1 unit of heparin/ml

Antiseptic solution

4 × 4 gauze sponges

Sterile drapes

Umbilical tape

Two curved mosquito hemostats

Scalpel (No. 11 blade) with handle

Two curved nontoothed iris forceps

Toothed forceps

Needle holder

Suture material on curved needle for securing catheter (4-0 silk or equivalent material)

Scissors

Tape to secure catheter

Soft limb restraints

Radiant warmer or other method to keep patient warm

(NOTE: Preassembled kits containing some of this equipment may be available.)

Patient Preparation

1. Place infant on radiant warmer.
2. Restrain extremities, check for adequate circulation throughout procedure.
3. Assemble the catheter and stopcock and prime with saline flush solution, leaving the flush syringe attached. If the catheter does not have a Luer-lok connector, you may cut the flared end of the catheter with scissors and insert an appropriately sized blunt-end needle to ensure a secure fit.
4. There are two recognized locations for UA placement. The recommended placement is high, between T6 and T9 (Barrington, 1999). However, low placement can be used if necessary. If the high position is not achieved, the catheter can also be withdrawn to the low position. Calculate the length of catheter to insert to achieve the desired catheter position (Shukla, Ped, & Ferrara, 1986):
   a. High line: T6 to T9
      i. UA catheter length (cm) = $[3 \times \text{body weight (kg)}] + 9$
   b. Low line: L3 to L4
      i. UA catheter length (cm) = body weight (kg) + 7

Procedural Steps

1. Prep the cord and surrounding abdominal wall with antiseptic solution. If the cord is long or still has a cord clamp attached, have a nonsterile assistant hold the cord out of the sterile field while it is prepped.
2. *Drape the area surrounding the cord in a sterile fashion.
3. *Place an umbilical tie loosely around the stump to control bleeding.
4. *If necessary to remove a cord clamp, cut the cord horizontally approximately 1 to 1.5 cm from skin with a scalpel inferior to the clamp.
5. Cannulate the vessel.
   a. Conventional method (transection of the artery)
      i. *Tighten the umbilical tape as needed to control bleeding.
      ii. *Identify the cord vessels (MacDonald, 2002a) (Figure 68-1). "The vein is usually a large, thin-walled, sometimes-gaping vessel that is easiest to identify at the 12 o'clock position. The arteries are smaller, white, and have a thicker lumen than veins. They may protrude slightly from cut surface" (MacDonald, 2002a).
      iii. *Using toothed forceps, grasp the cord stump close to the artery to be catheterized.
      iv. *Clamp two curved hemostats on each side of the cord to the Wharton's jelly. Everting the edges can sometimes help to expose the arteries and stabilize the cord. An assistant may be helpful.
      v. *Use one tip of the open, curved iris forceps and gently dilate the artery (Figure 68-2).
      vi. *Remove the forceps. Using both points of the closed forceps, introduce them into the lumen dilating the artery gently to a depth of 1 cm. Allow the forceps to open gently (Figure 68-3).
      vii. *Maintain forceps in this position for 15 to 30 seconds to dilate the vessel. Spending adequate time to ensure dilatation of the artery before catheter insertion greatly improves the chances of success (MacDonald, 2002a).
      viii. *Keeping curved iris forceps in the artery, grasp the catheter 1 cm from the tip with the curved iris forceps.
      ix. *Insert the catheter into the lumen of the artery between the prongs of the dilating forceps (Figure 68-4). Resistance is occasionally felt at 1 to 2 cm at the umbilical ring. Use gentle sustained pressure to bypass this ring. The umbilical tie may also need to be loosened. Do not force the catheter to advance.
      x. *After passing the catheter 5 cm, aspirate to verify intraluminal position. Blood should appear; if not, the catheter may be extraluminal. Clear the blood by injecting 0.5 ml of flush solution (MacDonald, 2002a).
      xi. Watch the blood–fluid interface for pulsation, which indicates arterial placement.
   b. Side-entry method (lateral arteriotomy)
   An alternative approach to the conventional method is a lateral arteriotomy (Bloom, Nelson, & Dirksen, 1986). Lateral arteriotomy is described as the

---

*Indicates portions of the procedure usually performed by a physician or are advanced practice nurse.

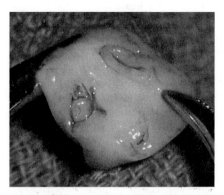

FIGURE 68-1 Vessels of the umbilical cord. The vein is thin walled and at the 12 o'clock position. The two arteries are smaller with thicker walls. (Photograph courtesy of Tamara Bleak.)

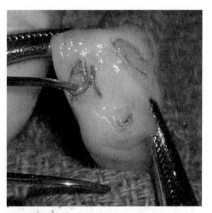

FIGURE 68-2 Using one tip of open curved forceps, gently probe to depth of 0.5 cm. (Photograph courtesy of Tamara Bleak.)

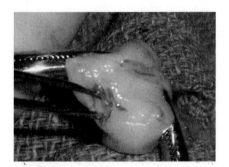

FIGURE 68-3 Allow the forceps to gently open and maintain this position for 15 to 30 seconds. (Photograph courtesy of Tamara Bleak.)

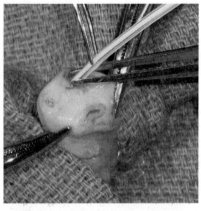

FIGURE 68-4 Using forceps, insert the catheter into the lumen of the artery between prongs of dilating forceps. (Photograph courtesy of Tamara Bleak.)

side-entry method and reported to be a more efficient method with less blood loss (Squire, Hornung, & Kirchhoff, 1990). This method requires a length of cord so the cord can be rolled over the mosquito clamp (Bloom et al., 1986; Squire et al., 1990).

   i. *Clamp the cord with mosquito hemostats horizontally approximately 2 cm above the skin with the nondominant hand.

   ii. *Firmly pull the cord toward the infant's head. This will cause traction on the arteries and immobilize them. The arteries are usually located in the 4-to-5 and 7-to-8 o'clock positions.

   iii. *Roll the cord 180 degrees over the hemostat toward abdominal wall.

   iv. *Approximately 1 cm up the cord from the abdominal wall, carefully incise down to an artery wall using a No. 11 scalpel blade (Figure 68-5).

   v. *Incise the artery halfway (Figure 68-6). The artery should remain stable with the traction held by the hemostat.

   vi. *A small drop of blood may appear on the artery where it has been partially incised. If necessary, use one tip of the open curved iris forceps to gently dilate artery. Insert both tips of the iris forceps in the closed position and dilate the artery by allowing the forceps to open gently (Figure 68-7).

   vii. *Insert the catheter into the lumen of the artery at a perpendicular angle to the artery wall; then direct it in a caudal direction (Figures 68-8 and 68-9).

6. *Advance the catheter to the desired distance as calculated previously.

7. *Secure the catheter by placing an anchor stitch in the substance of the cord while avoiding the other vessels in the cord and the skin. Tie the suture around the catheter to make sure it cannot move.

8. Loosen, do not remove, the umbilical tie so it can be retightened quickly in case of bleeding. If no bleeding occurs, the tie can be removed.

9. Secure to the catheter in a flat fashion to the abdomen with tape.

10. Obtain a radiograph for verification of placement.

Complications

1. Infection
2. Hemorrhage
3. Vasospasm
4. Perforation of vessel creating a false track within the artery or abdomen
5. Ischemia or infarction of lower extremities, bowel, or kidney
6. Air embolus

UMBILICAL VEIN CATHETERIZATION
Indications

1. Vascular access for emergency fluid and medication administration and laboratory sampling.
2. Central venous pressure monitoring.
3. Exchange transfusion.

---

*Indicates portions of the procedure usually performed by a physician or an advanced practice nurse.

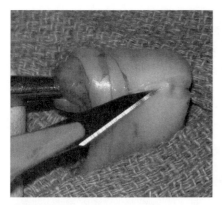

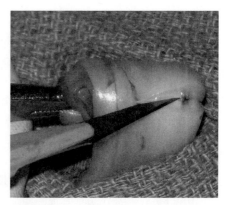

FIGURE 68-5 The umbilical cord is incised to the arterial wall. (Photograph courtesy of Tamara Bleak.)

FIGURE 68-6 The artery is incised halfway. Turn the scalpel over so the cutting side is away from the cord. Puncture the artery halfway through; pull the scalpel blade away from the cord. (Photograph courtesy of Tamara Bleak.)

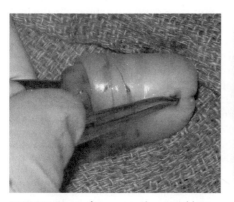

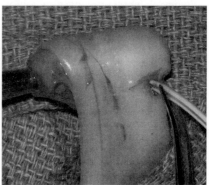

FIGURE 68-7 If necessary, the arterial lumen is dilated with iris forceps. (Photograph courtesy of Tamara Bleak.)

FIGURE 68-8 Place catheter into dilated lumen at a perpendicular angle. (Photograph courtesy of Tamara Bleak.)

Contraindications and Cautions

1. Contraindications for UV catheterization include omphalitis, omphalocele, necrotizing enterocolitis, and peritonitis.
2. It may not be possible to advance the catheter through the ductus venosus. Avoid vigorous attempts to advance the catheter.
3. Avoid hypertonic solutions when catheter tip is intrahepatic.
4. Do not advance catheter farther once it has been placed and secured and the sterile field has been broken.

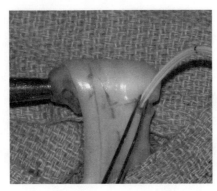

FIGURE 68-9 Advance catheter in a caudal direction. (Photograph courtesy of Tamara Bleak.)

5. Do not leave the catheter open to the atmosphere as there is a danger of air embolism (MacDonald, 2002b).
6. Obtain radiographic confirmation of catheter position before starting infusions. In an emergency, a radiograph is not needed if the catheter is in the low lying position.

Equipment

The equipment is the same as for UA catheter placement listed above with the following guidelines for umbilical catheter size:
- 5 Fr for most infants
- 3.5 Fr may be necessary for infants less than 1000 g

Patient Preparation

1. Prepare for the procedure as described for UA catheter insertion above.
2. Calculate the length of catheter to insert to achieve the desired catheter position (Shukla, Ped, & Ferrara, 1986). A low line is used if nonhypertonic solutions or resuscitation medications must be given quickly and there is no time confirm placement with a radiograph. If there is time for radiographic confirmation of placement, the preferred placement is high.
   a. Low line for resuscitation: advance 1 to 2 cm beyond the point at which good blood return is obtained. Measured from the anterior abdominal wall, depth of placement is usually 3 cm in a full-term infant.
   b. High line: T9 to T10, just above the right diaphragm. The depth of insertion is calculated using the following formula:

$$\frac{[3 \times \text{weight (kg)}] + 9}{2} + 1 = \text{UV catheter insertion depth in centimeters}$$

Procedural Steps

1. *Follow steps 1 through 4 above for the UA line procedure. The conventional method or side-entry method can be used to place a UV catheter.
2. *Firmly pull the cord toward the infant's feet. The vein is usually located at the 12 o'clock position. The vein is not as thick-walled as the arteries and is larger in size.
3. *Clear any clots with iris forceps.
4. *Grasp the catheter with forceps and insert it into the lumen of the vein aiming toward the right shoulder and advance it approximately 2 to 3 cm.
5. *Gently advance the catheter to the desired distance as calculated previously. If blood does not return easily, withdraw the catheter while maintaining gentle suction via a syringe. If the catheter has a clot on the tip, remove the clot and reinsert the catheter.
6. *Secure the catheter by placing an anchor stitch in the substance of the cord, avoiding the other vessels in the cord and the skin. Tie the suture around the catheter to ensure it does not move.
7. *Loosen, do not remove, the umbilical tie so it can be retightened quickly in the event bleeding occurs.
8. Secure the catheter in a flat fashion to the abdomen with tape.
9. Obtain a radiograph to verify placement.

Complications

1. Infection
2. Air embolism
3. Hepatic necrosis
4. Vessel perforation

---

*Indicates portions of the procedure usually performed by a physician or an advanced practice nurse.

REFERENCES

Barrington, K. J. (1999). Umbilical artery catheters in the newborn: Effects of position of the catheter tip (Cochrane Review). *The Cochrane Library.* Retrieved February 14, 2007, from http://www.cochrane.org/reviews/en/ab000505.html

Bloom, B. T., Nelson, R. A., & Dirksen, H. C. (1986). A new technique: Umbilical arterial catheter placement. *Journal of Perinatolology, 6,* 174.

MacDonald, M. (2002a). Umbilical artery catheterization. In M. G. MacDonald, & J. Ramasethu (Eds.), *Atlas of procedures in neonatology* (pp. 152-170). Philadelphia: Lippincott Williams & Wilkins.

MacDonald, M. (2002b). Umbilical vein catheterization. In M. G. MacDonald, & J. Ramasethu (Eds.), *Atlas of procedures in neonatology* (pp. 174-182). Philadelphia: Lippincott Williams & Wilkins.

Shukla, H., Ped, D., & Ferrara, A. (1986). A rapid estimation of insertional length of umbilical venous catheters in newborns. *American Journal of Disease of Children, 140,* 786.

Squire, S. J., Hornung, T. L., & Kirchhoff, K. T. (1990). Comparing two methods of umbilical artery catheter placement. *American Journal of Perinatology, 7,* 8-15.

Accessing Preexisting Central Venous Catheters

Robin A. Scott, RN, ND

There are many types of central venous catheters, including the Hickman/Broviac right atrial catheter, the Groshong catheter, the Leonard catheter, the peripherally inserted central catheter (PICC), and the hemodialysis catheter. Most are available in single- or multiple-lumen configurations (Table 69-1, Figures 69-1 and 69-2). Most patients carry an identification card that displays the manufacturer's name, model, and instructions. For the latest information, contact the manufacturer of the specific catheter.

INDICATIONS

To gain venous access in patients with preexisting central venous catheters to:
1. Administer intravenous (IV) fluids, medications, and blood products.
2. Obtain venous blood samples.
3. Administer parenteral nutrition.

CONTRAINDICATIONS AND CAUTIONS

1. Use only the in-line clamp provided on the line. Do not use hemostats because they may damage the catheter.
2. To prevent an air embolism in the event that the catheter is disconnected or damaged, clamp the catheter.
3. Catheter hubs and needleless caps should be cleaned daily (Tilton, 2006).
4. When available, needleless systems are recommended. Otherwise, use needles of 1 inch or shorter when inserting a needle into the male adapter plug of a central venous catheter because longer needles may puncture the catheter.
5. If administration of chemotherapy or other vesicant agents is anticipated, ensure patency of the catheter by aspirating blood before infusion. If there is any question of patency, evaluation by dye studies is recommended before infusion.
6. Rapid or forceful flushing may dislodge a clot into the central circulation.
7. Catheter access points should be cleansed with an alcohol pad four times during procedures: before attaching the initial saline flush to assess patency, before attaching infusion tubing or syringe, before attaching the flush syringe, and before attaching the heparin flush syringe, if appropriate (Hadaway, 2006).
8. Catheter flush protocols vary by institution; refer to institutional policies and procedures for flush solutions and protocols.
9. For administration of IV push medications or flush solutions, care must be taken to avoid excessive pressure on the syringe, which could rupture the catheter. Smaller syringes create higher pressures. Therefore, a syringe that is 10 ml or larger should be used for an IV push administration through any silicone elastomer catheter. Table 69-2 lists recommended flow rates.

TABLE 69-1
SELECTED CENTRAL VENOUS CATHETERS

Catheter Type/Name	Description of Catheter	Recommended Flush Protocol	Comments
Hickman, Broviac, Leonard	Tunneled, cuffed silicone catheter (see Figure 69-1). Surgically inserted usually in subclavian vein, may also use femoral access. Available in single-, double-, or triple-lumen configurations.	Flush with 5 ml of normal saline before and after medications and before transfusions. Flush with 10 ml of normal saline after discontinuing blood products or TPN. THEN Flush with 2.5 ml (Hickman or Leonard) or 1.5 ml (Broviac) of heparinized saline, or 5 ml (Hickman or Leonard) or 2 ml (Broviac) every 12 to 24 hours, or after each use. Appropriate heparin volume, concentration, and flushing are determined by the patient's medical condition and laboratory tests. Flush each lumen separately.	Check for closed clamp; do not flush vigorously or against resistance—catheter may rupture. If a needless system is not in use, change the injection cap every 7 days, after every 18 needle injections, or per hospital policy.
Groshong	Tunneled, cuffed silicone catheter, surgically inserted, usually in subclavian vein. Available in single- and double-lumen configurations. A three-way slit valve remains closed to prevent	Heparin is not necessary. Flush after each use or once weekly with 5 ml of normal saline. Flush with 20 ml of normal saline after each blood draw or after discontinuing blood or TPN administration.	Need to flush with enough turbulence to clear blood from closed-tip catheter. No clamp necessary, owing to the three-way valve. Infusion pressures should never exceed 25 psi.

Continued

TABLE 69-1
SELECTED CENTRAL VENOUS CATHETERS—cont'd

Catheter Type/Name	Description of Catheter	Recommended Flush Protocol	Comments
	air embolism and the backflow of blood (see Figure 69-2).	Pediatric flush volume: 2 ml for routine maintenance and 3 ml after blood aspiration.	
PICC (peripherally inserted central catheter)	Silicone or polyurethane catheter insertion site near the antecubital fossa and catheter tip threaded into the superior vena cava. Available in single- or double-lumen configurations.	5 ml heparinized saline every 12 hours or after each use. Flush each lumen separately. Flush lumens with 10 ml of normal saline after aspiration of blood. No heparin needed for Groshong, PICC; use normal saline solution as described above. For smaller-sized patients, decrease the amount of heparinized saline to 2 ml every 12 hours or 3 ml after aspiration of blood.	Avoid vigorous flushing. Do not flush against resistance; catheter may rupture. Infusion pressures should never exceed 25 psi. Do not use affected arm for venipuncture or blood pressures.
Hemodialysis catheter (Quinton, HEMED, Vas-Cath)	Silicone or polyurethane, usually subclavian or femoral access. Catheters maintained by dialysis personnel and not routinely used for IV therapy.	Heparin flush dose and strength should be by specific physician order only after flushing with 10 ml of normal saline. Typical concentration of heparin is 5000 units/ml; the total volume of heparin solution in each lumen should equal the internal volume of the lumen.	Aspirate heparin before use to avoid heparin-induced coagulopathy. Flush each lumen with 10 ml of normal saline and then Hep-Lock lumen per hospital protocol or physician order. Infusion pressures should never exceed 25 psi.

Data compiled from Bard Access Systems, 1994a, 1994b, 2000, 2002, 2003, 2006; Hurst & Keith, 2005; University of Colorado Hospital, 2005.

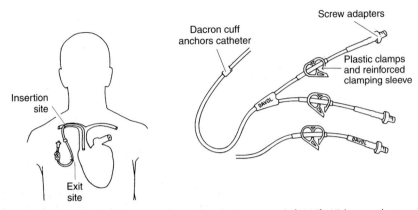

FIGURE 69-1 Schematic of tunneled catheter. (Courtesy Davol. [1994]. *Hickman subcutaneous ports and Hickman/Broviac catheters wall poster.* Cranston, RI: Author.)

EQUIPMENT

   10-ml syringe to withdraw blood for discard, or an extra blood-specimen collection tube if you are using a vacuum tube

   Sampling syringes for blood specimens

   Blood-specimen tubes

   Antiseptic swabs

   Normal saline solution for injection

   Heparin or saline flush, as needed (see Table 69-1 for recommended flush protocols)

PATIENT PREPARATION

Place the patient in a supine position and make sure that the catheter is clamped. For a PICC line, place the patient in any comfortable position.

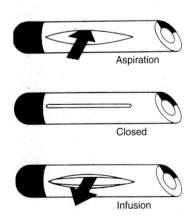

FIGURE 69-2 The Groshong three-position valve. (Courtesy Davol. [1994]. *Hickman subcutaneous ports and Hickman/Broviac catheters wall poster.* Cranston, RI: Author.)

TABLE 69-2

MAXIMUM FLOW RATES AND PRIMING VOLUMES FOR SELECTED CATHETERS AS RECOMMENDED BY THE MANUFACTURER

Catheter Type/Name/ Lumen Size	Maximum Flow Rate	Priming Volume
Power Hickman 8 Fr to 9.5 Fr	5 ml/sec	1.5 ml (8 Fr) to 1.3 ml (9.5 Fr)
Hickman 9.6 Fr (1.6 mm)	Greater than 500 ml/hr	0.15 ml
Hickman 7 Fr (0.8/1 mm)	Greater than 500 ml/hr	0.6 to 1.3 ml
Hickman 9 Fr (0.7/1.3 mm)	Greater than 500 ml/hr	0.6 to 1.3 ml
Hickman 12 Fr (1.6/1.6 mm)	Greater than 500 ml/hr	1.6 ml
Leonard 10 Fr (1.3/1.3 mm)	Greater than 500 ml/hr	1.3 ml
Broviac 6.6 Fr (1 mm)	Greater than 500 ml/hr	0.7 ml
Broviac 4.2 Fr (0.7 mm)	205 ml/hr	0.3 ml
Broviac 2.7 Fr (0.5 mm)	49 ml/hr	0.15 ml
Groshong 3.5 Fr (18 G)	500 ml/hr (PICC or tunneled)	0.13 ml
Per-Q-Cath PICC	Greater than 1,000 ml/hr	0.42 to 0.69 ml (varies based on lumen size)

Data modified from Bard Access Systems, 1994a, 1994b, 2000, 2002, 2003, 2006.

PROCEDURAL STEPS

Fluid Administration

1. Prepare the appropriate fluids and prime the tubing.
2. Clamp the catheter and cleanse the injection surface with alcohol.
3. Attach the primary tubing to the hub of the catheter.
4. Unclamp the catheter and adjust the IV flow to the prescribed rate.

Medication Administration

NOTE: For administration of IV push medications or flush solutions, care must be taken to avoid excessive pressure on the syringe, which could rupture the catheter. Smaller syringes create higher pressures. Therefore, a syringe that is 10 ml or larger should be used for an IV push administration through any silicone elastomer catheter. Table 69-2 lists recommended flow rates.

1. Check the compatibility of the prescribed medication with heparin. If the medication is potentially or actually incompatible with heparin, flush the catheter with 5 ml of normal saline solution for injection before administering the medication.
2. Flush the catheter with 5 ml of normal saline solution after the administration of the medication and before administering the heparin flush.

Troubleshooting (University of Colorado Hospital, 2005)

1. If resistance is met while flushing the catheter:
   a. Do not force the flush; remove any positive pressure devices on the line, and then attempt to aspirate.

    b. If able to aspirate, then flush with 10 ml of normal saline before flushing with appropriate flush solution. If unable to aspirate, notify the physician immediately.

2. If blood cannot be aspirated from the catheter:
    a. Use less negative pressure.
    b. Have the patient change position.
    c. Ask the patient to hold his or her breath or "bear down."

3. If air enters the catheter:
    a. Clamp the catheter.
    b. Turn the patient onto the left side.
    c. Administer oxygen.
    d. Notify the physician immediately.

Blood Sampling

NOTE: Using a heparinized catheter to collect blood samples for coagulation studies is not recommended. If coagulation studies are necessary for such an evaluation, use a separate peripheral site for venipuncture (ENA, 2005).

Blood sampling using a syringe

1. If a continuous IV infusion is running, stop the infusion for 1 minute before drawing the blood specimens.
2. Draw up 5 ml of normal saline into a 10-ml syringe. Draw up two 10-ml normal saline solution flushes and, if appropriate, heparin flush.
3. Clamp all lumens not being used for blood withdrawal. Clamp the catheter and remove the IV tubing or the male adapter plug.
4. Wipe adapter or positive pressure device with alcohol swab and attach syringe with 5 ml of normal saline. Unclamp the tubing and flush the line with the 5 ml of saline and then withdraw 5 ml of blood. Clamp the tubing, remove the syringe and discard the blood.
5. Attach 10-ml syringe, unclamp tubing, and aspirate gently. Forceful aspiration may collapse the catheter. To facilitate blood return, have the patient raise both arms, cough, perform the Valsalva maneuver, or change position.
6. Withdraw the amount of blood needed, clamp the tubing, remove the syringe, and transfer blood to the tubes with a transfer device.
7. After the blood is drawn, attach a 10-ml syringe prefilled with normal saline solution, unclamp the tubing, and flush the catheter with 10 to 20 ml of normal saline solution. Clamp the tubing and remove the syringe.
8. Attach the syringe containing heparin flush, unclamp the tubing, and flush the catheter with appropriate heparin flush, unless the line is a Groshong catheter or infusion is to be resumed.
9. Reestablish the IV fluids or administer an appropriate heparin flush through a new male adapter plug.

Blood sampling using a vacuum tube

NOTE: Vacuum tubes may collapse the catheter. If this occurs, use the syringe method as described previously.

1. When drawing blood specimens through a multiple-lumen catheter, use the largest lumen if it is known, or use the distal lumen. Avoid the lumen that is used for nutritional solutions (total parenteral nutrition).

2. Turn off all the running infusions for 1 minute before withdrawing blood specimens.
3. Leave the male adapter plug on the catheter. Clean the catheter injection port with an antiseptic solution.
4. Place the vacuum tube in the tube holder and insert the adapter or needle into the injection port of the catheter.
5. Withdraw 5 to 10 ml of blood into an extra tube and discard it.
6. Draw the appropriate number and types of tubes needed.
7. After the blood is drawn, flush the catheter with 10 ml of normal saline solution (20 ml for the Groshong catheter).
8. Reestablish IV fluids or administer an appropriate saline or heparin flush through the male adapter plug.

Dressing Application or Dressing Changes

1. Gauze dressings, when used, should be changed every 48 hours, and transparent dressings should be changed every 7 days or when dressing is loose, damp, or soiled. Gauze dressings under transparent dressings are considered gauze dressings and are changed every 48 hours (INS, 2006).
2. Perform hand hygiene. Don mask and clean gloves.
3. Remove previous dressing (if present) and inspect the access site. Notify the physician of swelling, redness, tenderness, or drainage from the site.
4. Dispose of old dressing and gloves. Perform hand hygiene.
5. Don new sterile gloves.
6. Cleanse the site for 30 seconds with appropriate solution per institutional policy, and allow area to dry completely (INS, 2006).
7. Apply an antimicrobial sponge to the access site per institutional policy.
8. Apply sterile transparent semipermeable membrane dressing to access site.
9. Tape the end of the catheter in place.
10. Date and initial the dressing.

AGE-SPECIFIC CONSIDERATION

Pediatric flush protocols vary according to catheter type and lumen size. Generally, lower flush volumes and infusion rates will be used for pediatric populations. Check your institution's protocols for specific rates and volumes. Table 69-1 also contains general guidelines for some catheters.

COMPLICATIONS

Table 69-3 lists complications associated with central catheters.

PATIENT TEACHING

These are preexisting central catheters, so patients should be familiar with self-care measures. Patient teaching should focus on handling catheter-related complications pertinent to the patient's presenting problem. If it is determined that the patient requires further training for home management of the catheter, a referral to a home health service or to the primary provider should be considered.

TABLE 69-3
IDENTIFICATION AND MANAGEMENT OF CENTRAL LINE COMPLICATIONS

Complication	Signs and Symptoms	Management
Infection	Redness, tenderness at site; may be pus or induration. May have fever, chills, or signs of sepsis.	Culture site (semiquantitative method). Blood culture through catheter and separate venipuncture. Antibiotics through catheter may resolve catheter-related bloodstream infections, but catheter may need to be removed to resolve infection. Do not remove except by physician order.
Infiltration or extravasation	Pain and/or swelling of the neck, shoulder, arm, and/or chest. Fluid may be visible at insertion site. Rate may slow or stop.	Note that blood return may still be present if fibrin sheath has formed. Stop IV or slow rate until patency is confirmed. Venography is diagnostic. Remove catheter only by physician order. If fibrin sheath is confirmed, thrombolytic therapy may be considered with or without catheter removal.
Central vein thrombosis	No blood return; slow flow rate; pain; redness; induration; or edema of shoulder, arm, or neck on affected side. Development of collateral circulation in chest, decreased venous emptying.	Stop or slow rate. Watch for infiltration. Venography is diagnostic. If thrombosis is confirmed, thrombolytic therapy may be considered with or without catheter removal.

Continued

TABLE 69-3
IDENTIFICATION AND MANAGEMENT OF CENTRAL LINE COMPLICATIONS—cont'd

Complication	Signs and Symptoms	Management
Pinch-off syndrome	Intermittent inability to aspirate blood return or infuse that is affected by a change in position of the arm or shoulder, caused by pinching of the catheter between the first rib and the clavicle.	Most common with silicone catheters. To confirm, order upright chest x-ray film and ask radiologist to check for pinch-off. If no blood return, venography will identify transection. If catheter is intact, may be used with caution. External rotation of shoulder may facilitate blood return. Do not irrigate against resistance. Catheter may need to be replaced; if it is nonfunctioning, contact the surgeon.
Damaged catheter	Catheter body or hub broken, cracked, or contaminated.	Immediately clamp catheter between break and body with a bulldog or other suitable clamp. Obtain repair kit (available from manufacturer). Repair according to repair-kit instructions. Ensure sterile technique. May be necessary to declot catheter following repair (see following text on Occlusion).
Occlusion	Inability to aspirate or infuse caused by occlusion by blood or precipitate. Note: Management of occlusion by precipitate other than blood is mostly anecdotal. Check with pharmacy for most current literature.	By history, confirm occlusion by blood, then declot. No blood work is necessary before declotting procedure. Recent ocular or cerebral bleed is a relative contraindication—check with physician first. (See Procedure 71: Declotting Central Venous Access Devices, for further information.)
Air embolism	Hypotension, pulse rapid and weak, cyanosis, changes in level of consciousness, shock, and auscultation of coarse machinery noise over the precordium.	Place patient in left Trendelenburg position, administer oxygen, and provide life support as needed. To avoid air embolism, place patient in Trendelenburg position for central line insertion or whenever line is disconnected.

REFERENCES

Bard Access Systems. (1994a). *Groshong® C.V. catheters: Nursing procedure manual*. Salt Lake City, UT: AuthorRetrieved December 3, 2006, from http://www.bardaccess.com/pdfs/nursing/ng-grosh-cath.pdf

Bard Access Systems. (1994b). *Hickman,® Leonard,® and Broviac® catheters: Nursing procedure manual*. Salt Lake City, UT: AuthorRetrieved December 3, 2006, from http://www.bardaccess.com/pdfs/nursing/ng-hick-leon-brov.pdf

Bard Access Systems. (2000). *Peripherally inserted central venous catheters (PICC): Nursing procedure manual*. Salt Lake City, UT: Author. Retrieved December 3, 2006, from http://www.bardaccess.com/pdfs/nursing/ng-siliradpicc-perqpluspicc.pdf

Bard Access Systems. (2002). *Long-term polyurethane hemodialysis/apheresis catheters: Nursing procedure manual*. Salt Lake City, UT: Author. Retrieved December 3, 2006, from http://www.bardaccess.com/pdfs/nursing/ng-hemodialysis.pdf

Bard Access Systems. (2003). *Poly Per-Q-Cath PICC, your partner in safety, product brochure*. Salt Lake City, UT: Author. Retrieved December 3, 2006, from http://www.bardaccess.com/pdfs/brochures/bro-polyperq.pdf

Bard Access Systems. (2006). *Power Hickman® central venous catheter, with AirGuard® valved introducer*. Salt Lake City, UT: Author.

Emergency Nurses Association (ENA). (2005). *Sheehy's manual of emergency care* (6th ed.). St. Louis: Mosby.

Hadaway, L. C. (2006). Keeping central line infection at bay. *Nursing, 36*, 58-64.

Hurst, S. M., & Keith, B. K. (2005). Innovative solutions: A collaborative effort of critical care oncology, the common ground of tubes and lines. *Dimensions of Critical Care Nursing, 24*, 37-40.

Intravenous Nurses Society (INS). (2006). Infusion nursing standards of practice. *Journal of Intravenous Nursing, 29*, S1-S79.

Tilton, D. (2006). Central venous access device infections in the critical care unit. *Critical Care Nursing Quarterly, 29*, 117-122.

University of Colorado Hospital. (2005). *University of Colorado Hospital policy and procedure: Lines, central venous* (revised March 2005). Denver: Author.

PROCEDURE 70

Accessing Implanted Vascular Port Devices

Robin A. Scott, RN, ND

An implanted port consists of a tunneled catheter attached to an injection port with a self-sealing septum (Figure 70-1). The device is implanted under the skin and must be accessed through the skin. Although most frequently used for venous access, implanted ports may also be placed intraarterially, epidurally, or intraperitoneally. Venous ports are usually located in the chest; however,

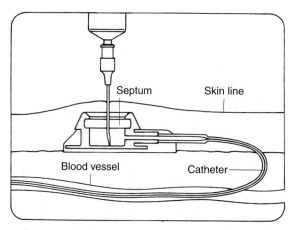

FIGURE 70-1 Implantable port configuration. (Courtesy Davol. *Davol implanted ports: Patient information.* Publication No. 99020 M [p. 4]. Cranston, RI: Author.)

some ports are located in the upper extremity, with the catheter insertion site in the basilic or cephalic vein and the tip threaded into a central vein, similar to a peripherally inserted central catheter (PICC). Catheter tip placement must be confirmed by aspiration of blood before the port is used. There are many brands of implanted ports, including one with the Groshong catheter attached. Many ports are available in single- or double-port or lumen configuration. Most septa are located on the top of the port. Patients may carry written information about their port.

INDICATIONS

To gain venous access in patients who have an implanted venous port to:
1. Administer intravenous (IV) fluids, medications, blood, or blood products.
2. Obtain samples of venous blood.
3. Perform routine heparin flushes to maintain catheter patency.

CONTRAINDICATIONS AND CAUTIONS

1. Use strict sterile technique to avoid infection because the patient would require a surgical procedure to have the device removed.
2. Use only noncoring or Huber point needles to access an implanted port because other needles may damage the port septum, leading to extravasation of fluids or medications (Nettina, 2005). Noncoring needles are available in 19-, 20-, or 22-G sizes and either in a straight configuration for one-time access or at a 90-degree angle with or without an attached extension set for continuous infusion (Figure 70-2). If blood samples are desired, use a 19-G noncoring needle.
3. Although the port is sutured in place, it is possible for it to flip over. Palpate the septum of the port to ensure that it is right side up before attempting needle insertion.
4. If the patient feels pain or an abnormal sensation at the port site during infusion, it may indicate that the medication has extravasated. The infusion should be stopped immediately until the port patency has been determined.

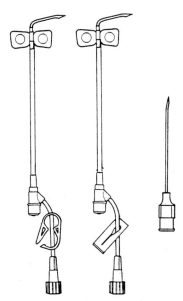

FIGURE 70-2 Noncoring (Huber) needle configuration. (Courtesy Pharmacia Deltec.)

A chest radiograph helps verify catheter placement if no blood return is obtained when the port is accessed. When port patency is uncertain, the only conclusive way to determine patency is to perform a cathetergram by injecting contrast dye into the port.

5. To administer whole blood or packed red blood cells, use a 19-G noncoring needle to access the port. It is usually necessary to use an infusion pump or add 50 ml of normal saline solution to the blood bag or run a normal saline solution concomitantly with the blood to maintain adequate flow rates.

6. For a routine heparin flush of the port, use 5 ml of heparin (100 units/ml). Use a 10-ml syringe for the flush.

7. To avoid an air embolism, the extension set should be clamped any time the IV line is disconnected.

8. The needle should be changed every 7 days or sooner if the flow rates decrease or blood return is absent (Karamanoglu et al., 2003).

9. When not accessed, the port should be flushed once per month with 5 ml of heparin, 100 units/ml, using a 10-ml syringe (University of Colorado Hospital, 2005). Ports placed in the hepatic artery are flushed weekly.

10. Observe the site and surrounding skin for any signs of swelling, redness, drainage, or increased temperature. Do not access the port if infection is suspected (University of Colorado Hospital, 2005).

11. Use a syringe 10 ml or larger for routine flushing and medication administration (Vanderbilt University Medical Center, 2005).

EQUIPMENT

Two pairs of sterile gloves
Mask(s)
One alcohol swab

Three antiseptic swab sticks

Noncoring or Huber needle

Luer-Lok T-extension set or short extension set, if this is not already attached to the needle

Bulldog or padded clamp, if not provided on the extension set

Sterile normal saline for injection

Two 10-ml syringes with needles

Dressing materials (if the port is to remain accessed), skin tapes, 4- to 5-cm transparent dressing, 2×2 sterile gauze dressings, tape

IV solution as prescribed, needleless adapter cap, or a male adapter plug

Blood specimen tubes, if needed

5 ml of heparin (100 units/ml) if heparin lock is needed

PROCEDURAL STEPS
Port Access

1. Apply a mask. Ask the patient to turn his or her head away from the port or apply a mask to the patient as well.
2. Prepare all supplies on a sterile field.
3. Assess the site for signs of infection. Do not access port if signs of infection are present; stop and notify the physician.
4. Expose the chest and identify the septum by palpating the outer perimeter of the port. The septum is located in the middle of the port.
5. Perform hand hygiene.
6. Using aseptic technique, fill the 10-ml syringes with sterile normal saline solution, attach the extension set to the noncoring needle, and prime the needle and extension setup with the normal saline solution to purge all air. Leave the syringe attached to the needle and extension set. Return the set to the sterile package to protect the needle, wings, and proximal portion of the extension against contamination.
7. Using sterile gloves, clean the skin over the port and any surrounding skin that will be covered by the final dressing per institutional protocol and allow to air dry (INS, 2006). Common site cleaning protocols include the following:
   a. Use an alcohol swab working from the center of the port outward in a clockwise direction followed with three povidone-iodine swab sticks in the same fashion.
   b. Scrub the area vigorously with a chlorhexidine applicator. Allow to air dry.
8. Change gloves.
9. Stabilize the port with the forefinger and thumb of nondominant hand (one on each side of the port). Insert the noncoring needle through the skin and into the middle of the septum. Hold the needle perpendicular to the port and apply continuous downward pressure. Do not twist, rock, or manipulate the needle sideways during or after the needle insertion, because this may core the septum and cause leaking from the port. Continue downward pressure on the needle until it hits the back of the septum and can go no farther (Figure 70-3).
10. Aspirate 5 ml of blood to confirm port patency. To facilitate blood return, have the patient raise his or her arms, cough, perform the Valsalva maneuver, or change position.

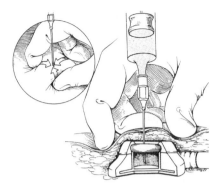

FIGURE 70-3 Accessing an implanted port. (Courtesy Davol. *Hickman subcutaneous port: use and maintenance.* Publication No. 11905 M [p. 6]. Cranston, RI: Author.)

11. If no blood return is obtained, the needle may be located at the side of the septum over the outer periphery of the port. If you are unable to achieve a blood return, remove the needle and try again with a new needle. If there is visual confirmation that the new needle is in the port, attempt to irrigate the port with normal saline solution. If there is no resistance when irrigating, and there is still no blood return, stop and report port access and findings to the physician. The provider may order radiographic studies or declotting procedures. (See Procedure 71: Declotting Central Venous Access Devices, for additional information.)

12. If blood is aspirated, flush port with 10 ml of normal saline. (If resistance is met during irrigation with 10 ml of normal saline, stop and report findings to the physician.).

13. Clamp the tube and remove the 10-ml syringe.

14. Clean the end of the extension tubing or needleless adapter cap with an alcohol swab. Attach primed IV tubing. Unclamp the port access tubing and proceed with the infusion (the IV fluid should drip freely by gravity if the needle is in the port) while monitoring the patient for signs of extravasation. To assess for extravasation, place the patient on his or her back and compare the breasts and both sides of the chest and neck. Observe for asymmetry, swelling, redness, or the patient's complaint of tenderness. A chest radiograph helps confirm the catheter's placement and rule out a catheter pinch-off or transection.

15. If the port is to remain accessed, apply a dressing as follows:
    a. Apply an antimicrobial sponge per institutional policy.
    b. Stabilize the needle and wings by placing a 2 × 2 sterile gauze pad under the angled needle to provide support as needed. To facilitate patient assessment, do not obscure the needle insertion site with the gauze dressing.
    c. Cover the entire area with a transparent semipermeable dressing, leaving only the end of the extension set with the clamp exposed.
    d. Label the dressing with the date of the insertion and the needle size.

Blood Sampling

NOTE: The use of a heparinized catheter for blood sampling for coagulation studies is not recommended if results are to be used to monitor anticoagulant therapy or to evaluate coagulopathy, because they may show falsely elevated levels (Prue-Owens, 2006). If coagulation studies are necessary for such an evaluation, use a separate peripheral site for the venipuncture. If the catheter must be used for coagulation studies, note this on the laboratory request form.

1. If a continuous IV infusion is running, stop the infusion for 1 minute, clamp the port access tubing, disconnect the IV infusion tubing, and attach a 10-ml syringe.
2. If no infusion is running, clean the end of the extension tubing or needleless adaptor cap with an alcohol swab and attach a 10-ml syringe.
3. Unclamp tubing and aspirate 6 ml of blood from the port (ENA, 2005). Clamp the tubing and discard the blood.
4. Clean the end of the extension tubing or needleless adaptor cap with an alcohol swab and attach the sampling syringe. Unclamp the tubing, and withdraw the amount of blood needed. Clamp the tubing, remove sampling syringe, and place blood in appropriate specimen tubes.
5. Clean the end of the extension tubing or needleless adaptor cap with an alcohol swab and attach a 10 ml-syringe filled with normal saline solution. Unclamp the tubing and flush the catheter with 10 ml of normal saline.
6. If no infusion is to be resumed, clean the end of the extension tubing or needleless adaptor cap with an alcohol swab, and flush the catheter with 5 ml of heparin (100 units/ml) using a 10-ml syringe. Clean the end of the extension tubing or needleless adaptor cap with an alcohol swab, and attach a sterile Luer-Lok cap.
7. If the infusion is to be resumed, after flushing with 10 ml of normal saline, clean the end of the extension set with an alcohol swab, and reattach the infusion tubing. Unclamp the tubing, and restart the infusion.

Removing the Needle from the Port

1. Perform hand hygiene.
2. Clean the end of the extension tubing or needleless adaptor cap with an alcohol swab and attach a 20-ml syringe filled with normal saline. Flush the port with 20 ml of normal saline solution for injection.
3. Clean the end of the extension tubing or needleless adaptor cap with an alcohol swab, and attach a 10-ml syringe containing 5 ml of heparin (100 units/ml). Flush the port with the 5 ml of heparin (100 units/ml).
4. Remove dressing, perform hand hygiene.
5. Don sterile gloves.
6. Stabilize the port with thumb and forefinger of your nondominant hand, and remove the needle according to the manufacturer's recommendations to make sure the needle retracts safely into the safety mechanism of the set (Univeristy of Colorado Hospital, 2005). Discard the needle in a sharps container.
7. Apply pressure over site until bleeding stops.
8. Apply dressing to site.

AGE-SPECIFIC CONSIDERATION

A smaller port and a shorter catheter are used for infants and children; therefore, there are lower blood discard volumes for laboratory draws and flushing volumes. Volumes should equal approximately two to three times the catheter or port volume, which can be found on the package insert. If the catheter volume is unknown, it is generally adequate to withdraw 5 ml of blood before the blood draw.

COMPLICATIONS

1. Infection
2. Medication or fluid extravasation
3. Catheter pinch-off syndrome and transection
4. Catheter occlusion (See Procedure 71, Declotting Central Venous Access Devices, for further information.)
5. Air embolism
6. Central venous thrombosis
7. Catheter rupture
8. Hematoma
9. Pneumothorax

PATIENT TEACHING

Ports are preexisting central catheters, so patients should be familiar with self-care measures. Patients should be reminded to have the catheter flushed monthly when not in use. Teach the patient about signs and symptoms of infection and extravasation, and reinforce that they should notify their health care provider immediately if they experience any of these symptoms. If it is determined that the patient requires further training for home management of the catheter, a referral to the home health service or the primary provider should be considered.

REFERENCES

Emergency Nurses Association (ENA). (2005). *Sheehy's manual of emergency care* (6th ed.). St Louis: Mosby.

Intravenous Nurses Society (INS). (2006). Infusion nursing standards of practice. *Journal of Intravenous Nursing, 29,* S1-S79.

Karamanoglu, A., Yumuk, P. F., Gumus, M., Ekenel, M., Aliustaoglu, M., Selimen, D., Sengoz, M., & Turhal, N. S. (2003). Port needles. *Journal of Infusion Nursing, 26,* 239-242.

Nettina, S. M. (2005). I.V. therapy. In K. Hanson (Ed.), *Lippincott manual of nursing practice* (8th ed., pp. 84-103). Philadelphia: Lippincott.

Prue-Owens, K. K. (2006). Obtaining blood samples for measurement of activated partial thromboplastin times. *Critical Care Nurse, 26*(1), 30-38.

University of Colorado Hospital. (March 2005). *University of Colorado Hospital policy and procedure: Lines, central venous.* Denver: Author.

Vanderbilt University Medical Center. (March 2005). *Vanderbilt University Medical Center policy and procedure: Implanted venous ports, care & maintenance.* CL 30–07.08 Nashville: Author.

Declotting Central Venous Access Devices

Ruth Altherr Rench, MS, RN, FAHA, and *Teresa L. Will, MSN, RN, CEN*

Tissue plasminogen activator is also known as *TPA, tPA, r-tPA, alteplase,* and *Cathflo Activase.*

INDICATION

TPA is indicated for the restoration of function to central venous access devices, as assessed by the ability to withdraw blood.

CONTRAINDICATIONS AND CAUTIONS

1. Known hypersensitivity to TPA or any component of the formulation is a contraindication.
2. Catheter dysfunction may be caused by many conditions other than thrombus formation, such as catheter malposition, mechanical failure, constriction of a suture, and lipid deposits or drug precipitates within the catheter lumen. These conditions should be ruled out before treatment with TPA is considered.
3. Avoid vigorous suction during attempts to determine catheter occlusion in order to avoid damage to the vessel wall or collapse of the catheter walls.
4. To prevent rupture of the catheter or expulsion of the clot into the systemic circulation, avoid excessive pressure when instilling TPA.
5. Bleeding is the most frequent adverse reaction associated with all thrombolytics in all approved indications. TPA use in this situation has not been studied in patients who are known to be at risk for bleeding events that may be associated with thrombolytics (Deitcher et al., 2002; Ponec et al., 2001). Exercise caution with patients who have active internal bleeding or have had any of the following:
   - Surgery (within 48 hours)
   - Obstetric delivery (within 48 hours)
   - Percutaneous biopsy of viscera or deep tissues (within 48 hours)
   - Puncture of noncompressible vessels (within 48 hours)
   - Thrombocytopenia
   - Hemostatic defects (e.g., severe hepatic or renal disease)
   - Any condition in which bleeding constitutes a significant hazard or would be particularly difficult to manage because of its location
   - High risk for embolic complications (e.g., venous thrombosis in the region of the catheter)
6. The use of TPA in patients with infected catheters may release a localized infection into the systemic circulation. Therefore, TPA should be used with caution in patients with known or suspected catheter-related infections.

EQUIPMENT

2-mg Cathflo Activase vial: contains 2.2 mg of TPA (which includes a 10% overfill)

Three 10-ml syringes

One three-way stopcock

10 ml of sterile water for injection (SWFI)

20 ml of normal saline (for catheter assessment and flushing)

Alcohol wipes

PATIENT PREPARATION

Perform a thorough assessment, to include:

1. Rule out external mechanical catheter obstruction
2. Rule out patient position–related mechanical catheter obstruction
3. Rule out obstruction due to lipid or drug precipitate
4. Review of cautions for TPA treatment

PROCEDURAL STEPS (Genentech, 1996)
TPA Reconstitution

1. Using a 10-ml syringe and aseptic technique, withdraw 2.2 ml of SWFI, and then inject the SWFI into the Cathflo Activase vial, directing the diluent stream into the powder. Slight foaming may occur; allow vial to stand until large bubbles dissipate.
2. Mix by gently swirling the vial contents until they are completely dissolved, which should occur within 3 minutes. Do not shake. The resulting solution should be a pale yellow to colorless transparent solution, which contains 1 mg/ml of Cathflo Activase.
3. Because Cathflo Activase contains no preservatives, it should be reconstituted immediately before use. The solution may be used for intracatheter instillation within 8 hours of reconstitution if it is stored at 2° to 30° C (36° to 86° F).

TPA Instillation (McKnight, 2004)

1. Using the same 10-ml syringe, administer the appropriate dose of solution from the reconstituted vial per Table 71-1. Instill the dose of Cathflo Activase into the occluded catheter. If resistance is met, never forcibly push the solution into the catheter, to avoid the risk of catheter rupture. If unable to instill the solution, use one of the following techniques to instill the Cathflo Activase.

TABLE 71-1
CATHFLO ACTIVASE DOSING

Patient Weight	Dose
30 kg or more	2 mg in 2 ml
Less than 30 kg	110% of the internal lumen volume of the catheter, not to exceed 2 mg in 2 ml

From Genentech. (2005). *Cathflo Activase (alteplase) 2 mg prescribing information.* San Francisco: Author.

a. Use the single 10-ml syringe containing the Cathflo Activase solution, which is attached directly to the hub of the catheter's dysfunctional lumen. After unclamping the catheter, gently pull back on the syringe plunger until it reaches the 8- or 9-ml mark and hold it to create negative pressure in the catheter. While holding the syringe in a vertical position to keep the solution at the syringe tip, slowly release the plunger and the negative pressure on the syringe. This will allow the Cathflo Activase solution to be drawn into the catheter. The procedure may need to be repeated in order to instill the dose of Cathflo Activase.

b. Use two 10-ml syringes and a three-way stopcock. In this technique, the syringe containing the Cathflo Activase is attached to the horizontal hub of the stopcock and an empty 10-ml syringe is attached to the vertical hub. After unclamping the catheter, turn the syringe off to the Cathflo Activase syringe and open to the empty syringe, gently aspirate the empty syringe until the plunger reaches the 8- to 9-ml mark. While holding the plunger on the empty syringe to create negative pressure, turn the stopcock open to the syringe containing the Cathflo Activase solution and allow it to be drawn into the catheter. Additional attempts to instill the complete dose of Cathflo Activase into the occluded lumen may be required.

2. Wait 30 minutes and then assess catheter function by attempting to withdraw blood. If the catheter is functional, then aspirate 4 to 5 ml of blood to remove the Cathflo Activase and residual clot and gently irrigate the catheter with 20 ml of 0.9% sodium chloride solution using a push–pause positive-pressure flushing technique.

3. If catheter function is not restored after 30 minutes, then relock the catheter and assess again after 120 minutes. At 120 minutes after the first instillation, again assess catheter function. If the catheter is functional, follow the same irrigation process described in step 2 above. If catheter function has not been restored, the 2-mg dose of Cathflo Activase may be repeated, following the same steps described above.

AGE-SPECIFIC CONSIDERATIONS

1. Cathflo Activase has been studied in a pediatric population aged 2 weeks to 17 years and is an FDA-approved therapy for the restoration of function to central venous access devices as assessed by the inability to withdraw blood.

2. Rates of serious adverse events and catheter function restoration are similar in both pediatric and adult patients.

3. In patients weighing less than 30 kg, the dose of Cathflo Activase is 110% of the internal lumen volume of the catheter, not to exceed 2 mg in 2 ml (see Table 71-1).

COMPLICATIONS

1. The most serious adverse events reported in the clinical trials were sepsis, gastrointestinal bleeding, and venous thrombosis. There were no reports of intracranial hemorrhage. No allergic-type reactions were observed in the patients treated with TPA (Deitcher et al., 2002; Ponec et al., 2001).

2. The goal is to prevent serious bleeding through careful screening. Assessment and prompt treatment are also critical to minimize the effects of bleeding when it does occur. Should serious bleeding occur (e.g., intracranial,

gastrointestinal, retroperitoneal, pericardial), treatment with Cathflo Activase should be stopped, and the drug should be withdrawn from the catheter.

PATIENT TEACHING

1. Report symptoms that occur with Cathflo Activase instillation.
2. Report any bleeding.

REFERENCES

Deitcher, M. R., Fesen, M. R., & Kiproff, P. M., et al. (2002). Safety and efficacy of alteplase for restoring function in occluded central venous catheters: Results of the Cardiovascular Thrombolytic to Open Occluded Lines trial. *Journal of Clinical Oncology, 20*(1), 317-324.

Genentech. (2005). *Cathflo ACTIVASE (alteplase) 2 mg prescribing information.* San Francisco: Author.

McKnight, S. (2004). Nurse's guide to understanding and treating thrombotic occlusion of central venous access devices. *MEDSURG Nursing, 13*(6), 377-382.

Ponec, D., Irwin, D., & Haire, W. D., et al. (2001). Recombinant tissue plasminogen activator (alteplase) for restoration of flow in occluded central venous access devices: A double-blind placebo-controlled trial: The Cardiovascular Thrombolytic to Open Occluded Lines (COOL) efficacy trial. *Journal of Vascular and Interventional Radiology, 12*(8), 951-955.

Blood Product Administration

Administration of Blood Products

Robin A. Scott, RN, ND

This procedure contains information on administering red blood cells (RBCs), whole blood, platelets, plasma, and cryoprecipitate.

See Procedures 73 to 76 for information regarding blood filters, massive transfusion, fluid warmers, and blood and fluid pressure infusers.

GENERAL PRINCIPLES (Rosenthal, 2004; Simmons, 2003; Simpson, 2006)

1. The intended recipient must be positively identified before a transfusion is started. This is the single most important step in preventing transfusion reactions.
2. Risks versus benefits need to be explained to the patient. Informed consent is required before a transfusion unless the patient's condition is emergent.
3. A filter designed to retain blood clots and particles must be used in the transfusion.
4. Verify patency of the patient's intravenous (IV) line (20- to 18-G or larger is preferred; however, RBCs can be administered through 22- to 25-G catheters).
5. Components should be mixed thoroughly before administration.
6. No medications or solutions should be added to, or transfused concurrently with, blood components except normal saline solution.
7. Lactated Ringer's solution or other electrolyte solutions containing calcium should never be administered concurrently with a blood component mixed with an anticoagulant containing citrate, because calcium binds to citrate.
8. If the integrity of any component is questioned on visual inspection, it should be returned to the blood bank for further evaluation.
9. If the blood component container is entered for any reason, the component expires after 4 hours at room temperature (20° to 24° C) or after 24 hours if refrigerated at 1° to 6° C (AABB, 2002).
10. All blood or blood components that are not used within 30 minutes must be stored in a monitored refrigerator that has been approved by the blood bank.
11. Blood components can be warmed if clinically indicated during massive transfusion or exchange; warming should be done through the use of an FDA-approved device that will not cause hemolysis.
12. Transfusion reactions can be life threatening and occur with exposure to even a small amount of blood; therefore, transfusions should be started slowly and vital signs should be obtained no more than 15 minutes after the transfusion is started.

13. Transfusions should be completed within 4 hours and before the expiration date/time of the blood component (AABB, 2002).

PATIENT PREPARATION

1. Obtain informed consent per the policy of the institution. Most policies waive consent in emergency situations but consider that the patient's religious beliefs may prohibit the administration of blood or blood products.
2. Obtain specimens for type and crossmatch as required.
3. Establish vascular access, preferably a 20-G or larger catheter.
4. Prime Y-type blood tubing with normal saline, which is indicated for most blood products. Ensure the filter is covered with blood.
5. Assess and document vital signs, including blood pressure, heart rate, respiratory rate, and temperature.

RED BLOOD CELLS

RBCs, or packed red blood cells (PRBCs), are prepared by removing approximately 250 ml of the plasma from whole blood; therefore, there are no significant amounts of clotting factors or platelets in RBCs. Each unit of RBCs contains 250 to 300 ml. One unit of RBCs can increase an average adult's hemoglobin by 1 g/dl, and hematocrit can increase by up to 2% to 3% (Rosenthal, 2004).

Indication

To increase the oxygen-carrying capacity of the circulatory system in the presence of acute or chronic blood loss (American Red Cross, 2003a).

Contraindications and Cautions

1. Removal of the plasma reduces the chance of adverse reactions from RBCs that might occur with the use of whole blood; however, transfusion reactions may still occur (Simpson, 2006).
2. Always have a second person check typing, crossmatching, expiration date, blood unit number versus unit number on the transfusion slip, and client identification. Document these data according to the hospital's policy. Most major or fatal transfusion reactions result from type mismatches caused by a clerical error, administration of blood to the wrong patient, or incorrect identification of the blood component (Beyea & Majewski, 2003). In emergency situations, O-negative blood can be administered until crossmatched blood is available; O-positive blood may be used in postmenopausal females and males of any age.
3. Monitor fluid balance carefully in patients at risk for fluid overload.
4. Do not allow the RBCs to stand at room temperature longer than 30 minutes before administration (Simpson, 2006).
5. Infusion time should not exceed 4 hours. The longer the RBCs are left at room temperature, the greater is the danger of bacterial proliferation and RBC hemolysis (Simpson, 2006).

Equipment

Blood administration set, Y type (170- to 260-micron filter) (American Red Cross, 2003a).

Procedural Steps

1. Check the expiration date on the blood.
2. Identify the patient according to institutional policy. With another person, compare the information on the blood record with the patient's identification bracelet.
3. Invert the RBCs gently several times to achieve suspension.
4. Close roller clamp on tubing.
5. Spike one tail of Y-type tubing with 0.9% normal saline solution, and prime the tubing.
6. Spike the second tail of the Y-type tubing with the RBC bag. Ensure the drip chamber is half full and the filter is covered with saline to prevent damage to the blood cells (Figure 72-1).
7. After cleaning the IV port with an alcohol swab, attach the Y tubing to the patient's IV site and open the roller clamp on the RBCs. A gentle squeeze on the filter helps start the flow of blood.
8. Infuse slowly for the first 15 minutes while observing the patient for reactions. Most serious reactions occur during this time. This step assumes that the patient is not in need of multiple, rapid, life-sustaining transfusions.
9. After 15 minutes, reassess the vital signs and adjust the flow rate to the desired speed if no signs of a transfusion reaction are noted.
10. Continue the assessments of the patient (always include the vital signs) throughout the transfusion as needed, according to the patient's condition, and the number of units being administered.

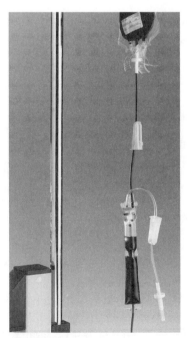

FIGURE 72-1 Red blood cells on Y-type tubing with upper chamber half full.

11. After the infusion is complete, reassess the vital signs and flush the tubing with normal saline solution. If the transfusion therapy is complete, either discontinue the IV or hang the prescribed solution with new IV tubing.

12. Continue to monitor vital signs for at least 1 hour post transfusion (Simpson, 2006).

Age-Specific Considerations (Simmons, 2003)

1. Fluid overload is of concern in both elderly and young patients. Assess lung sounds before and at the completion of the transfusion.

2. There is a risk of viral infection during a transfusion. Cytomegalovirus (CMV) infection can be found on white blood cells. Those at risk for CMV infection are premature infants and immunocompromised patients.

WHOLE BLOOD

Whole blood may be either stored or fresh. One unit of whole blood contains approximately 450 to 500 ml. Whole blood is rarely used in any hospital setting as blood components specific to the patient's needs, such as clotting factors, platelets, plasma, and RBCs, are used instead. Currently, the main use of whole blood is for massive transfusion (Rosenthal, 2004).

Indications (Simpson, 2006)

1. To increase the oxygen-carrying capacity of the blood.
2. To replace volume in a patient in shock.

Contradictions and Cautions (Rosenthal, 2004)

1. Whole blood has the same contraindications and cautions as RBCs.
2. Whole blood has a volume of 450-500 ml per unit and places the patient at a higher risk for fluid overload than RBCs.

Equipment, Procedural Steps, and Age-Specific Considerations

The equipment, procedural steps, and age-specific considerations for whole blood are identical to those for RBCs; see these sections in this procedure under Red Blood Cells.

ALBUMIN

Albumin is a circulating protein found in both the serum and the extravascular area. The primary function of albumin is the maintenance of normal colloid oncotic pressure. Albumin solutions are available in 5% and 25% solution concentrations (Baxter Healthcare Corporation, 2003).

Indications (Baxter Healthcare Corporation, 2003)

1. To replace volume after an acute loss, a therapeutic phlebotomy, or a plasma exchange.
2. To correct hypoalbuminemia.
3. May be used to improve intravascular volume in patients who have severe burns or who are developing signs of edema.
4. May be used in conjunction with a diruetic in patients with pulmonary edema or adult respiratory distress syndrome.

Contraindications and Cautions (Baxter Healthcare Corporation, 2003)

1. Reaction signs can include flushing, urticaria, fever, and nausea.
2. Albumin is very expensive when compared with the cost of crystalloid solutions.
3. If possible, hold angiotensin-converting enzyme (ACE) inhibitors for 24 hours before albumin administration.

Equipment

Use the vented administration set supplied with the glass vial of albumin.

Procedural Steps (Baxter Healthcare Corporation, 2003)

1. Check that the proper solution is being used (normal saline solution or D_5W).
2. Spike the bottle with a vented spike, close roller clamp on the tubing, and attach IV tubing to the vented spike opening.
3. Squeeze the drip chamber until the chamber is one-third full.
4. Open the regulating clamp and prime the IV tubing.
5. Attach tubing to the patient's IV access port after cleaning with an alcohol swab.
6. In patients experiencing hypovolemic shock, administer albumin at 1 to 2 ml/min. In other patients, administer at 2 to 4 ml/min for 5% albumin solutions and no faster than 1 ml/min for 25% albumin solutions.
7. Use of filters during albumin administration is determined by the manufacturer and institutional policy.

PLATELETS

Platelets play an important role in blood coagulation and thrombus formation. One unit of platelets can increase an average adult's platelet count by 5000 platelets per microliter (Rosenthal, 2004). Platelets are obtained through centrifugation of whole blood (Simpson, 2006).

Indication

To prevent or help in controlling bleeding due to thrombocytopenia.

Contraindications and Cautions

1. Platelets must be infused within 4 hours of their expiration time and date (Rosenthal, 2004).
2. Transfusion reactions are possible owing to the plasma in which the platelets are stored (Rosenthal, 2004).
3. Platelets must be transfused through a 170- to 220-micron filter. Do not use filters that were previously used to filter whole blood or PRBCs (Rosenthal, 2004).
4. Most adults do not require ABO crossmatching before platelet infusion, unless they have had multiple platelet infusions and have become resistant to pooled donor platelets (Rosenthal, 2004).
5. Infants and small children do require ABO crossmatching or reduced-volume ABO incompatible platelets (Rosenthal, 2004).
6. Contraindicated in heparin-induced thrombocytopenia (HIT) (Simpson, 2006).

Equipment

Blood administration set, Y type with filter
250-ml bag, or larger, of normal saline solution

Procedural Steps

1. Prime the blood administration set with a normal saline solution.
2. Check the platelet blood type versus the patient's blood type. It is not necessary to have the same ABO type, but it is preferred (American Red Cross, 2003b). Before exposure to Rh-positive platelets, anti–Rh-immune globulin should be administered to Rh-negative women who are of childbearing age (American Red Cross, 2003c).
3. Hang the platelet bag on one tail of the Y set.
4. Close the line roller clamp on the normal saline solution, and open the platelet line.
5. Run the infusion slowly for the first 15 minutes, as with other blood products, and watch closely for any transfusion reactions. After this, the infusion rate can be moved up to 4 to 8 ml/kg per hour according to the patient's tolerance (Rosenthal, 2004).
6. When the platelet pack is empty, close its roller clamp, open the normal saline solution, and flush the line to infuse all the platelets.
7. Document vital signs at 15 minutes into the infusion and again at the conclusion of the infusion.

FRESH FROZEN PLASMA

Fresh frozen plasma (also known as *FFP*, *FP*, or *frozen plasma*) contains all the components of plasma, including clotting factors and fibrinogen, of one unit of whole blood (American Red Cross, 2003b; Rosenthal, 2004).

Indications

1. To correct coagulation deficiencies for which specific factor concentrates are unavailable (American Red Cross, 2003b).
2. To correct a bleeding tendency of unknown cause or one associated with liver failure (American Red Cross, 2003b).
3. To correct coagulopathy and active bleeding, such as may occur during massive transfusion or in disseminated intravascular coagulation (American Red Cross, 2003b).
4. To reverse warfarin effect (American Red Cross, 2003b; Simmons, 2003).
5. Sickle cell crisis (American Red Cross, 2003b).

Contraindications and Cautions

1. FFP must be transfused as soon as possible after it is thawed, and it must be infused in less than 4 hours (AABB, 2002). After thawing, FFP must be stored at 4° C and used within 24 hours (Duguid et al., 2004;).
2. A filter (170- to 200-micron) must be used for FFP transfusion (Duguid et al., 2004).
3. FFP is not indicated solely for volume expansion (American Red Cross, 2003b; Rosenthal, 2004).
4. FFP must be ABO compatible (Rosenthal, 2004).

5. Thawed FFP should be yellow or light green in color and clear in appearance (Rosenthal, 2004).

Equipment

Blood administration set, Y type
Normal saline IV fluid

Procedural Steps

1. Identify the patient and the blood type and double check the unit of plasma with another person to ensure it is correct; it should be the same type. Document the double-checked data according to the institutional policy.
2. Inspect the bag for leaks and the color of the infusion (Duguid et al., 2004).
3. Prime the infusion set with normal saline.
4. Close the roller clamp on the normal saline solution and spike the plasma with the other tail of the Y set.
5. Open up the plasma, and regulate the drip rate.
6. Run the infusion slowly for the first 15 minutes, as with other blood products, and watch closely for any transfusion reactions.
7. Increase rate as prescribed.
8. Dosage is usually 10 to 15 ml/kg but may vary depending on clinical presentation (Duguid, et al., 2004).
9. Assess and document the vital signs after the initial 15 minutes of the infusion and again at the completion of the infusion.

CRYOPRECIPITATED ANTIHEMOPHILIAC FACTOR (CRYOPRECIPITATE)

Cryoprecipitate consists of clotting factor VIII (80 to 100 units), von Willebrand factor, fibrinogen (150 to 200 mg), and factor XIII suspended in 10 to 20 ml of plasma (American Red Cross, 2003a; Simpson, 2006).

Indications

1. To control bleeding by replacing clotting factors in the presence of the following (American Red Cross, 2003a; Simpson, 2006):
2. Factor VIII or factor XIII deficiency.
3. von Willebrand's disease.
4. Hypofibrinogenemia, disseminated intravascular coagulation.
5. Cryoprecipitate is also used as fibrin glue surgical adhesives. This use is not FDA approved (American Red Cross, 2003a).

Contraindications and Cautions (AABB, 2002)

1. Cryoprecipitate should not be used as a substitute for FFP.
2. Compatibility testing not required, but ABO-compatible plasma should used when possible. Rh type does not need to be considered.
3. Volume of infusion is dependent on clinical situation.
4. Infuse only at room temperature.
5. Use only a plastic syringe, because factor VIII may bind to the surface of a glass syringe.
6. Cryoprecipitate must be given through a filter.
7. Transfusion reactions can occur.

8. Infuse immediately after thawing, with complete infusion within 4 hours.

Equipment

Blood administration set, Y type with filter
Normal saline IV fluid

Procedural Steps

1. Initiate an IV line with normal saline solution and Y-type blood set at a keep-vein-open (KVO) rate.
2. Inspect the bag for leaks and examine the solution.
3. Mix by inverting bag gently several times.
4. Hang the cryoprecipitate on the other tail of the Y-type blood set. Cryoprecipitate dosing is based on the patient's plasma volume and the desired increase in factor VIII; multiple units are usually indicated (AABB, 2002).
5. Infuse slowly for the first 15 minutes and watch for a transfusion reaction. Then, adjust the drip rate to prescribed rate.
6. Flush the IV line with a normal saline solution after the cryoprecipitate is finished.
7. Assess and document the vital signs at 15 minutes into the infusion and immediately following the infusion.

Complications

1. Hemolytic-transfusion reactions occur due to incompatibility between donor and host (Simmons, 2003; Simpson, 2006) can be either immediate or delayed. Acute hemolysis can occur when recipient plasma antibodies react with the donor RBC antigens. Both acute and delayed hemolytic reactions are potentially life-threatening events.
   a. Signs and symptoms of hemolytic reactions occur almost immediately and include chills; apprehension; headache; fever; pain in the back, the abdomen, and the chest, or at the infusion site; respiratory distress; hypotension; peripheral circulatory collapse; tachycardia; hypotension; hemoglobinemia; hemoglobinuria; and shock (Simmons, 2003; Simpson, 2006).
   b. Stop the transfusion immediately. Prime new IV tubing with a normal saline solution, and replace the blood-filled tubing (Simmons, 2003; Simpson, 2006).
   c. Save the blood bag and the tubing, notify the blood bank, and follow your institution's policy regarding transfusion reactions.
   d. Contact the physician for further instructions. Some additional interventions may include placing a urinary catheter to track urine output more accurately, giving a diuretic, and sending a urine sample to the laboratory (Simpson, 2006).
   e. Administer IV fluids to achieve a urine output of 100 ml/hr to help prevent renal failure (Simpson, 2006).
   f. Treatment may include antihistamines, antipyretics, steroids, and fluid resuscitation.
2. Allergic reactions and fever occur in about 1 of every 100 units of blood. These usually occur as a result of the interaction of host antibodies with donor plasma proteins. An allergic reaction is most likely to occur with

administration of whole blood or plasma because the plasma contains many antibodies and antigens.

   a. Signs and symptoms commonly include a rash, urticaria, laryngeal edema, and pruritus. Less common reactions are dyspnea, wheezing, and occasionally anaphylaxis (Simpson, 2006).

   b. Stop the transfusion immediately (Simpson, 2006).

   c. Save the blood bag and the tubing, notify the blood bank, and follow your institution's policy for transfusion reaction.

   d. Contact the physician for additional interventions. Anticipate administration of an antihistamine such as diphenhydramine.

   e. Observe for anaphylaxis and prepare epinephrine as indicated.

3. Transfusion-related acute lung injury (TRALI) is the most common cause of transfusion-related deaths in recent years. The reaction activates the complement cascade and histamine release leading to pulmonary capillary permeability. This reaction occurs within 4 hours of the initiation of transfusions. Symptoms are the same as those for acute respiratory distress syndrome and may require intubation and mechanical ventilation (Wooldridge-King, 2005).

4. Graft-versus-host disease (GVHD) occurs when the blood product attacks the body's tissues. This phenomenon is particularly worrisome in the immunocompromised patient (Simmons, 2003). Signs and symptoms include erythematous rash, liver function abnormalities, and profuse diarrhea. Treatment includes immunosuppression with corticosteroids, fluid and electrolyte replacement, and symptomatic management (Simpson, 2006).

5. Febrile nonhemolytic transfusion reactions. This reaction is reflected by any increase in temperature greater than $1°$ C ($1.8°$ F) and may be accompanied by chills, headache, and flushing during or after transfusion. Treatment usually consists of stopping the transfusion of the IV line kept patent with normal saline. Administration of antipyretics and diphenhydramine may be ordered if allergic components are present. Blood samples should be drawn and crossmatching repeated (Simmons, 2003; Simpson, 2006).

6. Circulatory overload and pulmonary edema can occur, especially in older adults and patients with congestive heart failure. Close assessment of lung sounds, neck veins, and venous pressures is important in this patient population. Treatment may include administering diuretics and oxygen (Simmons, 2003; Simpson, 2006).

7. Hyperkalemia. As banked RBCs age, hemolysis occurs and potassium is released from the cells.

8. Hypocalcemia is another potential problem caused by a large amount of citrate-containing blood and blood products. Citrate chelates calcium and is a preservative used in many blood products. Normally, this problem is self-limiting and mild because citrate is quickly metabolized by the liver.

9. Infectious diseases, such as hepatitis, cytomegalovirus, Epstein-Barr virus, and human immunodeficiency virus may be transmitted via blood products. Bacterial contamination of donor blood is very rare, although immunosuppressive effects of blood transfusions may lead to increased infection rates after transfusion in immunocompromised patients, such as postoperative patients (Hall, Frawley, Griffith, Forestner, & Minei, 2003).

10. Hypothermia

PATIENT TEACHING

Report immediately any chills, itching, feeling of warmth, difficulty breathing, or pain in the back, abdomen, chest, or at the IV site.

REFERENCES

American Association of Blood Banks (AABB). (2002). *Circular of information for the use of human blood and blood components.* Retrieved September 30, 2006, from http://www.aabb.org/Documents/About_Blood/Circulars_of_Information/coi0702.pdf

American Red Cross, New England Region. (2003a). *Cryoprecipitate transfusion guidelines.* Retrieved September 25, 2006, from http://www.newenglandblood.org/professional/plasmaguide.htm

American Red Cross, New England Region. (2003b). *Plasma transfusion guidelines.* Retrieved September 25, 2006, from http://www.newenglandblood.org/professional/plasmaguide.htm

American Red Cross, New England Region. (2003c). *Platelet transfusion guidelines.* Retrieved September 25, 2006, from http://www.newenglandblood.org/professional/plateletguide.htm

Baxter Healthcare Corporation. (2003). *Albumin therapy: Ask an expert.* Retrieved September 29, 2006, from http://www.albumintherapy.com/us/en/ask.html

Beyea, S., & Majewski, C. (2003). Blood transfusion in the OR—Are you practicing safely? *AORN Journal, 78,* 1009-1010.

Duguid, J., O'Shaughnessy, D. F., Atterbury, C., Maggs, P. B., Murphy, M., Thomas, D., Yates, S., & Williamson, L. M. (2004). Guidelines for the use of fresh frozen plasma, cryoprecpitate and cryosupernatant. *The British Society for Haemotology, 126,* 11-18.

Hall, G. E., Frawley, W. H., Griffith, K. E., Forestner, J. E., & Minei, J. P. (2003). Allogenic blood transfusion increases the risk of postoperative bacterial infection: A meta-analysis. *Journal of Trauma, 54,* 908-914.

Rosenthal, K. (2004). Avoiding bad blood: Key steps to safe transfusions. *Nursing made incredibly easy, 25,* 20-28.

Simmons, P. (2003). A primer for nurses who administer blood products. *MEDSURG Nursing, 12,* 184-191.

Simpson, T. R. (2006). Transfusion therapy and blood and marrow stem cell transplantation. In S. M. Nettina, & E. J. Mills (Eds.), *Lippincott manual of nursing practice* (8th ed., pp. 962-978). Philadelphia: Lippincott Williams & Wilkins.

Wooldridge-King, M. (2005). Transfusion reaction management. In D. J. Lynn-McHale Wiegand, & K. K. Carlson (Eds.), *AACN procedure manual for critical care* (5th ed., pp. 1024-1030). Philadelphia: Saunders.

Blood Filters

Robin A. Scott, RN, ND

See Procedure 72 for information about specific blood components.

INDICATION

To remove and screen aggregates found in stored blood (clots and debris from blood components) (Moore, 2005; Simpson, 2006). All blood products should be administered through a standard filter (170 to 260 microns), which removes gross fibrin clots from the blood product (AABB, 2002; Simpson, 2006). Blood products may be filtered before release from the blood bank or may be released from the blood bank accompanied by the appropriate filter (Simpson, 2006).

TYPES OF FILTERS

1. *Standard filters:* 170- to 260-micron filter. Used during transfusion of all blood products (red blood cells, platelets, fresh frozen plasma, cryoprecipitate) to remove macroaggregates (clots and fibrin that accumulate during storage) (Savoia, 2003).
2. *Leukocyte-depletion filters:* Used for patients who require leukocyte-depleted products due to the need for multiple transfusions of platelets. These filters remove 80% to 95% of white blood cells from the platelets and may be used when the component was not leukocyte reduced by the blood supplier (AABB, 2002; Simpson, 2006).
3. *Microaggregate filters:* An approximately 40-micron filter, which may be used to remove microaggregates (fibrin, platelets, and white blood cells) during red blood cell transfusions; these filters also aid in the removal of cytomegalovirus (Simpson, 2006).

CONTRAINDICATIONS AND CAUTIONS

1. A standard blood filter should be changed at least every 12 hours; change the filter earlier if the flow rate is diminished (Northover, 2006).
2. Do not use a filter for platelet infusion if it has previously filtered red blood cells. The trapped cells can block the passage of the platelets (Northover, 2006; Rosenthal, 2004).
3. Standard blood filters can be flushed with normal saline (Northover, 2006).
4. Each standard blood filter may be used for up to 4 units of blood (Northover, 2006).
5. Do not prime leukocyte-reduction filters with 0.9% normal saline as this will interfere with its filtering function; the infusion set itself should be primed with normal saline (Southern Health, 2003).
6. Leukocyte reduction filters can be used for 1 to 2 units of blood, according to manufacturer's recommendations (Southern Health, 2003).

EQUIPMENT

Blood products as prescribed
Normal saline intravenous (IV) fluid
Y-type blood or solution set

PROCEDURAL STEPS (Wooldridge-King, 2005)

1. Spike one tail of Y-type tubing with 0.9% normal saline and prime the tubing.
2. Fill the drip chamber, the filter area, and the tubing from the normal saline solution bag. Clamp the patient line and the solution line.
3. Ensure that the filter is completely saturated with fluid so that it can function properly; this step helps avoid damage to the constituents of the blood or blood components.
4. Close the roller clamp to the patient.
5. Spike the other tail of the Y-type tubing with the blood or blood component bag.
6. Close the patient clamp and hold the blood bag and the filter upright, with the blood bag slightly above the level of the normal saline solution. Open the blood clamp slowly to allow the blood to enter the drip chamber.
7. Open the patient-line clamp to the desired rate.

COMPLICATIONS

1. All blood and blood components must be delivered through a filter to prevent inadvertant delivery of clots and debris (AABB, 2002; Simpson, 2006).
2. During rapid resuscitation, the filter may clog, making it necessary to change the filter or tubing sooner than recommended to achieve the desired flow rates (Northover, 2006).

REFERENCES

American Association of Blood Banks (AABB). (2002). *Circular of information for the use of human blood and blood components*. Retrieved February 17, 2007, from http://www.aabb.org/Documents/About_Blood/Circulars_of_Information/coi0702.pdf

Northover, S. (2006). *Administration of fresh blood products (clinical guideline)*. Melbourne, Australia: The Royal Children's Hospital.

Moore, J. M. (2005). Intravenous therapy. In L. Newberry, & L. M. Criddle (Eds.), *Sheehy's manual of emergency care* (6th ed., pp. 99-122). St Louis: Mosby.

Rosenthal, K. (2004). Avoiding bad blood: Key steps to safe transfusions. *Nursing made incredibly easy, 25,* 20-28.

Savoia, H. (2003). *Rationalising blood filters across Royal Children's Hospital (memorandum)*. Victoria, Australia: The Royal Women's Hospital.

Simpson, T. R. (2006). Transfusion therapy and blood and marrow stem cell transplantation. In S. N. Nettina (Ed.), *Lippincott manual of nursing practice* (8th ed., pp. 962-978). Philadelphia: Lippincott Williams & Wilkins.

Southern Health. (2003). *Use of blood filters (clinical protocol)*. Clayton, Australia: Author.

Wooldridge-King, M. (2005). Blood and blood component administration. In D. J. Lynn-McHale Wiegand, & K. K. Carlson (Eds.), *AACN procedure manual for critical care* (5th ed., pp. 991-999). Philadelphia: Saunders.

Massive Transfusion

Robin A. Scott, RN, ND

There is no standard definition of massive blood transfusion. The definition used often in the literature is the replacement of 10 units of blood over a 24-hour period or the replacement of a patient's circulating blood volume (Hardcastle, 2006). Other definitions may include the need for 4 units of packed red blood cells (PRBCs) within 4 hours with continued major bleeding, the transfusion of 50 units in 48 hours, or the tranfusion of 20 units in 24 hours and blood loss greater than 150 ml/min (Repine, Perkins, Kauvar, & Blackborne, 2006).

INDICATION

To treat severe hypovolemic shock secondary to blood loss. The goal of treatment is to restore circulating blood volume to a level that supports homeostasis, oxygen-carrying capacity, and oncotic pressure (Codner & Cinat, 2005).

CONTRAINDICATIONS AND CAUTIONS

1. There are no evidence-based guidelines on the procedural steps of massive transfusions (Hardcastle, 2006).
2. The patient's religious beliefs may prohibit administration of blood or blood products.
3. Warm all fluids to be administered during a massive transfusion (Mikhail, 2004).
4. Using systolic blood pressure as a lone indicator to guide resuscitation may lead to underresuscitation. Vasonconstriction secondary to catecholamine release during times of shock, pain, and hypothermia may result in normal blood pressure values despite persistent hypovolemia (Schulman, 2005).
5. If more than 4 units of uncrossmatched type O blood are transfused, the patient should continue to receive type O blood due to subsequent difficulty with compatibility testing. Whenever possible, type-and-crossmatch specimens should be drawn upon presentation prior to administration of blood products (Mikhail, 2004).
6. Peripheral IV access should be obtained using a 16-G or larger-bore IV catheter. If peripheral access is not successful, obtain central venous access with a large bore (6 Fr to 9 Fr) introducer (Sweeney, 2003).
7. Interossesous (IO) access is a viable option in patients of all ages. It may not be possible to aspirate marrow from the IO site; however, fluids should run freely through the line without use of a pump (Sweeney, 2003).
8. Due to the risk of complications, subclavian and internal jugular veins should not routinely be used for massive transfusion (Sweeney, 2003).

EQUIPMENT

Normal saline intravenous (IV) fluid

Blood products, as prescribed
IV catheters
IV tubing (Y-type blood or trauma tubing)
Fluid warmer
Pressure infuser or pressure bags

PATIENT PREPARATION

1. Make sure that a blood specimen has been sent for typing and crossmatching and that the patient has on an identification band with the information required by the blood bank (Mikhail, 2004).
2. Establish peripheral IV access using short, large-bore IV catheter. Central lines and venous cutdowns can also be used for rapid infusion of fluids (Schulman, 2005). (See Procedures 60 through 70.)
3. Prime the IV tubing (Y-type blood or trauma tubing with a 140-micron filter) with normal saline. Other types of IV tubing have smaller internal diameters and are unsuitable for massive transfusions. If the IV fluid is to be infused under pressure, the air in the fluid bag should be removed with a needle and a syringe to avoid an air embolism.
4. Set up the fluid warmer and pressure infuser (see Procedures 75 and 76). Blood and other fluids should be warmed using a fluid warmer to reduce the adverse effects of the rapid infusion of blood products (Mikhail, 2004). Alteration in the activity of red blood cells (RBCs) occurs at 46° C, so the majority of fluid warmers have a set point of 42° C (Smith, 2003).

PROCEDURAL STEPS

1. Give the initial crystalloid fluid bolus; adults can reach a hemoglobin level of less than 7 g/dl before requiring a transfusion of blood (Rudmann & Nicol, 2005).
2. If there is no response or the response is transient, repeat the fluid bolus and check with the blood bank on the availability of crossmatched blood.
3. Crystalloid fluids should be followed by type O blood products (negative for children and women of childbearing age and positive for men and women above childbearing age) when they become available from the blood bank (Malone, Hess, & Fingerhut, 2006).
4. When it is available, typed and crossmatched blood is preferred and next in order of preference is type specific blood (Mikhail, 2004).
5. Initially, uncrossmatched units can be transfused; these should be followed by type-specific blood within 10 minutes and then crossmatched blood within 40 minutes (Mikhail, 2004).
6. Recommendations for transfusion of coagulation components vary.
   a. Factors may be administered according to a 1:1:1 ratio—that is, for every unit of PRBCs transfused, 1 unit of fresh frozen plasma (FFP) and 1 unit of platelets will be transfused (Malone et al., 2006).
   b. Factors may be administered based on laboratory studies (Stapczynski & Martin, 2004):
      i. If the platelet count is less than 50,000/ml, platelet transfusion is warranted.
      ii. If the international normalized ratio (INR) is greater than 1.5, FFP may be given.

     iii. If fibrinogen level is below 100 mg/dl, it may be replaced with cryoprecipitate.

  c. The goal of replacement therapy should be a platelet count of greater than 50,000/ml and a reduction in prothrombin time (PT) to 15 seconds and in partial thromboplastin time (PTT) to 40 seconds (Malone et al., 2006).

7. Vital signs, skin perfusion, end-tidal carbon dioxide ($ETCO_2$), pulse oximetry, urine output, and temperature should be monitored often to assess the patient's response to fluid resuscitation.

8. After every 5 units of RBCs, send laboratory specimens for complete blood count (CBC), PT, PTT, and fibrinogen level to help guide the administration of additional blood products.

9. Document the use of a rapid infuser or warming device, blood loss, and infusion amounts.

10. Monitor vital signs every 5 to 15 minutes and temperature every 15 to 30 minutes (Schulman, 2005).

11. Check the patency of IV lines every 15 minutes (Schulman, 2005).

12. Monitor urine output, hematocrit, hemoglobin, and other cogulation studies every 30 to 60 minutes. Report urine output of less than 0.5 ml/kg per hour (Schulman, 2005).

13. After bleeding is controlled, maintenance of these factors can be achieved by transfusing 2 units of FFP for every 5 to 6 units of RBCs transfused while labs are pending. In addition, FFP should be administered when prothrombin time (PT) or activated partial thromboplastin time (aPTT) is greater than 1.5 times the laboratory control. Administer platelets when the patient's platelet count is less than 50,000; RBCs are to be transfused if hemoglobin is 10 g/dl and administer cryoprecitpitate when fibrinogen levels are less than 80 to 100 mg/dl (Mikhail, 2004).

AGE-SPECIFIC CONSIDERATIONS

1. In pediatric patients younger than 6 years, after two unsuccessful percutaneous IV attempts, IO access should be obtained (see Procedure 67). Suggested sites for IO access in children younger than 6 years are the proximal tibia and the distal femur (Sweeney, 2003).

2. Scalp veins should not be used (Sweeney, 2003).

3. The cardiovascular system of neonates can adapt better and withstand volume expansion better than those in adults (Rudmann & Nicol, 2005).

4. Neonates and pediatric patients are at risk for circulatory overload because of their small baseline blood volume.

5. The risk of a hyperkalemic cardiac arrest in pediatrics can be reduced by (Morray & Bhananker, 2005):

  a. Use the freshest PRBCs available. Avoid using whole blood.

  b. Do not irradiate the blood except when absolutely necessary (e.g., a premature baby or immunocompromised child). When irradiation is required, the time between irradiation and blood administration should be minimized.

  c. In high-risk situations (e.g., newborn or infant requiring greater than one blood volume, or with irradiated blood), measure the potassium in the blood to be transfused. If the potassium level is high, consider washing the cells in the cell saver and resuspending the cells in plasma before administration.

6. Children have different normal hematocrit values than adults. The volume of blood to be given must be calculated based on the child's blood volume per kilogram of body weight. In early infancy, the blood volume lies between 80 to 90 ml/kg. This level decreases to that of adults at age 1 year (70 to 75 ml/kg). Preterm infants may have an even higher ratio of 100 to 105 ml/kg (Rudmann & Nicol, 2005).

7. Due to the immaturity of the immune system, the neonate is at higher risk for developing transfusion-related infections (Rudmann & Nicol, 2005).

8. Decreases in renal function in the elderly necessitate close monitoring of renal function and urine output.

9. When treating the geriatric population, assess for comorbid conditions such as heart disease that may compromise the patient's ability to compensate for blood loss or tolerate large fluid loads given quickly.

10. The effect of hypovolemia and hypervolemia may be more pronounced in the elderly patient.

COMPLICATIONS

1. Coagulopathy. Coagulopathy is a result of hemodilution and hypothermia. Hemodilution of clotting factors due to the transfusion of multiple units of blood products as well as crystalloids and colloids can lead to hypercoagulable state in the body. In addition, stored PRBCs contain fewer clotting factors. Hypothermia slows the coagulation cascade (Hardy, de Moerloose, & Samama, 2004).

2. Dilutional thrombocytopenia may result from a decrease in platelet function in stored blood more than a few days old (Codner & Cinat, 2005).

3. Tranfusion-related acute lung injury (TRALI) (Codner & Cinat, 2005).

4. Hypothermia. Blood loss, environmental exposure, and infusion of crystalloids, colloids, and unwarmed blood products can lead to hypothermia. Hypothermia can cause decreased lactate and citrate metabolism, increased hemoglobin affinity for oxygen, and platelet dysfunction (Codner & Cinat, 2005).

5. Citrate toxicity. Each unit of PRBCs contains approximately 3 grams of citrate, which is normally metabolized by the liver within 5 minutes; however, in rapid transfusion, the liver may be unable to clear the level of citrate being introduced to the system (Codner & Cinat, 2005).

6. Hypocalcemia. Citrate binds to calcium in the body and may cause hypocalcemia (Codner & Cinat, 2005).

7. Hyperkalemia. The potassium concentration of blood increases as shelf-life increases and may result in hyperkalemia (Codner & Cinat, 2005).

8. Acid-base imbalance, especially metabolic acidosis. In the trauma patient, acidosis is caused by shock and poor oxygention, causing the body to use anaerobic metabolism for energy. This process results in the production and build up of lactic acid. Additionally, the citric and lactic acid levels increase over time in banked blood. Finally, stored PRBCs may also increase their affinity for oxygen, leading to poor tissue oxygenation. This may alter oxygen-carrying ability (Hardcastle, 2006).

9. Blood transfusions are a form of transplantation and can cause an immune response by the body (Codner & Cinat, 2005).

REFERENCES

Codner, P., & Cinat, M. (2005). Massive transfusion for trauma is apporpriate. *Trauma Care, 15*(3), 148-152.

Hardcastle, T. C. (2006). Complication of massive transfusion in trauma patients. *ISBT Science Series, 1*, 180-184.

Hardy, J. F., de Moerloose, P., & Samama, M. (2004). Massive transfusion and coagulopathy: Pathophysiology and implications for clinical management. *Canadian Journal of Anesthesia, 51*(4), 293-310.

Malone, D. L., Hess, J. R., & Fingerhut, A. (2006). Massive transfusion practices around the globe and a suggestion for a common massive transfusion protocol. *Journal of Trauma, 60*, S91-S96.

Mikhail, J. (2004). Massive transfusion in trauma: Process and outcomes. *Journal of Trauma Nursing, 11*(2), 55-61.

Morray, J. P., & Bhananker, S. M. (2005). Recent findings from the pediatric perioperative cardiac arrest registry. *ASA Newsletter, 69*(6), 10-12.

Repine, T. B., Perkins, J. G., Kauvar, D. S., & Blackborne, L. (2006). The use of fresh whole blood in massive transfusion. *Journal of Trauma, 60*, S59-S69.

Rudmann, S. V., & Nicol, K. K. (2005). Transfusion issues in selected patient populations. In S. V. Rudmann (Ed.), *Textbook of blood banking and transfusion medicine* (2nd ed., pp. 446-485). Philadelphia: Saunders.

Schulman, C. S. (2005). Massive infusion devices. In D. J. Lynn-McHale Wiegand, & K. K. Carlson (Eds.), *AACN procedure manual for critical care* (5th ed. pp. 1014-1023). St Louis: Saunders.

Smith, C. E. (2003). Current practices in fluid and blood component therapy in trauma. *Proceedings from the International Trauma Anesthesia and Critical Care Society (ITACCS) Seminar Panels, Massive Transfusion and Control of Hemorrhage in the Trauma Patient* (pp. 18-26). Baltimore: International Trauma Anesthesia and Critical Care Society. Available at http://www.itaccs.com/programs/Trans.pdf

Stapczynski, J. S., & Martin, G. A. (2004). Hematologic emergencies. In C. K. Stone, & R. Humphries (Eds.), *Current emergency diagnosis and treatment* (5th ed., pp. 788-823). San Francisco: McGraw-Hill.

Sweeney, M. N. (2003). Vascular access in trauma: Options, risks, benefits, complications. *Proceedings from the International Trauma Anesthesia and Critical Care Society (ITACCS) Seminar Panels, Massive Transfusion and Control of Hemorrhage in the Trauma Patient* (pp. 28-30). Baltimore: International Trauma Anesthesia and Critical Care Society. Available at http://www.itaccs.com/programs/Trans.pdf

Blood and Fluid Warmers

Andrew J. Bowman, RN, MSN, CEN, CTRN, CCRN-CMC, BC, CVN-I, FACCN, NREMT-P, and Jean A. Proehl, RN, MN, CEN, CCRN, FAEN

See Procedures 72, 73, 74, and 76 for information on blood products, blood filters, massive transfusion, and stand-alone pressure infusers.

INDICATIONS

Warming intravenous (IV) fluids and blood products is indicated in the following situations:

1. To prevent iatrogenic hypothermia when large quantities of IV fluid and blood products are administered.
2. To provide core rewarming and prevent additional heat loss in the presence of hypothermia.
3. To prevent coagulopathy in the trauma patient related to administration of unwarmed fluids and blood (Gin-Shaw & Jorden, 2006).

CONTRAINDICATIONS AND CAUTIONS

Hemolysis can occur with excessive warming (temperature greater than 42° C [107.6° F]) (AABB, 2005).

EQUIPMENT

IV fluid or blood as prescribed
Blood/fluid warmer
IV administration set compatible with warmer

PATIENT PREPARATION

1. Establish venous access (see Procedures 60 through 70).
2. Attach a short (20 cm or less) extension set to the IV cannula. This prevents the IV site from being disturbed when the blood tubing is being changed.

PROCEDURAL STEPS

†Level 1® Fluid Warmer (Figure 75-1) (Smiths Level 1, Inc., 2003a)

The Level 1® fluid warmer is a countercurrent heat exchanger; warmed fluid flows through a tube that surrounds the IV tubing.

1. Push the bottom end of the heat exchanger into the socket labeled "1."

---

†Refer to the Smiths Medical operator's manual, which contains specific information, including contraindications, warnings, precautions, and potential complications, for the safe and proper use of the product.

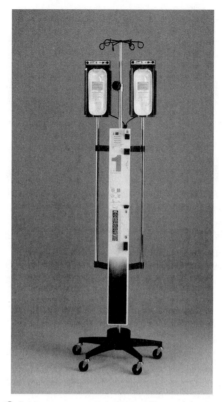

FIGURE 75-1 Level 1® fluid warmer, model 1200. (The model 1000 and 1025 are identical except that the model 1000 does not include the pressure infusers.) (Courtesy Smiths Level 1, Inc., Rockland, MA.)

2. Insert the heat exchanger into the guide. Slide the top socket, labeled "2," down over the top of the tube until it clicks.
3. Insert the filter/gas vent into its holder, labeled "3."
4. Plug in and turn on the machine. The display panel should have a green "system operational" indicator light.
5. Ensure that all the tubing connections are tight.
6. When infusing fluid under pressure, remove all the air from the fluid bag by withdrawing the air with a needle and a syringe to avoid an embolism.
7. Close all the IV clamps, spike the IV bag, and hang it on the IV pole.
8. Open the clamp above the drip chamber and squeeze the drip chamber until it is half full.
9. Open the last two clamps, remove the end cap, and prime the remaining tubing.
10. Close the distal clamp to cause the filter/gas vent to self-prime. Gently tap the filter or gas vent against the cabinet to remove all the trapped air.
11. Connect the system directly to the IV catheter to achieve the optimal flow rate. The Level 1 System 1000/1025/1200 can warm fluid to 37° to 42° C at a rate of up to 1 L/min (60,000 ml/hr).

12. When infusing blood products, replace the filter/gas vent or tubing set every 3 hours or sooner if the filter becomes clogged or the air is vented slowly.

13. To activate the pressure infuser (present on model 1025 and model 1200) (Smiths Level 1, Inc., 2003a), do the following:

   a. To prevent an air embolism, remove all the air from the IV bag with a 20-ml syringe and a needle, or use a needle to vent the air out of the injection port while squeezing the inverted bag. Spike the bag and prime the IV tubing. (The Smiths Level 1, Inc. model 1200 has an Integrated Air Detector System that automatically detects the presence of air in the infusion fluid, stops the flow of the fluid, and alerts personnel with audible and visual alarms. This should not preclude the air embolism precautions described above [Smiths Level 1, Inc., 2003b]). In addition, automatic air detector clamps can be obtained to augment your existing Smiths Level 1, Inc. 1025, 525, and 275 fast flow fluid warmers. See below for set-up information for the model 1200.

   b. Ensure that the venous access is made with a 14-G or larger cannula.

   c. Flip the toggle switch on the pressure infuser to the "off" position.

   d. Open the hinged latch on the right side of the infuser and hang the solution on the post at the top of the door. For blood or 500-ml bags of IV solution, use the post mounted on the inside of the door.

   e. Close the door and latch it. Open all the clamps in the IV tubing and close the clamp to the opposite spike tail.

   f. Flip the toggle switch to the "+" (on) position. Observe the pressure gauge to see whether a pressure of approximately 300 mm Hg is achieved. The pressure is not adjustable.

   g. When the fluid infusion is complete, flip the switch to the "−" (off) position and open the door. Remove the bag and repeat steps a through f. Manual decompression of the infuser bladder facilitates the insertion of a new IV bag.

14. PF-1 blood filter: The PF-1 is a 340-micron blood filter that prolongs the life of the 170-micron filter incorporated into the Level 1 tubing (Figure 75-2).

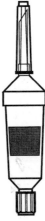

FIGURE 75-2 PF-1, 340-micron prefilter for blood. (Courtesy Smiths Level 1, Inc., Rockland, MA.)

Spike the blood bag with the PF-1 filter and then spike the PF-1 filter with the spike on the tubing set. Replace the PF-1 filter with each unit of blood.

15. Y-30 connector: Simultaneous infusion into two different IV sites can be achieved with the Y-30 connector. The Y-30 connector is added to the distal end of the tubing set and primed. The connector may be added even if two sites are not in use. Prime both tails and clamp off one. This ensures fast access to the warmed fluid if another site is obtained.

16. D-60HL tubing: Slow infusion rates increase the likelihood that much of the heat may be lost between the fluid warmer and the patient. The D-60HL tubing system, however, has a warm water jacket surrounding the full length of the tubing to allow the infusion of the warmed solution at rates as low as 75 ml/hr.

17. Troubleshooting alarms:
   a. The "check disposables" alarm indicates that a part of the tubing is not fully inserted into the warmer. Check the tubing at the points labeled "1," "2," and "3."
   b. The "add water" alarm signals a low water level in the circulating bath. Turn off the machine and remove the plug from the front of the machine. Add distilled water to the reservoir until it is full, as evidenced by the window in the front. (Sterile water is frequently distilled and may be used; however, the water does not need to be sterile.)
   c. The "over temperature" alarm signals excessive heating. Turn off the fluid warmer and remove it from service until it can be inspected and serviced.

†Level 1® H-1200 Fast Flow Fluid Warmer (Smiths Level 1, Inc., 2003b)

The Level 1® H-1200 warmer integrates pressure infusers, air detection, and automatic clamping in the presence of air.

1. Insert the bottom end of the heat exchanger into the block labeled "1" and push down to seat the heat exchanger firmly.
2. Slide the "2" block up and snap the heat exchanger into the guide. Slide the top socket, labeled "2," down over the top of the tube until it clicks.
3. Insert the gas vent/filter assembly:
   a. Open the "3" clamp slot door and slide the tubing up under the clamp slot door. Press the tubing into the clamp slot. Press the clamp slot door down to secure the tubing in the clamp slot.
   b. Align and insert the gas vent/filter assembly into the "4" block so as to prevent kinking of the tubing.
4. Make sure the toggle switch is in the off (−) position on both pressure chambers.
5. Press the green power on button.
   a. The air detector/clamp runs a power on test. All air detector/clamp indicators illuminate and an audible warning beeps.

---

†Refer to the Smiths Medical operator's manual, which contains specific information, including contraindications, warnings, precautions, and potential complications, for the safe and proper use of the product.

b. When the power on test is completed, the air detector/clamp enters unclamp mode; the unclamp LED lights up and the audible warning beeps every 5 seconds.

c. The green automatic operation indicator light on the Fluid Warmer display panel lights up.

d. If the disposable set/tubing is not correctly installed, the check disposables indicator illuminates and the audible alarm beeps. Confirm that each step of installation has been completed correctly.

6. Test the audible and visible alarms:

a. Press and hold the alarm test button on the Fluid Warmer's power and alarm test panel, and all visible alarm indicators will illuminate while the audible alarm signal beeps.

b. When the alarm test button is released, the over temperature alarm will continue to be active. To clear the over temperature alarm:

   i. Turn the Level 1® off and then turn it back on.

   ii. The air detector/clamp will run another power on test and go into unclamp mode. This is indicated by illumination of the yellow unclamp LED and beeping of the audible signal every 5 seconds. If the air detector/clamp does not go into unclamp mode, press the unclamp button.

7. Prime the disposable set/tubing:

a. Remove all the air from the IV bag with a 20-ml syringe and a needle, or use a needle to vent the air out of the injection port while squeezing the inverted bag. Alternatively, the bag can be spiked with the tubing, the spike withdrawn slightly from the bag, the air expressed, and the spike reinserted.

b. Ensure that all the tubing connections are tight. Close all the IV clamps, spike the IV bag, and hang it on the IV pole.

c. Open the clamp above the drip chamber and squeeze the drip chamber until it is one-third to one-half full.

d. Open the last two clamps, remove the end cap, and prime the remaining tubing.

e. Close the distal clamp to cause the filter/gas vent to self-prime.

8. Set the air detector/clamp to automatic operation (Figure 75-3):

a. Press the unclamp button on the air detector/clamp control panel; this should cause the yellow unclamp light to go off and the alarm to stop beeping.

b. The green automatic operation indicator lights up. Now the air detector/clamp will clamp the patient line if air is detected in the gas vent/filter assembly.

9. Test the air detector/clamp by pulling the top of the gas vent/filter assembly away from the air detector sensor. The following should occur:

a. Patient line is clamped shut and flow to the patient ceases.

b. Red clamped indicator lights up.

c. Audible alarm beeps.

10. Return system to normal operation:

a. Push the top of the gas vent/filter back into the "4" block.

b. Press the unclamp button on the air detector/clamp. The yellow unclamp button illuminates and the audible alarm beeps every 5 seconds.

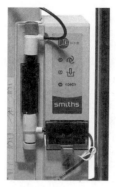

FIGURE 75-3 Level 1® Air Detector/Clamp with display panel. 1, Unclamp button indicator (yellow LED); 2, automatic operation LED indicator (green); 3, check tubing LED indicator (yellow); 4, clamped LED indicator (red). (Courtesy Smiths Level 1, Inc., Rockland, MA.)

     c. Press the unclamp button on the air detector/clamp control panel again; this should cause the yellow unclamp light to go off and the alarm to stop beeping.

     d. The green automatic operation indicator lights up.

11. Connect the system directly to the IV catheter to achieve the optimal flow rate. The Level 1® System 1000/1025 can warm fluid to between 37° and 42° C at a rate of up to 1 L/min (60,000 ml/hr).

12. See steps 12 through 17 above under Level 1® Fluid Warmer for information about pressurized infusion, various types of tubing and accessories, and troubleshooting.

†HotLine® Fluid Warmer (Smiths Level 1, Inc., 1998)

The HotLine uses a tubing half-set, which connects to the distal portion of any conventional IV tubing. Heating results from the warm water flowing around an inner lumen, which carries the IV fluids or blood. It is not considered a rapid infuser like the Smiths Level 1 infuser device described above.

1. Check the water level in the tank and plug the warmer into the power outlet.

2. Push the two extended tubes into the socket on the side of the warmer (Figure 75-4). A snap should be felt.

3. Turn on the power switch. If the warmer is functioning properly, a green "operating" light comes on and the water temperature gauge starts to increase.

4. The water flow should be visible in the outer lumen. Check to make sure that this lumen is fully primed before connecting it to the IV line.

5. Connect the IV tubing to the warmer set and prime the inner lumen with fluid.

6. Open and set the fluid rate with the roller clamp on the IV tubing set.

---

†Refer to the Smiths Medical operator's manual, which contains specific information, including contraindications, warnings, precautions, and potential complications, for the safe and proper use of the product.

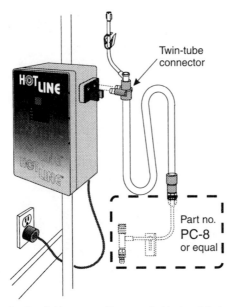

FIGURE 75-4 HotLine fluid warmer. (Courtesy Smiths Level 1, Inc., Rockland, MA.)

FloTem IIe (CVC/DataChem, Inc., 2000)

This warmer uses dry-heat technology that places IV tubing between metal heating plates (Figure 75-5).
1. Prime the IV tubing.
2. Place the tubing into the indented channel on the heating plate.
3. Close the warmer and turn on the power switch. The unit achieves the required temperature within 2 minutes.
4. A green power light is visible on the front of the unit along with the heated temperature of the fluid.
5. An audible alarm sounds if the temperature exceeds 41.5° C, and power to the coils is stopped. If the temperature reaches 42.5° C, the entire unit shuts off.

Warmflo® FW-538 Fluid Warmer (formerly Alton Dean) (Figure 75-6)
(Nellcor, 2002)

This warmer employs a stainless steel foil heat-exchange cassette. The cassette sits between two microprocessor-controlled heating plates.
1. The warmer displays specific operating instructions on the LCD screen. To start the warmer, press the "on" button and follow the instructions on the screen.
2. To remove the cassette, press the "eject" button and follow the instructions on the screen.
3. To turn the warmer off, press the "off" button and follow the instructions on the screen.
4. To change the temperature set point, press the "t" or "s" button.

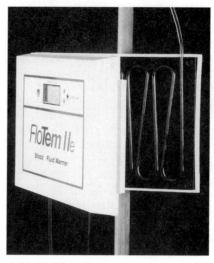

FIGURE 75-5 FloTem IIe blood and fluid warmer. (Courtesy CVC/DataChem, Indianapolis, IN.)

5. Fluid may be pressurized up to 500 mm Hg. For pressurized infusion, do the following:
   a. To prevent an air embolism, remove all the air from the IV bag with a 20-ml syringe and a needle, or use a needle to vent the air out of the injection port while squeezing the inverted bag. Spike the bag and prime the IV tubing.
   b. Place the IV bag in the infuser compartment and close and latch the door.
   c. Turn the toggle switch on the bottom of the infusor to the "+" (on) position. The pressure infuser can then be activated by the warmer at the appropriate time.

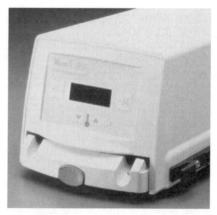

FIGURE 75-6 Warmflo blood and fluid warmer (formerly Alton Dean). (Courtesy Mallinckrodt Medical [Nellcor, division of Tyco], St. Louis.)

d. To increase the pressure, turn the regulator knob clockwise (right). To decrease infusion pressure, turn the regulator knob counterclockwise (left) one turn. Turn the toggle switch "off" and then "on" again to allow the pressure to stabilize. Repeat if necessary.

Thermal Angel (Figure 75-7) (Estill Medical Technologies, 2007)

This device is a battery-operated, portable in-line warmer. It is a disposable unit capable of warming fluids for 72 hours. The reusable battery must be charged before use—do not charge the battery while it is connected to the warming device.

1. Remove the female cap from the inlet end of the warming unit and connect the appropriate IV tubing (blood tubing, pump tubing, or primary set). Tighten until resistance is met without overtightening.
2. Remove the male cap from the outlet end of the device and connect a 9-inch IV extension tubing. Tighten until resistance is met without overtightening.
3. Connect the assembled tubing to the IV bag and prime the line.
4. Connect the male end of the power cable to the inlet end cap and connect the female end of the power cable to the battery.
5. The green LED will illuminate without blinking when the battery is properly connected.
6. Connect the extension set to the patient's IV site and begin the infusion.
7. Each battery will supply enough energy for warming 2 to 4 L of fluid or 1 to 3 units of blood. When the battery is depleted, another battery can be connected to the device to continue the warming. The warming device will operate for up to 72 continuous hours, at which point it will not respond to new batteries.

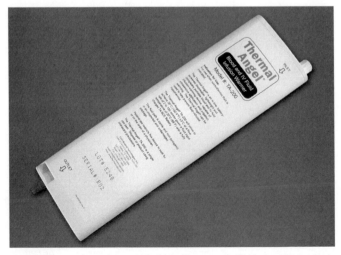

FIGURE 75-7 Thermal Angel TA-200. (Courtesy Estill Medical Technologies.)

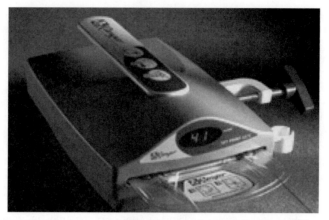

FIGURE 75-8 Ranger Blood/Fluid Warmer. (Courtesy of Arizant Healthcare.)

Ranger® Blood/Fluid Warming System (Figures 75-8 and 75-9)
Priming the fluid cassette

1. Slide the fluid-warming cassette into the slot in the warming unit.
2. Connect the short inlet line (A) on the Ranger Warming set to the fluid source.
3. Prime all tubing to purge air from the infusion line. Invert the bubble trap (D) while priming and fill it completely.

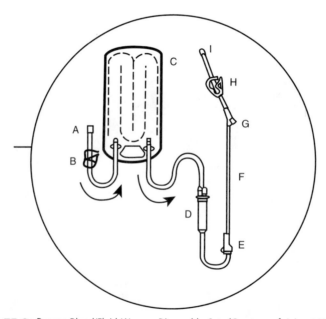

FIGURE 75-9 Ranger Blood/Fluid Warmer Disposable Set. (Courtesy of Arizant Healthcare.)

4. Turn the bubble trap right side up and continue priming the patient line (F).
5. Place the bubble trap into the holder on the warming unit.
6. Close all clamps.
7. Turn the warming unit "on."
8. Connect the tubing to the IV site and begin the infusion. Manual pressure bags may be used to speed the infusion

Removing air from the disposable set
1. Close the clamp (H) between the Injection port (G) and the patient connection (I).
2. Invert the bubble trap.
3. Insert a syringe into the injection port and aspirate air until the bubble trap and IV line are free of air.
4. Place the bubble trap right side up in the holder.
5. Open the clamp and continue infusion.

Removing the disposable set
1. Close the inlet clamp (B) and open the patient line clamps (E, H).
2. Disconnect the warming set from the fluid source.
3. Allow the fluid to flow into the patient if desired (this may take a few seconds).
4. Disconnect the warming set from the patient's IV and replace it with another IV line or a catheter cap.
5. Remove the fluid-warming cassette from the warming unit and discard.

AGE-SPECIFIC CONSIDERATIONS
1. Infants and children, because of the proportion of their surface area to their body weight (Cantor, 2006), and the elderly are especially susceptible to hypothermia. Blood and IV fluids should be warmed if rapid infusion is indicated.
2. Slower infusion rates (indicated for small children and the elderly) result in a loss of heat between the warmer and the patient. The Level 1 HotLine or the D-60HL tubing with the system 1000/1025/H-1200 can overcome this limitation.

COMPLICATIONS
1. Hemolysis
2. Sepsis
3. Air injection if a pressure infuser is used; this may occur if all the air is not removed from the bag before pressurization
4. Loss of fluid temperature prior to reaching the patient with either slow infusion rates or as the distance between the warmer and the patient increases

REFERENCES
American Association of Blood Banks (AABB). (2005). *Technical manual* (15th ed.). Arlington, VA: Author.

Cantor, R. M. (2006). Pediatric trauma. In J. A. Marx, R. S. Hockberger, & R. M. Walls (Eds.), *Rosen's emergency medicine: Concepts and clinical practice* (6th ed., pp. 328-343). St Louis: Mosby.

CVC/DataChem, Inc. (2002). *FloTem IIe Fluid Warmer: Instructions for use.* Indianapolis, IN: Author.

Estill Medical Technologies. (2007). *Thermal Angel® blood and IV fluid infusion warmer: TA-200 instructions.* Retrieved March 5, 2007, from http://www.thermalangel.com/html/products-thermalangelinstructions.html

Gin-Shaw, S. L., & Jorden, R. C. (2006). Multiple trauma. In J. A. Marx, R. S. Hockberger, & R. M. Walls (Eds.), *Rosen's emergency medicine: Concepts and clinical practice* (6th ed., pp. 300-316). St Louis: Mosby.

Nellcor. (2002). *Warmflo® Fluid Warming System.* Pleasanton, CA: Author. Available at http://www.nellcor.com/_Catalog/PDF/product/WarmFloBrochure.pdf

Smiths Level 1, Inc. (1998). *HotLine Fluid Warmer: Instructions for use.* Rockland, MA: Author.

Smiths Level 1, Inc. (2003a). *Level 1® Fluid Warmer instructions for use.* Rockland, MA: Author.

Smiths Level 1, Inc. (2003b). *H-1200 Fast Flow Fluid Warmer: Operator's manual.* Rockland, MA: Author.

PROCEDURE 76

Blood and Fluid Pressure Infusers

Andrew J. Bowman, RN, MSN, CEN, CTRN, CCRN-CMC, BC, CVN-I, FACCN, NREMT-P

The Level 1 (Smiths) blood and fluid warmer has an integrated pressure infuser on some models—see Procedure 75 for information and operating instructions.

INDICATION

To infuse blood products and/or intravenous (IV) fluids rapidly to treat intravascular volume deficit.

CONTRAINDICATIONS AND CAUTIONS

1. Remove all the air from the IV bag to prevent an air embolism.
2. Do not exceed 300 mm Hg of pressure because it may cause the bag to leak or rupture (Puget Sound Blood Center & Program, 2006).

3. Frequent assessment of blood pressure, pulse, skin temperature, capillary refill, urinary output, central venous pressure, or arterial pressure as available is required to evaluate the response to fluid resuscitation.
4. Because glass IV containers and some autotransfusion devices are not compressible, they cannot be used with pressure infusers.
5. Make sure that there are no in-line restrictions, such as small-bore T and Y adapters and stopcocks, in the IV tubing. If these connectors have small lumens, they restrict the flow.
6. Iatrogenic hypothermia may result from the rapid infusion of room temperature IV fluids or refrigerated blood products; warm the blood and IV fluids if rapid infusion is necessary (see Procedure 75).
7. Do not use a blood pressure cuff as a pressure device for delivering blood products. The cuff can cause uneven pressure on the bag, leading to rupture of the bag or damage to the contents (Puget Sound Blood Center & Program, 2006).
8. Many long-term implanted ports or tunneled catheters should not be used with pressure infusers; check the manufacturer's specifications before administering pressurized fluid through one of these devices.

EQUIPMENT
18-G needle
20-ml syringe
Pressure infuser (one of the following):
    Manual pressure bag
    Warmflo automatic pressure infuser (Nellcor, formerly Alton Dean)
    ZOLL Power Infuser® (ZOLL Medical)

PATIENT PREPARATION
1. Establish IV access, preferably with a 14-G or larger catheter (see Procedures 60 through 67). Use of a large-bore catheter prevents red blood cell hemolysis as the blood passes through the catheter. If the patient has a preexisting IV site, assess the site for signs of problems, such as redness, pain, and swelling.
2. Ensure that the IV tubing is large-bore tubing (blood or trauma tubing) compatible with the infusor to be used.

PROCEDURAL STEPS
Manual Bag (Figure 76-1)
1. To prevent an air embolism, remove all the air from the IV bag with a 20-ml syringe and a needle, or use a needle to vent the air out of the injection port while squeezing the inverted bag. Spike the bag and prime the IV tubing.
2. Invert and insert the IV bag through the lower opening of the pressure cuff.
3. Insert the loop at the top end of the pressure cuff through the eye of the IV bag.
4. Suspend the cuff and the solution bag by the strap on the IV pole.
5. Check the security of the IV tubing connections at the bag and at the IV site.
6. Inflate to the desired pressure but do not exceed 300 mm Hg. This is to prevent damage to the red blood cells, disruption of the delivery system, and complications at the IV site.

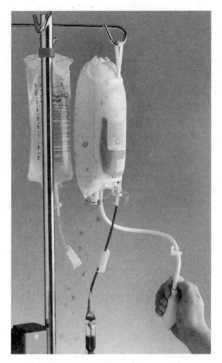

FIGURE 76-1 Manual pressure bag.

7. Maintain the desired pressure by squeezing the bulb pump as the fluid or blood is infused.
8. When the blood bag is empty, clamp the line and then flush any blood from the line with normal saline solution.
9. Remove the empty solution bag by releasing the pressure in the bag.
10. After removing the bag, finish deflating the pressure bag manually. This facilitates insertion of the next bag of solution.

Warmflo® Automatic Pressure Infuser (Figure 76-2) (Nellcor, 2003)

These devices require that a source of compressed gas be connected to the device.
1. To prevent an air embolism, remove all the air from the IV bag with a 20-ml syringe and a needle, or use a needle to vent the air out of the injection port while squeezing the inverted bag. Spike the bag and prime the IV tubing.
2. Turn the on/off switch to the "off" position.
3. Plug the air hose into the air or the oxygen outlet.
4. Open the door and hang the IV solution bag on the hang tab. If a 500-ml bag is being used, line up the bottom of the bag with the bottom of the door.
5. Close the door and lock it with the latch.
6. Hang the pressure infuser on an IV pole.
7. Turn the regulator knob to the left (counterclockwise) until it stops.
8. Turn the on/off switch to the "on" position. A hissing sound is heard as the air bladder behind the solution bag fills.

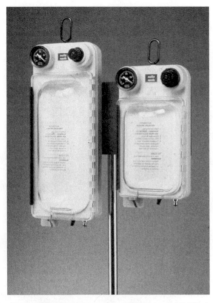

FIGURE 76-2 Warmflo Automatic Pressure Infuser. (Courtesy Mallinckrodt Medical [Nellcor, division of Tyco], St Louis, MO.)

9. While monitoring the pressure gauge, turn the regulator knob to the right (clockwise) until the desired pressure is reached.

10. If the pressure exceeds 300 mm Hg, or if you wish to decrease the pressure, keep the switch "on." Then turn the regulator knob to the left and observe the pressure reading in the gauge. Once the selected pressure is reached, turn the infuser toggle switch to "off" and then back to "on" and check the pressure reading. The gauge may need to be tapped lightly after an adjustment.

11. To increase the pressure (do not turn off the infuser), turn the regulator knob to the right until the desired pressure is reached. Do not exceed 300 mm Hg to prevent damage to the container or cells.

12. To remove the IV bag, turn the toggle switch to the "off" position. Open the door and remove the bag.

ZOLL Power Infuser® (Figure 76-3) (ZOLL Medical, 2006)

1. Set up and prime.
   a. Connect the bag, cartridge, and IV sets using standard IV bag spike with Luer-Lok connectors. When infusing blood products with the blood cartridge, always use an IV set that is designed for blood products and contains an appropriate screen or filter.
   b. Install the cartridge. Hold it at an angle and engage tab on the side of the cartridge; swing over rocker until the two pegs on the cartridge snap into the slots in the pump.
   c. Turn pump on for battery operation or connect optional power adapter.
   d. Hold down start/stop to prime entire IV set. Tap the cartridge to remove air bubbles and stop the pump.

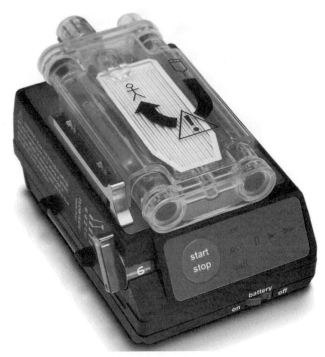

FIGURE 76-3 ZOLL Power Infuser. (Courtesy Infusion Dynamics a Division of ZOLL Medical, Plymouth Meeting, PA.)

2. Infuse IV fluids:
   a. Set the flow rate. The numbered settings (liters/hour) run continuously until stopped. BoLUS infuses approximately 250 ml in 2.5 minutes and then stops automatically.
   b. Press start/stop to begin infusion.
3. Change IV bag:
   a. Press start/stop to pause the pump.
   b. Close clamp on IV set.
   c. Change IV bag.
   d. Open clamp on IV set.
   e. Press start/stop to resume infusion.
4. End the infusion:
   a. Push to release cartridge.
   b. Gravity-driven infusion can continue with the cartridge inline.
   c. Turn off pump or unplug power adapter.
5. Troubleshooting:
   a. "Air" indicator illuminated and unit continues to alarm.
      i. Unit may have detected air as fluid exits the pump. If an air bubble is present, extract the air before resuming flow. Press start/stop to resume infusion. When using the crystalloid/colloid cartridge, this should only occur if the IV set has not been properly primed.

Under normal operation the cartridge should vent air entering the pump.

ii. Check if cartridge has been disconnected from the pump. Reinsert the cartridge. Press start/stop to resume infusion.

iii. Fluid being delivered does not have adequate salinity. Fluid must have a salinity level greater than 0.15%. Change fluid and press start/stop to resume infusion.

iv. Pump circuitry is adjusting to the IV fluid. This problem will correct itself 10 to 20 seconds after pump has been turned on and a primed cartridge has been installed or when switching from IV fluid to blood products in the same IV line. Press start/stop to resume infusion.

b. "Occ" indicator illuminated and unit continues to alarm.

i. Flow has become restricted between pump and patient. Check that clamps are open and that lines are not kinked.

ii. Confirm that IV catheter is of adequate size and properly positioned in vein. When infusing saline or lactated Ringer's, an 18-G peripheral IV catheter is recommended. When infusing blood or blood products, use of a 14- or 16-G peripheral catheter is recommended.

c. "Batt" indicator illuminated and unit continues to alarm. Batteries are low. Replace batteries or connect optional power adapter. Standard AAA alkaline batteries are recommended. Use only power adapters supplied by ZOLL Medical.

AGE-SPECIFIC CONSIDERATIONS

1. Elderly patients or those who have a chronic disease (renal or liver disease, heart failure) must be resuscitated cautiously with fluids because of their impaired ability to deal with a fluid overload. At the same time, elderly patients poorly tolerate hypotension and hypovolemia.
2. Neonates and pediatric patients are at risk for circulatory overload because of their small baseline blood volume.
3. Elderly and pediatric patients are at increased risk of iatrogenic hypothermia; warm the fluids if a rapid infusion is necessary (see Procedure 75).

COMPLICATIONS

1. Air embolization
2. Volume overload
3. Infiltration of IV fluid
4. Iatrogenic hypothermia can occur if unheated solutions are administered rapidly.

REFERENCES

Nellcor. (2003). *Warmflo® Pressure Infusor*. Pleasanton, CA: Author.

Puget Sound Blood Center and Program. (2006). *Blood and blood components reference manual*. Seattle: Author. Retrieved March 5, 2007, from http://www.psbc.org/bcrm/pdf/Regional_SectionB_RevB.pdf

ZOLL Medical. (2006). *ZOLL Power Infuser*. Retrieved March 5, 2007, from http://www.zoll.com/product_resource.aspx?id=791

General Principles of Autotransfusion

Deborah A. Upton, MSN, ARNP-BC, CEN

Autotransfusion is the collection and filtration of blood from an active bleeding site and reinfusion of that blood into the same patient for the maintenance of blood volume (Scott, 2005).

INDICATIONS

To return shed autologous blood to the patient with a massive hemothorax. The advantages of using autotransfused blood include warmth and immediately availability, perfect compatibility with the patient and no risk of transfusion reaction, no risk of blood-borne disease transmission to the patient, and decreased demand on the stored blood supply. Clinical situations may include:

1. Massive hemothorax.
2. Myocardial rupture.
3. Great vessel rupture.
4. Chest trauma where there is a known history of transfusion reactions.
5. Chest trauma where the patient, for religious or other reasons, refuses banked blood.

Some autotransfusion systems require assembly or in-line insertion into the chest-drainage system; therefore, consider routinely setting the autotransfusion component for patients who are at high risk for hemothorax. Otherwise, blood that drains immediately on chest-tube insertion may be lost to recovery. Some systems (Atrium & Argyle) offer the option of closed-loop collection and reinfusion.

CONTRAINDICATIONS AND CAUTIONS

1. If contamination of the pleural blood from gastrointestinal contents is suspected, the risk of sepsis is significant. When the possibility exists of a communication between the abdomen and the chest (e.g., diaphragmatic disruption from a gunshot or stab wound), the risks and benefits of auto-transfusion must be considered. Prophylactic broad-spectrum antibiotics are usually given if gastrointestinal contamination of autotransfused blood is suspected.
2. Wounds more than 4 hours old because of the potential for bacterial contamination (AABB, 2005a).
3. Reinfusion of collected blood should occur within 6 hours of initiating the collection (AABB, 2005a).
4. Autotransfusion is contraindicated in the presence of coagulopathy, malignant neoplasm, enteric contamination of thoracic cavity, or infection

(systemic, pulmonary, pericardial, or mediastinal) (Atrium Medical Corporation, 2006).

5. Only blood collected in the autotransfusion unit should be reinfused. Any collected in the chest-drainage device should not be reinfused. Blood collected by use of the Atrium system is an exception because it is collected in a sterile chamber and is later transferred to a bag for reinfusion.

PROCEDURAL STEPS

1. Insert a large-bore chest tube(s) (see Procedure 39).
2. Prepare the autotransfusion unit for blood collection (see Procedures 78 through 80).
3. Inject an anticoagulant into the collection unit (optional). The use of an anticoagulant is not mandatory because the blood is frequently defibrinated by friction in the pleural cavity. However, if blood loss and recovery are rapid, the blood may still clot. Anticoagulants do not dissolve clots; they prevent them. Hence, if clots form in the collection chamber, the blood is not available for autotransfusion. Some sources report no difficulty in autotransfusing blood without an anticoagulant (Purcell, 2004). If an anticoagulant is used, instill it as soon as possible during or before the blood collection. Common anticoagulant options include the following:
   a. Citrate phosphate dextrose (CPD) is a commonly used anticoagulant. One milliliter of CPD for every 7 ml of blood is recommended (AABB, 2005b). Because it is difficult to estimate the amount of blood in a patient's chest, one approach is to instill enough CPD to anticoagulate 1 unit of blood initially (60 ml). When 1 unit of blood has been collected (about 500 ml total volume of blood plus CPD), it may be reinfused, or additional CPD may be added to continue the collection. The CPD injection may be facilitated by the use of a volume-control intravenous chamber; run the desired amount of CPD into the chamber and then infuse the CPD via the intravenous tubing to the injection port.
   b. Citrate phosphate dextrose adenine (CPDA-1): 1 ml per 7 ml of blood is recommended (AABB, 2005b). Instill as described in step 3a above.
4. Collect blood.
5. When 500 to 1000 ml of blood has been collected, prepare for reinfusion (see Procedures 78 through 80).
6. A microfilter is suggested when infusing the collected blood to reduce the risk of microembolization and secondary pulmonary insufficiency (Purcell, 2004).
7. Ongoing evaluation of the patient who is being autotransfused includes evaluation of laboratory data to include hematocrit, prothrombin time (PT), partial thromboplastin time (PTT), platelet count, and arterial blood gases.

AGE-SPECIFIC CONSIDERATIONS

1. For pediatric patients, if an anticoagulant is used, instill a proportionately smaller amount (based on the amount you plan to collect before the recovery for reinfusion).
2. Notify the physician if bleeding exceeds 1 to 2 ml/kg per hour (Kadish, 2006).

COMPLICATIONS

1. Hematologic complications include decreased platelet count and fibrinogen level, prolonged PT and PTT, and red blood cell hemolysis. These complications usually occur with massive autotransfusion (greater than 1 to 1.5 times the patient's blood volume in pediatric patients). To avoid this complication, it has been recommended not to exceed 2000 ml of autotransfused blood (Atrium Medical Corporation, 2006; Purcell, 2004).
2. Nonhematologic complications include bacteremia and microembolism (Atrium Medical Corporation, 2006; Purcell, 2004).
3. Rapid reinfusion of citrate-containing blood can result in citrate toxicity, hypocalcemia, and myocardial depression. Signs and symptoms of citrate toxicity include tingling around the mouth, stomach cramps, arrhythmias, hypokalemia, alkalosis, circumoral cyanosis, and hypotension.

REFERENCES

American Association of Blood Banks (AABB). (2005a). *Guidance for standards for perioperative autologous blood collection and administration* (2nd ed.). Bethesda, MD: Author.

American Association of Blood Banks (AABB). (2005b). *Guidelines for blood recovery and reinfusion in surgery and trauma*. Bethesda, MD: Author.

Atrium Medical Corporation. (2006). *Chest drain autotransfusion (package insert)*. Hudson, NH: Author.

Kadish, H. (2006). Thoracic trauma. In G. R. Fleisher, S. Ludwig, & F. M. Henretig (Eds.), *Textbook of pediatric emergency medicine* (5th ed., pp. 1433-1452). Philadelphia: Lippincott Williams & Wilkins.

Purcell, T. B. (2004). Autotransfusion. In J. R. Roberts, & J. R. Hedges (Eds.), *Clinical procedures in emergency medicine* (4th ed., pp. 410-426). Philadelphia: Saunders.

Scott, J. (2005). Autotransfusion. In D. Lynn-McHale Wiegand, & K. K. Carlson (Eds.), *AACN procedure manual for critical care* (5th ed., pp. 121-124). St Louis: Saunders.

Autotransfusion Devices: Pleur-Evac

Deborah A. Upton, MSN, ARNP-BC, CEN

The information in this procedure should be used in conjunction with the information in Procedure 77.

Pleur-Evac and Sahara chest-drainage units are products of the Deknatel Product Group, Teleflex Medical OEM (Research Triangle Park, NC).

INDICATION
See Procedure 77.

CONTRAINDICATIONS AND CAUTIONS
See Procedure 77.

EQUIPMENT
Pleur-Evac chest-tube drainage system and autotransfusion unit
Blood tubing with filter
Suction setup
Anticoagulant (optional)
18-G needle (optional)
60-ml syringe or intravenous (IV) tubing with volumetric chamber (optional)

PATIENT PREPARATION
Insert a large-bore chest tube (see Procedure 39).

PROCEDURAL STEPS (Deknatel, 1997)
1. Prepare the chest-drainage unit (see Procedure 44).
2. Attach the autotransfusion bag if the unit is not ready for autotransfusion. The autotransfusion bag (A-1500) is attached to the side of the Pleur-Evac chest-tube drainage system. Use the foot hook and the ATS hanger on the side of the unit (Figure 78-1).
   a. Close the two white clamps on the top of the A-1500 replacement bag.
   b. Close the white clamp on the Pleur-Evac patient tubing and drain the blood distally from the tubing into the Pleur-Evac.
   c. Detach the red and the blue connectors.
   d. Remove the red protective cap from the collection tubing on the A-1500 replacement bag and connect it to the patient chest-drainage tubing using the red connectors.

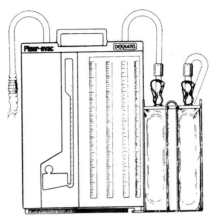

FIGURE 78-1 Pleur-Evac autotransfusion unit, set up to collect blood. (Courtesy Deknatel, Teleflex Medical OEM, Research Triangle, NC).

    e. Remove the blue protective cap from the tubing on the A-1500 replacement bag and connect it to the Pleur-Evac tubing using the blue connectors.

    f. Open all the clamps and make sure all the connections are airtight.

    g. Inject an anticoagulant into the collection bag (optional). A 60-ml syringe or a volumetric IV chamber can be used to instill the anticoagulant.

3. Collect blood.

4. To discontinue collection:

    a. Use the high-negativity relief valve to reduce excessive negativity.

    b. Close the white clamps on the patient tubing and on top of the autotransfusion bag.

    c. Detach all the red and the blue connectors.

    d. Attach the red and the blue connectors on top of the autotransfusion bag.

    e. Securely attach the red and the blue connectors by joining the patient tube (red) to the Pleur-Evac tube (blue).

    f. Open the white clamps on the patient tube so that the drainage can be collected in the Pleur-Evac. Failure to do this in a timely manner may result in tension pneumothorax.

    g. Remove the autotransfusion bag from the Pleur-Evac by removing the collection-bag frame from the hanger on the side of the unit. Disconnect the foot hook from the Pleur-Evac unit and slide the bag off the wire frame.

5. To change the autotransfusion bag, refer to preceding steps 2a through 2g.

6. Prepare for reinfusion (Figure 78-2) by doing the following:

    a. Invert the bag so that the spike port points upward, remove the protective cap, and insert a blood filter into the spike port by using a constant twisting motion (see Procedure 73).

    b. Remove the air from the bag. Keeping the unit inverted, squeeze all the air from the bag carefully through the filter and the drip-chamber assembly. Close the infusion set clamp, invert the autotransfusion bag, suspend it

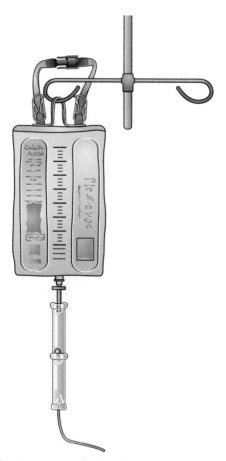

FIGURE 78-2 Pleur-Evac autotransfusion unit, set up for reinfusion of collected blood.

from an IV pole by using the plastic strap, open the infusion set, and flush the administration line carefully to remove all of the air.

7. Reinfusion: Attach the distal end of the infusion set assembly to the IV line and infuse the blood by using gravity or pressure. A pressure infuser that wraps around the bag is best suited for the A-1500 replacement bag when a pressure reinfusion is indicated. Be sure to remove all air from the bag before infusing under pressure.

AGE-SPECIFIC CONSIDERATION

Although the Pleur-Evac autotransfusion system is designed for adult use, it can be used for pediatric patients. The amount of anticoagulant used should be proportionate to the amount of blood that is anticipated to be collected prior to any reinfusion.

COMPLICATIONS

1. Refer to Procedure 77.

2. An air embolism is a potential complication during autotransfusion with this system. To reduce the risk of an air embolism, the collected blood must be properly prepared for reinfusion by removing all of the air from the blood bag before hanging it for reinfusion.

REFERENCE

Deknatel Product Group, Genzyme Surgical Products. (1997). *Pleur-Evac adult/pediatric single-use chest drainage unit: A-7000 (product insert)*. Research Triangle, NC: Teleflex Medical OEM.

PROCEDURE 79

Autotransfusion Devices: Argyle[†]

Deborah A. Upton, MSN, ARNP-BC, CEN

The information in this procedure should be used in conjunction with the information in Procedure 77.

INDICATION

See Procedure 77.

The Argyle autotransfusion system allows for the reinfusion of blood by using a continuous reinfusion method. This technique is generally not suitable for emergency department use, but it may be acceptable for a patient who belongs to a religious group, such as the Jehovah's Witnesses, that opposes blood transfusion.

CONTRAINDICATIONS AND CAUTIONS

See Procedure 77.

[†]Argyle is a registered trademark of Sherwood Medical (St. Louis, MO).

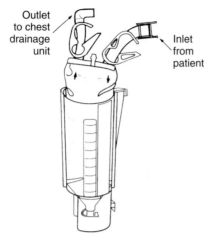

Outlet
to chest
drainage
unit

Inlet
from
patient

FIGURE 79-1 Autotransfusion accessory unit. (Courtesy Sherwood Davis & Geck, St Louis, MO.)

EQUIPMENT

Argyle autotransfusion chest-drainage unit (Thora-Seal III, Aqua-Seal, or Sentinel Seal)

Autotransfusion accessory unit (Figure 79-1)

Suction device setup

Anticoagulant of choice (optional)

18-G needle (optional)

60-ml syringe or intravenous (IV) tubing with volumetric chamber (optional)

Microembolus blood filter, IV pump, and blood-compatible pump tubing (continuous-infusion method only)

PATIENT PREPARATION

Insert a chest tube (see Procedure 39).

PROCEDURAL STEPS (Sherwood Medical, 1992a,b)

1. Prepare the chest-drainage unit as described in Procedure 45. The vacuum should not exceed −25 cm H_2O.
2. If not preattached, attach the autotransfusion unit to the chest-drainage unit by using the hooks and the Velcro closure. Connect the tubing so that the autotransfusion bag is in line between the patient and the chest-drainage unit (match the connectors: blue to blue and white to white) (Figures 79-2 and 79-3).
3. (Optional) Use a 60-ml syringe or IV tubing with a volumetric chamber to add an anticoagulant to the drainage-collection chamber through the injection port located on the top of the blood-collection bag.
4. Collect the blood.
5. Reinfusion via gravity includes the following steps:
   a. Close all the tubing clamps and detach the blue and the white connectors. Place a new autotransfusion unit in line, or reconnect the patient directly to the chest-drainage unit by connecting the blue and the white

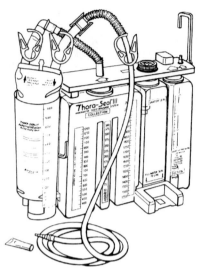

FIGURE 79-2 Thora-Seal III autotransfusion chest-drainage system. (Courtesy Sherwood Davis & Geck, St Louis, MO.)

connectors. Open all the clamps. Failure to do this in a timely manner may result in tension pneumothorax.

b. Attach the blue and the white connectors on the top of the autotransfusion bag. Remove the autotransfusion bag from the plastic tower.

c. Prime the blood tubing with saline solution (see Procedure 73).

d. Spike the port at the bottom of the autotransfusion bag with the primed blood tubing. Hang the bag on an IV stand.

e. Open the roller clamp and initiate the transfusion. If pressurized infusion is anticipated, remove all of the air from the autotransfusion bag. Reinfusion pressure should not exceed 150 mm Hg (see Procedure 76).

6. The continuous-reinfusion method includes the following steps:

a. When adequate blood has collected in the autotransfusion bag, prime the blood-compatible pump tubing with normal saline solution.

b. Spike the port at the bottom of the autotransfusion bag with the primed pump tubing.

c. Lower the IV pump as close to the level of the chest-drainage unit as possible. The chest-drainage unit must remain below the level of the patient's chest.

d. Set the pump to reinfuse the blood at a rate approximating the drainage rate. Monitor the amount of blood in the autotransfusion bag carefully and discontinue autotransfusion when there is 50 ml or less in the collection bag.

AGE-SPECIFIC CONSIDERATION

The Argyle autotransfusion system is designed for adult use, but it can also be used for pediatric patients. The amount of anticoagulant used should be proportionate to the amount of blood that is anticipated to be collected prior to any reinfusion.

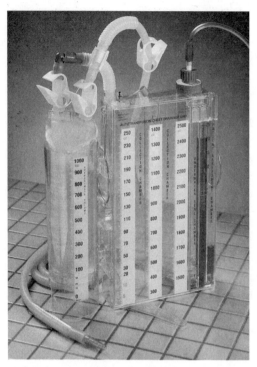

FIGURE 79-3 Sentinel Seal autotransfusion chest-drainage unit. (Courtesy Sherwood Davis & Geck, St Louis, MO.)

COMPLICATIONS

See Procedure 77.

An air embolism is a potential complication during autotransfusion with this system. To reduce the risk of an air embolism, the collected blood must be properly prepared for reinfusion by removing all of the air from the blood bag before hanging it for reinfusion.

REFERENCES

Sherwood Medical. (1992a). *Aqua-Seal autotransfusion accessory unit (instruction card)*. St Louis: Author.

Sherwood Medical. (1992b). *Thora-Seal III autotransfusion accessory unit (instruction card)*. St Louis: Author.

Autotransfusion Devices: Atrium

Deborah A. Upton, MSN, ARNP-BC, CEN

The information in this procedure should be used in conjunction with the information in Procedure 77.

INDICATION

See Procedure 77.

The Atrium autotransfusion system also allows for reinfusion of blood using a "closed-loop" technique. This technique is generally not suitable for emergency department use but may be acceptable to a patient who belongs to a religious group, such as the Jehovah's Witnesses, that opposes blood transfusion.

CONTRAINDICATIONS AND CAUTIONS

See Procedure 77.

EQUIPMENT

Atrium ATS chest-drainage unit
Atrium ATS blood-recovery bag (self-filling bag or in-line bag)
Suction setup
Sterile saline solution or sterile water (saline solution is recommended for all continuous ATS applications)
Anticoagulant of choice (optional)
18-G needle (optional)
60-ml syringe or intravenous (IV) tubing with volumetric chamber (optional)
Blood tubing and filter
IV pump, microembolus blood filter, blood-compatible pump tubing (closed-loop technique only)

PATIENT PREPARATION

Insert a chest tube (see Procedure 39).

PROCEDURAL STEPS (Atrium, 2006)

1. Prepare the Atrium blood-recovery chest-drainage unit as described in Procedure 46. Sterile saline solution is recommended for blood-recovery procedures. These units have an additional access line for autotransfusion (ATS access line), which allows access to the drainage unit without disconnecting the chest drain or interrupting the patient drainage (Figure 80-1).
2. (Optional) As soon as significant bloody drainage is noted, add the selected anticoagulant to the drainage-collection chamber or in-line blood collection

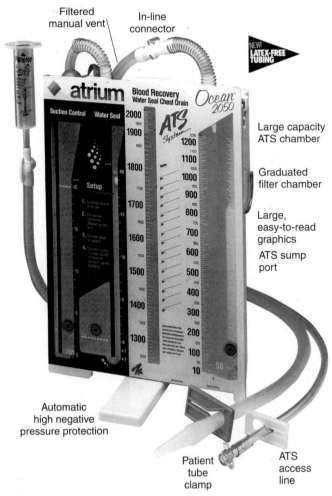

FIGURE 80-1 Atrium 2050 blood recovery system. (Courtesy Atrium, Hudson, NH.)

bag. To add anticoagulant to the chamber, swab the patient drainage tubing just proximal to the chest-drainage unit with an alcohol pad and inject the anticoagulant through the tubing 20-G or smaller needle. If an in-line blood collection bag is in use, add the anticoagulant through the injection site on the top of the ATS bag with an 18-G or smaller needle. Intravenous tubing with a volumetric chamber may be used to add the anticoagulant instead of a 60-ml syringe. The controlled doses for anticoagulant citrate dextrose (ACD), as recommended by the manufacturer, are noted in Table 80-1.

3. For self-filling ATS bags (Figure 80-2), do the following:
   a. Turn off the suction.
   b. Close the chest-drain ATS access-line clamp and remove the spike port cap before attaching the bag.

TABLE 80-1

MANUFACTURER'S RECOMMENDED DOSES OF ANTICOAGULANT CITRATE DEXTROSE-A

| | Amount of ACD-A | |
Blood Volume Expected	1:7 ratio	1:20 ratio
Low volume, 140-250 ml	20-35 ml	7-12.5 ml
Incremental volume, over 250 ml	14 ml/100 ml blood	5 ml/100 ml blood
Moderate volume, 250-500 ml	40-70 ml	12.4-25 ml
Large volume, 500-1000 ml	70-140 ml	70-140 ml

From Atrium (2006). *Atrium autotransfusion guide.* Hudson, NH: Author.

   c. Insert the ATS bag spike into the chest-drain ATS access line spike port by using a twisting motion. Position the ATS bag below the base of the chest drain to facilitate filling.

   d. Open both clamps and hold the ATS bag 2 to 4 inches below the base of the chest drain. Gently bend the bottom of the ATS bag upward to activate blood transfer.

   e. To disconnect the ATS bag, close both clamps, remove the ATS spike, and insert it into the ATS bag spike holder. Recap the ATS access line spike port and place the access line in the holder located on top of the chest drain. The ATS bag is ready for infusion.

   f. Turn on the suction.

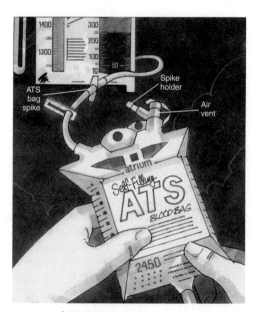

FIGURE 80-2 Autotransfusion blood recovery bag. (Courtesy Atrium, Hudson, NH.)

4. For in-line ATS bags (Figure 80-3):

    a. Open the patient tube clamp and move it next to the in-line connector for easy setup and visual checks.

    b. Close the patient-tube clamp and separate the connector by depressing the connector lock.

    c. Remove the cap from the female ATS-bag connector and insert it into the male patient-tube connector.

    d. Remove the second ATS-bag cap and insert the male ATS-bag connector into the female chest-drain connector.

    e. Open both in-line ATS-bag clamps before opening the patient-tube clamp. Open the patient-tube clamp after both ATS-bag clamps have been opened.

    f. To remove the in-line ATS bag from the chest drain, close the patient-tube clamp and both ATS bag clamps. Disconnect the chest-drain side first, and then disconnect the patient-side connector. Place the male patient-tube connector into the female chest-drain connector and open the patient-tube clamp. Failure to do this is a timely manner may result in tension pneumothorax. Reconnect the ATS-bag connectors to each other. The ATS bag is ready for reinfusion.

5. Reinfusion requires the following steps:

    a. Prime the blood tubing with saline solution (see Procedure 73).

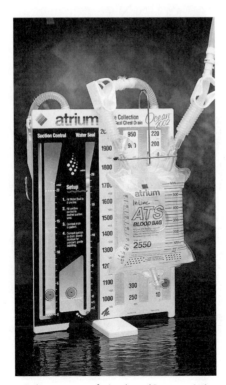

FIGURE 80-3 In-line autotransfusion bag. (Courtesy Atrium, Hudson, NH.)

b. Invert the ATS bag with the spike port pointing up and remove the teth-
ered cap. Insert the blood filter spike into the ATS-bag spike port by using
a firm twisting motion. Hang the ATS bag on an IV stand.

c. Open the air vent and initiate the transfusion.

d. Do not squeeze or otherwise attempt to pressurize the bag.

6. The closed-loop technique (not usually used in the emergency department)
(Figure 80-4) requires the following steps:

a. For direct reinfusion of shed autologous blood via a blood-compatible
infusion pump, a microembolus blood filter and a nonvented, blood-
compatible IV pump tubing are required. Position the IV pump as close
to the chest-drainage unit as possible. Prime the tubing with saline
solution according to the directions of the pump manufacturer, spike
the ATS access line with the blood-tubing setup, and connect it to an
injection port on a preexisting IV site. Program the pump to deliver
the blood at approximately the same rate that it is draining from the
chest.

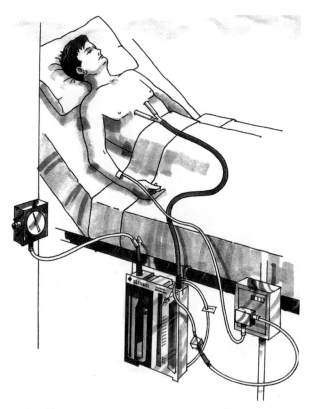

FIGURE 80-4 Closed-loop setup using an intravenous infusion pump. (Courtesy Atrium,
Hudson, NH.)

AGE-SPECIFIC CONSIDERATION

The Atrium autotransfusion system is designed for adult use, but it can also be used for pediatric patients. The amount of anticoagulant used should be proportionate to the amount of blood that is anticipated to be collected prior to any reinfusion.

COMPLICATIONS

See Procedure 77.

REFERENCE

Atrium. (2006). *Atrium autotransfusion guide*. Hudson, NH: Author.

Electrical Therapy

Defibrillation

Mike D. McMahon, RN, BSN

Defibrillation is also known as *direct-current countershock, electrical counter-shock therapy, unsynchronized cardioversion,* or *defib.* The word *defibrillate* refers to an effect on the heart (deplorizing all myocardial cells simultaneously) and is not synonymous with delivery of a shock from a defibrillator. This section deals only with manual use of defibrillators; see Procedure 83 for information on the automatic external defibrillator.

Since 1996, external defibrillators have been available with two different types of energy waveforms: the monophasic and the biphasic. In a monophasic defibrillator, the electrical current travels in one direction between the paddles or electrodes. In a defibrillator that has a biphasic waveform, the electrical current starts in one direction and then reverses direction part way through (Figure 81-1). This allows the peak current delivered by a biphasic shock to be lower than the same peak current delivered by a monophasic shock. The majority of currently produced defibrillators now exclusively use some form of biphasic energy waveforms. The American Heart Association (AHA) (2005) has not made a recommendation for optimal biphasic defibrillation energy levels, but biphasic shock energies of 200 joules (J) or less are safe and effective. "The consensus is that it is reasonable to use 150 J to 200 J for the initial shock with a biphasic truncated exponential waveform or 120 J with a rectilinear biphasic waveform" (AHA, 2005, p. IV-208). Other studies have provided data demonstrating good results for cardioversion of atrial fibrillation and defibrillation of ventricular fibrillation with biphasic shocks up to 360 J (Jain & Wheelan, 2002).

INDICATIONS

1. To terminate ventricular fibrillation.
2. To terminate pulseless ventricular tachycardia.

CONTRAINDICATIONS AND CAUTIONS

1. Rapid defibrillation is crucial to increase the patient's chance of survival. For each minute that passes, there is a 7% to 10% reduction in successful defibrillation (AHA, 2005).
2. Successful defibrillation depends on the metabolic state of the myocardium. Factors that affect the metabolic state include severe hypothermia, hypoxia, acidosis, and electrolyte imbalances.
3. Transthoracic impedance, or resistance, to current flow can affect the ability to defibrillate the myocardium. Factors that determine transthoracic impedance include:
   a. Energy level: More current flows with higher energy levels. The AHA (2005) recommends that the first defibrillation attempt be performed at 360 J if a monophasic device is used. For the biphasic device, use the

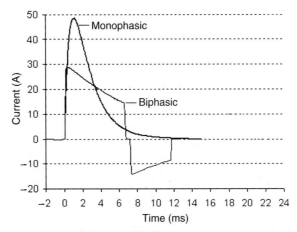

FIGURE 81-1 Monophasic and biphasic defibrillation waveforms. The monophasic waveform is generated from a 200-J shock and reaches a peak current of 48 amps. The biphasic waveform is generated from a 150-J shock and its peak current is 28 amps. (Modified from Walker, R. G., Melnick, S. B., Chapman, F. W., et al. [2003]. Comparison of six clinically used external defibrillators in swine. *Resuscitation, 57,* 73–83.)

device-specific level, typically 120 to 200 J. For second and subsquent shocks, use the same or higher energy level. Perform CPR for 2 minutes between each shock.

b. Electrode or paddle size: For adults, the defibrillation electrodes or paddles range from 8.5 to 12 cm in diameter. The total area of the two electrodes should not exceed 150 cm^2.

c. Correct electrode or paddle placement is an important factor in determining the success of defibrillation.

d. The more shocks delivered and the shorter the interval between shocks, the lower is the transthoracic impedance. However, it is now understood that the incremental benefit of immediate additional shocks is low. Resumption of CPR has greater benefit than immediately delivering additional shocks (AHA, 2005).

e. Delivering shocks during exhalation lowers impedance.

f. Use of a conductive gel lessens the transthoracic impedance. Too little conductive gel may result in skin burns, whereas too much conductive gel may lead to arcing of the current between the paddles. Disposable defibrillation electrodes are manufactured with a gel coating, which is the conductive medium.

4. Remove transdermal medication patches or ointments from the patient's chest because they may also allow an inappropriate path for the current.

5. The defibrillation electrodes should be placed at least 1 inch away from an implantable medical device (AHA, 2005). Damage can occur if the generator is directly defibrillated. The generator may also absorb the discharged current and thus reduce the chance of successful defibrillation.

6. Defibrillation may become necessary during noninvasive pacing. This may require turning off the pacemaker before the external defibrillation can be

performed. Most devices that provide both noninvasive pacemakers and defibrillation disable the pacemaker function when defibrillation is selected. If pacing electrodes have already been applied, hard paddles should neither touch the disposable electrodes nor lie on top of them.

7. An implantable cardioverter-defibrillator (ICD) is an implanted electronic device used in patients who are at high risk for ventricular fibrillation or ventricular tachycardia. An ICD is designed to monitor cardiac rhythms and deliver countershocks if ventricular fibrillation or ventricular tachycardia is identified. If ventricular tachycardia or ventricular fibrillation is present despite an ICD, an external shock should be given immediately. Place the paddles or electrodes at least 1 inch from the ICD. The internal ICD electrodes may cover a section of the epicardium and interfere with the current flow to the heart. If shocks delivered up to 360 J or clinically equivalent biphasic shocks fail to defibrillate the patient, change the paddle or defibrillation electrode placement to an alternative site (anteroposterior or axillary-axillary).

8. Hypothermia. On initial presentation, ventricular fibrillation should be treated with defibrillation. If there is no success with the initial shock, rewarming should be started. Most attempts at defibrillation are unsuccessful when the patient's core temperature is below 28° to 30° C (82.4° to 86° F) (Danzl, 2006).

EQUIPMENT

Cardiac monitor/defibrillator
Electrocardiogram (ECG) electrodes
ECG cable
Strip-chart recorder
Strip-chart recording paper
Disposable defibrillation electrodes or hard paddles
Defibrillation gel or pads (if paddles are used)

PATIENT PREPARATION

1. Remove the patient from wet or metallic surfaces.
2. If possible, quickly obtain a hard copy of the preshock rhythm.

PROCEDURAL STEPS

1. Identify ventricular fibrillation or pulseless ventricular tachycardia through a three-lead ECG monitoring system (lead I, II, or III), through the disposable defibrillation electrodes, or through hard paddles ("quick look").
2. Turn on the defibrillator, making sure the synchronized selection is off.
3. Select an energy level. The first defibrillation is performed with 360 J (monophasic) or 150 J to 200 J with a biphasic truncated exponential waveform or 120 J with a rectilinear biphasic waveform.
4. Charge the defibrillator.
5. Ensure the proper placement of the paddles or the defibrillation electrodes on the chest (Figure 81-2).
   a. Defibrillation electrodes: Disposable defibrillation electrodes are manufactured with a gel coating. The AHA (2005) recommends placing the anterior electrode to the right of the upper sternal border below the clavicle, and the apex electrode to the left of the nipple line with

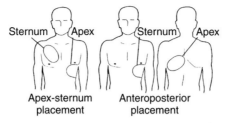

Sternum — Apex   Sternum — Apex

Apex-sternum   Anteroposterior
placement   placement

FIGURE 81-2 Placement options for defibrillation paddles or electrodes; apex-sternum or antero-posterior placement may be used. (Courtesy Medtronic Emergency Response Systems, Redmond, WA.)

the center of the electrode in the midaxillary line. The anteroposterior placement is also acceptable for defibrillation, but this may take more time, because the patient must be turned for placement of the posterior electrode. The anterior electrode is placed over the precordium, and the posterior electrode is placed behind the heart at the left scapular line at the inferior angle of the scapula. Ensure proper placement for an adequate adherence to the chest wall.

b. Paddles: Apply the conductive gel on the hard paddles, rubbing the paddles together to spread the gel over the surfaces of both paddles. Ensure the proper paddle placement and exert 25 to 30 pounds of pressure on each paddle. The goal is to ensure the maximal contact between the chest wall and the paddle. Be sure that there is no path of gel between the paddles; otherwise, an energy arc may occur.

6. Say "Clear" loudly, and visually assess that all personnel have no direct or indirect contact with the patient.

7. Deliver a countershock by depressing both discharge buttons simultaneously, or, in the case of disposable electrodes, press the shock button on the device.

8. Immediately resume CPR for 2 minutes or five cycles.

9. Observe the rhythm. If ventricular fibrillation or pulseless ventricular tachycardia persists, deliver another shock at the same or higher energy level. Restart CPR for 2 minutes and then deliver a third shock at same or higher energy level if the second shock is unsuccessful, and proceed with advanced cardiac life-support recommendations. If an organized rhythm results from the defibrillation, check the pulse and obtain a hard copy of the postshock rhythm.

AGE-SPECIFIC CONSIDERATIONS

1. Ventricular fibrillation is rare in infants and children, but it can occur as a result of respiratory arrest. Two J per kilogram is the initial energy delivered to defibrillate, and the strength should be doubled for repeated shocks (AHA, 2005). The AHA (2005) states that biphasic energy settings should be the same as for monophasic defibrillators. There are inadequate data to recommend effective lower doses.

2. For infants and children who weigh more than 10 kg, the AHA recommends using adult electrodes or paddles because the smaller pediatric electrodes increase transthoracic impedance (AHA, 2005).

3. In children and infants, regardless of the electrode or paddle size, they must not touch each other (AHA, 2005).
4. If hard paddles are used, enough pressure should be applied to the paddles so that complete contact with the chest wall is ensured.
5. Neonatal and pediatric patients may be propped on their side and an antero-posterior paddle placement may be used (AHA, 2005). This may be helpful if only adult paddles or disposable electrodes are available.

COMPLICATIONS

1. Skin irritation, redness, or burns may result if an inadequate conductive medium is used or if there are multiple countershocks.
2. Arcing of the current may occur if the defibrillation gel is spread across the chest wall.
3. A current literature search does not yield any references to bystander death due to contact with a patient during defibrillation. However, there have been documented cases of harm requiring hospitalization.

REFERENCES

American Heart Association (AHA). (2005). American Heart Association guidelines for cardio-pulmonary resuscitation and emergency cardiovascular care. *Circulation, 112*(suppl. IV). Available online at www.circulationaha.org

Danzl, D. F. (2006). Accidental hypothermia. In J. A. Marx, R. S. Hockberger, & R. M. Walls, et al. (Eds.), *Rosen's emergency medicine: Concepts and clinical practice* (6th ed., pp. 2236-2254). St Louis: Mosby.

Jain, V. C., & Wheelan, K. (2002). Successful cardioversion of atrial fibrillation using 360-joules biphasic shock. *American Journal of Cardiology, 90*, 331-332.

PROCEDURE 82

Synchronized Cardioversion

Mike D. McMahon, RN, BSN

Synchronized cardioversion is also known as *cardioversion, direct-current synchronized countershock,* and *electrical synchronized countershock therapy.* The goal of synchronized cardioversion is to deliver a defibrillation shock outside the relative refractory period of the electrocardiogram (ECG) cycle (Barnason, 2003), protecting the patient from going into ventricular fibrillation.

Cardioversion may be performed with either a monophasic or a biphasic waveform (see Procedure 81). The cardioversion energies given below are all monophasic. If the defibrillator is a biphasic unit, use the clinically equivalent energy dose as provided by the manufacturer. Jain and Wheelan (2002) presented three case studies in which 360 joules (J) of biphasic energy was used without adverse effects.

INDICATIONS

1. To terminate ventricular tachyarrhythmias in a patient who has a pulse. Patients who are stable are given oxygen and antiarrhythmic medications as the first line of treatment. Synchronized cardioversion is used if these methods fail (AHA, 2005). Patients who are unstable with signs and symptoms related to tachycardia, including chest pain, dyspnea, decreased level of consciousness, low blood pressure (systolic less than 90 mm Hg), pulmonary congestion, congestive heart failure, ischemia, or infarction, are prepared for immediate synchronized cardioversion if the ventricular rate is greater than 150 beats per minute (bpm). A brief trial of antiarrhythmic medications is sometimes used during set-up for the cardioversion. When the ventricular rate is less than 150 bpm, synchronized cardioversion is used after failed trials of medications according to Advanced Cardiac Life Support (ACLS) guidelines. Wide-complex tachycardias of uncertain type may be treated in similar fashion.
2. In the stable patient with narrow-complex supraventricular tachycardia, cardioversion is used only if medication administration and vagal maneuvers fail to convert the rhythm to a normal sinus rhythm.
3. To terminate atrial fibrillation and atrial flutter. Synchronized cardioversion is used as a first-line therapy for atrial rhythms with a rapid ventricular response (more than 100 bpm) accompanied by clinical distress (AHA, 2005). See cautions for patients who have had atrial fibrillation and atrial flutter for longer than 48 hours.

CONTRAINDICATIONS AND CAUTIONS

1. Airway protection may be necessary, especially when the patient is sedated. Intubation equipment and materials must be readily available.
2. The hemodynamic status must be monitored continuously. A sudden deterioration may warrant rapid synchronized cardioversion or an unsynchronized countershock.
3. Premedication with sedative and analgesic medications is warranted if the patient's condition permits.
4. Remove any transdermal medication patches or ointment from the chest because they may allow an inappropriate path for the current.
5. Digoxin or quinidine toxicity increases the risk of ventricular tachycardia and ventricular fibrillation after cardioversion. Patients receiving a maintenance dose of digoxin therapy can be safely treated with low-dose energy (50 J or less) cardioversion (Bolton, 2004).
6. If the patient is stable, electrolyte imbalances should be corrected before synchronized cardioversion is administered. Hypokalemia can predispose patients to postshock arrhythmias after cardioversion (Hambach, 2005).

7. Cardioversion is not used as the first-line treatment of stable atrial fibrillation and atrial flutter in a patient with onset of the arrhythmia longer than 72 hours prior because there is a risk of embolization of a mural thrombus (Yealy & Delbridge, 2006). Options include rate control with medication, consultation with the patient's primary care provider, and a search for atrial clots.
8. If the patient's condition permits, intravenous access should be established before this procedure (see Procedure 60).
9. Paddle or electrode placement must be modified if the patient has a permanent pacemaker or an implanted cardioverter-defibrillator (ICD). Place the paddles or electrodes at least one inch from the implanted device (AHA, 2005). The internal ICD electrodes may cover a section of the epicardium and interfere with the current flow to the heart. If shocks delivered up to 360 J or clinically equivalent biphasic shocks fail to convert the rhythm, change the paddle or electrode placement to alternative sites (anteroposterior or axillary-axillary).

EQUIPMENT

Cardiac monitor/defibrillator with synchronization capability
ECG electrodes and cable
Strip chart recorder and paper
Disposable defibrillation electrodes or hard paddles
Defibrillation gel or pads
Supplies and equipment for resuscitation (i.e., a crash cart)

PATIENT PREPARATION

1. When the patient's condition permits, a standard 12-lead ECG should be obtained (see Procedure 56). If this is not possible, obtain a hard-copy rhythm strip. Allow the patient access to the bathroom to empty his or her bladder. Remove dentures to prevent them from obstructing the patient's airway (Barnason, 2003).
2. Administer sedation, analgesia, or both as prescribed.
3. Remove any transdermal medication patches or ointment from the patient's chest.
4. Remove the patient from any wet or metallic surfaces.

PROCEDURAL STEPS

1. Turn on the monitor/defibrillator.
2. Attach the monitor leads and ensure the proper display of the patient's rhythm.
3. Depress the SYNC button to activate the synchronized mode. Note that the default setting in some defibrillators can be set to the synchronized mode after each attempt. Other machines need to be reset to deliver a subsequent synchronized countershock.
4. Look for markers on the QRS complex that indicate that the defibrillator is in the SYNC mode (Figure 82-1).
5. Adjust the R-wave gain on the monitor to ensure that SYNC markers occur on each QRS complex.
6. Select an energy level of 100 J or a clinically equivalent biphasic level as prescribed.

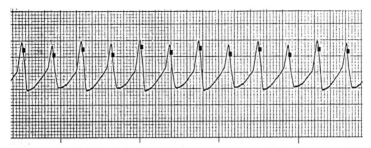

FIGURE 82-1 Appropriate SYNC marker placement on the QRS complex. (Courtesy Medtronic Emergency Response Systems, Redmond, WA.)

7. Position the electrodes or paddles on the patient (Figure 82-2).
   a. Defibrillation electrodes: Disposable defibrillation electrodes are pregelled. The AHA (2005) recommends placing the anterior electrode to the right of the upper third of the sternum below the clavicle and the apex electrode to the left of the nipple line below the axilla. An anteroposterior placement is also acceptable. The anterior electrode is placed over the precordium, and the posterior electrode is placed behind the heart at the left scapular line at the inferior angle of the scapula. Ensure the proper placement for adequate adherence to the chest wall. Success rates of cardioversion using anteroposterior versus anterolateral have been studied. Use of the anteroposterior electrode placement has been seen to lower the energy requirement and increase the overall success (Fuster et al., 2001). But a study by Siaplaouras et al. (2005) found no difference between the two electrode placement sites.
   b. Paddles: Apply a conductive gel on the hard paddles and rub the paddles together to spread the gel over the surfaces of both paddles. Make sure that the paddles are placed correctly and that each paddle is receiving 25 to 30 pounds of pressure. The goal is to ensure the maximal contact between the chest wall and the paddle. Be sure that there is no path of gel between the paddles; otherwise, an energy arc may occur.
8. Charge the defibrillator, and say "Clear" loudly. Visually confirm that no personnel have direct or indirect contact with the patient.
9. Deliver a countershock by depressing the discharge button until the energy is delivered. When using paddles, depress both of the discharge buttons

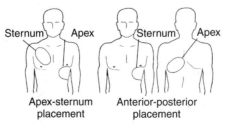

FIGURE 82-2 Placement options for paddles or electrodes; apex-sternum or anteroposterior placement may be used. (Courtesy of Medtronic Emergency Response Systems, Redmond, WA.)

simultaneously and hold them down until discharge occurs; this may take several milliseconds.

10. Check the monitor. If an arrhythmia persists, increase the energy level to 200 J or a clinically equivalent biphasic level and deliver another shock. A third shock at 300 J or a clinically equivalent biphasic level and a fourth shock at 360 J or a clinically equivalent biphasic level are recommended if the rhythm does not convert (AHA, 2005). Remember to check that the SYNC mode is active after each attempt. Some defibrillators can be set to remain in SYNC mode after each discharge. If cardioversion is successful, record the vital signs, obtain a hard copy of the postshock rhythm, and repeat the 12-lead ECG.

11. If the patient has an implanted pacemaker or ICD, the device should be interrogated after the cardioversion to verify functionality (Fuster et al., 2001).

AGE-SPECIFIC CONSIDERATIONS

1. The pediatric patient with a tachyarrhythmia may present with a history of poor feeding, tachypnea, pallor, and lethargy (Corrall, 2004).

2. For pediatric patients, the initial energy level is 0.5 to 1 J/kg; the dose is doubled for subsequent shocks. The AHA (2005) states that biphasic energy settings should be the same as for monophasic defibrillators. There are inadequate data to recommend effective lower doses.

3. Paroxysmal supraventricular tachycardia is the most common rapid rate arrhythmia seen in children. Ventricular tachycardia and atrial fibrillation and flutter are common in children and are usually related to congenital or rheumatic heart disease or to dilated cardiomyopathy (Corrall, 2004).

4. If vascular access is available, consider treating the pediatric patient with unstable supraventricular tachycardia first with adenosine before cardioversion (Primm & Reamy, 2002).

5. For infants and children who weigh more than 10 kg, the AHA recommends using adult electrodes or paddles because the smaller pediatric electrodes increase transthoracic impedance (AHA, 2005).

6. In children and infants, regardless of the electrode or paddle size, they must not touch each other (AHA, 2005).

7. If you are using hard paddles for a pediatric patient, apply enough pressure to the paddles so there is complete contact with the chest wall.

8. Neonatal and pediatric patients may be propped on their side and an anteroposterior paddle placement may be used (AHA, 2005). This may be helpful if only adult paddles or disposable electrodes are available.

COMPLICATIONS

1. Inappropriate sensing of the QRS complex may result in improper timing of the discharge of the current. This may result in ventricular tachycardia or fibrillation, especially if the current is delivered while superimposed on a T wave. An unsynchronized countershock at 200 J or a clinically equivalent biphasic shock should be given immediately if ventricular fibrillation occurs. If this is needed, make sure that the SYNC function is turned off or there will be a delay in delivering the defibrillation shock.

2. Burns may occur if the conductive medium is insufficient or excessive. Proper pressure applied to the paddles and proper positioning decrease this risk. The risk of burns increases with multiple shocks. Ambler, Zideman, & Deakin (2005) found that placing 5% ibuprofen cream on the electrode site 2 hours before an elective cardioversion reduced pain and inflammation.

3. A pulmonary embolus is a rare complication that usually occurs in a patient who has been in chronic atrial fibrillation. This risk can be minimized with anticoagulant therapy administered before cardioversion.

4. Embolic cerebrovascular events occur rarely as a result of cardioversion, but they are also a risk in conditions for which synchronized cardioversion is undertaken, especially if the atrial wall motion is compromised.

5. A current literature search does not yield any references to bystander death due to contact with a patient being defibrillated. Gibbs et al. (1990) documented cases of harm requiring hospitalization.

6. Muscle soreness may be experienced by some patients.

7. Transient elevations in creatine kinase (CK) and lactate dehydrogenase may be noted, but more specific cardiac markers, such as CK-MB and troponin, are rarely abnormal (Bolton, 2004).

8. Transient ST-segment elevation may be noted after cardioversion. These changes typically resolve within 5 minutes (Bolton, 2004).

PATIENT TEACHING

1. Explain the procedure as the delivery of a small electrical impulse to the heart. Patients need to be aware of the possibility that multiple attempts may be necessary.

2. Inform patients that this procedure is performed while they are awake (unless general anesthesia is used) but that sedation with medication produces a relaxed and usually drowsy state and that some medications also result in amnesia for the event.

3. Patients do want to know how the shock feels. Some patients report a brief, very sharp pain. The sedative usually erases the memory of this pain.

4. After effects may include redness of the skin and minimal soreness of the chest wall.

5. Patients who are discharged from the emergency department should be instructed to seek emergency care promptly if they experience chest pain, shortness of breath, lower-extremity swelling, dizziness, weakness, or changes in vision or speech.

REFERENCES

Ambler, J. J., Zideman, D. A., & Deakin, C. D. (2005). The effect of topical non-steroidal anti-inflammatory cream on the incidence and severity of cutaneous burns following external DC cardioversion. *Resuscitation, 65*(2), 173-178.

American Heart Association (AHA). (2005). American Heart Association guidelines for cardiopulmonary resuscitation and emergency cardiovascular care. *Circulation, 112*(suppl. IV). Available online at www.circulationaha.org

Barnason, S. (2003). Cardiovascular emergencies. In Emergency Nurses Association & L. Newberry (Eds.), *Sheehy's emergency nursing* (5th ed., pp. 450-604). St Louis: Mosby.

Bolton, E. (2004). Disturbances of cardiac rhythm and conduction. In J. E. Tintinalli, G. D. Kelen, & J. S. Stapszynski (Eds.), *Emergency medicine* (pp. 179-202). New York: McGraw-Hill.

Corrall, C. J. (2004). Pediatric heart disease. In J. E. Tintinalli, G. D. Kelen, & J. S. Stapszynski (Eds.), *Emergency medicine* (pp. 758-769). New York: McGraw-Hill.

Fuster, V., Ryden, L. E., & Asinger, R. W., et al. (2001). ACC/AHA/ESC guidelines for the management of patients with atrial fibrillation: Executive summary. *Journal of the American College of Cardiology, 38,* 1231-1265.

Gibbs, W., Eisenberg, M., & Damon, S. K. (1990). Dangers of defibrillation: Injuries to emergency personnel during patient resuscitation. *American Journal of Emergency Medicine, 8,* 101-104.

Hambach, C. (2005). Cardioversion. In D. J. Lynn-McHale Wiegand, & K. K. Carlson (Eds.), *AACN procedure manual for critical care* (5th ed., pp. 248-257). St Louis: Saunders.

Jain, V. C., & Wheelan, K. (2002). Successful cardioversion of atrial fibrillation using 360-joules biphasic shock. *American Journal of Cardiology, 90,* 331-332.

Primm, P. A., & Reamy, R. R. (2002). Cardiopulmonary resuscitation. In G. R. Strange, W. Ahrens, & S. Lelyvled, et al. (Eds.), *Pediatric emergency medicine: A comprehensive guide* (pp. 18-27). New York: McGraw-Hill.

Siaplaouras, S., Buob, A., Rotter, C., Bohm, M., & Jung, J. (2005). Randomized comparison of anterolateral versus anteroposterior electrode position for biphasic external cardioversion of atrial fibrillation. *American Heart Journal, 150*(1), 150-152.

Yealy, D. M., & Delbridge, T. R. (2006). Dysrhythmias. In J. A. Marx, R. S. Hockberger, & R. M. Walls, et al. (Eds.), *Rosen's emergency medicine: Concepts and clinical practice* (6th ed., pp. 1199-1246). St Louis: Mosby.

PROCEDURE 83

Automated External Defibrillator Operation

Mike D. McMahon, RN, BSN

INDICATION

Automated external defibrillators (AEDs) are for use on patients who are in cardiac arrest. They differ from manual defibrillators in that the device, not the user, makes the decision to deliver the shock, thus allowing a minimally trained individual to treat a sudden cardiac arrest. They use voice and visual promps to guide less experienced rescuers. The American Heart Association (AHA) (2005)

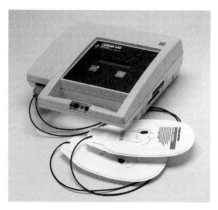

FIGURE 83-1 LIFEPAK 500. (Courtesy Medtronic Emergency Response Systems, Redmond, WA.)

has set a high-priority goal to increase survival in sudden cardiac arrest by recommending that the first shock be delivered within 5 minutes of activating Emergency Medical Services. Further, it is a Class I recommendation that hospitals be able to provide defibrillation within 3 minutes from time of collapse. AEDs are now present in many public locations and on most airplanes.

CONTRAINDICATIONS AND CAUTIONS

1. Most standard AEDs are for use in patients who are older than age 8 or weigh more than 25 kg. See Age-Specific Considerations for exceptions.
2. AEDs are designed for use in patients who are in cardiac arrest. When used in AED mode, do not place the device on a patient who is conscious or has a pulse or respirations. AEDs cannot differentiate from a cardiac rhythm that is generating a pulse from one that is not. Some models can monitor patients' electrocardiogram (ECG) and display waveforms on a screen.
3. Place the defibrillation pads in the same positions as for manual defibrillation (see Procedure 81). Place the anterior electrode to the right of the upper sternal border below the clavicle, and the apex electrode to the left of the nipple line with the center of the electrode in the midaxillary region. The device's algorithms for determining shockability are based on these positions.
4. Some AEDs are fully automatic and do not have a SHOCK button. These devices deliver defibrillation energy to the patient without the user pressing any buttons. Make sure that no one is touching the patient while the device is preparing to delivery energy.

EQUIPMENT

AED (Figure 83-1)
Disposable defibrillation electrodes

PATIENT PREPARATION

1. Remove the patient from any standing water, and expose and dry the chest.
2. Remove any transdermal patches or ointments from areas where the defibrillation electrodes are to be attached.

PROCEDURAL STEPS

Currently, many different AEDs are available. Devices range from those with three-button function (POWER, ANALYZE, SHOCK) to those that are always on and deliver energy without user intervention. Most devices also allow the user to customize functions of the defibrillator to meet local requirements. Users may be able set a range of energy to be delivered, change the time between series of shocks, and choose what, if any, verbal commands will be delivered by the device. Some devices can be used in AED mode only, and others allow the user to override the automated function and manually deliver a shock for defibrillation. For specific details, see the manufacturer's operating instructions for each device.

The AHA (2005) recommends the following steps for the operation of an AED:

1. Start cardiopulmonary resuscitation (CPR) until an AED is available. If no one witnessed the arrest, provide CPR for 2 minutes/five cycles of CPR before the first shock is delivered.
2. Power on the AED.
3. Attach the electrode pads to the patient in the standard apex-sternum locations. If the patient has an implanted pacemaker or an implanted cardioverter-defibrillator, place the electrodes at least 1 inch away from the device (AHA, 2005).
4. Analyze the rhythm.
5. Clear the victim and press the SHOCK button (if advised).
6. Immediately start CPR for 2 minutes/five cycles.
7. Repeat steps 4-6 until advanced life support providers take over or the arrest victim begins to move.

AGE-SPECIFIC CONSIDERATION

Currently, many AED manufacturers have devices or accessories that are cleared by the U.S. Food and Drug Administration (FDA) for use in children age 1 to 8. Medtronic Emergency Response Systems and Philips Medical Systems (Figure 83-2) have AEDs that use specially designed electrodes (attenuated) to

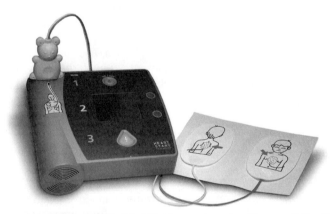

FIGURE 83-2 Heartstream FR2 with pediatric use electrodes. (Courtesy Philips Electronics.)

reduce the defibrillation energy delivered by the AED to the patient by approximately one-third the set charge. Because the AED continues to deliver a full charge, pediatric nonattenuated defibrillation electrodes should not be used with an AED. This will lead to full energy (120 to 360 joules [J]) being delivered to the pediatric patient. ZOLL Medical AEDs sense that a pediatric defibrillation electrode is attached and reduce the energy level in the AED.

The AHA (2005) recommends using an AED that can accommodate the pediatric patient, if available. If unavailable, then the recommendation is to use a standard AED.

While AEDs are not approved for use in infants (younger than age 1), Atkins and Jorgenson (2005) and Bar-Cohen (2005) report on a 4-month-old infant who received a 50-J shock with a successful outcome.

COMPLICATIONS

1. Skin irritation, redness, or burns may result if the defibrillation pads are not completely adhered to the patient's chest or if the patient receives multiple shocks.
2. A current literature search does not yield any references to bystander death due to contact with a patient during defibrillation. There have been documented cases of harm requiring hospitalization (Gibbs, Eisenberg, & Damon, 1990).
3. Using pediatric AED electrodes on an adult patient may prevent successful defibrillation because less energy is delivered. Conversely, using anything but the specially designed AED pediatric electrodes on the pediatric patient will deliver full energy to the patient.
4. AEDs make a shock decision based on cardiac rhythms only, they do not detect perfusion. Some instances of pulsatile ventricular tachycardia and even patient movement may cause the device to reach a shockable decision. This can lead to inappropriate defibrillation of a patient who may not need it.

REFERENCES

American Heart Association (AHA). (2005). American Heart Association guidelines for cardiopulmonary resuscitation and emergency cardiovascular care. *Circulation, 112*(suppl. IV). Available online at www.circulationaha.org

Atkins, D. L., & Jorgenson, D. B. (2005). Attenuated pediatric electrode pads for automated external defibrillator use in children. *Resuscitation, 66*(1), 31-37.

Bar-Cohen, Y., et al. (2005). First appropriate use of automated external defibrillator in an infant. *Resuscitation, 67*(1), 135-137.

Gibbs, W., Eisenberg, M., & Damon, S. K. (1990). Danger of defibrillation: Injuries to emergency personnel during patient resuscitation. *American Journal of Emergency Medicine, 8*, 101-104.

Emergency Management of the Patient with an Implantable Cardioverter-Defibrillator

Mike D. McMahon, RN, BSN

Implantable cardioverter-defibrillators (ICDs) are also known as automatic implantable cardioverter-defibrillators (AICDs). First brought into service in 1980, now more than 50,000 units are implanted each year. These devices have become a standard of care for patients who are at high risk for sudden cardiac arrest and sustained ventricular tachycardia. The devices currently available (dual chamber) combine the functions of an internal defibrillator and that of an implanted pacemaker. Additional models are being developed for the treatment of tachycardiac rhythms originating in the atrium. The patient or family usually carries information about the specific device that is in place.

The devices are connected to cardiac lead wires and continually monitor the electrocardiogram (ECG) cycle. Because the defibrillation leads are in direct contact with the myocardium, lower energy levels are needed. ICDs can be set to deliver up to approximately 30 joules (J) of biphasic energy if the patient goes into ventricular fibrillation, but most patients need only 15 to 20 J to restore the heart rhythm to normal sinus. These devices are also capable of delivering lower energy for cardioversion and antitachycardic pacing (Niemann, 2006).

INDICATIONS

Patients who have ICDs may present to the emergency department under the following circumstances:

1. After cardiac arrest with successful defibrillation by the device. Treat patients who have had a cardiac arrest and undergone successful resuscitation the same as any other arrest patient. The cardiology department should be notified so that the ICD event can be downloaded. If the patient is conscious, solicit information about the number of shocks delivered, any symptoms preceding the defibrillation, and the patient's activity around the event (Bessman, 2004).

2. In cardiac arrest, with the device having functioned properly but the heart rhythm not converted to a perfusing rhythm. If the patient arrives in cardiac arrest and the ICD has stopped its defibrillation function, external defibrillation may be needed. ICDs shut down the defibrillation function after a set number of defibrillations according to a preprogrammed algorithm. Place the

defibrillation pads or electrodes at least 1 inch away from the implanted device (AHA, 2005). The epicardial patches used in older ICDs may protect the heart from external defibrillation, and alternate (anteroposterior or axillary-axillary) positions may be needed. Current models use transvenous electrodes, eliminating the need for epicardial patches (Niemann, 2006).

3. Successful and unsuccessful correction of tachycardic rhythms. The underlying tachycardic rate may fall out of the range to which the ICD is programmed to respond.

4. Inadvertent firing of the defibrillator. This can be related to external stimuli, such as poorly grounded electrical equipment (Sabaté, Moure, Nicholás, Sed, & Navarro, 2001). Gold (2000) has found that chest wall muscle movement, such as hand gripping, Valsalva maneuver, and deep breaths, can cause the ICD to discharge.

5. Another problem not related to the ICD, for which the patient may undergo procedures that could damage or disrupt the device.

CONTRAINDICATIONS AND CAUTIONS

1. Strong magnetic fields, such as from magnetic resonance imaging (MRI), cause the ICD to not respond in the event that the patient has a rhythm of ventricular fibrillation or ventricular tachycardia. Additionally, MRI energies may cause the unit or the leads to heat up and cause cardiac injury. Multiple case studies have been published (Gimbel, Kanal, Schwartz, & Wilkoff, 2005; Roguin, Donahue, Bomma, Bluemke, & Halperin, 2005; Wollmann et al., 2005) where patients with ICDs had no complications when undergoing MRI scanning. However, the FDA (Faris & Shein, 2005) cautions that more controlled studies are required before any changes in the "approval for labeling that endorses the general or limited use of MRI for pacemaker or ICD patients."

2. Electrocautery devices can damage the ICD. Make sure that everyone is aware of the patient's implanted device.

3. The epicardial pads in older ICDs can shield the heart, making external defibrillation more difficult. Higher external defibrillation energy or alternate pad/paddle placement may be needed to convert the patient's heart rhythm.

4. The ICD may need to be deactivated in the postresuscitation period. This is to prevent discharge due to recurrent ventricular dysrhythmias caused by metabolic changes during the arrest (Niemann, 2006).

EQUIPMENT

ECG monitor
12-lead ECG
Doughnut-shaped (round) magnet
External cardiac defibrillator

PROCEDURAL STEPS
Deactivating the ICD

Placing a doughnut-shaped magnet on top of the pulse generator can inhibit the defibrillation component of most ICDs. Second-generation devices require that the magnet be placed on the generator for 30 seconds, and then the magnet can be removed. Third-generation devices require that the magnet remain on the device for the entire time that the defibrillation function is stopped (Bessman, 2004). The underlying pacemaker functions in the ICD are not affected by the magnet (Reilly, Morton, & Vojtko, 2005).

1. To deactivate an ICD, place a doughnut-shaped magnet over the ICD pulse generator.
2. The magnet will stop the device from delivering defibrillation energy, but it will not stop the pacemaker function of the device.
3. After the magnet is removed, 12-lead electrocardiography should be performed to record the current state of the device.
4. All patients require follow-up with their cardiologist to check out the functions of the device.

COMPLICATIONS

With the defibrillation function turned off, no defibrillation shocks will be delivered if the patient goes into ventricular fibrillation or tachycardia. An external monitor/defibrillation should always be present when this procedure is performed.

PATIENT TEACHING
ICD and Electrical Appliances

Patients may have questions about devices that they should avoid or around which caution is recommended. The following list is condensed from websites created by Medtronic, St. Jude Medical Center and Guidant (2007). Patients should be directed to contact their cardiologist for any concerns they may have regarding their ICD.

Medical Equipment

Most medical equipment is safe for use around patients who have an ICD. This includes most diagnostic x-ray types, including fluoroscopy, dental and chest x-ray machines, computed tomography scans, mammography, and ultrasonic dental cleaners.

The following procedures should be avoided until the patient's cardiologist has been consulted:
- MRI
- Electrical nerve and muscle stimulators (transcutaneous electrical nerve stimulation units)
- Diathermy
- Electrocautery
- Lithotripsy, if the ICD is in the treatment field

General Household and Office Items

- Any household item in good repair is safe to use. The items should have three prongs or polarized prongs (i.e., one prong is larger than the other).
- Do not put magnets or products containing magnets close to the ICD.
- Avoid bringing power tools like drills or saws close to the chest area.
- When working with tools or appliances, be careful in situations in which you could be injured if you become dizzy or receive a therapeutic shock from your ICD.

Security Systems

- Walk through the screening areas at a normal pace and do not linger in these areas.
- If you are being searched with a hand wand, ask the screener to avoid the ICD.
- If dizziness or weakness occurs, move away from the screening devices.

Industrial Areas

- Large industrial equipment, such as generators, electric motors, and arc welders, often generate strong electromagnetic fields that can interfere with an ICD.
- Make sure that the equipment is properly grounded before working near it.

ICD and End-of-life Issues

Patients who present to the emergency department with a history of ICD implantation should be encouraged to discuss their end-of-life requests with their cardiologist and family. Stein (2006) describes an elderly man who suffered a life-ending head injury, but because he had an ICD, the patient received multiple defibrillation shocks. Berger (2005) discusses ethical issues surrounding patients with ICDs. He explains that patients with do-not-resuscitate orders may still benefit from an ICD if the arrhythmia is from a primary cardiac condition.

REFERENCES

American Heart Association (AHA). (2005). American Heart Association guidelines for cardiopulmonary resuscitation and emergency cardiovascular care. *Circulation, 112*(suppl. IV). Available online at www.circulationaha.org.

Berger, J. T. (2005). The ethics of deactivating implanted cardioverter defibrillators. *Annuals of Internal Medicine, 142*(8), 631-634.

Bessman, E. S. (2004). Invasive monitoring, pacing techniques, and automatic and implantable defibrillators. In J. E. Tintinalli, G. D. Kelen, & J. S. Stapczynski (Eds.), *Emergency medicine* (6th ed., pp. 132-138). New York: McGraw-Hill.

Faris, O. P., & Shein, M. J. (2005). Government viewpoint: U.S. Food & Drug Administration: pacemaker, ICDs and MRI. *Journal of Pacing and Clinical Electrophysiology, 28*(4), 268-269.

Gimbel, J. R., Kanal, E., Schwartz, K. M., & Wilkoff, B. L. (2005). Outcome of magnetic resonance imaging (MRI) in selected patients with implantable cardioverter defibrillators (ICDs). *Journal of Pacing and Clinical Electrophysiology, 28*(4), 270-273.

Gold, M. R. (2000). ICD therapy in the new millennium. *Cardiology Clinics, 18,* 375-387.

Guidant. (2007). *ICDs.* Retrieved January 19, 2007, from http://www.guidant.com/products/AICD.shtml.

Medtronic. (2007). *Defibrillators (ICDs).* Retrieved January 19, 2007, from http://www.medtronic.com/patients/heart.html.

Niemann, J. T. (2006). Implantable cardiac devices. In J. A. Marx, R. S. Hockberger, & R. M. Walls, et al. (Eds.), *Rosen's emergency medicine: Concepts and clinical practice* (6th ed., pp. 1246-1258). St Louis: Mosby.

Reilly, D. N., Morton, P. G., & Vojtko, K. (2005). Implantable cardioverter-defibrillator. In D. J. Lynn-McHale Wiegand, & K. K. Carlson (Eds.), *AACN procedure manual for critical care* (5th ed., pp. 314-323). Philadelphia: Saunders.

Roguin, A., Donahue, J. K., Bomma, C. S., Bluemke, D. A., & Halperin, H. R. (2005). Cardiac magnetic resonance imaging in a patient with implantable cardioverter-defibrillator. *Journal of Pacing and Clinical Electrophysiology, 28*(4), 336-338.

Sabaté, X., Moure, C., Nicolás, J., Sed, M., & Navarro, X. (2001). Washing machine associated 50 Hz detected as ventricular fibrillation by an implanted cardioverter defibrillator. *Journal of Pacing and Clinical Electrophysiology, 24*(8), 1281-1283.

St. Jude Medical Center. (2007). *Learn more about ICDs.* Retrieved January 19, 2007, from http://www.stjudemedical.com/4.0/4.3/4.3.shtm.

Stein, R. (2006, December 19). Implantable heart devices save lives, may worsen deaths. Retrieved February 21, 2007, from http://archives.seattletimes.nwsource.com.

Wollmann, C., Grude, M., Tombach, B., Kugel, H., Heindel, W., Breithardt, G., Böcker, D., & Vahlhaus, C. (2005). Safe performance of magnetic resonance imaging on a patient with an ICD. *Journal of Pacing and Clinical Electrophysiology, 28*(4) 339-342.

Cardiac Pacing

Transcutaneous Cardiac Pacing

Mike D. McMahon, RN, BSN

Transcutaneous cardiac pacing is also known as *TCP, noninvasive cardiac pacing, external cardiac pacing, precordial cardiac pacing, temporary pacing,* and *external transthoracic pacing.*

INDICATIONS

1. To provide emergency pacing in patients with hemodynamically unstable bradycardias (Class I recommendation according to the American Heart Association [AHA], 2005):
   a. Signs and symptoms of hemodynamic instability include systolic blood pressure lower than 80 mm Hg, altered mental status, angina, acute myocardial infarction, chest pain, shortness of breath, congestive heart failure, and pulmonary edema (AHA, 2005).
   b. Simultaneous initiation of TCP and pharmacologic therapy may stabilize the patient more rapidly.
   c. TCP may be used as a prophylactic treatment in patients who have a high risk of atrioventricular block (Bolton, 2004)
   d. TCP is no longer recommended by the AHA (2005) for treatment in patients who have bradyasystolic cardiac arrest.
2. To increase heart rate in patients with a myocardial infarction who may present with bradycardia-dependent life-threatening ventricular rhythms (Hollander & Diercks, 2004).
3. To provide overdrive pacing in patients with supraventricular and ventricular tachycardias that are resistant to pharmacologic therapy or electrical cardioversion.
   a. TCP is a Class IIa intervention for overdrive pacing of tachycardias refractory to drug therapy or electrical cardioversion when serum magnesium concentration is normal (AHA, 2005).

CONTRAINDICATIONS AND CAUTIONS

1. Misinterpreting a fine ventricular fibrillation as asystole may lead to inappropriate pacing when defibrillation is indicated.
2. TCP is contraindicated in severe hypothermia because the bradycardia may be physiologic as a result of a decreased metabolic rate (AHA, 2005).
3. TCP is relatively contraindicated in bradyasystolic arrest that lasts longer than 20 minutes because the chance of success is low.
4. Check the manufacturer's guidelines regarding the length of time the pacing electrodes may be used for continuous pacing.

5. Never cut the pacing electrodes.

EQUIPMENT

Transcutaneous pacemaker with monitor
Multifunction cable or pacing cable
Pacing electrodes
Electrocardiogram (ECG) cable
ECG electrodes
Monitor recorder paper
Advanced life support equipment
Sedatives or analgesics as indicated

PATIENT PREPARATION

1. A simple explanation of the purpose and procedure for TCP should be given to the conscious patient. A description of the sensations, including discomfort, that are associated with TCP, and the sedation and analgesia options may be discussed. The sensation at low-current levels has been described as a superficial tingling and at high current levels as a deep thumping. The patient may require continuous reassurance and/or sedation during the procedure.
2. Administer sedatives or analgesics as indicated and prescribed.
3. Place the ECG electrodes on clean, dry skin. Lead II gives a clearer picture of the pacing artifact (see Procedure 55). The ECG cable must be connected for the pacemaker to operate in the demand mode.
4. Obtain a hard-copy strip of the baseline rhythm along with vital signs.

PROCEDURAL STEPS

1. Following the manufacturer's recommendations, attach the multifunction or pacing electrodes in either the anterior-anterior (sternum-apex) position (Figure 85-1) or the anteroposterior position (Figure 85-2). The skin should be clean and dry. Remove lotions and ointments with soap and water, and dry the skin completely afterward. No other cleaning agents should be used. Excessive hair should be clipped rather than shaved. Shaving causes micro-abrasions and increases the likelihood of skin burns. The electrodes should not be placed over wires, drains, dressings, ECG electrodes, implanted cardioverter-defibrillators, pacemakers, or medication patches. Rolling the

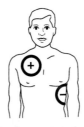

FIGURE 85-1 Sternum-apex electrode placement. In female patients, position the negative electrode under the breast. (Modified from illustrations supplied by Medtronic Physio-Control Corporation, Redmond, WA.)

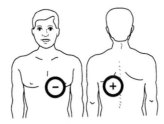

FIGURE 85-2 Anteroposterior electrode placement. In female patients, position the negative electrode under the breast. (Modified from illustrations supplied by Medtronic Physio-Control Corporation, Redmond, WA.)

electrodes onto the skin decreases the amount of air trapped beneath and improves electrical conduction. Press firmly on the adhesive area around the periphery to increase adherence. Press gently on the gelled area to remove any trapped air and to ensure good skin coupling.

2. Select the pacing mode (demand or asynchronous). In some pacemakers, the mode is automatically "demand" if the ECG cable is attached. It switches to "asynchronous" when the ECG electrodes or cable is removed.

   a. *Demand mode.* The demand mode is used when the patient has an underlying rhythm. The pacemaker delivers a pacing stimulus only when the patient's intrinsic heart rate falls below the preset rate. Correct sensing of the intrinsic R wave must be ensured. Some pacemakers mark each sensed R wave, whereas others flash a symbol each time an R wave is sensed. The sensitivity is increased by increasing the ECG gain until all intrinsic R waves are seen.

   b. *Asynchronous mode.* The asynchronous (fixed rate) mode should be used only in emergency situations when the patient has no underlying rhythm or when an ECG cannot be obtained (ZOLL Medical Corporation, 2006). In this mode, the pacemaker disregards the patient's intrinsic rhythm and delivers a pacing stimulus at the preset rate. There is a risk that a lethal arrhythmia may be generated if the pacing stimulus occurs during the vulnerable period of ventricular repolarization (Bessman, 2004).

3. Select the pacing rate. The rate range is typically 60 to 100 beats per minute (bpm).

4. Set the output (mA) on zero and turn on the pacemaker.

   a. For a patient in a comprised hemodynamic state, but not in arrest, determine the capture threshold and set the maintenance pacing output. Beginning at zero milliamperes (mA), increase the output until the electrical capture is seen. Electrical capture is evidenced by a wide QRS complex (greater than 0.12 msec) and broad T wave following the pacing artifact (Figure 85-3). Capture thresholds typically range from 40 to 80 mA. Maintenance pacing outputs should be set about 10% above the threshold (ZOLL Medical Corporation, 2006).

   b. For patients without a pulse, the device should be set to maximum output when it is turned on. If capture of the heart rate is achieved at the

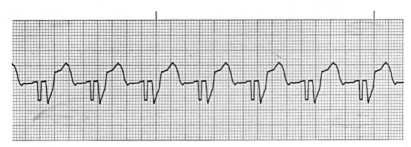

FIGURE 85-3 Electrical capture. Each pacing spike is followed by a wide QRS.

maximum energy, the device should be turned down until loss of capture occurs and then increased to 110% of capture energy (threshold).

5. Hypoxia, acidosis, pericardial effusion, and tamponade may lead to higher capture thresholds (Del Monte & Gamrath, 1996). The identification of electrical capture may be difficult in the presence of ECG signal distortion (Figure 85-4). An artifact increases in size as the current is increased. Positioning the ECG electrodes as far as possible from the pacing electrodes may reduce the signal distortion. Sometimes changing the lead being monitored minimizes the distortion (Del Monte & Gamrath, 1996).

6. Assess the patient for mechanical capture by palpating a pulse. A Doppler, a pulse oximeter, or both may also assist in identifying and confirming the mechanical capture (Del Monte & Gamrath, 1996).

7. Document the electrical capture with a rhythm strip indicating the pacemaker settings. Document the mechanical capture with vital signs.

8. Assess the patient's comfort level. Most patients have difficulty tolerating pacing currents above 50 mA. Sedation and analgesia should be used for conscious patients.

9. TCP is a bridge to a more definitive treatment. The patient should be prepared for the insertion of a transvenous pacemaker. See Procedure 86.

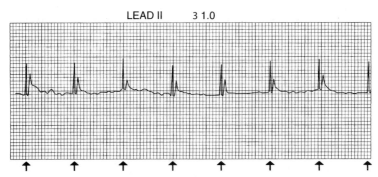

FIGURE 85-4 Signal distortion. Each pacing spike is followed by a signal-distortion artifact that must be distinguished from electrical capture. (From Del Monte, L., & Gamrath, B. [1996]. *Noninvasive pacing: What you should know* [2nd ed., p. 25]. Redmond, WA: Medtronic Physio-Control Corporation.)

AGE-SPECIFIC CONSIDERATIONS

1. Severe bradycardias in children are usually the result of airway compromise and respiratory insufficiency (Fish, Kannankeril, & Johns, 2006). These issues should be addressed before pharmacologic agents or pacing is attempted.
2. Minimal heart rates indicating possible need for pacing are the following (Conway, 1997):
   a. Infant: less than 55 bpm
   b. Child: less than 45 to 50 bpm
   c. Adolescent: less than 40 bpm
3. Consider using TCP in children who have primary bradycardia secondary to congenital or acquired heart disease (AHA, 2005).
4. As with adults, discomfort during TCP is a major drawback to its use. Sedation and artificial ventilation should be considered.
5. Smaller-sized pacing electrodes are available for patients who weigh less than 15 kg (ZOLL Medical Corporation, 2006). However, the smaller the pacing electrode, the higher the resistance. Therefore, using a larger electrode is beneficial as long as the adherence is good and the electrodes do not touch.
6. Placement of pacing electrodes in the pediatric population does not differ from that in the adult population (AHA, 2005; Primm & Reamy, 2002). Be sure that the pacing electrodes do not touch; use of the smaller pacing electrodes or an anteroposterior position may be necessary to ensure this in infants and small children.
7. Pediatric patients are at a higher risk for skin breakdown when TCP is used for longer than 30 minutes. In newborns and infants, the area under the pads should be inspected regularly for signs of thermal damage to the skin (ZOLL Medical Corporation, 2006).

COMPLICATIONS

1. Failure to capture is evidenced by pacer spikes that do not induce the wide QRS of an electrical capture (Figure 85-5). A capture threshold may change over time and should be determined frequently when the patient is dependent on a pacemaker (Del Monte & Gamrath, 1996).
2. Undersensing occurs when the pacemaker does not sense an intrinsic QRS and delivers a pacing spike. Failure to sense is recognized by competition between the pacing rhythm and the intrinsic rhythm and by a short interval between the native QRS and the pacing spike (Figure 85-6). If the pacer fails to recognize all the intrinsic QRS complexes, it operates as if it were in the asynchronous mode.

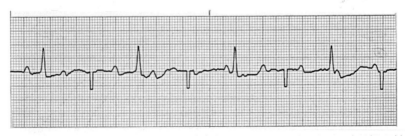

FIGURE 85-5 Failure to capture. Pacing stimuli fail to capture in a patient in complete heart block.

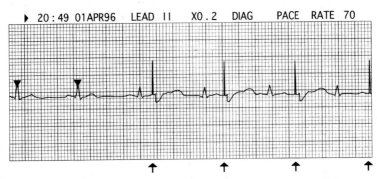

FIGURE 85-6 Undersensing. The first two QRS complexes are sensed, but the remaining QRS complexes are not of sufficient amplitude to be detected. The pacemaker fires even though the patient's intrinsic rate is greater than the set pace rate. (From Del Monte, L., & Gamrath, B. [1996]. *Noninvasive pacing: What you should know* [2nd ed., p. 29]. Redmond, WA: Medtronic Physio-Control Corporation.)

3. Oversensing is due to an inappropriate inhibition of the pacing by electrical signals from outside the heart (Figure 85-7). Extracardiac electrical signals include muscle artifact and electromagnetic signals in the environment. These may be corrected by decreasing the ECG size, which decreases the sensitivity to the native QRS. If the problem persists, it may be necessary to operate the pacemaker in the asynchronous mode to obtain reliable pacing (Del Monte & Gamrath, 1996).
4. Loss of the ECG monitoring leads causes the pacing device to default to asynchronous mode. This can lead to pacing energy being delivered during the heart's vulnerable period.

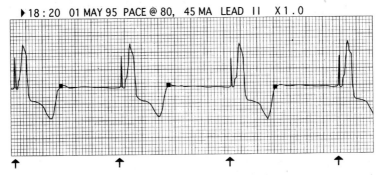

FIGURE 85-7 Oversensing. The set rate is 80, but the actual paced rate is 45. Note the sense marker on the T wave, which inappropriately inhibits the pacemaker. The next paced pulse is late, which disrupts the timing cycle of the pacemaker. (From Del Monte, L., & Gamrath, B. [1996]. *Noninvasive pacing: What you should know* [2nd ed., p. 29]. Redmond, WA: Medtronic Physio-Control Corporation.)

5. Prolonged pacing (longer than 2 hours) in patients with poor peripheral perfusion can result in burns. Monitor the skin under the electrodes frequently (ZOLL Medical Corporation, 2006).

PATIENT TEACHING

1. Report increasing discomfort related to the pacing impulses.
2. Touching the patient during TCP does not cause any harm. A small shock hazard does exist, and the pacing energy can be felt.
3. Some pacing devices continue to deliver pacing energy when the electrodes are removed from the patient. As in item 2, there is a shock hazard, but there is no risk of harm to the user.

REFERENCES

American Heart Association (AHA). (2005). American Heart Association guidelines for cardiopulmonary resuscitation and emergency cardiovascular care. *Circulation, 112*(Suppl IV). Available online at www.circulationaha.org

Bessman, E. S. (2004). Invasive monitoring, pacing techniques, and automatic and implantable defibrillators. In J. E. Tintinalli, G. D. Kelen, & J. S. Stapczynski (Eds.), *Emergency medicine* (6th ed., pp. 132-138). New York: McGraw-Hill.

Bolton, E. (2004). Disturbances of cardiac rhythm and conduction. In J. E. Tintinalli, G. D. Kelen, & J. S. Stapczynski (Eds.), *Emergency medicine* (6th ed., pp. 179-202). New York: McGraw-Hill.

Conway, S. P. (1997). Pediatric pacemakers for patients with complete heart block. *Dimensions of Critical Care Nursing, 16*(1), 29-39.

Del Monte, L., & Gamrath, B. (1996). *Noninvasive pacing: What you should know* (2nd ed.). Redmond, WA: Physio-Control Corporation.

Fish, F. A., Kannenkeril, P. J., & Johns, J. A. (2006). Disorder of cardiac rhythm. In B. P. Fuhrman, & J. J. Zimmerman (Eds.), *Pediatric critical care* (pp. 365-393). Philadelphia: Mosby.

Hollander, J. E., & Diercks, D. B. (2004). Intervention strategies for acute coronary syndromes. In J. E. Tintinalli, G. D. Kelen, & J. S. Stapczynski (Eds.), *Emergency medicine* (6th ed., pp. 352-359). New York: McGraw-Hill.

Primm, P. R., & Reamy, R. R. (2002). Cardiopulmonary resuscitation. In G. R. Strange, W. R. Ahrens, S. Lelyveld, & R. W. Schafermeyer (Eds.), *Pediatric emergency medicine* (pp. 18-27). New York: McGraw-Hill.

ZOLL Medical Corporation. (2006). ZOLL M *Series operator's guide*. Burlington, MA: Author. Retrieved February 18, 2007, from http://www.zoll.com/product_manuals.aspx

Temporary Transvenous Pacemaker Insertion

Patricia A. DeWitt, RN, MSN

INDICATIONS

1. To maintain an adequate heart rate in the presence of hemodynamically compromising bradycardias, including complete heart block, symptomatic second-degree block, symptomatic sick-sinus syndrome, drug-induced bradycardias, permanent pacemaker failure, temporary epicardial pacemaker failure, postoperative cardiac surgery, idioventricular bradycardias, symptomatic atrial fibrillation with slow ventricular response, refractory bradycardia during resuscitation of patients who are in hypovolemic shock, and bradyarrhythmias with malignant ventricular escape mechanisms, or acute bifascicular or trifascicular block (Overbay & Criddle, 2004).
2. To maintain an adequate heart rate if transcutaneous pacing is ineffective (AHA, 2005).
3. To provide pacing in anterior myocardial infarction if heart rate is less than 40 beats per minute (bpm) or if there are symptoms of low cardiac output, associated angina, or ventricular irritability (Rosendorff, 2005).
4. To suppress or terminate supraventricular tachycardia or ventricular tachycardia (VT) refractory to pharmacologic therapy or electrical cardioversion.
5. To diagnose arrhythmias by simultaneous recording of surface electrocardiogram (ECG) and either atrial or ventricular electrograms or both (Preuss & Wiegand, 2005).
6. To provide a bridge to permanent pacing.
7. To suppress bradycardia-induced incessant VT in patients with prolonged QT syndrome (Rosendorff, 2005).
8. To manage tachyarrhythmias with overdrive pacing (Rosendorff, 2005).
9. Prophylaxis for a cardiac diagnostic or interventional procedure (Becker, 2005).

CONTRAINDICATIONS AND CAUTIONS

1. Transcutaneous pacing is preferred for standby pacing (see Procedure 85) (Rosendorff, 2005).
2. Asynchronous pacing is contraindicated in patients who have an intrinsic rhythm.
3. Overdriving ventricular tachycardias using high-rate burst pacing is contraindicated in the ventricle because it may result in life-threatening arrhythmias. In some temporary pacer models, a high rate of burst pacing can be achieved only in the asynchronous mode and may result in R-on-T, leading to

ventricular fibrillation. Care must be taken to correctly identify the origin of pacing wires.

4. Transvenous pacing is relatively contraindicated in a bradyasystolic arrest that lasts longer than 20 minutes because the chance of success is low (AHA, 2005).

5. Right-sided heart catheterization, i.e., floating a pacemaker wire through the right heart, may induce transient right bundle-branch block (Rosendorff, 2005).

6. Pacing a severely hypothermic patient who is bradycardic may precipitate ventricular fibrillation secondary to irritation. Bradycardia may be physiologic in these patients because of decreased metabolic demand. The hypothermic ventricle, once fibrillating, is resistant to defibrillation (AHA, 2005).

7. Because of the risk of infection, temporary transvenous pacing should be avoided if permanent pacing is expected.

8. If permanent pacing will be required, it is best to avoid the subclavian approach for temporary wire placement because it is commonly used for permanent lead placement.

9. Temporary atrial pacing with a J-shaped catheter requires fluoroscopy for positioning and traction on the lead to maintain stability.

10. Electrical safety precautions include the following:
    a. Use properly grounded hospital equipment.
    b. Insulate metal parts on the generator or pacing catheter.
    c. Wear gloves when handling the exposed terminal wires.
    d. Do not touch other electronic equipment and the patient or the pacing system simultaneously.
    e. Use adaptors for shrouded electrode pins to articulate with older model pacemakers.

11. Safety considerations related to catheter-generator connector compatibility include the following:
    a. The Food and Drug Administration (FDA) requires that all temporary transvenous pacing catheter pins be shrouded to protect against insertion into electrical outlets.
    b. When assembling a pacing system for your institution or an individual patient, assure that all pacing components are compatible and fit properly.

12. Safety considerations related to generator malfunction include the following:
    a. Older devices may be prone to malfunction and require vigilance when attached to patients.
    b. The Medtonic 5388 has been reported to turn on spontaneously due to a loosened internal part (Parekh & Alston, 2004).
    c. Annual preventative maintenance per biomedical engineering is required.

13. Safety considerations related to human error or generator design include the following:
    a. Some pulse generators go through a self-test when turned on. If another key is pushed during the self-test the pacer will lock and become inoperable.

b. Reactivate a frozen pacer (Medtronic 5388) by removing the battery and reinserting it (Kleinman, Baumann, & Andrus, 2001).

EQUIPMENT

Percutaneous sheath introducer kit (jugular, subclavian, or femoral insertion site; the introducer needs to be 1 Fr size larger than the pacing wire; i.e., a 6-Fr introducer can accommodate a 5-Fr bipolar balloon-tipped catheter)

Cutdown tray (brachial insertion site only)

Sterile towels and drapes

Sterile gowns, gloves, masks, and caps for everyone at the bedside (recommended)

Temporary pacemaker generator (single or dual chamber)

Extension cables

9-volt battery

Pacing lead (a balloon-tipped, flow-directed, bipolar catheter is usually used; unipolar and pacing pulmonary artery catheters are also available)

12-lead ECG with a male-to-male connector or an alligator clip

Cardiac monitor/defibrillator/pacemaker

Advanced life support equipment

Fluoroscopy equipment (optional)

PATIENT PREPARATION

1. Place the patient on continuous ECG monitoring (see Procedure 55).
2. Obtain a baseline 12-lead ECG (see Procedure 56).
3. Position the patient on the fluoroscopy table, if applicable.

PROCEDURAL STEPS

1. Ensure the generator, extension cables and pacing catheter are compatible.
2. Clip the hair at the insertion site. Avoid shaving because it increases the risk of infection.
3. Don a mask, a gown, a cap, and sterile gloves.
4. *Prepare the skin with a povidone-iodine or chlorhexidine gluconate solution and drape the area with sterile towels.
5. *Insert the introducer via the percutaneous or the cutdown technique (see Procedures 62 through 66). In an emergency situation, the preferred approach is the percutaneous technique via the subclavian site or the internal jugular insertion site, both of which offer ease and speed of insertion. The right internal jugular approach provides a straight line into the right ventricle. There are risks associated with the subclavian insertion site, including bleeding due to an inadvertent puncture of the subclavian artery and pneumothorax. The brachial-vein approach site is problematic because the catheter tends to be unstable and the patient experiences discomfort. The femoral site carries the greatest risk of thrombosis, phlebitis, and infection.
6. *Insert the pacemaker catheter using one of the following techniques:
   a. Emergency placement: The pacemaker and the extension cable are attached to the pacing catheter. The tip, or the distal electrode, of the

---

*Indicates portions of the procedure usually performed by a physician or an advanced practice nurse.

pacing catheter is connected to the negative pole of the pacemaker. The ring, or the proximal electrode, is connected to the positive pole of the pacemaker. The pacemaker is turned on and advanced blindly. Contact with the right ventricular endocardium is indicated by capture. The right internal jugular approach is used because it provides the straightest route to the right ventricle (Figure 86-1).

b. Urgent insertion via ECG monitoring: Place the limb electrodes of the 12-lead ECG in the standard positions. The V1 electrode is connected with alligator clips or a male-to-male connector to the distal electrode of the pacing catheter. The standardization of the ECG machine may have to be decreased to half or quarter standard because the electrical activity sensed at the tip of the pacing catheter is of greater magnitude when it is recorded internally. As the pacemaker tip approaches and enters the right atrium, the P wave becomes larger. When the catheter tip enters the right ventricle, the P wave diminishes in size and the QRS complex becomes larger. When the tip of the pacing catheter is against the wall of the right ventricle, the P wave disappears and the QRS complex becomes very large and shows ST-segment elevation. ST elevation is the marker of catheter position against the right ventricular wall (Figure 86-2).

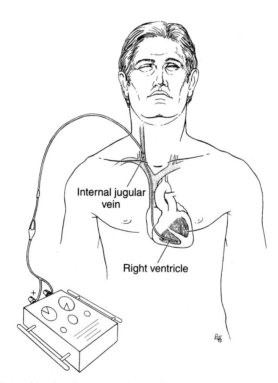

FIGURE 86-1 Internal jugular placement and setup for temporary transvenous pacing. (Courtesy of P. Rosen. M.D.)

c. Fluoroscopic insertion: Proper positioning of the patient and the fluoroscope is necessary for tracking the advancement of the catheter tip; therefore, continuous communication between the physician and the assistant is essential. The desired final catheter position is in the right ventricular apex. Most rigid catheter or brachial insertions require the use of a fluoroscope for safe and proper placement in the right ventricle. The confirmation of the catheter position by ECG may be made as described previously in step 5b.

d. Real-time ultrasound using the subcostal view has been reported to aid in the insertion of temporary pacing catheters and to evaluate mechanical capture (Tang & Euerle, 2005). It is used in a similar fashion to fluoroscopy. Echocardiography may also be useful in identifying catheter misplacement (Aguilera, Durham, & Riley, 2000).

7. Every 5 minutes, monitor the patient's tolerance of the procedure, vital signs, and rhythm. If the pacing catheter induces ventricular ectopy

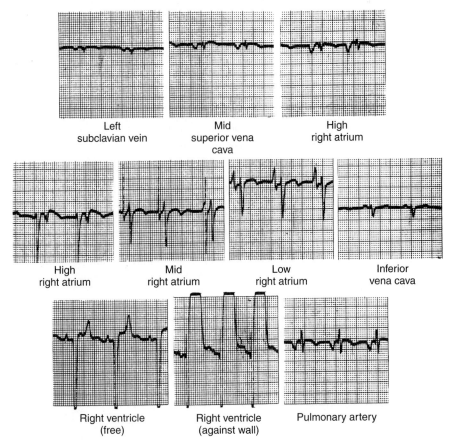

FIGURE 86-2 Pacemaker placement by electrocardiographic monitoring. (From Bing, O. H. L., Mc Dowell, J. W., Hantman, J., et al. [1972]. Pacemaker placement by electrocardiographic monitoring. *New England Journal of Medicine, 287,* 651.)

during the insertion, inform the physician. Antiarrhythmic medication and a defibrillator should be available to treat ectopy that does not abate by withdrawing the catheter from the right ventricle.

8. When the endocardial placement is achieved with ECG or fluoroscopic guidance, connect the pacing catheter to the generator directly or via a connecting cable. The distal electrode, or the tip, is connected to the negative terminal of the pacemaker. The proximal electrode, or the ring, is attached to the positive terminal of the pacemaker. The electrode lead pins on the catheter are protected by a shrouded pin. The shrouded pin requires a universal adapter to connect with older pacemakers and pacemaker cables (Figure 86-3).

9. The pacing mode and the pacemaker settings are directed by the physician, and the pacemaker is turned on. The pacemaker rate is set higher than the patient's intrinsic rate. An initial rate of 80 beats/min is selected for most patients. The mode of pacing is determined by the type of catheter used and the clinical situation. See Figures 86-4, 86-5, and 86-6 for examples of pacemakers.

   a. Demand pacing: In patients with an intrinsic, perfusing rhythm or who have been stabilized with transcutaneous pacing, the demand mode is used. Sensitivity settings may be the default settings of the specific pacemaker, or they may be set manually. The default ventricular sensitivity setting is usually about 2 millivolts. This sensitivity ensures that even a small native QRS can be sensed by the pacemaker. The mA output is increased until continuous capture is achieved, which is the threshold. The maintenance pacing output is set at 1.5 to 2 times the threshold output required to achieve capture (Figure 86-7).

   b. Asynchronous pacing: In cases where over-sensing prevents appropriate pacing, the physician may choose to pace asynchronously. This is dangerous and can result in ventricular fibrillation in the event of an R-on-T pacing impulse. The milliampere (mA) setting in this mode should be at the maximum, which is 20 to 25 mA, depending on the model of generator used. The milliamperes may be reduced after capture is achieved. Newer models of pacemakers have an EMERGENCY ON that automatically turns on the pacemaker in the asynchronous mode at a rate of 80 mA with maximal output settings. Older models require that the settings be adjusted manually. See Figures 86-4, 86-5, and 86-6 for examples of pacemakers.

10. Assess the patient's response to pacing by continuously monitoring the ECG and checking for a palpable pulse, assessing vital signs, neurologic status, and urine output.

**Step 1. Insert and secure
adaptor to cable**

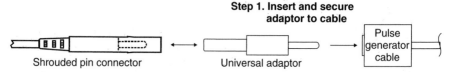

Shrouded pin connector   Universal adaptor

FIGURE 86-3 Pacing catheter shrouded pin connector inserts into the universal adaptor. The universal adaptor converts the connection to an unshrouded pin, which articulates with most pulse generators. (Courtesy Edwards Lifesciences LLC, Irvine, CA.)

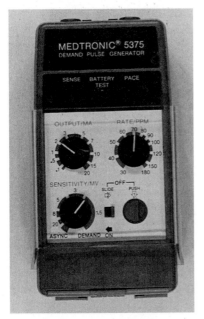

FIGURE 86-4 An example of an older-model single-chamber temporary pacemaker.

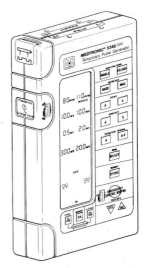

FIGURE 86-5 An example of key pad–controlled, dual-chamber, temporary pacemaker with rapid atrial pacing capacity. (Courtesy Medtronic, Inc. [1993]. *Pulse generator model 5346 technical manual* [p. 2]. Minneapolis, MN.)

1. Pace/sense LEDs
2. Lock/unlock key
3. Lock indicators
4. Rate dial
5. Atrial output dial
6. Ventricular output dial
7. Menu parameter dial
8. Parameter selection key
9. Menu selection key
10. Pause key
11. Power on key
12. Power off key
13. Emergency/asynchronous pacing key
14. Lower screen
15. Ventricular output graphics
16. Atrial output graphics
17. Upper screen
18. Rate graphics
19. Setup indicators
20. DDI indicator
21. Low battery indicator
22. Setup labels

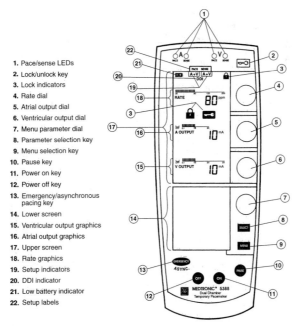

FIGURE 86-6 An example of a dial- and key pad–controlled, dual-chamber temporary pacemaker. (Courtesy Medtronic, Inc. [1996]. *Dual chamber temporary pacemaker model 5388 technical manual* [p. 3-3]. Minneapolis, MN.)

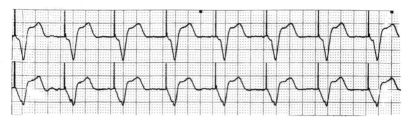

FIGURE 86-7 Ventricular capture in a single-chamber pacemaker. Each pacing spike is followed by a wide QRS complex.

TABLE 86-1
NORMAL PEDIATRIC HEART RATES

Age	Heart Rate (bpm)
First week	90-160
1-3 weeks	100-180
1-2 months	120-180
3-5 months	105-185
6-11 months	110-170
1-2 years	90-165
3-4 years	70-140
5-7 years	65-140
8-11 years	60-130
12-15 years	65-130
16 years and older	50-120

BPM, Beats per minute. From Doniger, S. J., & Sharieff, G. Q. (2006). Pediatric dysrhythmias. *Pediatric Clinics of North America, 53,* 85–105.

11. *Secure the pacing catheter to the skin with a suture.
12. Place a sterile dressing over the insertion site.
13. Secure the pacing leads by looping and taping them to the outside of the dressing. Secure the generator to the patient, and ensure electrical safety as mentioned in the Contraindications and Cautions section.
14. Obtain a chest radiograph to verify the lead placement and evaluate the patient for a pneumothorax or hemothorax.

AGE-SPECIFIC CONSIDERATIONS

1. In children, bradycardia is defined as a heart rate slower than the lower limit of normal for the patient's age. See Table 86-1 for normal ranges by age (Doniger & Sharieff, 2006).
2. Severe bradycardias in children usually result from hypoxia or hypoventilation. Oxygenation, airway patency, and ventilation should be addressed

---

*Indicates portions of the procedure usually performed by a physician or an advanced practice nurse.

before pharmacologic agents are used or pacing is attempted (Doniger & Sharieff, 2006).

3. A common cause of significant bradycardia in children is acquired or congenital complete heart block. Other causes may be vagal stimulation, acidosis, and elevation of intracranial pressure (Doniger & Sharieff, 2006).

COMPLICATIONS
Related to the Patient Pacer Interface

1. Failure to achieve capture is evidenced by pacer spikes that fail to induce a wide QRS complex (Figure 86-8). The capture threshold may change over time and should be determined frequently when the patient is pacemaker dependent.

2. Undersensing occurs when the pacemaker does not sense an intrinsic QRS and delivers a pacing spike. Failure to sense is recognized by competition between the paced rhythm and the intrinsic rhythm and by a short native QRS-to-pacing spike interval (Figure 86-9). If the pacer fails to recognize all the intrinsic QRS complexes, it operates as if it is in the asynchronous mode.

3. Oversensing is due to an inhibition of pacing by extracardiac or cardiac electrical signals (Figure 86-10). Extracardiac electrical signals include muscle artifact and electromagnetic signals in the environment. Inappropriate cardiac signals include P waves (cross talk) and T waves. These may be corrected by increasing the numerical millivolt sensitivity setting, thereby decreasing the sensitivity to the inappropriate electrical

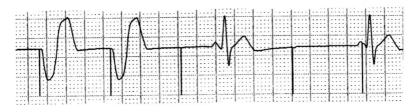

FIGURE 86-8 Intermittent failure to capture. Some pacing spikes are not followed by wide QRS complexes. (Courtesy Medtronic, Inc. [1996]. *Temporary pacing workshop instructor guide* [overhead S-5]. Minneapolis, MN.)

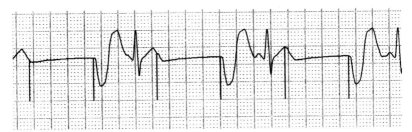

FIGURE 86-9 Undersensing. The pacer fails to sense the intrinsic beats (beats 2 and 4) and fires prematurely. The pacer also does not capture, because the spike has fallen during the refractory period. (Courtesy Medtronic, Inc. [1996]. *Temporary pacing workshop instructor guide* [overhead S-6]. Minneapolis, MN.)

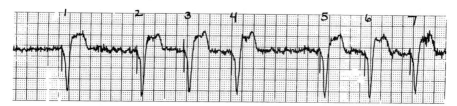

FIGURE 86-10 Oversensing. Pacing spikes 2 and 5 occur late because of oversensing of myopotentials. (Courtesy Medtronic, Inc. [1996]. *Temporary pacing workshop instructor guide* [overhead S-7]. Minneapolis, MN.)

signals. If the problem persists, it may be necessary to operate the pacemaker in the asynchronous mode to obtain reliable pacing. This solution is used during cautery to maintain pacing.

Related to Insertion

1. Hemothorax and pneumothorax are associated with subclavian and jugular insertion.
2. Bleeding that is difficult to control may be associated with femoral and subclavian insertion.
3. Myocardial perforation, which may lead to cardiac tamponade or diaphragmatic pacing. This is more common with brachial or femoral catheters and is more likely with rigid catheters.
4. Myocardial irritability, which may cause ventricular arrhythmias
5. Transient bundle branch block.
6. Failure to achieve capture because of malpositioning of the catheter in the inferior vena cava or the pulmonary artery.
7. Arterial trauma and air embolism.

Related to Catheter Maintenance

1. Local myocardial edema and inflammation, causing an increase over time in the threshold to achieve capture.
2. For long-term temporary pacing, the femoral vein should be avoided in order to prevent infection.

Related to Equipment

1. Generator or battery failure, or both, possibly resulting in failure to fire, capture, or sense.
2. Lead displacement, possibly resulting in failure to sense or capture. This is usually associated with brachial and femoral insertion.
3. Poor connections, possibly resulting in failure to fire, sense, or capture.

PATIENT TEACHING

1. Bed rest and restriction of movement at the hip are required with femoral insertion. Immobilization of the arm is required with brachial insertion. Other insertion sites do not require movement or position restrictions.
2. Do not move or manipulate the pacemaker or the wire.
3. Report dizziness, lightheadedness, or weakness immediately.

REFERENCES

Aguilera, P. A., Durham, B. A., & Riley, D. A. (2000). Emergency transvenous cardiac pacing placement using ultrasound guidance. *Annals of Emergency Medicine, 36,* 224-227.

American Heart Association (AHA). (2005). Management of symptomatic bradycardia and tachycardia. *Circulation, 112,* 67-77.

Becker, D. E. (2005). Temporary transvenous pacemaker insertion (perform). In D. J. Lynn-McHale Wiegand, & K. K. Carlson (Eds.), *AACN procedure manual for critical care* (5th ed., pp. 340-361). Philadelphia: Saunders.

Kleinman, B., Baumann, M., & Andrus, C. (2001). Faulty design resulting in temporary pacemaker failure. *Chest, 120,* 684-685.

Overbay, D., & Criddle, L. (2004). Mastering temporary invasive cardiac pacing. *Critical Care, 24*(3), 25-32.

Parekh, S. D., & Alston, T. A. (2004). Temporary pacemaker who wouldn't quit. *Anesthesiology, 101,* 810.

Preuss, T., & Wiegand, D. L. (2005). Atrial electrograms. In D. J. Lynn-McHale Wiegand, & K. K. Carlson (Eds.), *AACN procedure manual for critical care* (5th ed., pp. 296-303). Philadelphia: Saunders.

Rosendorff, C. (2005). *Essential cardiology: Principles and practice* (2nd ed.). Tofowa, NJ: Humana Press, Inc.

Tang, A., & Euerle, B. (2005). Emergency department ultrasound and echocardiography. *Emergency Medicine Clinics of North America, 23,* 1179-1194.

Invasive Hemodynamic Monitoring

Central Venous Pressure Measurement

June F. Stacey, RN, BSN, CEN

Central venous pressure is also known as *CVP* or *right atrial pressure (RAP)*.

INDICATIONS

1. To monitor volume status and right ventricular function. CVP monitoring is most helpful in patients without preexisting cardiopulmonary disease (Mickiewicz, Dronen, & Younger, 2004).
2. To guide the administration of fluids, diuretics, and vasoactive drugs when other invasive monitoring options are not available. CVP is a key monitoring parameter used to guide resuscitation as part of early goal-directed therapy (EGDT) for severe sepsis (Dellinger et al., 2004).
3. To assist in the diagnosis of cardiac tamponade (Mickiewicz et al., 2004).

CONTRAINDICATIONS AND CAUTIONS

1. Increases in CVP may occur as a result of increased cardiac output, right ventricular infarct or failure, increased vascular volume, cardiac tamponade, tension pneumothorax, constrictive pericarditis, or pulmonary hypertension. Falsely elevated CVP measurements may occur in the setting of a pneumothorax, positive-pressure ventilation, or chronic obstructive pulmonary disease.
2. Inaccurate readings can be caused by dislocation of the tip of the central line from the superior vena cava or improper manometer or transducer positioning. Zero the transducer whenever the patient's position is changed.
3. Decreases in CVP may be due to any condition that decreases preload such as hypovolemia, drug-induced vasodilation, or shock of any etiology.

EQUIPMENT
Manometer
CVP water manometer
Intravenous (IV) fluid and tubing
Skin marker

Transducer
Cardiac monitor with hemodynamic monitoring capability
Pressure transducer cable
Pressure tubing with continuous flush device and transducer

Pressure extension tubing (extra length of pressure tubing if planning to mount transducer on IV pole)

Two or three three-way stopcocks

Dead-end caps for stopcocks

250- or 500-ml bag of flush solution per institutional policy (normal saline or heparin solution)

Pressure infusion bag or cuff

Pole with transducer mount

Level (optional)

Skin marker

PATIENT PREPARATION

1. See Procedures 62 through 65 for information about central line insertion. Preexisting central venous lines or ports, without a valve (i.e., Groshong), may be used for initial evaluation of CVP until another central line is inserted (Gilboy & Tanabe, 2006).
2. Place the patient in the supine position with the head of the bed flat or elevated no more than 30 degrees.
3. Locate and mark the phlebostatic axis with the skin marker to ensure that the same zero reference point is used for consistent measurements. The phlebostatic axis is found by locating the junction of the fourth intercostal space and the midaxillary line (Figure 87-1).

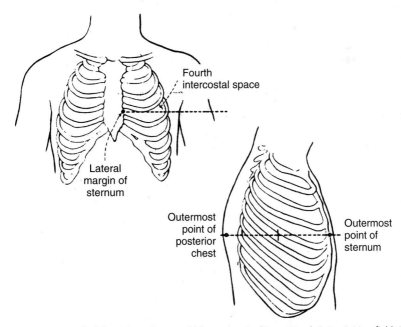

FIGURE 87-1 Level of the right atrium or phlebostatic axis. (From Wood, S. L., & Mansfield, L. W. (1976). Body position upon pulmonary artery capillary wedge pressures in noncritically ill patients. *Heart and Lung, 5,* 84.)

PROCEDURAL STEPS

Manometer

1. Turn the stopcock off to the manometer and flush the tubing with IV fluid (Figure 87-2, *A*).
2. Attach the manometer tubing to the central venous line and flush to ensure patency.
3. Position the zero mark on the water manometer (not the base of the manometer) at the phlebostatic angle. The manometer can be either secured to an IV pole or hand held at the point of reference.
4. Turn the stopcock off to the patient and open it between the IV solution and the manometer. Allow the manometer to fill slowly with IV fluid up to the 25-cm level. Note that the faster the IV fluid is running, the faster the manometer fills. Avoid letting the fluid run out the top of the manometer, because contamination of the manometer may result (Figure 87-2, *B*).
5. Turn the stopcock off to the IV fluid and open between the patient and manometer. This causes the fluid level to fall and fluctuate with respirations (Figure 87-2, *C*).
6. Take the CVP reading when the fluid level stabilizes. The reading should be taken from the base of the meniscus at the end of expiration. If the patient is spontaneously breathing, the fluid in the manometer slightly drops with inspiration; end-expiration is seen when the fluid in the manometer rises. In a ventilated patient, the fluid height in the manometer increases during inspiration and drops at end-expiration.
7. Turn the stopcock off to the manometer and run the IV fluids through the central venous line as prescribed
8. Document the reading and the patient's position.
9. Normal CVP ranges from 6 to 12 cm H_2O (Mickiewicz et al., 2004). When monitoring CVP, the trend is more significant than a single reading.

Transducer

1. Assemble the pressure tubing and transducer and zero the transducer as described in Procedure 88: Arterial Line Insertion and Monitoring. The transducer setup will convert the pressure in the right atrium to an electrical signal that can be viewed on the monitor.
2. The transducer can be patient- or pole-mounted. In order to obtain accurate measurements, the transducer must also be placed at the level of the phlebostatic axis and zeroed.
3. Observe the CVP values and waveform. If the patient is spontaneously breathing, note the pressure at the end of inspiration. In a ventilated patient, note the pressure at the end of expiration.
4. Document the reading and the patient's position.
5. Normal CVP ranges from 6 to 12 cm H_2O (1 mm Hg equals 1.3595 cm H_2O) (Mickiewicz et al., 2004). When monitoring CVP, the trend is more significant than a single reading.

AGE-SPECIFIC CONSIDERATIONS (Nichols et al., 2006)

1. CVP catheters are indicated for children with large blood loss or with fluid shifts or those requiring vasoactive drugs. They may be placed in the internal jugular, subclavian, or femoral vein.

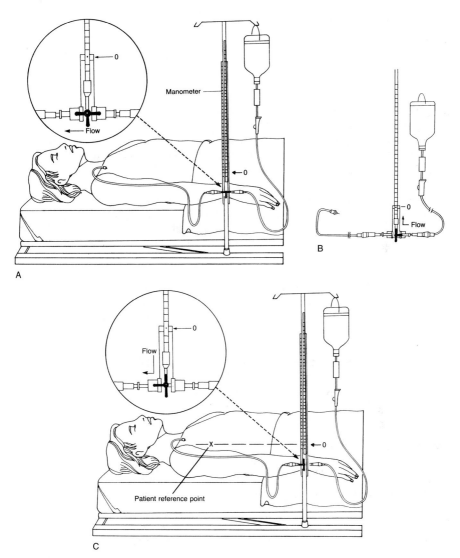

FIGURE 87-2 Simple manometry setup to measure CVP at the bedside. **A,** The stopcock is opened to direct flow to the patient to maintain catheter patency. The tubing is always flushed before connecting to the CVP catheter. **B,** The stopcock is opened to allow fluid to flow into the manometer to 25 cm H_2O. **C,** The stopcock is then opened to the patient and the water level allowed to stabilize before reading the value. Note that the zero mark on the manometer (not the base of the manometer) is at the phlebostatic axis. (From Mickiewicz, M., Dronen, S. C., & Younger, J. G. [2004]. Vascular techniques and volume support. In J. R. Roberts & J. R. Hedges (Eds.), *Clinical procedures in emergency medicine* [4th ed., p. 441]. Philadelphia: Saunders.)

2. Normal CVP values in infants are difficult to define. Healthy infants usually have values between –2 and 4 mm Hg. Infants and children with congenital heart or respiratory diseases will have readings between 2 and 6 mm Hg. Elevated pressures may indicate cardiac dysfunction, increased intrathoracic pressure, or volume overload. Note that the normal values listed above for adults are in cm H_2O, not mm Hg; 1 mm Hg equals 1.3595 cm H_2O.
3. Because veins are small in infants and children, cannulation may be difficult and arterial puncture is a risk.
4. Proper positioning and zeroing of the transducer are especially important in children because minute changes can be a significant finding.

COMPLICATIONS

1. As with other procedures using central venous catheters, complications may include infection, phlebitis, venous thrombosis, and air embolism.
2. Occlusion of the catheter caused by improper positioning of the stopcock results in slowing or cessation of IV fluid administration through the central venous line.
3. Hemorrhage may result from disconnection of the tubing from the central venous catheter.
4. Inaccurate readings may result from air bubbles in the circuit, a transducer that is not correctly calibrated (zeroed), malposition of the catheter tip, increased intrathoracic pressure (positive pressure ventilation, coughing, tension pneumothorax, or Valsalva maneuver), occlusions of catheter or tubing, inaccurate reference point, readings at the wrong phase of respiration, or readings by different observers (Mickiewicz et al., 2004).

PATIENT TEACHING

Report any tubing disconnections or blood in the tubing immediately.

REFERENCES

Blot, F., & Laplance, A. (2000). Accuracy of totally implantable ports, tunneled, single- and multi-lumen central venous catheters for measurement of central venous pressure. *Intensive Care Medicine, 26*, 1837-1842.

Dellinger, R. P., Carlet, J. M., Masur, H., Gerlach, H., Calandra, T., & Cohen, J., et al. (2004). Surviving sepsis campaign. *Critical Care Medicine, 32*, 858-873.

Gilboy, N., & Tanabe, P. (2006). Can different types of central venous catheters be used to obtain central venous pressures in an emergent situation? *Advanced Emergency Nursing Journal, 28*, 269-274.

Mickiewicz, M., Dronen, S. C., & Younger, J. G. (2004). Central venous catheterization and central venous pressure monitoring. In J. R. Roberts, & J. R. Hedges (Eds.), *Clinical procedures in emergency medicine* (4th ed., pp. 413-446). Philadelphia: Saunders.

Nichols, D. G., Ungerleider, R. M., Spevak, P. J., Greely, W. J., Cameron, D. E., Lappe, D. G., & Wetzel, R. C. (2006). *Critical heart disease in infants and children* (2nd ed.). St Louis: Mosby.

Arterial Line Insertion and Monitoring

Lucinda W. Rossoll, RN, MSN, CCRN, CEN

An arterial line is also known as an *A-line* or an *art line.*

INDICATIONS

1. To monitor arterial pressure accurately and continuously in patients who are, or who have the potential to become, hemodynamically unstable.
2. To monitor the response to vasoactive drugs.
3. To facilitate frequent sampling of arterial blood gases (ABGs) and other laboratory specimens.
4. To determine derived hemodynamic parameters, such as the mean arterial pressure (MAP). This is helpful for calculating and monitoring cerebral perfusion pressure.

CONTRAINDICATIONS AND CAUTIONS

1. Knowledge and understanding of the arterial line monitoring system, the waveforms, and how to obtain accurate values is necessary when assisting with insertion and monitoring of the A-line.
2. Significant blood loss may occur if the tubing is disconnected.
3. Close patient monitoring is necessary for any patient with an A-line in place, and monitoring alarms should always be enabled to alert the nurse of hemodynamic changes or system malfunction.
4. Avoid A-line insertion in extremities with injuries that may compromise distal circulation.

EQUIPMENT

Arterial catheter or 18- to 20-G, 1- to 2-in intravenous (IV) catheter
Sterile gloves
Antiseptic solution
Lidocaine 1% (without epinephrine) for local anesthesia
3-ml syringe for lidocaine
18-G, 1½-in needle (to draw up lidocaine)
25-G, ½-in needle (to administer lidocaine)
250- to 500-ml bag of flush solution, normal saline or heparinized saline, per institutional policy
Cardiac monitor with invasive monitoring capability
Recorder (preferably analog recorder)
Pressure transducer cable

†Microdrip IV tubing

†Pressure tubing with continuous flush device

†Pressure transducer (if not already part of the pressure tubing setup)

†Pressure extension tubing

†Long pressure extension tubing (for pole-mounted transducer)

†Two or three (three-way) stopcocks (number used depends on how blood draws are performed, i.e., one- or two-stopcock method)

†Dead-ender nonvented caps for stopcock ports

Pressure-infuser bag or cuff

Armboard

Pole-mounted transducer holder (optional)

Level (optional)

4-0 nylon sutures

Dressing supplies per institutional protocol, e.g., tincture of benzoin, adhesive tape or surgical tape closures, and transparent occlusive dressing

Blood drawing supplies: ABG syringe, blood tubes as needed, vacutainer holder with Luer adaptor, and one or two 10-ml syringes (supplies needed depend on laboratory studies ordered and blood draw technique (see steps 12a and 12b). (Indicates equipment that may come prepackaged in a pressure tubing and transducer set)

PATIENT PREPARATION

1. Establish cardiac monitoring (see Procedure 55).
2. Check with the physician regarding the site to be cannulated. The radial, ulnar, brachial, or femoral arteries are commonly selected. The radial artery is usually used for arterial pressure monitoring because it generally has good collateral circulation, is easily accessible, is not prone to contamination by products of elimination, and does not require extremity immobilization, which restricts patient movement, as the other sites frequently do. Collateral circulation to the hand may be assessed before insertion of the radial or ulna line by use of the Allen's test (Procedure 19) or a Doppler ultrasound device (Procedure 49).
3. Position the extremity in extension.

PROCEDURAL STEPS

1. Turn on the hemodynamic monitor and attach the transducer cable. Set the scale on the 200–mm Hg range. NOTE: The range may be adjusted to adapt to extreme pressures.
2. Prepare the pressure monitoring system as follows (Figure 88-1):
   a. Spike the flush solution with the IV pressure tubing and remove all air from the bag. Attach the flush solution to the microdrip IV tubing portion of the pressure tubing set and fill the drip chamber half full to prevent air from entering the system.
   b. If you do not use preassembled transducer and tubing sets:
      i. After spiking the flush solution and flushing the IV tubing, attach the IV tubing to the transducer.
      ii. If the transducer is to be patient mounted, attach two stopcocks onto the transducer and add the short extension tubing to the end. If extra

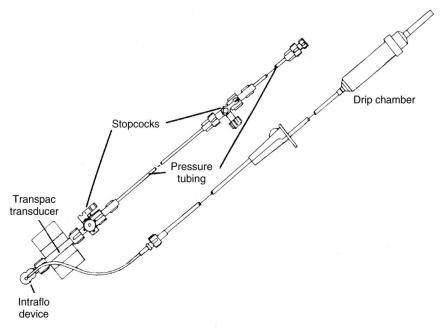

FIGURE 88-1 Preassembled disposable transducer and tubing for pressure monitoring. (Courtesy Abbott Critical Care Systems, North Chicago, IL.)

length is needed for the transducer to reach the patient, add extension tubing between the IV tubing and transducer.

iii. If the transducer is to be pole mounted, add a stopcock onto the transducer and add a long piece of pressure extension tubing, then add the two stopcocks and the short pressure tubing.

c. Prime the tubing and the transducer to remove all the air from the system. This is accomplished by opening the roller clamp and activating the flush device (pigtail or squeeze mechanism) according to the manufacturer's directions. Work down the tubing and flush each stopcock until all air is flushed through the fenestrated (vented) cap. Replace the vented caps with nonvented caps on each side port of the stopcock as the stopcock is flushed. Continue until all the air is removed from the system and all the stopcocks are flushed. Inspect the entire system, especially the transducer, for air, which may result in a dampened waveform. Tapping any bubbles that adhere to the tubing or within the transducer will release them so they can be flushed out of the nearest stopcock. The flush device, also known as the continuous-flow device, allows a flow rate of 3 to 5 ml/hr (usual rate is 3 ml/hr) to maintain patency of the system. Turn each stopcock on to both the patient and the transducer.

d. Place the flush solution in the pressure bag and pressurize it to 300 mm Hg. This step is not performed before step c, because the increased pressure causes rapid flushing and increased turbulence, which may trap air bubbles in the system and cause a damped waveform.

    e. Attach the transducer cable(s) to the transducer(s) and monitor.

    f. Position the transducer. If the patient-mounted option is being used, keep the transducer on the same plane as the right atrium to reflect central arterial pressure. Leveling the transducer to the tip of the arterial catheter will reflect transmural pressure at that point in the artery (Preuss & Wigand, 2005). For a pole-mounted transducer, secure the transducer on the IV pole at the level of the right atrium so that the stopcock at the air-fluid interface (the same stopcock that is used to open the system to atmospheric pressure) is at the level of the phlebostatic axis (use a level to guide placement). The phlebostatic axis is found by locating the junction of the fourth intercostal space and the midaxillary line (see Procedure 87, Figure 87-1).

    g. Zero balance the transducer. Zero balancing the system to the atmospheric pressure negates the effects of the atmospheric pressure. To prevent erroneous pressure readings, zero the system before and after the pressure system is attached to the patient, with any significant change in the waveform and the values, whenever the system is disconnected, and at the beginning of each shift. To zero, turn the stopcock next to the transducer off to the patient and open to air (this is known as the air-fluid interface). Zero the monitor according to the manufacturer's directions. Once the monitor is zeroed, flush the open stopcock port and replace the dead-end cap. Turn the stopcock on to the patient and on to the transducer. Some monitors also need to be calibrated; if this is the case, do so according to the manufacturer's directions.

3. *Cleanse the insertion site with antiseptic solution. Infiltrate the insertion site with a local anesthetic (optional).

4. *Cannulate the artery with the catheter and remove the inner wire. Allow the catheter to back fill with blood (Figure 88-2).

5. Connect the pressure tubing to the catheter and secure it tightly via the Luer-Lok connection.

6. Activate the flush device to clear the line of any blood resulting from the backflow.

7. *Suture the catheter in place.

---

*Indicates portions of the procedure usually performed by a physician or an advanced practice nurse.

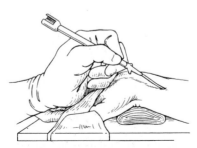

FIGURE 88-2 Insertion of a radial artery cannula. (Courtesy of P. Rosen, M.D.)

8. Cleanse the site with an antiseptic solution, apply tincture of benzoin or other skin preparation around the insertion site (optional), use adhesive tape to secure the catheter in place, and cover with a sterile or occlusive dressing (as per institutional policy). Stabilize the extremity with an armboard as needed.

9. Observe and record the arterial pressure waveform (Figure 88-3) on the monitor and note the digital blood pressure reading. Many protocols require checking the cuff pressure to ensure the accuracy of the arterial measurement. In low-flow states, such as hypotension, lower pressure readings are obtained with a cuff pressure rather than A-line pressures, and higher cuff pressure readings are obtained in high-flow states, such as sepsis. Darovic (2004) cautions against the inconsistent practice of accepting

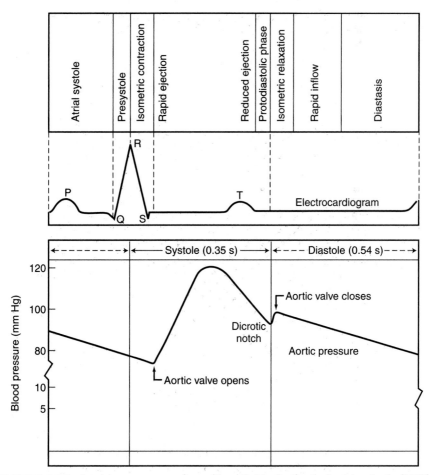

FIGURE 88-3 Arterial pressure waveform. (From Smith, R. N., & de Asla, R. A. [1988]. Instrumentation. In M. R. Kinney, D. R. Packa, & S. B. Dunbar [Eds.], *AACN's clinical reference manual for critical care nursing* [2nd ed., p. 48]. St Louis: Mosby.)

a cuff pressure reading one time and an A-line pressure another. There is no need to correlate cuff pressures with monitor pressures if the square wave shows an optimally damped system. See square wave information under Complications, number 3.

10. Maintain a continuous display of the pressure tracings. Set the monitor to view systolic, diastolic, and mean pressure readings. This allows for early detection of hemodynamic changes in the patient or catheter disconnection.

11. Turn on the monitor alarms to limits determined by the patient's clinical condition, physician order, or institutional protocol.

12. To withdraw blood for laboratory analysis from an open withdrawal system, use either the one-stopcock or the two-stopcock method.

   a. Two-stopcock method
      i. Clean the stopcock with alcohol and attach a 10-ml syringe to the stopcock most distal to the insertion site (distal stopcock). Clean the proximal stopcock with alcohol and attach the heparinized ABG syringe, the blood-drawing syringe, or vacutainer holder with Luer adaptor.
      ii. Turn the distal stopcock off to the transducer and turn it on to the patient. Withdraw 10 ml of blood to clear the flush solution from the line (or other amount per institutional protocol). Turn the stopcock off to the 10-ml syringe.
      iii. Turn the proximal stopcock off to the transducer and on to the patient. Withdraw 1 ml of blood into the ABG syringe or designated volume into the draw syringe or withdraw blood through vacutainer holder with adaptor directly into the tube. Turn the stopcock off to the ABG syringe/blood-drawing syringe or vacutainer holder. Remove the ABG syringe and purge any air before capping it and placing it on ice or remove draw syringe and place blood in appropriate tubes.
      iv. Reinfuse the blood in the 10-ml clearing syringe (optional). Turn the distal stopcock off to the transducer, turn it on to the patient, reinfuse the blood slowly, and turn the stopcock off to the syringe port. If reinfusion is not desired, leave the stopcock closed, remove the 10-ml clearing syringe, and discard it.
      v. Flush both stopcocks as described in Procedural Step 2c, clean with alcohol, and cap them with sterile dead-end caps.

   b. One-stopcock method
      i. Clean the stopcock closest to the catheter site with alcohol and attach a 10-ml syringe.
      ii. Turn the stopcock off to the transducer and turn it on to the patient. Withdraw 10 ml of blood to clear any flush solution from the line (per institutional protocol). Turn the stopcock off to the 10-ml syringe. Remove and discard the 10-ml syringe.
      iii. Clean the stopcock with alcohol and attach the heparinized ABG/blood-draw syringe or vacutainer holder with Luer adaptor to the port. Turn the stopcock off to the transducer and turn it on to the patient. Withdraw 1 ml of blood into the ABG syringe or designated volume into the blood-draw syringe or withdraw blood through vacutainer holder with adaptor directly into the appropriate tubes. Turn

the stopcock off to the ABG/blood-draw syringe or vacutainer holder. Remove the ABG/blood-draw syringe. Place blood from draw syringe into appropriate vacutainers. If an ABG was drawn, purge any air before capping it and placing it on ice.

iv. Flush the stopcock as described in Procedural Step 2c, clean with alcohol, and cap it with a sterile dead-end cap.

AGE-SPECIFIC CONSIDERATIONS

1. In the pediatric population, the radial artery is most commonly used, other sites include the femoral, dorsalis pedis, posterior tibial, or brachial arteries (Darovic, 2002).
2. In infants, catheter patency may be maintained with a 1- to 3-ml/hr infusion of flush solution. Use a volume-controlled infusion pump instead of a pressure bag to avoid accidental fluid overload.

COMPLICATIONS

1. An air embolism can be introduced into the circulation if the tubing and transducer are not flushed properly before connection to the cannula. If air bubbles persist despite tight connections, check the flush device and stopcocks for cracks.
2. Severe blood loss, or exsanguination, may occur if the connections are not tightly secured or the catheter is dislodged.
3. Damping of the waveform may occur if the cannula lodges against the vessel wall or if there is clot formation, kinking of the catheter, or inadequate pressure on the pressure bag (Figure 88-4). Slight readjustment of the cannula may free it from its position against the vessel wall. If a clot is suspected, aspirate with a syringe to attempt to remove the clot. Never inject into the line because a clot may become dislodged into the circulation. If air is entrapped in the transducer and cannot be cleared, replace the transducer assembly. To ensure accurate and consistent pressure readings:
   a. Level and zero the transducers as outlined in procedural steps 2e and 2f. Inaccurate pressure readings may occur if the transducer is placed incorrectly. If the transducer is above the level of the right atrium, the pressure reading will be falsely low. If the transducer is below the level of the right atrium, the pressure reading will be falsely elevated. To prevent inaccurate pressure readings, level before and after the pressure system is attached to the patient, any change in bed height, any significant change in the waveforms and their values, whenever the system is disconnected, and at the beginning of each shift.

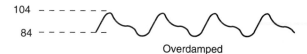

Overdamped

FIGURE 88-4 Damping of arterial waveform. The systolic pressure is falsely low, the diastolic pressure is falsely elevated, and the dicrotic notch is obscured. (From Darovic, G. O. [Ed.], *Hemodynamic monitoring* [3rd ed]. Philadelphia: Saunders.)

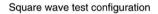

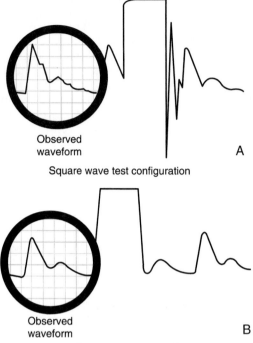

A

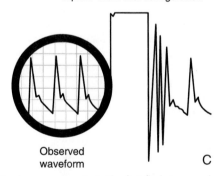

B

C

FIGURE 88-5 A, Optimal square wave test. The fast flush trace ends with a small undershoot, followed by a small overshoot, and the oscillations cease before the next patient waveform. **B,** Overdamped square wave. The fast flush trace slowly returns to the next patient waveform without any oscillations. **C,** Underdamped square wave. The fast flush trace has oscillations that continue into the next waveform. (From Darovic, G. O. [Ed.], *Hemodynamic monitoring* [3rd ed]. Philadelphia: Saunders.)

   b. Check the dynamic response. The dynamic response is used to ensure that the monitoring system is accurately reproducing the patient's pressure signal at the monitor. This is achieved by evaluating the square wave. With the pressure bag inflated to 300 mm Hg, activate and release the fast flush quickly.
      i. The system is optimally damped when the resulting waveform exceeds the upper limits of the scope followed by a negative deflection and a small overshoot. It then returns to the patient's pressure waveform (Figure 88-5, *A*).
     ii. The system is overdamped if the fast flush results in a waveform that does not exceed the upper limits of the scope, followed by a slow return to the baseline (Figure 88-5, *B*). This gives a false-low systolic pressure. The most common cause is a stopcock or inadequate pressure on the system, allowing the blood to back up.
    iii. The system is underdamped if the fast flush results in a waveform that goes above and below the limits of the scope, with several more positive and negative deflections occurring before returning to baseline. If the system is underdamped, it gives falsely elevated systolic values. This can be due to excessive catheter length, fast heart rate, or high pressures that cause a "ringing" in the system (Figure 88-5, *C*). Commercial devices that attach to the pressure system are available to assist in controlling underdamping.
     iv. If the system is underdamped or overdamped and cannot be corrected, monitor the mean arterial pressure because this measurement is not affected by catheter movement within the vessel or by poor dynamic response and will provide a reliable trend.
4. Infection may occur if poor aseptic technique is used, if there are openings in the system that allow entrance and promote growth of bacteria (e.g., blood not cleared from the port after the blood is drawn or after failure to apply sterile dead-end caps to the unused ports) or if the catheter is left in for a prolonged period of time. Stopcocks should be cleaned with alcohol prior to connecting a syringe or cap.
5. Median nerve damage may occur if the wrist remains dorsiflexed.
6. A hematoma, with possible nerve compression at the insertion site, may occur.

PATIENT TEACHING

1. Use care when moving about in bed so as not to disconnect the system.
2. Report any disconnections or dampness around the site immediately.

REFERENCES

Darovic, G. O. (2002). *Hemodynamic monitoring* (3rd ed.). Philadelphia: Saunders.
Darovic, G. O. (2004). *Handbook of hemodynamic monitoring* (2nd ed.). Philadelphia: Saunders.
Preuss, T., & Wiegand, D. J. L. (2005). Single- and multiple-pressure transducer systems. In D. J. Lynn-McHale Wiegand, & K. K. Carlson (Eds.), *AACN procedure manual for critical care* (5th ed., pp. 591-601). Philadelphia: Saunders.

Pulmonary Artery Catheter Insertion

Lucinda W. Rossoll, RN, MSN, CCRN, CEN

The pulmonary artery (PA) catheter is also known as a *Swan-Ganz catheter* or a *flow-directed, balloon-tipped, thermodilution catheter.* Pulmonary artery occlusive pressure (PAOP) is also known as *pulmonary capillary wedge pressure* (PCWP), *pulmonary artery wedge* (PAW), or *wedge pressure.* It is reflective of left ventricular end-diastolic pressure (LVEDP). Catheters with more than the standard four ports are available and are used to provide additional proximal ports, fiberoptic monitoring of mixed venous oxygen saturation (SvO_2), pacemaker insertion, measurement of ejection fraction, monitoring of cardiac output (CO), and various combinations of the above.

INDICATIONS

1. To provide a continuous and reliable method of monitoring right atrial, PA, and pulmonary wedge pressures in hemodynamically unstable patients and patients with pulmonary or cardiac conditions. This information may help determine underlying pathology, for example, with septic shock there is hypotension with low systemic and peripheral vascular resistance and high cardiac output.
2. To determine cardiac output using the thermodilution method.
3. To obtain mixed venous samples for analysis of an intrapulmonary shunt, an intracardiac shunt, and oxygen consumption.
4. To monitor interventions such as the titration of vasoactive and inotropic medications and the administration of fluids and diuretics.

CONTRAINDICATIONS AND CAUTIONS

1. There are no absolute contraindications for insertion of a PA catheter. Caution should be used in patients with prolonged bleeding times, hypercoagulable states, mechanical tricuspid valve, left bundle-branch block, or recurrent sepsis.
2. Knowledge and understanding of the hemodynamic monitoring system, the PA catheter, and the waveforms, as well as how to accurately obtain readings from the waveforms, are essential when assisting with the insertion and monitoring of the PA catheter.
3. Never inflate the balloon with greater than 1.5 ml of air. To obtain the PAOP, inflate the balloon with only as much air as needed to obtain a "wedge" waveform. Never leave the balloon inflated.

EQUIPMENT

Level

Pressure-infuser bag or cuff

†8.5-Fr or one that is one size larger than the selected PA catheter (most introducers come with a side port for continuous fluid administration)

†Percutaneous sheath

†Sterile drapes

†Suture

†Lidocaine 1% (without epinephrine) for local anesthesia

†3-ml syringe (for lidocaine)

†18-G 1½-in needle (to draw up lidocaine)

†25-G ½-in needle (for administration of lidocaine)

†Scalpel

Intravenous (IV) fluid and tubing of choice for the side port (and proximal port of the PA catheter if two transducers are not used)

Antiseptic solution

250- to 500-ml bag of flush solution, normal saline or heparinized saline, per institutional policy

Pressure transducer cable(s) (the number needed depends on the number of waveforms to be monitored continuously)

Pole-mounted transducer holder

‡Pressure tubing with continuous flush device

‡Pressure transducer(s) (the number needed depends on the number of waveforms to be monitored continuously)

‡Pressure extension tubing

‡Two stopcocks (three-way)

‡Nonvented (dead-end) caps for stopcock ports

Cardiac monitor with hemodynamic monitoring capability

Recorder (preferably analog recorder)

Cardiac output monitor with thermodilution setup

Indelible felt-tip marker

Sterile caps, gloves, gowns, and masks

Dressing supplies per institutional protocol, e.g., tincture of benzoin, adhesive tape or surgical tape closures, and transparent occlusive dressing

Cardiopulmonary resuscitation equipment, including a temporary pacemaker (may be a transcutaneous pacemaker)

Antiarrhythmic agent (if prescribed by physician) for possible IV use in the event of an arrhythmia

PA catheter (size and port configuration per physician preference) (Figure 89-1)

Sterile basin (optional, see Procedural Step 7)

Sterile water or normal saline (optional, see Procedural Step 7)

PATIENT PREPARATION

1. Establish cardiac monitoring (see Procedure 55).
2. Establish a peripheral IV line because there is the potential for cardiac arrhythmias during catheter insertion (see Procedure 60).

---

†Indicates equipment that may come in a prepackaged introducer kit.

‡Indicates equipment that may come prepackaged in a pressure tubing and transducer set.

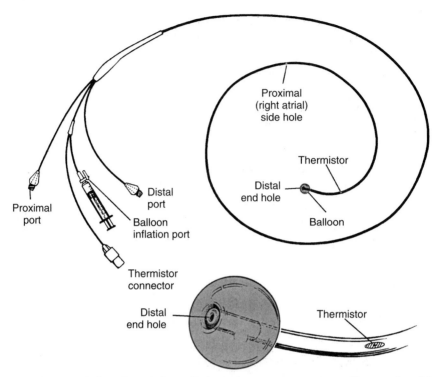

FIGURE 89-1 A flow-directed thermodilution pulmonary artery catheter. (Courtesy Spacelabs Medical, Inc, Issaquah, WA.)

3. Position the patient. For an internal jugular (IJ) or subclavian insertion, the patient should be placed in a slight Trendelenburg position with a rolled towel under the shoulder on the side in which the catheter will be inserted. For a femoral vein insertion, the patient should be in the supine position. Infrequently, a median basilic vein or a lateral cephalic vein in the antecubital fossa may be used.

4. Mark the phlebostatic axis with the felt-tip marker to ensure that the same zero reference point is used for consistent measurements. The phlebostatic axis is found by locating the junction of the fourth intercostal space and the midaxillary line (see Procedure 87, Figure 87-1).

PROCEDURAL STEPS

1. Turn on the hemodynamic monitor and attach the transducer cable. Set the scale on the 40- to 60-mm Hg range. The range may be adjusted to adapt to extreme pressures.

2. Assemble and flush the pressure monitoring system as outlined in steps a–c (Figure 89-2). One or two transducers may be used, depending on the number of pressures that need to be monitored.

   a. Spike the flush solution with the IV pressure tubing and remove all air from the bag. Attach the flush solution to the pressure tubing set, and fill the drip chamber half full to prevent air from entering the system.

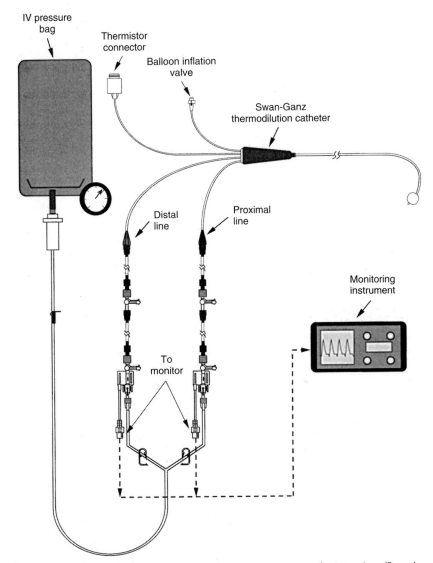

FIGURE 89-2 Monitoring system set up to monitor two pressures at the same time. (From Arone, M. [2001]. Single and multiple pressure transducer systems. In D. J. Lynn-McHale & K. K. Carlson (Eds.), *AACN procedure manual for critical care* [4th ed., p. 477]. Philadelphia: Saunders.)

   b. Prime the tubing and the transducer to remove all the air from the system. This is accomplished by opening the roller clamp and activating the flush device (pigtail or squeeze mechanism) according to the manufacturer's directions. Work down the tubing and flush each stopcock until all air is flushed through the fenestrated cap. Replace the vented caps with non-vented caps on each side port of the stopcock as the stopcock is flushed. Continue until all the air is removed from the system and all the stopcocks are flushed. Inspect the entire system, especially the transducer, for air, which may result in a dampened waveform. Tapping bubbles that adhere to the tubing sides or within the transducer will release them so they can be flushed out of the nearest stopcock. The flush device, also known as the continuous-flush device, allows a flow rate of 1-5 ml/hr (usual rate is 3 ml/hr) to maintain patency of the system. Turn each stopcock on to the patient and on to the transducer.

   c. Place the flush solution in the pressure bag and pressurize it to 300 mm Hg. This step is not performed before step 3, because the increased pressure causes rapid flushing and increased turbulence, which may entrap air bubbles in the system and cause a damped waveform.

3. Attach the transducer cable(s) to the transducer(s) and monitor.

4. Level the transducer(s). Inaccurate pressure readings may occur if the transducer is placed incorrectly. If the transducer is above the level of the right atrium (RA), the pressure reading will be falsely low. If the transducer is below the level of the RA, the pressure reading will be falsely elevated. To prevent inaccurate pressure readings, level before and after the pressure system is attached to the patient, any change in bed height, any significant change in the waveforms and their values, whenever the system is disconnected, and at the beginning of each shift. Using a level to guide placement, secure the transducer to the pole, so that the stopcock at the air-fluid interface (the same stopcock that is used to open the system to atmospheric pressure) is at the level of the phlebostatic axis.

5. Zero balance the transducer. Zero balancing the system to the atmospheric pressure negates the effects of the atmospheric pressure. To prevent erroneous pressure readings, zero the system before and after the pressure system is attached to the patient, with any significant change in the waveforms and the values, whenever the system is disconnected, and at the beginning of each shift. To zero, turn the stopcock next to the transducer off to the patient and open to air (this is known as the air-fluid interface) and remove the nonvented cap. Zero the monitor according to the manufacturer's directions. Once the monitor is zeroed, flush the open stopcock port, clean it with alcohol, and replace the nonvented cap. Turn the stopcock on to the patient and on to the transducer. Some monitors may also need to be calibrated; if this is the case, do so according to the manufacturer's directions.

6. Place the sterile sheath over the catheter before testing the balloon. This protects the balloon from damage during placement of the sheath. The sheath allows the catheter to be repositioned and may prevent contamination of the PA catheter.

7. Check the catheter balloon for leaks by attaching the inflation syringe to the balloon port and inflating it to the recommended inflation volume, usually 0.8 to 1.5 ml of air. The balloon should inflate symmetrically and have no air leaks (i.e., stay inflated). If a right-to-left shunt is suspected, extra caution is warranted to prevent an air embolism. In this instance, the inflated balloon may be tested for an air leak by placing it into a basin of sterile water and looking for air bubbles.

8. Connect the proximal and distal lumens of the catheter to the pressure tubing and flush the catheter to remove the air.

9. Don sterile gowns, masks, and gloves.

10. *Cleanse the insertion site with an antiseptic solution.
11. *Infiltrate the insertion site with local anesthetic.
12. *Cannulate the vein by using the technique required for that particular insertion site, and insert the introducer (see Procedures 62 through 65). Attach IV fluid and tubing to the side port of the introducer, if present.
13. *Advance the catheter through the introducer about 15 to 20 cm until it is in the RA, where the RA waveform can be seen (Figure 89-3). Inflate the balloon at this point. Advance the catheter through the RV and into the PA, which is identified by the development of a dicrotic notch (see Figure 89-3). Continue to advance the catheter to a distal branch of the PA, as evidenced by the PCOP or PCWP waveform.
14. Monitor and record the distal lumen waveform during insertion. Keep the physician informed of the catheter's location in the heart, and document the pressures in each location. Table 89-1 lists normal adult pressures.
15. After the PAOP is measured, take the syringe off the balloon port to allow the balloon to deflate passively, and position the stopcock so that the balloon cannot be inflated accidentally. The balloon must be deflated so that it does not obstruct the distal blood flow and cause a pulmonary infarct.
16. Observe the ECG tracing for arrhythmias during the insertion. Premature ventricular contractions (PVCs) and ventricular tachycardia are frequently observed as the catheter passes through the RA to the right ventricle (RV). These usually resolve if the catheter is withdrawn or when it has passed through the RV.
17. *Suture the introducer in place and document the number of centimeters that the catheter is inserted at the level of the introducer. The catheter is marked with a thin black line for each 10 cm, and there is a thick black line for every 50 cm.
18. Obtain a chest radiograph to check the catheter placement and to rule out a pneumothorax. If the catheter needs to be repositioned, manipulate it within the sterile sleeve and recheck the placement with a radiograph.
19. To ensure accurate and consistent pressure readings:
    a. Level and zero the transducers as outlined above (steps 4 and 5).
    b. The pressure readings may be taken in the supine position with the head of the bed positioned from 0 to 45 degrees (Lynn-McHale & Preuss, 2001). The air-fluid interface in the transducer must remain level with the phlebostatic axis if the position is changed.
    c. Take the readings at end expiration when the intrapleural and atmospheric pressures are about the same. This provides a more consistent and accurate reading.
    d. The dynamic response is used to ensure that the monitoring system is accurately reproducing the patient's pressure signal at the monitor. This is achieved by evaluating the square wave. With the pressure bag inflated to 300 mm Hg, activate the fast flush quickly. If the system is optimally damped, the resulting waveform exceeds the upper limits of the scope, followed by a negative deflection and a small overshoot.

---

*Indicates portions of the procedure usually performed by a physician or an advanced practice nurse.

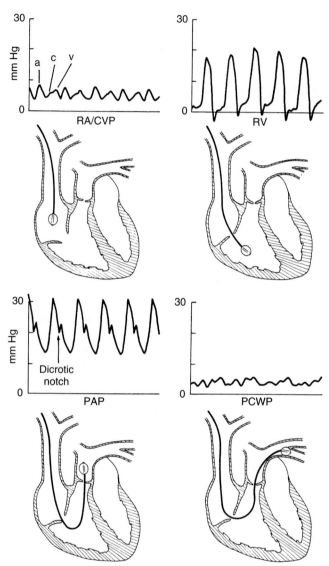

FIGURE 89-3 Right-sided heart pressures and waveforms. Pulmonary artery pressures and waveforms. (Courtesy Abbott Critical Care Systems, Morgan Hills, CA.)

TABLE 89-1
NORMAL ADULT PRESSURES

Parameter	Normal Adult Range
Cardiac index	2.5-4.2 L/min/m^2
Cardiac output	4-8 L/min
Mixed venous oxygen	60%-75%
Pulmonary artery pressure	15-30/6-12 mm Hg
Pulmonary artery occlusive pressure	Mean 4-12 mm Hg
Right atrium pressure	Mean 0-8 mm Hg
Right ventricle pressure	25–30/0-8 mm Hg
Systemic vascular resistance	770-1500 dyne/sec/cm^{-5}

Data from Darovic, G. O. (2004). *Handbook of hemodynamic monitoring* (2nd ed.). Philadelphia: Saunders.

It then returns to the patient's pressure waveform (see Procedure 88, Figure 88-5, *A*).

e. The system is overdamped if the fast flush results in a waveform that does not exceed the upper limits of the scope, followed by a slow return to the baseline (see Procedure 88, Figure 88-5, *B*). This gives a false-low systolic pressure. The most common cause is a stopcock or inadequate pressure on the system, allowing the blood to back up.

f. The system is underdamped if the fast flush results in a waveform that goes above and below the limits of the scope, with several more positive and negative deflections occurring before returning to baseline. If the system is underdamped, it gives falsely elevated systolic values. This can be due to excessive catheter length, fast heart rate, or high pressures that cause a "ringing" in the system (see Procedure 88, Figure 88-5, *C*). Commercial devices that attach to the pressure system are available to assist in controlling underdamping.

20. Maintain a continuous display of all pressure tracings. This allows for early detection of hemodynamic changes in the patients or catheter malposition. Digital readings of PAOP reflect the mean pressure.

21. Connect the thermistor connector to the cardiac output computer to obtain cardiac output by the thermodilution method. Inject a bolus of cold or room-temperature fluid per institutional protocol into the RA through the proximal port of the catheter. The temperature change in the blood, when sensed by the thermistor over a period of time, gives the cardiac output in liters per minute. The volume and temperature of the injectate and the number of injections are according to institutional protocol.

22. Measurements of mixed venous blood may be performed by continuous monitoring with an oximetric, fiberoptic catheter or by sampling the blood from the distal port of the catheter. To obtain a mixed venous sample, aspirate 2.5 times the dead space (approximately 3 ml) from the distal lumen of the catheter to clear the lumen of the flush solution.

Attach an arterial blood-gas syringe to the catheter and obtain the sample. Slow aspiration is imperative while the lumen is cleared and while the sample is obtained to avoid mixing the mixed venous blood sample with oxygenated blood from the pulmonary circulation. Flush the lumen after sampling to clear the catheter of blood and to prevent clotting of the lumen.

AGE-SPECIFIC CONSIDERATIONS

1. For children who weigh less than less than 20 kg, use a 5-Fr, 70 cm catheter (6 Fr introducer); for children weighing 20 kg or more, use a 7- to 7.5-Fr, 110 cm catheter (7.5 or 8 Fr introducer) respectively (Graves, 2007). In very small children, the injectate port of the catheter may not be in the RA, and a shorter catheter may be needed.
2. The volume of air need to inflate the balloon varies with catheter size, most manufacturers supply a syringe that limits it to the correct amount. The 5-Fr catheter requires 0.5 ml of air and the 7-Fr and 7.5-Fr catheters require 1.5 ml of air (Graves, 2007).
3. A PA catheter may be indicated in a pediatric patient who has sepsis or who is in shock that does not respond to fluid therapy and inotropic support, as well as to monitor the effects of a new drug that may cause cardiovascular instability. A PA catheter may be indicated in a child with pulmonary hypertension, but the risk of PA rupture must be weighed against the benefit of the information gathered.
4. Caution should be used in children with intracardiac shunting lesions, tricuspid or pulmonary valve dysfunction, ventricular arrhythmias that could be exacerbated by PA placement, RV to PA discontinuity or placement of an RV to PA conduit to establish continuity (Graves, 2007).
5. Normal resting values in children are not the same as those in adults, and they are dependent on the age of the child.
6. The small lumens in the 5-Fr catheter are easily occluded by fibrin, making it imperative to maintain a continuous flush system at all times.
7. Most complications related to the use of a PA catheter in children are similar to those in adults but the risk of thrombosis and infection appear to be higher (Darovic, 2002).

COMPLICATIONS

1. A pneumothorax may result from internal jugular or subclavian insertion.
2. A hemothorax or hematoma may result from vascular damage. If a hematoma appears on one side of the neck, observe the patient for airway obstruction and do not attempt cannulation on the opposite side of the neck.
3. An air embolism may occur during the time of insertion or if there is a loose connection anywhere in the system.
4. Cardiac arrhythmias may occur (as previously discussed). In a patient with a preexisting left bundle-branch block, irritation of the right bundle branch may result in right bundle-branch block and lead to complete heart block. If the waveforms and pressure values indicate that the catheter has migrated back into the RV, inflate the balloon to cushion the tip of the catheter. This protects the RV from irritation by the catheter resulting in arrhythmias. Notify the physician, who may advance the catheter or order that it be pulled back into the RA.

5. PA perforation may occur during insertion of the catheter if it is advanced too far with an underinflated balloon or if the balloon is overinflated during PAOP measurement. Inflate the balloon slowly and stop when the PAOP waveform appears. Use caution in patients with high PA pressures when obtaining PAOP, because the high pressures may drive the PA catheter into the smaller vessels, resulting in infarction and/or hemorrhage.

6. Pulmonary infarction may result from frequent or prolonged PAOP measurements or migration of the catheter. The balloon should not be inflated for longer than three cycles, the time it takes to obtain the measurement. If the waveforms and pressure values indicate that the catheter had migrated into "wedge" position, reposition the patient and/or have the patient cough. If the catheter is still wedged, make sure the balloon is deflated and pull the catheter back to the PA position. Notify the physician. Do not flush the wedged PA catheter as this could lead to rupture of the PA.

7. Damage to the intracardiac structures may occur if the balloon is withdrawn while inflated.

8. Cardiac tamponade may occur if the RA or RV is perforated.

9. The balloon may rupture if there have been multiple inflations or if the catheter has been in place for a prolonged period of time. If the balloon ruptures, withdraw the air until blood is seen in the syringe and then close off the port. The catheter should be removed because the pieces of the ruptured balloon may come free and produce an embolus. In a patient with a right-to-left shunt, there is a greater chance for an air embolism to occur if the balloon ruptures. Use carbon dioxide to inflate the balloon in this situation because carbon dioxide is easily dispersed in the blood if the balloon should rupture (Hazinski, 2002). If an air embolism is suspected, place the patient in the left lateral Trendelenburg position, have the patient perform the Valsalva maneuver, and administer high-flow oxygen.

10. Infection or sepsis may occur in a catheter left in for a prolonged period of time.

11. Thrombus formation may occur on the catheter tip or around the catheter and may lead to venous occlusion.

12. Endocarditis may occur during a prolonged PA catheter insertion.

13. Knotting or coiling of the catheter may occur. This is more frequent with the small-sized catheters or during a prolonged insertion time.

14. Neurovascular compromise may occur from a catheter inserted femorally or peripherally. Monitor the peripheral pulses.

15. Heparin-induced thrombocytopenia may result from continuous heparin infusion. Non-heparinized PA catheters are available.

16. Perforation of pulmonary or tricuspid valve (Graves, 2007).

PATIENT TEACHING

1. Request assistance for position changes so that the catheter is not displaced.
2. Report any tubing disconnections or dampness around the site immediately.

REFERENCES

Daily, E. K., & Schroeder, J. S. (1994). *Techniques in bedside hemodynamic monitoring* (5th ed.). St Louis: Mosby.

Darovic, G. O. (2002). *Hemodynamic monitoring* (3rd ed.). Philadelphia: Saunders.

Darovic, G. O. (2004). *Handbook of hemodynamic monitoring* (2nd ed.). Philadelphia: Saunders.

Graves, D. (2007). Flow-directed pulmonary artery catheter: Insertion, assist. In J. T. Verger, & R. M. Lebet (Eds.), *AACN procedure manual for acute and critical pediatric care* (pp. 433-442). Philadelphia: Saunders.

Hazinski, M. F. (2002). Pediatric evaluation and monitoring considerations. In G. O. Darovic (Ed.), *Hemodynamic monitoring: Invasive and noninvasive clinical applications* (3rd ed.). Philadelphia: Saunders.

Lynn-McHale, D. J., & Preuss, T. (2001). Pulmonary artery catheter insertion (assist) and pressure monitoring. In D. J. Lynn-McHale & K. K. Carlson (Eds.), *AACN procedure manual for critical care* (4th ed., pp. 439-456). Philadelphia: Saunders.

Neurologic Procedures

Positioning the Patient with Increased Intracranial Pressure

Ruth L. Schaffler, RN, PhD, ARNP, CEN

OVERVIEW

Positioning the patient properly is important to minimize increased intracranial pressure (ICP) in the presence of a head injury, brain lesion, stroke, or other neurologic disorder. Normal ICP is 0 to 10 mm Hg. ICP above 15 mm Hg is elevated; a level above 20 mm Hg is considered intracranial hypertension; and levels above 25 mm Hg should be avoided. Proper positioning facilitates cerebrospinal fluid (CSF) and venous drainage from the head via jugular veins and the vertebral venous plexi, thus reducing ICP (Fan, 2004; McLeod, 2004; Price, Collins, & Gallagher, 2003).

Head elevation reduces ICP; however, this practice has been challenged. Some investigators argue that although head elevation lowers ICP, it also contributes to decreased cerebral perfusion pressure (CPP); others rationalize that a horizontal position increases cerebral blood flow (CBF) (Fan, 2004). Data suggest a moderate approach of head elevation between 15 and 30 degrees reduces ICP significantly without impairing CPP (Fan, 2004). Adequate blood flow to the brain is dependent on the CPP, which is the difference between the systemic mean arterial pressure (MAP) and the ICP: CPP = MAP − ICP. Normal MAP levels range from 80 to 100 mm Hg. Autoregulation keeps the cerebral blood flow stable when CPP is between 50 and 150 mm Hg. When CPP decreases, autoregulation may be lost and cerebral blood flow will decrease. In the presence of a traumatic brain injury, a CPP of 50-70 mm Hg is recommended for adult patients (Brain Trauma Foundation, 2007). Elevating the head of the bed more than 40 degrees may contribute to postural hypotension and decreased cerebral perfusion (McLeod, 2004).

INDICATIONS

1. To minimize increased ICP in the presence of a head injury, a brain lesion, or other neurologic disorders
2. To facilitate venous drainage from the head

CONTRAINDICATIONS AND CAUTIONS

1. Avoid the prone and Trendelenburg positions. Some controversy exists as to whether the patient should be placed in a flat position, and ICP monitoring

may be indicated. Types of monitoring devices available may include bolts or screws, cannulas, and fiberoptic probes) (see Procedure 92).

2. Head elevation is commonly used to reduce ICP; however, research has challenged this practice. Although head elevation lowers ICP, it also contributes to decreased CPP; a horizontal position increases CPP. A moderate approach of head elevation between 15 and 30 degrees can reduce ICP significantly without impairing CPP. Consult with the physician to determine if head elevation is indicated.

3. When head elevation must be interrupted, restore it promptly—that is, during transport after computed tomography (CT) scan or after endotracheal intubation (two common reasons the patient may be flat for a procedure).

4. Elevating the head of the bed more than 40 degrees may contribute to postural hypotension and decreased cerebral perfusion.

5. Minimize noxious stimuli. Warn the patient before you touch him or her, explain the procedures, and use gentle movements. Do not jar the bed, make loud noises, or use bright lights.

6. Plan turning or positioning activities separately from other nursing interventions. Allow at least 15 minutes between each activity to avoid a cumulative effect of ICP increases.

7. Head elevation is contraindicated in hypotensive patients because it further compromises CPP.

8. Spinal alignment should be maintained until the patient's spine has been cleared of fracture per institutional protocol.

9. Plan for cervical CT scan when brain CT is being done. Prompt clearance of the cervical spine permits earlier removal of boards and collars, which impede access and cause skin pressure problems.

PATIENT PREPARATION

1. Place the patient in a supine position.
2. Maintain the head in a neutral position without flexion, extension, or rotation.
   a. If a cervical collar is used, be sure that it does not obstruct venous return through the jugular veins.
   b. Towel rolls or foam blocks can be used to support the head if necessary.
3. The patient's head should remain in a neutral position without rotation to the left or right, flexion, or extension of the neck.

EQUIPMENT

Stretcher or hospital bed
Towel rolls or foam blocks (optional)
Cervical collar (optional)

PROCEDURAL STEPS

1. Place the bed or stretcher in the prescribed position.
2. Align the torso and the lower extremities. Extreme hip flexion may increase intraabdominal pressure, which can also increase ICP. Legs should be flexed no more than 90 degrees at the hip.
3. A padded footboard at the end of the stretcher or bed can prevent the patient from sliding or shifting positions when the head of the bed is elevated (Figure 90-1).

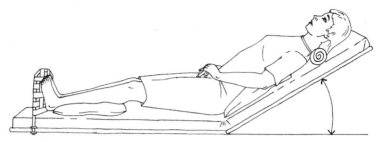

FIGURE 90-1 Head of the bed elevated to 30 degrees.

4. Padded side rails may be needed for seizure precautions.
5. Reposition the patient every 2 hours. Logroll the patient while maintaining head and neck alignment. Ensure the legs are flexed no more than 90 degrees at the hip while the patient is side-lying. Movement of the patient should be slow and purposeful (Kerr & Crago, 2004).
6. If the patient must remain on a backboard or cannot flex at the hips, use a reverse Trendelenburg position at a 15-degree angle to elevate the patient's head (Figure 90-2). Make sure the board cannot slide off the foot of the stretcher or bed. Backboards are rescue and transport devices not suited for long-term care. Earliest possible safe removal is necessary and should have priority in planning care.

AGE-SPECIFIC CONSIDERATIONS
Pediatrics
1. Children are predisposed to head trauma because their head-to-body ratio is greater, their brains are less myelinated, and their cranial bones are thinner than in adults (Brain Trauma Foundation, 2003). Emergency personnel must be aware of the potential for intracranial complications when assessing and managing children with head trauma.
2. The use of restraints and immobilization devices to maintain body position may compound the patient's agitation and lead to increased ICP, especially in young children.
3. If using the Glasgow Coma Scale for neurologic assessment of children under the age of 2 years, a full verbal score can be assigned if the child cries after stimulation (Brain Trauma Foundation, 2003).
4. A CPP of 40 mm Hg or higher is recommended in children with traumatic brain injury (Brain Trauma Foundation, 2003).

Geriatrics
1. Age-related physiologic changes result in a decline in function of all organ systems and may predispose the elderly to trauma.
2. Undertriage has been reported in the literature (Scheetz, 2005). Vital signs, used as a measure of physiologic response to injury, may be altered due to underlying disease or the use of certain medications. Confusion, which is used as a measure of cerebral perfusion, may be mistaken for dementia.
3. Cognitive impairment may be associated with altered function or reduced complaints of pain.

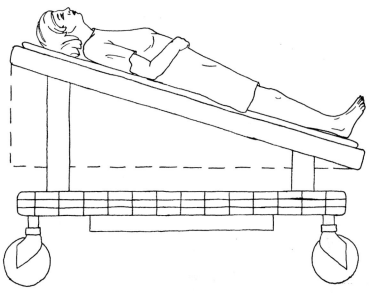

FIGURE 90-2 Reverse Trendelenburg position.

COMPLICATIONS

1. Neck flexion or extension, or rotation of the head to the left or right, increases ICP by obstructing venous outflow.
2. Abnormal posturing may be stimulated by the position of the head in relation to gravity or by excessive noxious stimuli.
3. Pooling of secretions or skin breakdown may occur if the patient is not turned every 2 hours. Consider a nasopharyngeal airway as a protective conduit for pharyngeal suctioning to minimize noxious stimuli. Presence of a basilar skull fracture may alter the airway plan, however.
4. Turn and move the patient gently. Pain or agitation can increase ICP.

PATIENT TEACHING

1. Conscious patients should report increasing headache, nausea, or visual disturbances.
2. Explain that positioning is used along with other interventions to control the intracranial pressure. The position is to be changed every 2 hours.
3. Family members should be advised not to give the patient additional fluids or to change the position of the bed without asking the nurse.

REFERENCES

Brain Trauma Foundation. (2000). *Management and prognosis of severe traumatic brain injury.* Retrieved December 6, 2006, from www2.braintrauma.org/guidelines

Brain Trauma Foundation. (2003). *Guidelines for the acute medical management of severe traumatic brain injury in infants, children, and adolescents.* Retrieved December 8, 2006, from www2.braintrauma.org/guidelines

Brain Trauma Foundation. (2007). *Guidelines for the management of severe traumatic brain injury*. Retrieved July 26, 2007 from www2.braintrauma.org/guidelines

Fan, J. (2004). Effect of backrest position on intracranial pressure and cerebral perfusion pressure in individuals with brain injury: A systematic review. *Journal of Neuroscience Nursing, 36*(5), 278-288.

Kerr, M., & Crago, E. (2004). Acute intracranial problems. In S. Lewis, M. Heitkemper, & S. Dirksen (Eds.), *Medical-surgical nursing: Assessment and management of clinical problems* (pp. 1491-1524). St Louis: Mosby.

McLeod, A. (2004). Traumatic injuries to the head and spine 2: Nursing considerations. *British Journal of Nursing, 13*(17), 1041-1049.

Price, A., Collins, T., & Gallagher, A. (2003). Nursing care of the acute head injury: A review of the evidence. *Nursing in Critical Care, 8*(3), 126-133.

Scheetz, L. (2005). Relationship of age, injury severity, injury type, comorbid conditions, level of care, and survival among older motor vehicle trauma patients. *Research in Nursing & Health, 28*, 198-209.

PROCEDURE 91

Lumbar Puncture

June F. Stacey, RN, BSN, CEN

Lumbar puncture is also known as *LP*, *spinal tap*, or *spinal puncture.*

INDICATIONS

1. To assist in the diagnosis of meningitis or encephalitis in febrile patients exhibiting an acute alteration in mental status.
2. As part of fever work-up in a febrile infant less than 3 months old without any obvious source of infection.
3. To assist in the diagnosis of subarachnoid hemorrhage (SAH). If SAH is highly suspected and computed tomography (CT) of the head results are negative, LP may be required for diagnosis.
4. To instill medication, blood, or radiopaque contrast material into the subarachnoid space for the diagnosis or treatment of central nervous system (CNS) disorders.
5. To measure cerebrospinal fluid (CSF) pressure.
6. To assist with the diagnosis acute or chronic demyelinating diseases (e.g., Guillain-Barré, multiple sclerosis, transverse myelitis), malignancies (e.g., meningeal carcinomatosis), or unexplained neurologic disorders when the CT scan is negative (e.g., altered level of consciouness, polyneuropathy) (German & O'Brien, 2003).

CONTRAINDICATIONS AND CAUTIONS

1. If a LP is performed in the presence of elevated intracranial pressure, supratentorial or foramen magnum herniation may occur due to changes in the pressure gradient between the supratentorial and lumbar spaces when CSF is removed. Herniation may lead to serious injury or death. A computed tomography (CT) scan should precede the LP in a patient with a history of a progressive deterioration of mental status, a worsening headache, localizing neurologic signs, or papilledema (Euerle, 2004).
2. Positioning patients with excessive neck flexion may cause respiratory compromise. The risk is higher in sedated patients and children (due to their increased neck flexibility and shorter, narrower airways). In these populations, monitor respiratory status with pulse oximetry and/or end-tidal CO_2 (see Procedures 21 and 24). End-tidal CO_2 via side-stream capnography will provide earlier warning of hypoventilation or airway compromise than pulse oximetry.
3. Performing a LP in an anticoagulated or thrombocytopenic patient may result in a spinal epidural hematoma.
4. A superficial infection at the puncture site could cause meningitis or an epidural or subdural empyema. LP through infected tissue is contraindicated.

EQUIPMENT

Sterile drape and towels

Gauze dressings

21- to 25-G, 2.5- to 3-in spinal needle with stylet (longer needles may be necessary for obese patients). Atraumatic spinal needles are preferred (see Figure 91-1)

1% lidocaine with epinephrine

25-G, ⅝-in needle and 21- or 22-G, ½- and 1-in needles for anesthetic infiltration

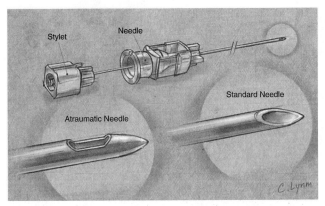

FIGURE 91-1 Two types of lumbar puncture needles are available—the atraumatic (Sprotte or Pajunk) needle and the standard (Quinke) needle. The atraumatic needle descreases the incidence of post-procedure headache. (From Straus, S., Thorpe, K., & Holroyd-LeDuc, J. [2006]. How do I perform a lumbar puncture and analyze the results to diagnose bacterial meningitis? *JAMA, 296,* 2016.)

3- to 5-ml syringe
Manometer with three-way stopcock (extension tubing optional)
Four collection tubes
Adhesive gauze patch
Antiseptic solution
(Preassembled kits containing all or some of these supplies are available.)

PATIENT PREPARATION

1. Obtain a blood glucose level to rule out symptomatic hypoglycemia (neuro-glycopenia) and as a baseline to compare with CSF glucose level.
2. Assist the patient into a lateral decubitus position, with the shoulders and pelvis perpendicular to the stretcher. The patient should flex or curl the back and maintain this position to separate the lumbar spine segments (Figure 91-2). It may help to provide a small pillow for the head. Infants, children, and uncooperative adults may require assistance to maintain this position.
3. If the patient has bony deformities or is obese, a sitting position with head and arms resting over a padded bedside table may help to identify landmarks. This position can be maintained during the LP. The initial opening pressure measurement is not valid in the sitting position due to the vertical column of CSF in the spinal canal. Patients with bony deformities may need fluoroscopic guidance for the puncture.
4. When time allows, a topical anesthetic, such as EMLA, may be used over the insertion site and the next lower level as an alternate site (see Procedure 135).

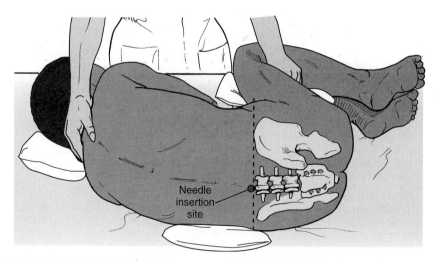

Needle
insertion
site

FIGURE 91-2 Positioning for lumbar puncture. Flexing the patient's back opens up the spaces between the vertebrae. The needle is inserted between the third and fourth lumbar vertebrae. (From Black, J., & Hawks, J. [2005]. *Medical-surgical nursing* [7th ed., p. 2044]. Philadelphia: Saunders.)

PROCEDURAL STEPS

1. *Palpate the back to identify the spinous process levels. The levels of L3-4, L4-5, or L5-S1 can be used safely, because they avoid the spinal cord, which ends at the level of L2-3. The posterior iliac crest is even with L3-4. The site may be marked with an indentation from a fingernail or a skin marker.

2. *Cleanse the back in a circular fashion with an antiseptic solution.

3. *Attach the sterile drape to the patient's back with the adhesive strips.

4. *Infiltrate the skin and the subcutaneous tissue with the anesthetic solution via the 25-gauge needle. Infiltrate the interspinous spaces with the anesthetic solution at the intended puncture site via the 22-gauge needle.

5. *Identify the intended puncture site and insert the spinal needle at the midline with the bevel parallel to the axis of the spine. The needle is often angled slightly cephalad. The patient will feel pressure but should not feel pain.

6. *A pop may be felt once the needle passes the ligamentum flavum, and it is advisable at this point to remove the stylet and to check for the CSF every 2 mm or so to avoid passing through the subarachnoid space into the ventral epidural space. If the epidural space is entered, the patient may feel pain from the puncture of a nerve root or there may be bleeding from puncture of the plexus of veins that forms a ring around the spinal cord. This is termed a traumatic tap, but it is not a patricularly dangerous problem in a patient with normal coagulation (Euerle, 2004).

7. *Once CSF is noted at the hub of the needle, attach the manometer and the three-way stopcock to measure CSF opening pressure. Extension tubing may be used between the needle and the manometer to allow greater flexibility, but the manometer should be placed so that the zero mark is at the level of the hub of the spinal needle. The patient should be asked to relax and may extend the legs as this does not meaningfully affect the opening pressure reading (Euerle, 2004). Have the patient breathe quietly, and read the pressure when it comes to a rest and fluctuates only slightly with each breath. Normal CSF pressure is 50 to 200 mm H_2O (German & O'Brien, 2003).

8. *Collect CSF specimens in the four collection tubes. Fluid from the manometer may be drained into the first tube. Usually, 1 to 2 ml is placed in each tube. Each institution determines which tests will be performed on the different tubes. Generally, if the fluid in the first tube is bloody, it is discarded or held. Cell counts with differential, protein, and glucose are done on tube 2 or 3. Gram stain with culture and sensitivity is done on tube 3 or 4 in order to lessen the chance of skin contamination. Viral testing, cytology or other specialized studies may be done on tube 4 as indicated. If a traumatic tap is suspected, a comparison cell count may also be done on tube 4. The CSF specimens should be transported to the laboratory

---

*Indicates portions of the procedure usually performed by a physician or an advanced practice nurse.

TABLE 91-1

BASIC DIFFERENTIATION OF CEREBROSPINAL FLUID FINDINGS IN VIRAL AND BACTERIAL MENINGITIS

	Viral	Bacterial
WBC	Elevated, lymphocytes predominant	Very high, neutrophils predominant
Protein	Normal-to-mild increase	High
Glucose	Usually normal	Low, less than 60% of serum glucose

WBC, White blood cell.

promptly to prevent cell lysis, which may cause false results (Chernecky & Berger, 2004).

Normal CSF findings include the following (German & O'Brien, 2003):

- Opening pressure: 50 to 200 mm H_2O
- Clear, colorless fluid
- White blood cell count: less than 5/mm^3 with no neutrophils
- Total protein: 15 to 45 mg/dl (adults). Numerous processes elevate the protein level, including blood in the CSF, but levels above 500 mg/dl are uncommon and usually indicate meningitis, subarachnoid bleeding, or spinal tumor (Euerle, 2004).
- Glucose is normally 60% to 70% of the blood glucose level; a decreased level may implicate disease of the CNS and is a useful indicator in differentiating viral from bacterial meningitis (Table 91-1).

9. *Reinsert the stylet and slowly remove the spinal needle. Apply pressure to the site with a gauze pad, and then apply the adhesive gauze pad.

10. The patient should remain flat for at least 2 hours. Prone positioning may help reduce CSF leakage and thereby decrease the likelihood of post-LP headache.

11. Observe the patient for any changes in the level of consciousness (in case of worsening meningitis or possible herniation), altered motor or sensory status in the lower extremities, bladder dysfunction (spinal subdural hematoma), or complaints of headache.

AGE-SPECIFIC CONSIDERATIONS

1. Use 1.5-inch spinal needle for infants and toddlers. A 3.5-inch spinal needle can be used for children older than age 12 (German & O'Brien, 2003).

2. When positioning children, avoid excessive neck flexion, because this may occlude the airway and lead to respiratory compromise or arrest. A nurse should be in the room with the infant or toddler during the procedure, and oxygen saturation and/or end-tidal CO_2 should be monitored. Excessive neck flexion may also impede CSF return.

---

*Indicates portions of the procedure usually performed by a physician or an advanced practice nurse.

3. The infant may be placed in the upright position with the thighs against the abdomen and the neck flexed forward. The assistant should hold an arm and leg with each hand for stabilization (ENA, 2004).
4. Struggling, agitatation, or crying may falsely elevate CSF pressures and sedation should be considered. The upper limit of normal is 50 mm H_2O in neonates and 85 mm H_2O in infants and young children (Euerle, 2004).
5. Avoid ketamine because it can increase intracranial pressure (Zorc, 2001) and random movements.

COMPLICATIONS

1. To differentiate between a traumatic tap and an SAH, compare the cell count of the first tube with that of the last tube. If there is a decrease in the number of red blood cells, it is likely a traumatic tap rather than an SAH. Xanthochromia is a yellow-orange discoloration of the CSF, which typically indicates an SAH of several hours' duration and can help differentiate prior bleeding from a traumatic tap (Euerle, 2004).
2. A spinal subdural hematoma may occur in thrombocytopenic patients or in elderly patients whose CSF was removed too rapidly or in too large a volume.
3. Headache, thought to be caused by leakage of fluid through the dural puncture site, is the most common complication following LP and occurs in 5% to 40% of patients. A smaller-diameter needle will decrease the chance of post-procedure headache due to smaller puncture hole in the dura. A blood patch (injection of autologous blood into the epidural space) is a highly successful treatment for prolonged postprocedural headaches (Euerle, 2004). Atraumatic spinal needles reduce the incidence of postprocedural headaches (Thomas, Jamieson, & Muir, 2000).
4. Although extremely rare, transtentorial or foramen magnum herniation may occur (Euerle, 2004).
5. A spinal epidural hematoma occurs rarely in anticoagulated patients.
6. In a dry tap, no CSF is obtained.
7. An infection is usually related to an inadequate aseptic technique or a puncture through irritated or infected tissue. A local infection, meningitis, or epidural or subdural empyema may result.

PATIENT TEACHING

1. Monitor temperature and report it if it is greater than 38.3° C (101° F).
2. Take an analgesic or a prescribed medication for headache. Report a severe or prolonged headache.
3. Remain flat for at least 2 hours after the procedure. A prone position may help prevent a spinal headache.
4. Increase fluid intake to help replace CSF and prevent spinal headache.

REFERENCES

Chernecky, C., & Berger, B. (2004). *Laboratory tests and diagnostic procedures* (4th ed.). St Louis: Saunders.

Emergency Nurses Association (ENA). (2004). *Emergency nursing pediatric course* (3rd ed.). Des Plaines IL: Author.

Euerle, B. (2004). Spinal puncture and cerebrospinal fluid examination. In J. R. Roberts, & J. R. Hedges (Eds.), *Clinical procedures in emergency medicine* (4th ed., pp. 1197-1222). Philadelphia: Saunders.

German, J. O., & O'Brien, J. O. (2003). Lumbar puncture. In J. L. Pfenninger, & G. C. Fowler (Eds.), *Procedures for primary care* (2nd ed., pp. 1649-1653). St Louis: Mosby.

Thomas, S. R., Jamieson, D., & Muir, K. (2000). Randomized controlled trial of atraumatic versus standard needles for diagnostic lumbar puncture. *British Medical Journal, 321,* 986-990.

Zorc, J. J. (2001). Lumbar puncture. In J. G. Goepp, & M. A. Hostetler (Eds.), *Procedures for primary care pediatricians* (pp. 43-47). St Louis: Mosby.

PROCEDURE 92

Intracranial Pressure Monitoring

Reneé Semonin Holleran, RN, PhD, CEN, CCRN, CFRN, CTRN, FAEN

Intracranial pressure (ICP) monitoring can be accomplished through the use of bolts and intraventricular catheters.

INDICATIONS

To measure ICP, which allows for calculation of cerebral perfusion pressure (CPP). CPP is an important indicator of cerebral blood flow. ICP monitoring may be useful in patients with the following conditions (American Association of Neurological Surgeons, 2000; Preuss, 2005; Salim & Khoo, 2002):

1. Severe head injury (Glasgow Coma Scale score of 7 or less) in patients who are hemodynamically unstable and computed tomography (CT) cannot be obtained because of prolonged resuscitative or operative interventions

2. Severe head injury with normal CT scan in the presence of two or more of the following: age over 40 years, unilateral or bilateral motor posturing, systolic blood pressure less than 90 mm Hg

3. Severe head injury in patients in whom CT/magnetic resonance imaging (MRI) demonstrates diffuse injury

4. Anoxic event that may contribute to secondary cerebral injury (e.g., near-drowning)

5. To monitor the effects of specific interventions (hyperventilation, diuresis) on the patient's ICP/CPP

CONTRAINDICATIONS AND CAUTIONS

1. Severe coagulopathy and chronic coagulopathy (hemophilia, von Willebrand disease) are absolute contraindications to ICP monitor insertion because of the high risk of intracranial hemorrhage (Salim & Khoo, 2002).
2. Relative contraindications include infection, open wounds of the scalp and skull near the planned insertion site, and immunosuppression. Small or effaced ventricles are a relative contraindication for ventriculostomy (Salim & Khoo, 2002).
3. The resuscitation process may make it difficult to set up and obtain accurate ICP readings, and other resuscitation priorities may preclude placement of an ICP monitoring device in the emergency department.
4. Kinked tubing, air bubbles, catheter movement, failure to properly zero the transducer, and loose connections can contribute to inaccurate readings.
5. An intraventricular catheter (IVC) can become occluded with blood or brain tissue and cease to function.
6. A fiberoptic or pressure-sensing ICP monitor is easily damaged and cannot be calibrated once inserted.

EQUIPMENT

Razor or hair clippers
Antiseptic solution
Sterile drapes and towels
No. 11 scalpel
Local anesthetic
10-ml syringe; 18-, 25-, and 27-G needles for local anesthesia (optional)
Twist drill
Nonbacteriostatic saline
3-ml syringe
Three-way stopcock and nonvented caps
Analgesics and sedatives as prescribed
ICP monitoring system options:
    Fiberoptic system requires a stand-alone monitor or microprocessor and a preamp connector cable to connect the microprocessor to the bed side monitor in addition to the CSF collection system
    Sensor system requires a microprocessor sensor cable and a monitoring cable to connect to the monitor at the bedside in addition to the CSF collection system
    Transducer and cable for specific monitoring system being used
Monitor, calibrated, with ICP monitoring setup
Suture, needle carrier, scissors
Topical antibiotic
Sterile occlusive dressing

PATIENT PREPARATION

1. A conscious patient requires sedation and/or analgesia for this procedure. At a minimum, the area of insertion should be anesthetized with a local anesthetic.

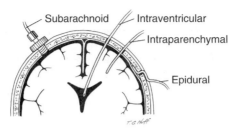

FIGURE 92-1 Sites for intracranial pressure monitoring. (From Youmans, J. R. [1996]. *Youmans' neurological surgery* [4th ed., p. 505]. Philadelphia: Saunders.)

2. Perform and document a baseline neurologic assessment, including the Glasgow Coma Scale score and motor and sensory responses. Calculate and record the patient's mean arterial pressure (MAP).

3. Consider using restraints to prevent the patient from dislodging the monitor (see Procedure 190).

4. Calibrate the monitoring equipment according to the manufacturer's recommendations.

5. Place the patient in a supine position.

6. Administer analgesia and sedation as prescribed.

7. *Cleanse the site with an antiseptic solution, shave or clip hair, and infiltrate the site with a local anesthetic. There are five common places that an ICP monitor may be placed inside of the head, as well as many access devices available (Figure 92-1). The location and type of device are determined by the neurosurgeon after consideration of the advantages and disadvantages of each (Table 92-1).

PROCEDURAL STEPS

1. *Incise down to the skull. Use a small twist drill to make a hole in the skull, aiming toward the ipsilateral medial canthus (see Procedure 93).
   Place the monitor as follows (Salim & Khoo, 2002):
   a. *Ventricular catheter: Penetrate the dura and insert the ventricular catheter with the stylet in place through the brain tissue until it is in the ventricle. Remove the stylet. Free flow of cerebrospinal fluid (CSF) confirms placement.
   b. *Subarachnoid bolt: Insert the bolt into the subarachnoid space.
   c. *Subdural monitor: Place the catheter or the fiberoptic monitor in the subdural space.
   d. *Epidural monitoring: Place the epidural sensor between the skull and the dura.
   e. *Intraparenchymal monitoring: Penetrate the dura and insert the sensor catheter into the brain tissue to a predetermined distance.

2. *Irrigate the wound gently to remove blood and bony debris.

---

*Indicates portions of the procedure usually performed by a physician.

TABLE 92-1

ADVANTAGES AND DISADVANTAGES OF DIFFERENT INTRACRANIAL MONITOR
LOCATIONS

Site	Advantages	Disadvantages
Epidural	Low infection risk Decreased risk of brain injury	Cannot drain CSF Readings may be inaccurate because it can become wedged against the skull Affected by fever Diaphragm can rupture
Subarachnoid	Easy and quick to insert Useful for patient with cerebral edema when the ventricles cannot be accessed	Cannot drain CSF May become occluded May dampen and give unreliable readings Brain tissue can herniate into the bolt
Intraventricular	Most likely to display whole-brain pressures Allows for drainage and sampling of CSF Accurate and reliable readings Contrast can be injected for studies	Highest risk of infection CSF drainage requires constant nursing monitoring Takes longer to insert and has more potential for injury to brain tissues More difficult to insert CSF will leak at the drainage site

CSF, Cerebrospinal fluid.
Data from Barker, E. [2002]. Intracranial pressure and monitoring. In E. Barker (Ed.), *Neuroscience nursing: A spectrum of care* (2nd ed., p. 393). St Louis: Mosby.

3. Attach the device to the calibrated monitoring system. Observe for an appropriate waveform (Figure 92-2). A ventricular drainage system requires that the sliding graduated-flow chamber be set at zero. The transducer is then aligned with a reference point at the anatomic level of the foramen of Monro. This is a point lateral to the canthus of the eye or the top of the ear (Figure 92-3). Consult with the neurosurgeon for specific positioning information. For fluid-coupled monitors, the transducer may be zeroed before or after insertion. Fiberoptic and sensor systems must be zeroed before insertion.

4. Once a good waveform is established, assist with wound closure and apply an antibiotic ointment and a sterile occlusive dressing.

5. Monitor and document the ICP.
   a. Document the initial ICP, quality of the waveform, and appearance of the cerebrospinal fluid. Normal ICP is 1 to 15 mm Hg (50 to 200 cm H_2O). However, like blood pressure, ICP is a dynamic, not static, number.
   b. Calculate the CPP (CPP = MAP − ICP). Normal CPP is greater than 60 to 70 mm Hg. The usual target CCP is 50-70 mm Hg in the brain-injured

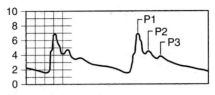

FIGURE 92-2 Normal intracranial pressure waveform at a rapid chart speed. The waveform should resemble an arterial blood pressure waveform. P1 is the percussion wave, P2 is the tidal wave, and P3 is the dicrotic wave. (From Youmans, J. R. [1996]. *Youmans' neurological surgery* [4th ed., p. 497]. Philadelphia: Saunders.)

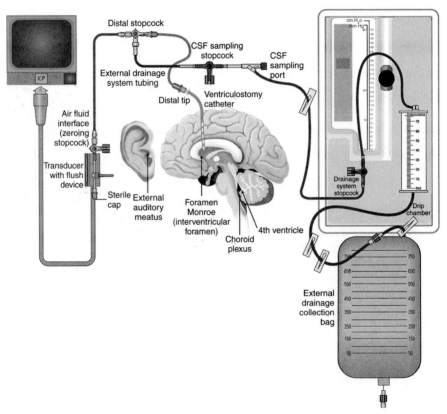

FIGURE 92-3 External ventricular drainage system for intracranial pressure monitoring and cerebral spinal fluid drainage. (Preuss, D. N. [2005]. Neurologic drainage and pressure monitoring systems. In D. J. Lynn-McHale Wiegand and K. K. Carlson [Eds.], *AACN procedure manual for critical care* [5th ed., p. 759]. St Louis: Mosby.)

patient (Brain Trauma Foundation, 2007). Consult with the neurosurgeon for patient-specific goals.

c. The ICP waveform should fluctuate with respirations and heartbeats.

AGE-SPECIFIC CONSIDERATIONS

1. Neonates and infants with open sutures may not benefit from ICP monitoring because of their thin and pliable skulls (Bergsneider & Becker, 1995).
2. In infants and small children, the occipital or coronal approach is recommended because of their open sutures, fontanelles, and thin skull bones (Montague, 1990).
3. In children with an internal shunt, a shunt reservoir can be used to measure ICP as well as drain cerebrospinal fluid (Montague, 1990).
4. Normal ICP varies with age as follows:
   - Newborns, 0.7 to 1.5 mm Hg
   - Infants, 1.5 to 6 mm Hg
   - Children, 3 to 7.5 mm Hg (Vernon-Levett, 2001).

COMPLICATIONS

1. Iatrogenic epidural hematoma (Salim & Khoo, 2002).
2. Occlusion of a ventricular catheter by blood or brain tissue can occur. If the blockage is distal to a port that can be used for flushing, flush the system away from the patient and toward the drainage bag. If the blockage is proximal to the drainage port, notify the physician.
3. If a break in the sterile system occurs, notify the physician.
4. If a dampened waveform appears, check for the presence of air bubbles or loose connections. Flush the system with solution in the direction away from the patient and toward the drainage bag. Check that all connections are intact.
5. If the ICP waveform is lost or the catheter is not draining, check that all equipment is functioning. Recalibrate the monitor. If the waveform is still inadequate, notify the physician.
6. Monitor for signs and symptoms of infection, including fever, redness, or drainage at the insertion site; headache; nuchal rigidity; or seizures.

PATIENT TEACHING

1. Remain in a supine position so the monitor functions accurately. Do not touch or manipulate the ICP device.
2. Allow visitors to talk to and touch the patient, but try to keep external stimulation to a minimum.

REFERENCES

American Association of Neurological Surgeons (AANS). (2000). The Brain Trauma Foundation: Joint Section on Neurotrauma and Critical Care. Guidelines for the management of severe traumatic brain injury. *Journal of Neurotrauma, 17*, 6-7.

Bergsneider, M., & Becker, D. (1995). Intracranial pressure monitoring. In S. Ayers, A. Grenvick, & P. R. Holbrook (Eds.), *Textbook of critical care* (3rd ed., pp. 311-315). Philadelphia: Saunders.

Brain Trauma Foundation. (2007). Guidelines for the management of severe traumatic brain injury. Retrieved July 26, 2007 from http://www2.braintrauma.org/guidelines/

Montague, D. (1990). Intracranial pressure measurements. In Blumer, J. (Ed.), *A practical guide to pediatric intensive care* (pp. 879-887). St Louis: Mosby.

Preuss, D. N. (2005). Neurologic drainage and pressure monitoring systems. In D. J. Lynn-McHale Wiegand, & K. K. Carlson (Eds.), *AACN procedure manual for critical care* (5th ed.. pp. 756-767). St Louis: Mosby.

Salim, A., & Khoo, L. (2002). Intracranial pressure monitoring. In W. C. Shoemaker, G. C. Velamahos, & D. Demetriades (Eds.), *Procedures and monitoring for the critically ill.* Philadelphia: Saunders.

Sullivan, J. (2002). Intracranial bolt insertion (pp. 551-560). In D. J. Lynn-McHale & K. K. Carlson (Eds.), *AACN procedure manual for critical care* (4th ed.). Philadelphia: Saunders.

Vernon-Levett, P. (2001). Intracranial dynamics. In M. A. Q. Curley, & P. A. Maloney-Harmon (Eds.), *Critical care nursing of infants and children* (2nd ed., pp. 323-368). Philadelphia: Saunders.

PROCEDURE 93

Burr Holes

Daun A. Smith, RN, MSN

Burr holes are also known as *skull trephination* or *twist drill holes.*

INDICATIONS

1. To place an intracranial pressure (ICP) monitoring device (see Procedure 92).
2. To relieve increased ICP in a patient with a suspected epidural or subdural hematoma when the following conditions exist:
   a. The patient is nonresponsive to conventional first-line interventions to decompress the brain tissue and prevent brain herniation (such as occurs in hyperventilation or hyperosmolar or diuretic therapy), and
   b. The patient also exhibits a rapidly deteriorating neurologic status manifested by a unilateral dilated and fixed pupil and contralateral hemiparesis or hemiplegia, and
   c. An operating room and/or a neurosurgeon is not available, and transport time is lengthy (Donovan, Moquin, & Ecklund, 2006).

CONTRAINDICATIONS AND CAUTIONS

1. Therapeutic burr holes are rarely placed in the emergency department. The optimal environment for hematoma evacuation is in the controlled atmosphere of an operating room.
2. Make sure there is a secure and patent airway before inserting the burr holes; intubation is preferred (Donovan et al., 2006).
3. Patients with hemophilia who are taking anticoagulants or who have other known or suspected coagulopathies require special treatment. Obtain

baseline coagulation studies and prepare to administer vitamin K and fresh frozen plasma to decrease intracranial bleeding.

4. Therapeutic burr holes should not be attempted in patients who have intracranial hematomas without signs of tentorial herniation, such as flaccid extremities and bilateral fixed, dilated pupils, or when a neurosurgeon is immediately available.

5. If a therapeutic burr hole is successful in releasing a hematoma, the patient's mental status may lighten and he or she may become combative. Be prepared to administer sedatives and analgesics.

EQUIPMENT

Burr hole or craniotomy tray, which includes the following:
Hand drill with bits (or twist drill) and drill stop
Knife handle with No. 10, 11, or 15 blade
Two curved hemostats
Dural suction tip
Scalp or dural hook
Self-retaining retractors
Sterile towels and drapes
(NOTE: Disposable trays are commercially available.)
Local anesthetic with epinephrine (optional)
Syringes and needles for local anesthesia
Electric hair clippers or razor
Antiseptic solution
Gauze dressings
Hemostatic agents (Gelfoam)
Bone wax
Monopolar disposable coagulator
Suture material
3-0 chromic gut
4-0 nylon

PATIENT PREPARATION

1. Insert a gastric tube to decompress the stomach and help prevent aspiration (see Procedure 98).

2. Intubate the patient orally to ensure a patent airway (Ghandhi & Penney, 2004).

3. Maintain cervical spine precautions if injury has not been ruled out. If no cervical spine precautions are needed, place the patient in the supine position with the head of the bed elevated 15 to 20 degrees (Simon & Brenner, 2002). For a therapeutic burr hole, turn the head so that the side of the head with the dilated pupil is parallel to the floor and is on the upper side (Donovan et al., 2006). Pupillary changes occur on the same side as the hematoma in most patients. If possible, place a sandbag or rolled towel under the patient's shoulder to help prevent kinking of the neck and venous outflow obstruction, which may increase ICP (Figure 93-1).

4. Shave or clip the hair at the insertion site. If an epidural hematoma is suspected after trauma, a temporal burr hole is usually attempted first on the

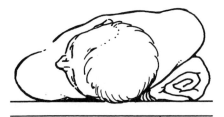

FIGURE 93-1 Patient position for emergency temporal burr hole. (From Winfield, J. [1992]. Emergency temporal burr hole in patients with clinical signs of progressive tentorial herniation. In M. S. Jastremski, M. Dumas, & L. Penalver (Eds.), *Emergency procedures* [p. 219]. Philadelphia: Saunders.)

side of the dilated pupil. Burr holes for intracranial monitoring devices are usually placed through the top of the head.

5. Cleanse the insertion site with an antiseptic solution.
6. Administer sedatives or paralytics as prescribed.
7. Administer broad-spectrum antibiotic as prescribed (Ghandhi & Penney, 2004).

PROCEDURAL STEPS

1. *Anesthetize the site with a local anesthetic (optional depending on the level of consciousness of the patient).
2. *Drape the area to provide a sterile field.
3. *Palpate the superficial temporalis artery to determine its course through the skin. The temporal burr hole site is located just above the root of the zygomatic arch and one finger breadth anterior to the external ear (Simon & Brenner, 2002) (Figure 93-2).

---

*Indicates portions of the procedure usually performed by a physician.

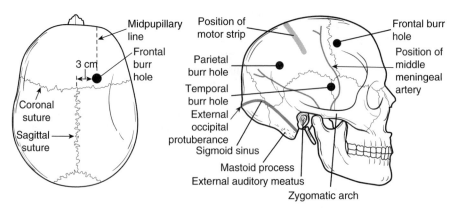

FIGURE 93-2 Placement of burr holes and incision sites. (From Reichman, E., & Simon, R. [2004]. *Emergency medicine procedures* [p. 886]. New York: McGraw-Hill.)

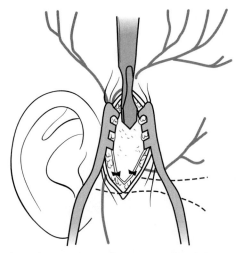

FIGURE 93-3 Use of a self-retaining retractor to expose burr hole site. (From Reichman, E., & Simon, R. [2004]. *Emergency medicine procedures* [p. 887]. New York: McGraw-Hill.)

4. *Using the scalpel, make a 3- to 4-mm vertical skin incision at the site. Minimal bleeding is usually encountered and may be controlled by the application of direct pressure with a gauze dressing.

5. *Expose the burr hole site and place a self-retaining retractor (Figure 93-3). Spreading the self-retaining retractor usually results in a complete hemostasis. If bleeding continues, hemostats or a cautery can be used to stop the sources of the bleeding (Donovan et al., 2006).

6. *Using either the standard hand-held drill or a twist drill with a drill stop (Figure 93-4), introduce the drill bit perpendicular to the site and rotate the drilling in a clockwise motion to penetrate to the inner table of the skull. At this site, the skull is 3 to 8 mm thick and has three layers, so the drilling passes through three stages (difficult, easy, then difficult again) as it approaches the inner table (Donovan et al., 2006).

7. *Using a saline-filled syringe, gently irrigate the bone dust from the site.

8. *Inspect the extradural site for a hematoma. Dark red, clotted blood usually indicates an epidural hematoma. Use the dural suction tip to assist in evacuating the clotted material (Figure 93-5). If the exposed dura begins to pulsate, the procedure is finished and the incision may be closed (Donovan et al., 2006).

9. *If bright red blood is present, an active bleed is likely and it should be located and clamped until further intervention can be provided. Gelfoam strips may also be placed as a temporary measure to promote hemostasis.

10. *A bluish tinge usually indicates a subdural hematoma. Insert the dural hook through the outer layer of the dura, pull it upward, and incise with a No. 11 blade to release the accumulated blood. Suction may be needed to evacuate

---

*Indicates portions of the procedure usually performed by a physician.

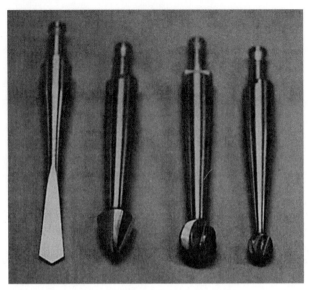

FIGURE 93-4 Hand-held twist drill. Chisel drill bit. (From Reichman, E., & Simon, R. [2004]. *Emergency medicine procedures* [p. 884]. New York: McGraw-Hill.)

the clot. Use a low-vacuum setting to prevent damage to the brain tissue. If bleeding continues, small pieces of Gelfoam may be applied to the area.

11. *If no clot is seen, repeat the procedure at one of the other sites.

12. Apply a loose gauze dressing over the site and prepare the patient for transport to the operating room or a tertiary care facility for definitive treatment.

13. Assess and document the neurologic status.

_____

*Indicates portions of the procedure usually performed by a physician.

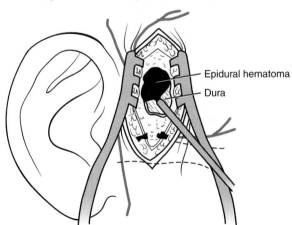

FIGURE 93-5 Once the extradural space is entered, a hematoma may be visualized. Use suction to remove any clots or hemorrhaging present. (From Reichman, E., & Simon, R. [2004]. *Emergency medicine procedures* [p. 887]. New York: McGraw-Hill.)

COMPLICATIONS

1. Potential damage to the underlying brain tissue if the drill is advanced too far while the burr hole is being placed. This can usually be prevented by use of a drill stop.
2. Infection or subdural empyema
3. Laceration of an artery or sinus perforation
4. Broken drill bit
5. False-positive or false-negative tap
6. Release of a tamponaded epidural may result in further bleeding and patient deterioration.

REFERENCES

Donovan, D. J., Moquin, R. R., & Ecklund, J. M. (2006). Cranial burr holes and emergency craniotomy: Review of indications and technique. *Military Medicine, 171,* 12-19.

Ghandhi, Y., & Penney, D. (2004). Burr holes. In E. F. Reichman, & R. R. Simon (Eds.), *Emergency medicine procedures* (pp. 881-889). New York: McGraw-Hill.

Simon, R., & Brenner, B. (2002) *Emergency procedures and techniques* (4th ed.). Baltimore: Williams & Wilkins.

PROCEDURE 94

Tongs or Open-back Halo for Cervical Traction

Daun A. Smith, RN, MSN

Tongs for cervical spine traction are also known as *Gardner-Wells tongs, skull tongs, caliper traction,* or *tongs.*

INDICATIONS

1. To reduce and stabilize an unstable cervical spine secondary to fracture, subluxation, dislocation, arthritis, or neoplasm
2. To provide continuous traction and stabilization for an unstable cervical spine

CONTRAINDICATIONS AND CAUTIONS

1. Pins should not be inserted over skull fractures or through infected tissue (Ghandhi & Penney, 2004).

2. The cervical collar should be kept in place during tong or halo application. When the traction is established and cervical spine films have been cleared, the hard cervical collar may be removed (Botte et al., 1995).
3. Addition or deletion of traction weights should be supervised by a physician.
4. Avoid sudden movements of the traction apparatus, patient, or bed.
5. Cervical tongs and open-back halos usually take 24 hours to become seated. The stability of the device should be assessed and documented frequently for the first 24 hours.
6. Airway management of the patient with tongs or halo will be problematic. If there is potential for deterioration, early plans should be made for alternative rescue airway management such as a supraglottic airway (laryngeal mask airway) or rigid or flexible fiberoptic laryngoscopy and the equipment for the rescue airway should be readily available. Suction should always be readily available.
7. A clear plan and tools for access through a halo vest should CPR be needed must be known and taped to the vest.
8. Atlanto-occipital dislocations should not be managed by skeletal traction (Ghandhi & Penney, 2004; Hosalkar et al, 2005).
9. If magnetic resonance imaging (MRI) is anticipated, be sure the cervical tongs or the halo apparatus are safe with the use of MRI.
10. There is insufficient evidence to make strong recommendations about specific pin care techniques (Holmes & Brown, 2005). Options include:
    a. Chlorhexidine solution may be the most effective agent for cleaning the site (Holmes & Brown, 2005).
    b. Gauze dressing around the pin
    c. Antibiotic ointment around the pin entrance and exit
    d. No dressing or ointment to sites

EQUIPMENT

Razor or clippers
Antiseptic solution
Sterile gauze dressings
Syringes and needles for local anesthetic
Local anesthetic for infiltration
Sterile open-back halo ring in appropriate size with sterile halo pins and halo torque wrenches
or
[†]Sterile cervical tong set
Bed with pulley or traction system attached (e.g., Roto-Rest bed, Stryker frame)
Weights in assorted sizes: 1, 2, 3, 5 lb
Weight holder, usually a C- or an S-hook

[†]NOTE: Various tongs are available for insertion. This procedure discusses the Gardner-Wells tongs. Gardner-Wells tongs feature spring-loaded points for assisting in cervical traction (Gardner, 1973) and are easily placed on the patient in the emergency department (Figure 94-1). Tong selection is usually by physician preference or availability. Open-back halo traction devices are also easily applied in the emergency department and may be attached to traction via a pulley or

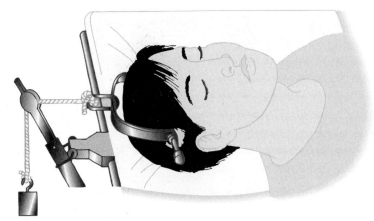

FIGURE 94-1 Gardner-Wells tongs. (From Black, J., & Hawks, J. [2005]. *Medical-surgical nursing* [7th ed., p. 2218]. Philadelphia: Saunders.)

immediately fitted to a halo vest in the stable patient. If MRI is anticipated, be sure the cervical tongs or the halo apparatus are safe with the use of MRI.

PATIENT PREPARATION

1. Assess and document neurologic status.
2. Shave or clip a small area of hair from the scalp at selected sites for tong or halo pin insertion.
3. Cleanse the area with an antiseptic solution.
4. *Infiltrate the pin insertion sites with a local anesthetic.
5. Instruct the patient to report immediately any increased pain, paresthesia, or difficulty in breathing during or after the insertion.
6. Consider sedation so that the patient may be comfortable yet remain awake enough that peripheral neurologic status may be monitored during the application of the immobilization device (see Procedure 177).

PROCEDURAL STEPS
Gardner-Wells Tongs

1. *Apply the points of tongs below the temporal ridges and in line with the external auditory meatus. Tighten each side alternately until the spring-loaded mechanism extends approximately 1 mm on each side (Figure 94-2). This indicates a squeezing pressure of 30 pounds (Simon & Brenner, 2002).
2. *Gently rock the tong back and forth to ensure that it is securely seated in the scalp (Ghandhi & Penney, 2004).
3. *Connect the S-hook on the tongs to the pulley rope. Cervical flexion and extension may be obtained by adjusting the height of the pulley.
4. *Place the desired amount of weight onto the weight holder. Ten pounds is usually needed for the head, and an additional 5 lbs per disc space is required

---

*Indicates portions of the procedure usually performed by a physician or an advanced practice nurse.

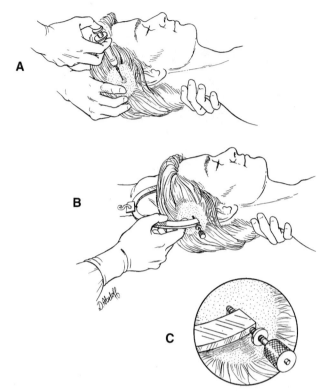

FIGURE 94-2 A, Anesthetizing the insertion site. **B,** Placement of Gardner-Wells tongs. **C,** Indicator of spring-loaded pins extends 1 mm on each side when a squeeze pressure of 30 lbs has been obtained. (Courtesy of P. Rosen, M.D.)

for reduction (Ghandhi & Penney, 2004). Additional weight may be needed to overcome severe muscle spasm in the neck or upper back.

5. Obtain a radiograph to check alignment 5 to 10 minutes after each weight or position change (Ghandhi & Penney, 2004).

6. To prevent rotation of the head, place sandbags under the projecting points of the tongs. This is especially important in odontoid fractures (Simon & Brenner, 2002).

7. Perform pin site care according to institutional guidelines.

Open-back Halo

1. *Measure the patient's head circumference, and select the appropriate-sized halo according to the manufacturer's guidelines.

2. *Select pin sites. Anterior pins should be placed 1 cm above the lateral third of each eyebrow. Posterior pins should be placed in the lateral occipital areas at approximate positions of 4 o'clock and 8 o'clock (mid forehead = 12 o'clock)

---

*Indicates portions of the procedure usually performed by a physician or an advanced practice nurse.

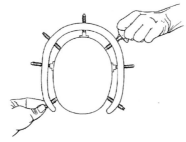

FIGURE 94-3 Insertion of halo pins until "finger-tight." (Courtesy Ace Medical Company, El Segundo, CA.)

3. *Keep the halo sterile so that contamination does not occur as each pin is passed through the ring and into the skin and the skull.
4. *Place the halo using positioning pins or padding, so that there is approximately 1 cm of clearance from the head below the equator of the skull but above the top of the ear.
5. *Insert the four skull pins and turn until finger-tight, as perpendicular to the skull as possible (Figure 94-3).
6. *Advance each pin through the skin into the skull using torque wrenches. During the anterior pin placement, the patient's eyes should be closed (to prevent difficulty in closing the eyes after the pin placement). Tighten diagonally opposite pairs of pins at alternating 2 inches per pound intervals until the desired torque of 8 inches per pound is reached (the torque wrenches stop functioning when the desired pressure is reached) (Figure 94-4).
7. *Gently place pin locks or locknuts according to the manufacturer's guidelines.

---

*Indicates portions of the procedure usually performed by a physician or an advanced practice nurse.

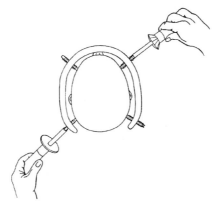

FIGURE 94-4 Tightening alternate halo pins with torque wrenches. (Courtesy Ace Medical Company, El Segundo, CA.)

8. Apply traction as described for the Gardner-Wells tongs.
9. Obtain postprocedure cervical spine films.
10. Perform pin site care according to institutional guidelines.

AGE-SPECIFIC CONSIDERATIONS

1. Less weight is needed for traction in small children; 1 to 2 lbs may be adequate for upper cervical injuries. Be careful not to use excessive weight, which may result in overdistraction.
2. Patient cooperation in remaining immobile is paramount. In children, cooperation must be obtained in a manner appropriate to the child's developmental level (see Procedure 191).

COMPLICATIONS

1. Pin loosening
2. Infection
3. Pin site pain
4. Penetration of the skull and dura
5. Loss of immobilization
6. Dysphagia
7. Bleeding at pin sites
8. Nerve injury secondary to excessive traction or inadequate traction
9. Sensory deprivation secondary to restrictions from the halo device

PATIENT TEACHING

1. Report nausea immediately.
2. Report increased pain at the insertion site, neck, or across the shoulders.
3. Avoid sudden movements because mobility of the neck and head is severely restricted.

REFERENCES

Bott, M. J., Byrne, T. P., Abrams, R. A., & Garfin, S. R. (1995). The halo skeletal fixator: Current concepts of application and maintenance. *Orthopedics, 39*, 543.

Gardner, W. (1973). The principle of spring loaded points for cervical fraction. *Journal of Neurosurgery, 39*, 543.

Ghandhi, Y., & Penney, D. W. (2004). Skeletal traction (Gardner-Wells tongs) for cervical spine dislocations and fractures. In E. F. Reichman, & R. R. Simon (Eds.), *Emergency medicine procedures* (pp. 913-918). New York: McGraw-Hill.

Holmes, S. B., Brown, S. J. Pin Site Care Expert Panel. (2005). Skeletal pin site care: National Association of Orthopedic Nurses guidelines for orthopedic nursing. *Orthopedic Nursing, 24*(2), 99-107.

Hosalkar, H., Cain, E. L., Horn, D., Chin, K. R., Dormans, J. P., & Drummond, D. S. (2005). Traumatic atlanto-occipital dislocation in children. *Journal of Bone and Joint Surgery, 87A*, 2480-2488.

Simon, R. R., & Brenner, B. E. (2002). *Emergency procedures and techniques* (4th ed.). Baltimore: Williams & Wilkins.

Abdominal and Genitourinary Procedures

Diagnostic Peritoneal Lavage

Jean A. Proehl, RN, MN, CEN, CCRN, FAEN

Diagnostic peritoneal lavage (DPL) is also known as *belly tap*, *peri dial*, *peri lavage*, and *peritoneal lavage*.

INDICATIONS

1. To help diagnose intraabdominal bleeding or viscous perforation in hemody-namically unstable patients, especially those who are unable to contribute to the physical examination because of paralysis, unconsciousness, or intoxica-tion or in patients in whom the examination is equivocal because of lower rib, pelvis, or lumbar spine fractures.
2. To evaluate patients at risk for intraabdominal trauma who are about to undergo lengthy anesthesia for nonabdominal surgical or radiographic procedures.
3. To assess patients with undiagnosed hypotension after trauma.
4. To help diagnose intraabdominal bleeding or viscous perforation in hemody-namically stable patients when computerized tomography (CT) or ultrasound is not available.
5. To provide core rewarming for moderately to severely hypothermic patients (temperature less than 32° C [90° F]).

CONTRAINDICATIONS AND CAUTIONS

1. CT or ultrasonography of the abdomen is performed instead of peritoneal lavage in most situations.
2. If abdominal surgery is already indicated because of physical examination or clinical presentation, there is no need to perform peritoneal lavage.
3. The open technique is preferred to decrease the risk of iatrogenic injury; the Seldinger technique is an acceptable alternative for physicians trained in the technique (ACS, 2004).
4. Multiple prior abdominal surgeries increase the risk of adhesions, which may cause the intestines to adhere to the abdominal wall and result in viscous perforation when the catheter is introduced.
5. The open technique with a supraumbilical insertion site is preferred for preg-nant patient or pelvic fractures (ACS, 2004; Nagy, 2004).
6. Pelvic fractures may cause false-positive results if the catheter enters a pelvic hematoma. Therefore, the open technique with a supraumbilical insertion site should be chosen in this situation (ACS, 2004).
7. Peritoneal lavage does not rule out retroperitoneal injuries, perforation of a hollow viscus, or diaphragmatic disruption.
8. Morbid obesity, advanced cirrhosis, advanced pregnanacy, and preexisting coagulopathy are relative contraindications to DPL (ACS, 2004; Marx & Isenhour, 2006).

EQUIPMENT

Razor or clippers
Antiseptic solution
Scalpel (No. 10, 11, or 15)
Mosquito forceps
Gauze sponges
1% lidocaine (with epinephrine)
10-ml syringe, 18-G or 25-G to 27-G needles for local anesthesia
1000 ml of warmed (36.6° to 37.7° C [98° to 100° F]) normal saline or lactated
   Ringer's solution
Peritoneal dialysis catheter (with or without trocar) or catheter, dilator, and
   spring-wire guide assembly
Nonvented intravenous (IV) tubing without a backcheck valve or cystoscopy
   tubing
Sterile drapes or towels
20-ml syringe
Blood collection tubes (optional, for transport of lavage specimens to the
   laboratory)
Needle holder
4-0 nylon suture
Antibiotic ointment
Adhesive tape
(NOTE: Preassembled kits containing much of this equipment are available.)

PATIENT PREPARATION

1. Insert an indwelling urinary catheter (Procedure 104) to decompress the
   bladder and to prevent bladder perforation when the catheter is introduced.
   If a catheter cannot be inserted for some reason, the open technique should
   be used (Nagy, 2004).
2. Insert a gastric tube (Procedure 98) to decompress the stomach and to prevent stomach perforation during catheter insertion.
3. If possible, complete any abdominal radiographs before the procedure,
   because air may enter the abdomen and confuse any future abdominal films.
4. Place the patient in the supine position.
5. *Shave the abdomen or clip the hair and cleanse it with antiseptic solution.
   The usual site for catheter insertion is midline, one third of the distance
   between the umbilicus and the symphysis pubis. The umbilical or supraumbilical areas may also be used.

PROCEDURAL STEPS

1. *Drape the abdomen with sterile towels.
2. *Infiltrate the insertion site with lidocaine. In general, lidocaine with epinephrine is used to help control bleeding at the site. Absolute hemostasis at the
   site is essential to help prevent false-positive results.
3. *Insert the catheter into the peritoneal space via open or Seldinger (closed)
   technique.

---

*Indicates portions of the procedure usually performed by a physician or an advanced practice
nurse.

a. Open technique (ACS, 2004). Incise through the abdominal skin and the subcutaneous tissue to the fascia. Elevate the wound edges with clamps and incise the fascia down to the peritoneum. Nick the peritoneum and insert the catheter into the peritoneal cavity. Advance the catheter caudally into the pelvis.

b. Seldinger (closed) technique (ACS, 2004). Elevate the skin on both sides of the intended needle insertion site with fingers or forceps and insert an 18-G needle attached to a syringe into the abdomen. Remove the syringe and thread the guidewire through the needle until resistance is met or only 3 cm of wire is exposed. Remove the needle while leaving the wire in place. Incise the skin adjacent to the wire and thread the lavage catheter over the wire and into the abdomen. Remove the wire while leaving the catheter in place.

4. *For core rewarming or cooling, insert two catheters; one is used to infuse constantly and the other is used to drain the solution. This is more time efficient than infusing and draining via the same catheter.

5. If the lavage is for diagnostic purposes, attach a 20-ml syringe and aspirate. If 10 ml or more of gross blood is obtained the test is considered positive (ACS, 2004; Marx & Isenhour, 2006; Nagy, 2004).

6. Attach the primed IV tubing to the catheter (Figure 95-1). The IV tubing should not contain a backcheck valve because this prevents the fluid from being siphoned out of the abdomen. If the tubing is vented, the fluid may

---

*Indicates portions of the procedure usually performed by a physician or an advanced practice nurse.

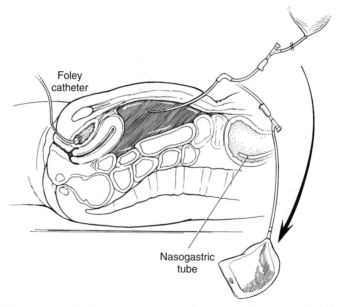

FIGURE 95-1 Lavage catheter in peritoneal space. (From Rosen, P., Chan, T. C., Vilke, G. M., & Sternbach, G. [2001]. *Atlas of emergency procedures.* [p. 111]. St Louis: Mosby.)

leak from the vent, or a water seal may form and prevent fluid return. Cystoscopy tubing allows much faster infusion and drainage. To connect the catheter to the cytoscopy tubing, push the end of the connecting tubing into the sleeve of the cystoscopy tubing. Tying a suture around the distal end of the sleeve of the cystoscopy tubing tightens the connection (optional).

7. Infuse 1 L of sterile warmed normal saline solution or lactated Ringer's solution. Room temperature solutions may cause or worsen hypothermia. Stopping the infusion before the drip chamber is dry facilitates siphoning of the fluid. Monitor urinary catheter and chest-tube drainage for evidence of lavage fluid because this may assist with a diagnosis of diaphragm or bladder rupture.

8. If the patient's condition allows, leave the fluid in the peritoneal space for 5 to 10 minutes. Palpate the abdomen or gently rock the patient from side to side to help distribute the fluid throughout the peritoneal cavity.

9. Lower the IV bag to the floor and allow the fluid to siphon out of the abdomen. If the fluid does not return, make sure the appropriate tubing has been used. If necessary, cut off a backcheck valve or vent and drain the fluid into a basin. Then try repositioning the patient. The physician may reposition the catheter or insert another catheter to facilitate drainage. Additional fluid may also be instilled to encourage fluid return. Adequate fluid return is 30% or more of the infused volume (ACS, 2004). Any fluid left in the abdomen is absorbed through the peritoneum and should be added to the patient's parenteral fluid intake.

10. Obtain laboratory specimens from the IV bag when the fluid return is finished. Visual inspection of the fluid is not accurate. Commonly ordered tests include red blood cell (RBC) count, white blood cell (WBC) count, and Gram's stain. The fluid is placed in the same specimen tubes that would be used if the tests were being performed on blood. Some laboratories also accept the fluid in the IV bag or syringes. Recommended diagnostic tests and positive findings vary from source to source but commonly include the following (ACS, 2004; Marx & Isenhour, 2006):
    - RBC count 100,000/mm^3 or greater (except in stab wounds to the lower chest or gunshot wounds, where 5,000 to 10,000/mm^3 may be considered positive)
    - WBC count 500/mm^3 or greater
    - Bacteria or food fibers present on Gram's stain

11. *Remove the catheter and suture the wound. If a laparotomy is indicated, the wound should not be sutured, and a sterile dressing should be applied. If the findings are equivocal, the catheter may be left in place, the wound sutured, and the lavage repeated 2 to 3 hours later.

12. Place a thin layer of an antibiotic ointment and a dry sterile dressing over the wound.

---

*Indicates portions of the procedure usually performed by a physician or an advanced practice nurse.

AGE-SPECIFIC CONSIDERATIONS

1. Children require sedation and analgesia. If a child is too young to cooperate with the procedure without deep sedation, DPL should not be performed. The patient should undergo CT scanning or, if the patient is unstable, DPL in the operating room under general anesthesia (Henneman, 1997).
2. Because distressed children tend to swallow air, which leads to stomach distention, it is essential that a gastric tube be inserted before the dialysis catheter is inserted.
3. An infraumbilical approach is used for most children, one-third the distance from the umbilicus to the pubic symphysis. Because the bladder may extend well into the abdominal cavity, a supraumbilical approach (1 to 2 cm above the umbilicus) is used for infants and small children (King & Henretig, 2000).
4. Infuse 10 to 20 ml/kg, but no more than 1000 mL, of warm normal saline solution or lactated Ringer's solution in children. Infusing additional fluid may interfere with respirations (ACS, 2004; King & Henretig, 2000).
5. Withdrawal of any significant amount of blood is positive for a child under 8 years of age. For an older child or adolescent, 5 to 10 ml of blood is considered a positive result (King & Henretig, 2000).
6. Trocars are not used in children.

COMPLICATIONS

1. Perforation of abdominal organs or blood vessels, resulting in peritonitis or hemorrhage.
2. False-positive results may result from bleeding at the insertion site, bleeding within the muscle sheath, or pelvic fractures and lead to a negative laparotomy.
3. Inadequate fluid return or false-negative results as a result of incorrect catheter placement.
4. Wound infection or dehiscence, hematoma.
5. Evisceration or incisional hernia.

PATIENT TEACHING

1. Keep the wound clean and dry, and observe for signs of infection.
2. Have the sutures removed in 8 to 10 days.
3. Notify the nursing or medical staff if abdominal pain, tenderness, rigidity, or fever increases.

REFERENCES

American College of Surgeons (ACS). Committee on Trauma. (2004). *Advanced trauma life support for doctors* (7th ed.). Chicago: Author.

Henneman, P. L. (1997). Diagnostic peritoneal lavage. In R. A. Dieckmann, D. H. Fiser, & S. M. Selbst (Eds.), *Pediatric emergency and critical care procedures* (pp. 604–606) (pp. 604-606). St Louis: Mosby.

King, C., & Henretig, F. M. (2000) *Pocket atlas of pediatric emergency procedures*. Philadelphia: Lippincott Williams & Wilkins.

Marx, J. A., & Isenhour, J. (2006). Abdominal trauma. In J. A. Marx, R. S. Hockberger, & R. M. Walls, et al. (Eds.), *Rosen's emergency medicine: Concepts and clinical practice* (6th ed., pp. 489-514). St Louis: Mosby.

Nagy, K. (2004). Diagnostic peritoneal lavage. In E. F. Reichman, & R. R. Simon (Eds.), *Emergency medicine procedures* (pp. 478-489). New York: McGraw-Hill.

Paracentesis

June F. Stacey, RN, BSN, CEN

INDICATIONS

1. To obtain peritoneal fluid for analysis, to aid in the diagnosis of new-onset ascites, or to diagnose infection in a patient with ascites.
2. To promote comfort and improve cardiorespiratory and gastrointestinal status by relieving intraabdominal pressure (Hu & White, 2003).

CONTRAINDICATIONS AND CAUTIONS

1. Coagulopathies, thrombocyctopenia, and portal hypertension with abdominal collateral circulation increase the chance of bleeding and hemorrhage.
2. Use caution in patients with multiple prior abdominal surgeries and adhesions as the intestines may be adhered to the abdominal wall which could result in viscous perforation during introduction of the needle.
3. An open supraumbilical or ultrasound-assisted approach is preferred during a second- and third-trimester pregnancy (Marx, 2004).
4. Use caution in patients with infection at the insertion site.

EQUIPMENT

Antiseptic solution
Sterile drapes/towels
2-in sterile needle with inner trocar or 2-in intravenous (IV) catheter with stylet, size 10-G, 12-G, or 14-G
3-ml syringe with 18-G and 27-G, 1½-in needles for local anesthesia
1% lidocaine with epinephrine
10-ml syringe
60-ml Luer-Lok syringe
Scalpel, No. 11 blade
Sterile gauze sponges
Four empty 1000-ml vacuum bottles or other drainage collection container (e.g., bag, bottle)
Three-way stopcock
Nonvented IV tubing without a backcheck valve, or 36-in pressure tubing
Four sterile tubes or cytology bottles for specimen collection
Male-to-male IV tubing connecter
Sterile dressing/tape/antibiotic ointment
(NOTE: Preassembled trays with some or all of these supplies are available.)

PATIENT PREPARATION

1. Have the patient void immediately before the procedure or if the patient is unable to void, place an indwelling catheter (see Procedure 104) to

decompress the bladder and prevent perforation of the bladder during introduction of the needle.

2. Position the patient in an upright postion to faciliate fluid accumulation in the lower abdomen. This can be accomplished by sitting the patient in a chair, on the side of the bed or in high Fowler's position. Alternatively, a lateral decubitus position may be used if the patient is unable to tolerate being upright for the procedure.

PROCEDURAL STEPS

1. Cleanse the abdomen with antiseptic solution.
2. *Drape the abdomen with the sterile drapes or towels.
3. *Infiltrate the insertion site with lidocaine.
4. * Make an incision midline 2 cm below the umbilicus. In a patient with midline scarring, the incision can be made in either lower quadrant medial to the anterior superior iliac crest and 4 to 5 cm cephalad (Marx, 2004).
5. *Attach a 10-ml syringe to the catheter. The needle or IV catheter is inserted slowly in 5-mm increments through the abdominal wall until peritoneal fluid is aspirated. Avoid continuous aspiration during insertion as this may pull the bowel toward the needle. Remove the inner trocar or stylet.
6. Fluid may be drained by gravity drainage, by aspiration with 60-ml syringe, or by vacuum drainage.
   a. The paracentesis kit may come with a bag and tubing for fluid drainage by gravity, or IV tubing connected to a collection device may be attached to the needle. NOTE: Nonvented IV tubing should be used because fluid may leak from the vent in vented tubing. The IV tubing should not contain a backcheck valve because this will prevent the drainage of the fluid.
   b. A three-way stopcock may be attached to the needle and fluid aspirated with a 60-ml syringe.
   c. Pressure tubing may be attached to the paracentesis needle or catheter to drain the fluid using a vaccuum bottle. Attach a needle to the other end of the tubing using a male-to-male adapter. Insert the needle into the bottle to remove the fluid by vacuum. The vacuum may collapse regular IV tubing.

   Some sources cite concerns about potential hemodynamic compromise due to rapid removal of large volumes of ascitic fluid, but there have also been reports of 6 L being removed in 15 minutes without complications. Some practitioners may administer colloids to maintain intravascular volume, but this is not recommended for paracentesis volumes of less than 5 L (Marx, 2004).
7. Collect laboratory specimens in sterile containers. Commonly ordered laboratory tests include a differential cell count, albumin assay, and cultures (Marx, 2004).
8. When the needle is withdrawn, apply antibiotic ointment and dressing as per institutional dressing protocol.
9. Monitor the patient during and after the procedure. Watch for and report bleeding, fluid leakage, or scrotal edema. Check vital signs often to detect

---

*Indicates portions of the procedure usually performed by a physician or an advanced practice nurse.

hypotensive complications early. Vital signs are recommended every half hour for 2 hours after the procedure, then hourly for 2 hours, then every 4 hours for 24 hours.

AGE-SPECIFIC CONSIDERATION

An older patient may not be able to tolerate sitting up in a chair or on the side of the bed for the period of time needed for procedure and may need to be placed in high or semi-Fowler's or lateral decubitus position.

COMPLICATIONS

1. Perforation of blood vessels or abdominal organs (bladder, bowel, or stomach) resulting in hemorrhage or peritonitis
2. Infection at insertion site
3. Shock secondary to fluid and electrolyte shifts
4. Leaking of peritoneal fluid at the puncture site. If leakage continues after applying direct pressure to the site for five minutes a suture may be placed at the site (Hu & White, 2003).

REFERENCES

Hu, K., & White, B. (2003). Abdominal paracentesis. In J. L. Pfenninger, & G. C. Fowler (Eds.), *Procedures for primary care* (2nd ed., pp. 749-752). St Louis: Mosby.

Marx, J. A. (2004). Peritoneal procedures. In J. R. Roberts, & J. R. Hedges (Eds.), *Clinical procedures in emergency medicine* (4th ed., pp. 841-859). Philadelphia: Saunders.

PROCEDURE 97

Intraabdominal Pressure Monitoring

Lucinda W. Rossoll, RN, MSN, CCRN, CEN

Intraabdominal pressure (IAP) can be measured directly with an intraperitoneal catheter or indirectly via a gastric balloon or urinary bladder pressure measurement (the gold standard). The bladder acts as a pressure reservoir, a compliant structure that reflects pressure changes. There is a significant correlation between bladder pressure and abdominal pressure. Abdominal compartment syndrome (ACS) is defined as a condition in which end-organ dysfunction or damage results from untreated intraabdominal hypertension (IAH) (Cheatham, 2006). IAH occurs when the contents of the abdomen expand secondary to increased organ volume, tumor, blood, fluid, or a change in abdominal wall compliance. This leads to decreased venous return, decreased cardiac output, and dysfunction of the organs contained in the abdominal cavity. When IAP pressure is greater than 15 mm Hg, renal dysfunction can occur. IAH is defined as sustained or repeated IAP of 12 mm Hg or greater or an abdominal perfusion pressure (APP) that is 60 mm Hg or less (Cheatham, 2006). APP is a calculated by subtracting the IAP from the mean arterial pressure (MAP). Normal IAP is less than 5 mm Hg. IAP is categorized by severity according pressure (Wolfe & Gallagher, 2006):

Grade I = 12 to 15 mm Hg
Grade II = 16 to 20 mm Hg
Grade III = 21 to 25 mm Hg
Grade IV = greater than 25 mm Hg

INDICATIONS

IAP monitoring is indicated for any condition that may produce elevated pressures in the abdomen, such as blunt abdominal trauma, abdominal aortic aneurysm rupture, bleeding, large hematoma, abdominal packing, bowel obstruction, abscess, peritonitis, visceral edema, ascites, tumors, burn eschar, or use of a pneumatic antishock garment.

CONTRAINDICATIONS AND CAUTIONS

Bladder pressure may not be accurate in a patient with a small or noncompliant bladder or a patient in Trendelenburg or reverse Trendelenburg position.

EQUIPMENT

500- to 1000-ml bag of normal saline
Cardiac monitor with hemodynamic monitoring capability
Pressure transducer cable
Intravenous (IV) tubing
Pressure tubing, 12-in
Pressure transducer (if not already part of the pressure tubing setup)
Pressure extension tubing
Long pressure extension tubing (for pole-mounted transducer)
Four-way stopcock or two three-way stopcocks
Dead-ender caps (nonvented) for stopcock ports
Pressure-infuser bag or cuff
Pole-mounted transducer holder (optional)
Level (optional)
60-ml Luer-Lok syringe
18-G needle or IV catheter
Clamp
Povidone-iodine pads, swab sticks, or alcohol pad
Urinary catheter with closed drainage bag

PATIENT PREPARATION

1. Insert a urinary bladder catheter (see Procedure 104).

2. Place patient in a supine position, as flat as possible to negate downward pressure of abdominal organs that may falsely elevate pressure readings.

PROCEDURAL STEPS

1. Prepare the pressure monitoring system as follows (Figure 97-1):
   a. Spike the normal saline solution with the IV tubing.
   b. Attach the four-way stopcock or the two three-way stopcocks (connected together) to the pressure transducer and attach the IV tubing to the stopcock. If two three-way stopcocks are used, one side port is the air-fluid interface and the other holds the 60-ml syringe.
   c. Attach the pressure tubing to the other end of the transducer.
   d. Attach the 18-G needle to the pressure tubing.
   e. Attach the 60-ml syringe to the side port of the stopcock.
   f. Flush the stopcock, pressure tubing, and transducer with normal saline.
   g. Cap each port with a nonvented cap after flushing.
2. Level the air side of the stopcock (air-fluid interface) to the top of the symphysis pubis.
3. Turn on the monitor and select either the 30- or the 60-mm Hg scale.
4. Connect transducer to the monitor and zero balance the transducer. Zero balancing the system to the atmospheric pressure negates the effects of the atmospheric pressure. To prevent erroneous pressure readings, zero the system before and after the pressure system is attached to the patient,

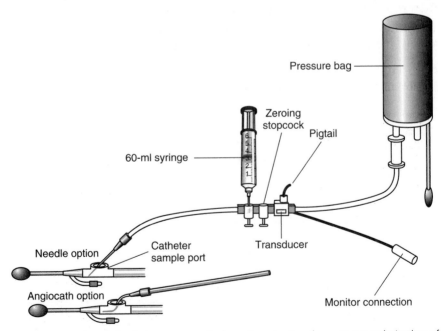

FIGURE 97-1 Intraabdominal pressure monitoring setup using two threeway stopcocks in place of a four-way stopcock. (From Gallagher, J. J. [2005]. Intraabdominal pressure monitoring. In D. J. Lynn-McHale Wiegand & K. K. Carlson [Eds.], *AACN procedure manual for critical care* [5th ed., p. 894]. Philadelphia: Saunders.)

with any significant change in the waveform and the values, whenever the system is disconnected, and at the beginning of each shift. To zero, turn the four-way stopcock off to the patient and open to the transducer and to air (air-fluid interface). Zero the monitor according to the manufacturer's directions. Once the monitor is zeroed, flush the open stopcock port and replace the dead-ender cap. Turn the stopcock on to the patient and on to the transducer.

5. Clamp the drainage bag tubing distal to the sampling port.
6. Cleanse the port with alcohol.
7. Insert the 18-G needle into the sampling port of the drainage tubing or insert the 18-gauge IV catheter and thread the catheter into the port.
8. Instill 50 ml of sterile normal saline into the urinary catheter through the sampling port.
9. Briefly release the clamp to allow fluid from the bladder to fill the tubing and remove air from the system.
10. Run a strip of the waveform and read the mean IAP at end-expiration.
11. Document the reading and patient position (flat or supine).
12. Remove the needle and unclamp the drainage system. If an IV catheter is used, it may be left in place.

COMPLICATION

Urinary tract infection

REFERENCES

Cheatham, M. L. (2006). Consensus definitions for intra-abdominal hypertension and abdominal compartment syndrome. *Critical Connections*, *5*(1), 7.

Wolfe, T., & Gallagher, J. (2006). Intra-abdominal hypertension: Pitfalls, prevalence, and treatment options. *AACN News*, *23*(10), 12-17.

Insertion of Orogastric and Nasogastric Tubes

Lucinda W. Rossoll, RN, MSN, CCRN, CEN

Orogastric and nasogastric tubes are also known as *Levin, Lavacuator, Salem sump, Ewald, enteric,* or *feeding tubes.*

NOTE: This procedure does not address the insertion of small-bore feeding tubes. Different procedures are required for insertion and verification of placement with these tubes.

INDICATIONS

1. To decompress the stomach through the removal of air or gastric contents
2. To instill fluid and/or medications into the stomach
3. To facilitate clinical diagnosis through analysis of gastric contents

CONTRAINDICATIONS AND CAUTIONS

1. In the presence of head trauma, maxillofacial injury, or anterior fossa skull fracture, there is the potential for inadvertent penetration of the brain via the cribriform plate or ethmoid bone if the tube is inserted nasally. In these instances, the orogastric route is used.
2. Caution should be used when inserting the tube in a patient with a potential cervical spine injury; the patient's head should be manually immobilized for this procedure.
3. If the patient has esophageal varices, there is a risk of inadvertent esophageal rupture and hemorrhage as a result of tube placement.
4. The smallest possible tube appropriate to the intervention or task should be used, because smaller tubes place less stress on the esophageal sphincter.
5. Do not irrigate a Salem sump tube through the blue air vent.
6. If tetracaine is used for intranasal anesthesia, the dose should not exceed 20 mg (Clinical Pharmacology On-Line, 2006).
7. Spray medications used for posterior pharyngeal anesthesia should not exceed 2 seconds of application time. Systemic absorption of benzocaine can have serious adverse effects, including death (FDA, 2006).
8. The traditional method of instilling air while auscultating over the epigastrium is not reliable as the sound produced cannot distinguish between placement in the bronchus, pleural space, or gastrointestinal tract (Cirgin Ellett, 2004). Metheny and Titler (2001) report that there is little scientific evidence to support the use of this method and that the literature contains numerous reports of its ineffectiveness.

EQUIPMENT

60-ml catheter-tip syringe

Water-soluble lubricant gel or 2% lidocaine gel

Bite block or oral airway (for oral placement)

Tongue blade

pH test strips

Emesis basin

Cup of water with straw (optional)

1-in tape, benzoin, or commercial tube holder

Specimen container (optional)

Capnometer or colormetric end-tidal CO_2 (ETCO$_2$) detection device (optional)

Connector from a 5-mm endotracheal tube (if capnography is used to verify placement)

Orogastric or nasogastric tube (Figure 98-1)

NOTE: The type and the size of the tube chosen relate to the size of the patient and the reason for the tube placement. Large-bore tubes are desirable for rapid removal of gastric contents. Smaller-bore tubes are chosen for diagnostics and for removal of air and gastric secretions.

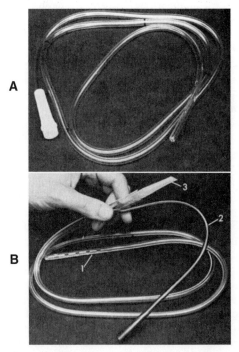

FIGURE 98-1 Two varieties of gastric tubes. **A,** Large-bore tube (Lavacuator, Levin, or Ewald tube). **B,** Salem sump tube: *1,* gastric end with suction eyes; *2,* air vent tube; *3,* adaptor to connect gastric lumen to suction. (From Samuels, L. E. [2004]. Nasogastric and feeding tube placement. In J. R. Roberts & J. R. Hedges [Eds.], *Clinical procedures in emergency medicine* [4th ed., p. 794]. Philadelphia: Saunders.)

The single-lumen tube (Levin) is nonvented; it is used for gastric decompression, lavage, or feeding and should not be attached to suction. The double-lumen tube (Salem sump tube) is chosen if constant air flow and controlled suction force are desired.

Optional for nasopharyngeal anesthesia: Atomizer or mucosal atomization device (MAD; Wolfe Tory Medical, Inc., Salt Lake City, UT) with a 10-ml syringe. Anesthetic (tetracaine, lidocaine, benzocaine) and vasoconstrictor (oxymetazoline, phenylephrine) sprays as prescribed.

PATIENT PREPARATION

1. Position alert patients in an upright or high Fowler's position. Position obtunded or unconscious patients head down, preferably lying on the left side.
2. If the nasogastric route is to be used, choose the largest naris. Have the patient occlude one nostril at a time and take a breath through the open nostril; select the nostril with the best air flow.
3. Estimate the length of the tube needed to reach the stomach by measuring the tube either from the tip of the nose to the earlobe and down to the xiphoid process or from the tip of the nose to the umbilicus. Mark the length (Figure 98-2).

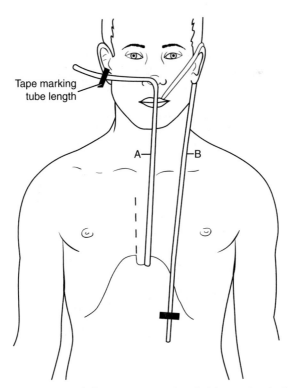

Tape marking tube length

A———B

FIGURE 98-2 Measurement of the nasogastric tube. (Reichman, E., & Simon, R. (2004). *Emergency medicine procedures* [p. 415]. New York: McGraw-Hill).

4. The obtunded or unconscious patient requiring gastric lavage for drug over-dose should be intubated to prevent aspiration.
5. If prescribed, apply a topical anesthetic to reduce pain during tube placement. If using lidocaine jelly, it may be applied to the inside of the nose with a cotton swab 2 to 5 minutes before insertion (DHMC, 2004). Alternatively, anesthetics, such as benzocaine, tetracaine, or lidocaine, with or without a vasoconstrictor, such as oxymetazoline, may be sprayed into the nose and posterior pharynx with an atomizer (Ducharme & Matheson, 2003; Wolfe, Fosnocht, & Linscott, 2000). Do not exceed a 2-second spray of anesthetic. Systemic absorption of benzocaine can have serious adverse effects, including death (FDA, 2006).

PROCEDURAL STEPS

1. Nasogastric placement
   a. Curve the tube by wrapping the end of the tube (4 to 6 inches) around a finger.
   b. Lubricate the tip of the tube, choose the largest naris, and thread the tube through the naris, with the curved end pointing downward. Aim down and back toward the pharynx with the patient's head flexed forward (Figure 98-3).
   c. When the tube reaches the nasopharynx, resistance may be felt. Apply gentle pressure downward to advance the tube. Try to rotate the tube to see whether it will advance. Do not force the tube. If tshe tube still meets resistance, withdraw the tube and try the other side.
   d. When the tube reaches the pharynx, the patient should flex the head forward. Flexing forward is desirable for tube passage in an alert, unconscious, or obtunded patient because it closes off the upper airway to facilitate insertion.
   e. Advance the tube while the patient swallows (either mimicking swallowing or swallowing a small amount of fluid from a cup or straw) until the previously noted level or mark is reached. If the patient coughs, gags, or begins to choke, pull back the tube to let the patient rest. If the patient

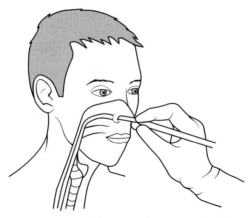

FIGURE 98-3 Placement of a nasogastric tube.

continues to gag, use a tongue blade to check the back of the pharynx to see if the tube is coiled in the back of the pharynx. If tracheal or bronchial intubation is suspected, withdraw the tube before reattempting insertion.

2. Orogastric placement
   a. In an uncooperative patient, place an oral airway or bite block in the mouth before attempting to place the tube. This prevents the patient from biting the tube and obstructing the flow or severing the tube.
   b. Lubricate the tip of the tube and pass it through the lips and over the tongue, aiming down and back toward the pharynx with the patient's head flexed forward (Figure 98-4).
   c. Advance the tube while the patient swallows (either mimicking swallowing or swallowing a small amount of fluid from a cup or straw) until the previously noted mark is reached.

3. Verify the tube position. Use the 60-ml syringe to aspirate gastric contents, and assess the appearance of the aspirate. Gastric contents may be cloudy, grassy green, straw, tan, brown, clear, or off-white (Metheny & Titler, 2001). Test the pH of the aspirate. Gastric pH usually has an acidic range of 1 to 5 (Metheny & Titler, 2001). If either of these findings is not consistent with gastric placement, an additional method of verification is recommended. Additional methods include:
   a. Detection of $ETCO_2$ using a capnometer or a colormetric $ETCO_2$ detector. A colormetric detector is as accurate as capnography for detecting carbon dioxide when a gastric tube is placed (Burnes, 2006). The absence of $ETCO_2$ verifies that the tube is not in the respiratory tract; however, it does not verifiy where in the gastrointestinal tract the tube terminates. This method may be used during tube insertion or after tube insertion.
      i. Insert the ETT connector into distal end of the gastric tube and attach the $ETCO_2$ device.

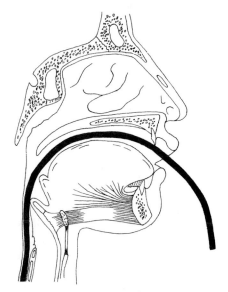

FIGURE 98-4 Placement of an orogastric tube.

    ii. Observe the $ETCO_2$ device. If a CO_2 waveform appears when using a capnometer or the CO_2 level is 15 mm HG or higher, remove the tube. When using a colormetric device, leave it in place for 1 minute. If the color does not change, indicating no CO_2 is present, the tube is correctly placed. If the color turns tan or yellow, indicating the presence of CO_2, remove the tube.

  b. Chest radiograph may be used when patient is at risk for malposition of the tube or other methods are inconclusive. Patients at high risk for malposition include intubated patients and those with an altered level of consciousness.

NOTE: The traditional method of instilling air while auscultating over the epigastrium is not reliable because the sound produced cannot differentiate between placement in the bronchus, pleural space, or gastrointestinal tract (Cirgin Ellett, 2004; Metheny & Titler, 2001).

4. Center and secure the tube in place with adhesive tape or with a gastric tube holder. Do not tape the tube to the forehead because this places undue pressure on the nares, resulting in tissue ulceration.

AGE-SPECIFIC CONSIDERATIONS

1. Nasogastric tubes should not be placed in infants because they are obligate nose breathers; use the orogastric route instead.

2. The diameter of the air passages of the nasopharynx is smaller in children, and their tongues are disproportionally large for the oral cavity.

3. Children in distress swallow large amounts of air. This can result in gastric distention, which can compromise an efficient abdominal examination as well as effective ventilation; therefore gastric decompression is a high-priority intervention.

4. Gastric dilation is common in children after traumatic injury and in children being ventilated via bag-mask and may compromise ventilation or lead to vomiting and aspiration.

COMPLICATIONS

1. Hypoxia, cyanosis, or respiratory arrest as a result of inadvertent intubation of the trachea or bronchus

2. Cardiac compromise as a result of vagal response secondary to gagging

3. Injury to the spinal cord if movement occurs during tube insertion in a patient with a spinal injury

4. Intracranial placement if a tube is placed through the nose in a patient with head or facial fractures

5. Nasal irritation or skin erosion, rhinorrhea, sinusitis, esophagitis, esophago-tracheal fistula, gastric ulceration, or pulmonary and oral infections from prolonged tube placement

6. Epistaxis from trauma during tube insertion

7. Vomiting and aspiration resulting in aspiration pneumonia secondary to a gagging response as the tube is passed

8. Aspiration secondary to incorrect tube position. Reassess tube position before instilling any medication, feeding, or irrigating.

9. Pharyngeal paralysis, vocal cord paralysis, and rupture of esophageal varices

PATIENT TEACHING

1. Report any respiratory difficulty or displacement of the tube immediately.
2. Do not manipulate or reposition the tube.

REFERENCES

Burns, S. M. (2006). Detection of inadverdent airway intubation during gastric tube insertion: Capnography versus a colormetric carbon dioxide detector. *American Journal of Critical Care, 15*(2), 188-193.

Cirgin Ellett, M. L. (2004). What is known about methods of correctly placing gastric tubes in adults and children? *Gastroenterology Nursing, 27*(6), 253-259.

Clinical Pharmacology On-Line. (October 2006). Tetracine. *Clinical Pharmacology On-Line*, Version 6.10. Retrieved December 6, 2006, from www.http://cponline.hitchcock.org

Dartmouth-Hitchcock Medical Center (DHMC). (2004). *Nasogastric or orogastric tube: Insertion, verification, & monitoring (adult critical care policy/procedure)*. Lebanon, NH: Author.

Ducharme, J., & Matheson, K. (2003). What is the best topical anesthetic for nasogastric insertion? A comparison of lidocaine gel, lidocaine spray and aromized cocaine. *Journal of Emergency Nursing, 29*(5), 427-430.

Food & Drug Administration (FDA). (2006). *FDA Public Health Advisory: Benzocaine sprays marketed under different names, including Hurricaine, Topex, and Cetacaine*. Retrieved February 17, 2007, from http://www.fda.gov/cder/drug/advisory/benzocaine.htm

Metheny, N. A., & Titler, M. G. (2001). Assessing placement of feeding tubes. *American Journal of Nursing, 101*(5), 36-45.

Wolfe, T. R., Fosnocht, D. E., & Linscott, M. S. (2000). Atomized lidocaine as topical anesthesia for nasogastric tube placement: A randomized, double-blind, placebo-controlled trial. *Annals of Emergency Medicine, 35*, 421-425.

PROCEDURE 99

Gastric Lavage for Gastrointestinal Bleeding

Joni Hentzen Daniels, MSN, RN, CEN, CCRN

In a gastrointestinal (GI) emergency, the primary clinical concern should be hemodynamic stability. The overall mortality of GI bleeding is approximately 10% and has not changed significantly since the 1960s (Henneman, 2006).

INDICATIONS

1. To control an acute upper-GI hemorrhage when other interventions are not immediately available. Other interventions may include electrocoagulation,

injection sclerotherapy, photocoagulation (laser technology), vasoactive infusion (usually vasopressin), octreotide infusion, and transcatheter embolization.

NOTE: Gastric lavage is still being performed to control acute GI hemorrhage, but its therapeutic value has not been proved. In many facilities, emergency departments have access to endoscopy units capable of performing esophagogastroduodenoscopy, the primary method of identifying the site of upper GI hemorrhage (Yuan, Padol, & Hunt, 2006).

2. To remove irritating gastric secretions and prevent nausea and vomiting through gastric decompression.
3. To obtain information on the site and rate of bleeding.
4. To help evacuate clots (Maltz, 2003).

CONTRAINDICATIONS AND CAUTIONS

1. In the presence of GI hemorrhage, irrigation can knock the clot off a bleeding vessel and cause further bleeding, resulting in shock.
2. If the patient has a gag reflex but is obtunded or if the patient does not have a gag reflex, there is risk of aspiration if vomiting occurs during lavage. Endotracheal intubation should be considered in order to protect the airway.
3. Airway protection by an endotracheal tube is not absolute. Assurance of gastric placement of the lavage tube is necessary before instilling anything in a patient who is confused, obtunded, sedated, or resisting the procedure (see Procedure 98).
4. Patients with symptoms suggestive of a perforated viscus (e.g., severe pain, abdominal ridgidity) should have a radiograph to exclude the presence of free air. If perforation is present, lavage should not be performed.
5. Controversy exists regarding the use of iced or room-temperature solution. Some authors believe that iced solution causes a local vasoconstriction, resulting in decreased bleeding and in clot formation. Others maintain that cold temperatures stimulate hydrochloric acid production, thereby adding to gastric irritation. Iced solutions may cause hypothermia and prolong bleeding times; room-temperature solutions have been shown effective in clearing the stomach and promoting hemostasis (Maltz, 2003).
6. The traditional method of instilling air while auscultating over the epigastrium to verify tube placement is not reliable as the sound produced cannot distinguish between placement in the bronchus, pleural space or gastrointestional tract (Cirgin Ellett, 2004). Metheny and Titler (2001) report that there is little scientific evidence to support the use of this method and that the literature contains numerous reports of its ineffectiveness. See Procedure 98 for additional information about verifying tube placement.

EQUIPMENT

Gastric tube (usually a large 26 Fr to 32 Fr gastric lavage tube)
Irrigation tray
Adhesive tape
Lubricating jelly (lidocaine gel may be used if ordered for patient comfort)
Cetacaine spray (may be ordered to locally numb the throat for comfort)
60-ml catheter-tip syringe

Tincture of benzoin
Normal saline or tap water
Bite block
Suction equipment

PATIENT PREPARATION

1. Protect the patient's airway from aspiration by endotracheal intubation if indicated (see Procedures 8 through 11).
2. Have suction equipment readily available.
3. Place the patient on the cardiac monitor and pulse oximeter (see Procedures 55 and 21) and assess the vital signs every 5 to 10 minutes.
4. Insert at least one large-bore intravenous line; two lines are preferred. Send blood samples for type and crossmatch as indicated (see Procedures 60 and 58).
5. Insert a gastric tube in the mouth or nose using lubricating jelly and topical anesthetics and verify gastric placement (see Procedure 98). If the gastric tube is inserted via the mouth, a bite block with a hole for the tube to pass through is preferable.
6. Place the patient in left lateral decubitus position with the bed in Trendelenburg position or semi-Fowler's position.

PROCEDURAL STEPS

1. Pour normal saline or tap water into an irrigation container.
2. Draw up the solution using a 60-ml syringe and inject it into the gastric tube. Alternatively, use a preassembled lavage setup (see Procedure 100). Infuse approximately 200 to 300 ml.
3. Aspirate or drain the solution from the stomach and discard it into a measured basin.
4. Repeat until active bleeding stops or until the patient is transferred to endoscopy.
5. Measure the volumes of irrigant and aspirant, and document as intake and output.

AGE-SPECIFIC CONSIDERATIONS

1. Older persons are far more likely than younger adults to experience significant morbidity and death from untreated GI conditions or emergencies. Most deaths reulting from GI bleeding occur in patients over the age of 60 (Henneman, 2006). Patient complaints may include vomiting blood or passing blood in the stool but may also be less obvious with complaints of dizziness, weakness, or syncope.
2. Beware of patients on β-blockers. β-Blockers prevent tachycardia, thereby preventing normal compensatory responses and potentially masking symptoms of hypovolemia.
3. Lower GI bleeding requiring admission is more common in children than adults (Henneman, 2006).

COMPLICATIONS

1. Perforation of esophageal varices

2. Mallory-Weiss tear resulting from repeated vomiting, a sharp increase in intraabdominal pressure from overdistention of the stomach, or aggressive insertion of the lavage tube
3. Aspiration of gastric contents into an unprotected airway
4. Systemic hypothermia if the lavage is prolonged or large quantities of cold irrigant are used

REFERENCES

Cirgin Ellett, M. L. (2004). What is known about methods of correctly placing gastric tubes in adults and children? *Gastroenterology Nursing, 27*(6), 253-259.

Henneman, P. L. (2006). Gastrointestinal bleeding. In J. A. Marx, R. S. Hockberger, & R. M. Walls, et al. (Eds.), *Rosen's emergency medicine: Concepts and clinical practice* (6th ed., pp. 220-227). St Louis: Mosby.

Maltz, C. (2003). Acute gastrointestinal bleeding. *Best practice of medicine*, February 2003, 1–19. Retrieved August 31, 2006, from http://merck.micromedex.com/index

Metheny, N. A., & Titler, M. G. (2001). Assessing placement of feeding tubes. *American Journal of Nursing, 101*(5), 36-45.

Yuan, Y., Padol, I. T., & Hunt, R. H. (2006). Peptic ulcer disease today. *Nature Clinical Practice Gastroenterology & Hepatology, 3*(2), 80-89.

PROCEDURE 100

Gastric Lavage for Removal of Toxic Substances

Robin A. Scott, RN, ND, and *Jean A. Proehl, RN, MN, CEN, CCRN, FAEN*

Gastric lavage for removal of toxic substances is also known as *gastric decontamination, orogastric lavage, gastric emptying,* and *stomach pumping.*

INDICATION

To assist in the removal of toxic substances or poisons from the stomach, thereby decreasing drug availability and absorption in the body. The effectiveness of gastric lavage is time dependent and is most effective when the procedure is completed within 60 minutes of ingestion (Heard, 2005). Gastric lavage should not routinely be used in managing poisoned patients; instead, gastric lavage should be consider for use in patients who have ingested a potentially life-threatening amount of poison (AACT & EAPCCT, 2000). Lavage can remove drugs either in whole or fragments; however, the amount of drug recovered from the stomach can vary widely (Bartlett & Muller, 2003). Contact your Poison Control Center using the national access number, 1-800-222-1222, for current recommendations regarding the treatment of specific ingestions.

CONTRAINDICATIONS AND CAUTIONS

1. Clinical studies cannot confirm the benefits of gastric lavage as a stand-alone treatment for poisoned patients. The amount of ingested substance that is retrieved using gastric lavage is on average very low, approximately 30% (Bartlett & Muller, 2003).
2. If a patient is unable to protect the airway, then gastric lavage should not be performed unless the patient is intubated (Heard, 2005).
3. Lavage is contraindicated for patients who have ingested a corrosive material or sharp objects (AACT & EAPCCT, 2000).
4. Lavage is contraindicated in patients who have ingested a substance that may cause seizures or abrupt central nervous system depression unless the patient is intubated (Heard, 2005).
5. Gastric lavage may propel stomach contents into the small intestine, which increases the chance of drug absorption (AACT & EAPCCT, 2000).
6. Patients at risk for gastrointestinal bleeding or perforation secondary to pathology, recent surgery, or other medical history should not undergo gastric lavage (AACT & EAPCCT, 2000).
7. Airway protection by an endotracheal tube is not absolute. Careful assessment of gastric placement of the lavage tube is necessary before instilling fluid, especially in a patient who is confused, obtunded, sedated, or resisting the procedure.
8. The gastric lavage procedure is complete when pill fragments are no longer seen in the lavage fluid; however, there is no clearly defined endpoint for the procedure in cases where pill fragments are not seen in the lavage fluid (Heard, 2005).
9. The traditional method of instilling air while auscultating over the epigastrium to confirm tube placement is not reliable as the sound produced cannot distinguish between placement in the bronchus, pleural space or gastrointestinal tract (Cirgin Ellett, 2004). Metheny and Titler (2001) report that there is little scientific evidence to support the use of this method and that the literature contains numerous reports of its ineffectiveness. See Procedure 98 for additional information about verifying tube placement.

EQUIPMENT

Pharyngeal suction equipment
Bite block
Cardiac and pulse oximetry monitoring equipment
Orogastric tube
- 36 to 40 Fr for adults (Heard, 2005)
- 24 to 32 Fr for children

60-ml irrigating syringe with catheter tip
Lavage tubing setup (commercially available or may be constructed with Y-cystoscopy tubing, suction extension tubing, and enema bags)
Tubing clamps

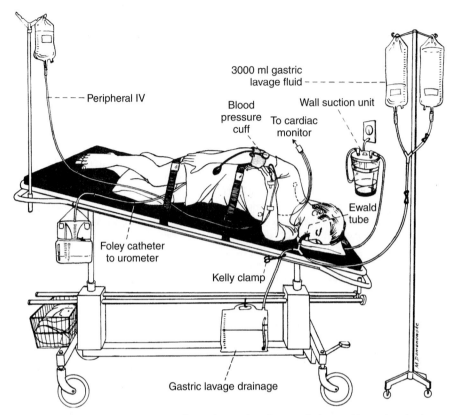

FIGURE 100-1 Correct positioning for patient undergoing gastric lavage. The patient is shown uncovered with side rails down for illustration purposes only. The patient should be covered to maintain body temperature and preserve privacy; side rails should be up for safety. (From Luckman, J., & Sorenson, K. [1987]. *Medical-surgical nursing: A psychophysiologic approach* [3rd ed., p. 1934]. Philadelphia: Saunders.)

Tap water or warm normal saline (Heard, 2005)
Endotracheal intubation supplies and restraints (as indicated and prescribed)
Activated charcoal (if indicated and prescribed)

PATIENT PREPARATION

1. Set up pharyngeal suction equipment (see Procedure 29).
2. Initiate pulse oximetry monitoring (see Procedure 21) and cardiac monitoring (see Procedure 55).
3. Restrain the patient as indicated and prescribed (see Procedure 190).
4. Obtain intravenous access (Procedure 60).
5. Assess the patient's level of consciousness, gag reflex, and ability to maintain airway. Remove dental appliances. Request endotracheal intubation if indicated (Procedures 8 through 11).
6. Assemble the lavage tubing and prime it with fluid.

7. Insert a large-bore orogastric tube and verify tube placement according to Procedure 98. Place a bite block to keep the patient from biting the tube.

PROCEDURAL STEPS

1. Aspirate the stomach contents and save the initial sample for a toxicology screen.
2. Unclamp the tubing between the fluid bag and the patient, and instill 200–300 ml of warmed fluid (Heard, 2005). Warming the fluid helps prevent hypothermia and may increase the efficacy of emptying (Gorelick, 1997). Reclamp the tubing.
3. Unclamp the tubing between the patient and the drainage source, and allow the fluid to drain into the bucket by use of gravity. If no fluid returns, use the syringe to pull the fluid and the particles gently through the tube. Position change may assist with fluid return. Do not use continuous suction to remove the fluid because this may result in gastric mucosal damage. Keep a running tally of the fluid input and output.
4. Repeat steps 1 and 2 until the fluid return is clear of stomach contents. If no gastric contents return, it is likely that the substance is in the small intestine or that large pill fragments are present and cannot traverse the tube.
5. If prescribed, instill activated charcoal before removing the lavage tube.

AGE-SPECIFIC CONSIDERATIONS

1. Children are more prone to the vagal stimulation associated with endotracheal and gastric intubation and gastric lavage; monitor the heart rate carefully and consider premedication with atropine.
2. Use 10-ml/kg aliquots of warmed fluid for children. Do not use tap water to lavage a child's stomach because children are more prone to electrolyte imbalances such as hyponatremia (AACT & EAPCCT, 2000). Use saline in gastric lavage of children to decrease risk of electrolyte imbalances (Blazys, 2000).
3. Ensure fluids are warm to decrease the risk of hypothermia, especially in children who are at higher risk of hypothermia (AACT & EAPCCT, 2000).

COMPLICATIONS

1. Tracheal placement of lavage tube (AACT & EAPCCT, 2000)
2. Aspiration
3. Pneumonia
4. Hypoxia
5. Stomach, esophageal, and throat injuries
6. Laryngospasm (AACT & EAPCCT, 2000)
7. Fluid and electrolyte imbalances (AACT & EAPCCT, 2000)
8. Vagal stimulation leading to bradycardia (Bartlett & Muller, 2003)
9. Hypothermia (AACT & EAPCCT, 2000)

REFERENCES

American Academy of Clinical Toxicology (AACT) and European Association of Poison Centres and Clinical Toxicologists (EAPCCT). (2000). Position statement: Gastric lavage. *Journal of Clinical Toxicology, 38,* 689-690.

Bartlett, D., & Muller, A. (Eds.). (2003). The ABCs of gastric decontamination. *Journal of Emergency Nursing, 29*, 576–577.

Blazys, D. (2000). Use of lavage in treating overdose: Are we still using lavage when treating a patient who has overdosed? *Journal of Emergency Nursing, 26*, 343-345.

Cirgin Ellett, M. L. (2004). What is known about methods of correctly placing gastric tubes in adults and children? *Gastroenterology Nursing, 27*(6), 253-259.

Gorelick, M. (1997). Gastric emptying. In R. A. Dieckmann, D. H. Fiser, & S. M. Selbst (Eds.), *Pediatric emergency and critical care procedures*. St Louis: Mosby.

Heard, K. (2005). Gastrointestinal decontamination. *Medical Clinics of North America, 89*, 1067-1078.

Metheny, N. A., & Titler, M. G. (2001). Assessing placement of feeding tubes. *American Journal of Nursing, 101*(5), 36-45.

PROCEDURE 101

Whole Bowel Irrigation

Andrew J. Bowman, RN, MSN, CEN, CTRN, CCRN-CMC, BC, CVN-I, FACCN, NREMT-P

Whole bowel irrigation (WBI) involves having a patient drink, or be given via a nasogastric or orogastric tube, a solution of an electrolyte-balanced polyethylene glycol solution (GoLYTELY, NuLYTELY, etc). This solution is delivered at a rate of up to 2 L/hr in an effort to mechanically flush the gastrointestinal (GI) tract and reduce absorption of certain ingested agents. Although WBI should not be used as a routine approach to GI decontamination in patients with an ingested toxin, its use should be considered for potentially toxic ingestions of sustained-release preparations or enteric-coated drugs, especially for patients who present more than 2 hours after ingestion (AACT & EAPCCT, 2004). The hypothetical endpoint is the presence of a clear rectal effluent (Krenzelok, 2002). Although volunteer studies show a decrease in drug bioavailability after WBI (Erickson AKS, Gussow, & Williams, 2001), there is no conclusive evidence that WBI improves the outcome for the poisoned patient (AACT & EAPCCT, 2004). Contact your Poison Control Center using the national access number, 1-800-222-1222, for current recommendations regarding the treatment of specific ingestions.

INDICATIONS

To decontaminate the GI tract when other methods are ineffective or inadequate. Indications for WBI may include the following (AACT & EAPCCT, 2004; Erickson et al., 2001; Farmer & Chan, 2002; Krenzelok, 2002; McLaughlin, 2005):

1. Substances that are not well bound by activated charcoal (e.g., iron, lithium, lead, zinc)
2. Medications that are slowly released over 12 to 24 hours (sustained-release preparations), especially when serum drug levels continue to rise or the patient continues to deteriorate
3. Massive ingestions with a significant delay in presentation
4. Toxic solid object (e.g., drug-filled packets or vials, or condoms filled with heroin or cocaine such as those found in body packers)
5. Presence of pharmacobezoars (as may be seen with aspirin ingestion)

CONTRAINDICATIONS AND CAUTIONS

1. WBI is contraindicated in the presence of significant GI hemorrhage, bowel obstruction, perforation, ileus, absent gag reflex, uncontrollable intractable vomiting, hemodynamic instability, or compromised unprotected airway (AACT & EAPCCT, 2004; McLaughlin, 2005).
2. Nausea and bloating are common; vomiting with aspiration is a risk. Anal irritation and discomfort secondary to diarrhea are common (AACT & EAPCCT, 2004; McLaughlin, 2005).
3. The patient must remain sitting on a commode or bedpan for a prolonged time, so this procedure is not appropriate for patients who may be clinically unstable or at risk for a depressed level of consciousness (AACT & EAPCCT, 2004).
4. Aggressive use of antiemetics may be required to control vomiting. Metoclopramide or ondansetron may be used (AACT & EAPCCT, 2004).
5. Polyethylene glycol electrolyte solution decreases the adsorptive capacity of activated charcoal and therapeutic drugs (AACT & EAPCCT, 2004).
6. The traditional method of instilling air while auscultating over the epigastrium to confirm tube placement is not reliable as the sound produced cannot distinguish between placement in the bronchus, pleural space, or gastrointestinal tract (Cirgin Ellett, 2004). Metheny and Titler (2001) report that there is little scientific evidence to support the use of this method and that the literature contains numerous reports of its ineffectiveness. See Procedure 98 for additional information about verifying tube placement.

EQUIPMENT

Small-bore gastric tube (if indicated), minimum of 12 Fr for an adult (AACT & EAPCCT, 2004)
Enteral feeding bag (if indicated)
Bedside commode or bedpan
2 to 8 L of a polyethylene glycol–balanced electrolyte solution (PEG-EBS) (e.g., GoLYTELY, Colyte)

PATIENT PREPARATION

1. Insert a gastric tube if the patient is unwilling or unable to drink the pre-scribed amount of solution (see Procedure 98). Most patients have difficulty drinking an adequate amount of solution at the required rate, and gastric intubation facilitates the procedure (AACT & EAPCCT, 2004).
2. Place the patient on a commode; an upright posture aids in evacuation of the bowel (AACT & EAPCCT, 2004). If the patient cannot sit on a commode, a bedpan may be used with the patient's head elevated.

PROCEDURAL STEPS

1. Administer the PEG-EBS either orally or by gastric tube at 1 to 2 L/hr (AACT & EAPCCT, 2004; Krenzelok, 2002; McLaughlin, 2005). Start at the lower amount and increase to 2 L/hr as the patient tolerates it.
2. If vomiting occurs, slow the administration rate, and gradually increase the rate as tolerated. Antiemetics may be prescribed to control vomiting.
3. Continue administration of the solution until the rectal effluent is clear. This process varies in time according to the substance and amount being removed. If a radiopaque substance (iron, lithium) was ingested, con-tinue until there is no radiographic evidence of toxin remaining in the GI tract.

AGE-SPECIFIC CONSIDERATIONS

1. The pediatric dose for WBI is 500 ml/hr (25 ml/kg/hr) for children aged 1 to 6 years and 1 L/hr for children aged 6 to 12 years (AACT & EAPCCT, 2004; Erickson et al., 2001).
2. Children are more prone to hypothermia; warm the fluid to 37° C (98.6° F) to help avoid this complication.

COMPLICATIONS

1. Aspiration, nausea, vomiting, abdominal cramping, bloating, or distention (AACT & EAPCCT, 2004). These effects can be decreased by keeping the head of the bed elevated or slowing the rate of administration. Consider administering an antiemetic (AACT & EAPCCT, 2004; Kulig, 2001). Metoclopramide is recommended if an antiemetic is indicated because improves GI mobility (Holstege & Baer, 2004).
2. Hypoglycemia may occur if WBI use exceeds 6 hours.
3. Rectal irritation can be decreased by discouraging the patient from wiping until the procedure has been completed.

PATIENT TEACHING

1. Sitting up on the commode is important to help move material through the bowel. Notify the nurse immediately if dizziness or light-headedness occurs. If this procedure is used for someone who must lie in the bed, the copious amounts of liquid stool it produces require frequent linen change.
2. Frequent wiping may cause rectal irritation; try not to wipe until the entire procedure is finished.
3. The procedure may take 4 to 6 hours to complete (Erickson et al., 2001).
4. Additional liquid bowel movements may occur after completion of WBI (AACT & EAPCCT, 2004).

REFERENCES

American Academy of Clinical Toxicology (AACT) and European Association of Poison Centres and Clinical Toxicologists (EAPCCT). (2004). Position paper: Whole bowel irrigation. *Clinical Toxicology*, *42*, 843-854.

Cirgin Ellett, M. L. (2004). What is known about methods of correctly placing gastric tubes in adults and children? *Gastroenterology Nursing*, *27*(6), 253-259.

Erickson, T., Aks, S., Gussow, L., & Williams, R. (2001). Toxicology update: A rational approach to managing the poisoned patient. *Emergency Medicine Practice*, *3*(8), 1-28.

Farmer, J., & Chan, S. (2003). Whole bowel irrigation for contraband bodypackers. *Journal of Clinical Gastroenterology*, *37*(2), 147-150.

Holstege, C. P., & Baer, A. B. (2004). Decontamination of the poisoned patient. In J. R. Roberts, & J. R. Hedges (Eds.), *Clinical procedures in emergency medicine* (4th ed., pp. 824-840). Philadelphia: Saunders.

Krenzelok, E. (2002). New developments in the therapy of intoxications. *Toxicology Letters*, *127*, 299-305.

Kulig, K. (2001). Gastrointestinal decontamination. In M. Ford, K. Delaney, L. Ling, & T. Erickson (Eds.), *Clinical toxicology* (pp. 34-41). Philadelphia: Saunders.

McLaughlin, S. (2005). Toxicologic emergencies. In S. Mahadevan, & G. Garmel (Eds.), *An introduction to clinical emergency medicine* (pp. 531-542). Cambridge, England: Cambridge University Press.

Metheny, N. A., & Titler, M. G. (2001). Assessing placement of feeding tubes. *American Journal of Nursing*, *101*(5), 36-45.

PROCEDURE 102

Balloon Tamponade of Gastroesophageal Varices

Jean A. Proehl, RN, MN, CEN, CCRN, FAEN

Balloon tubes for the tamponade of gastroesophageal varices are also known as *Sengstaken-Blakemore (SB) tube, Minnesota (MN) tube,* and *Linton-Nachlas (LN) tube.*

INDICATIONS

1. To temporarily control severe bleeding from gastroesophageal varices or Mallory-Weiss tears unresponsive to other interventions or when other interventions are unavailable or contraindicated.

2. To control bleeding from the rectum, uterus, or aortoesophageal fistula. These uses are uncommon and are not addressed in this procedure.

CONTRAINDICATIONS AND CAUTIONS

1. Because of the potential for serious complications, including death, more conservative measures, such as pharmacologic therapy (using octreotide, vasopressin and nitroglycerin, somatostatin) or endoscopic treatments (sclerotherapy, banding), are usually attempted first.
2. Absolute contraindications include a history of esophageal stricture, recent surgery of the gastroesophageal junction, or if the bleeding has already stopped based on the appearance of gastric aspirate (Attar, 2004).
3. Nasal insertion is more difficult and is associated with more complications; therefore, the oral route is preferred (Attar, 2004). A history of transsphenoidal hypophysectomy is an absolute contraindication to nasal insertion (Day, 2005). Relative contraindications to nasal insertion include coagulopathy or a history of nasal trauma, deformity, or surgery.
4. Caution should be exercised in the presence of esophageal pathology (e.g., strictures, cancer, caustic ingestion) or significant concurrent medical problems (respiratory or congestive heart failure, arrhythmias).
5. Note that air insufflation with simultaneous auscultation over the epigastric region is not an accurate or reliable method for assessing the placement of gastric tubes. Chong (2005) reported three fatal cases of esophageal rupture associated with inflation of the gastric balloon after using only auscultation to verify tube placement.
6. Air is usually used to inflate the balloons because using water makes the balloon heavy and increases the risk of pressure necrosis of the mucosa (Attar, 2004). Also, water is more difficult to remove if emergency deflation of the balloon(s) becomes necessary (Attar, 2004). However, some physicians use water or water mixed with a radiographic contrast solution (Christensen, 2004).
7. To avoid introducing particulate matter, which may obstruct a balloon lumen, use a clean syringe to inflate the balloons.
8. Never deflate the gastric balloon while the esophageal balloon is inflated; this may result in upward tube migration and airway obstruction.
9. Spray medications used for posterior pharyngeal anesthesia should not exceed 2 seconds of application time. Systemic absorption of benzocaine can have serious adverse effects including death (FDA, 2006).

EQUIPMENT

Gastroesophageal balloon tube (Figure 102-1). Options include the following:
- SB, a triple-lumen, double-balloon tube. One lumen functions as a gastric tube, another is used to inflate or deflate the gastric balloon, and the third is used to inflate or deflate the esophageal balloon.
- MN, a quadruple-lumen tube. It is the same as an SB tube, but it also has a lumen that terminates just proximal to the esophageal balloon. This lumen is attached to suction to remove oropharyngeal secretions that accumulate in the esophagus.
- LN, a modified Linton tube with a larger gastric balloon and a port to drain the esophagus.

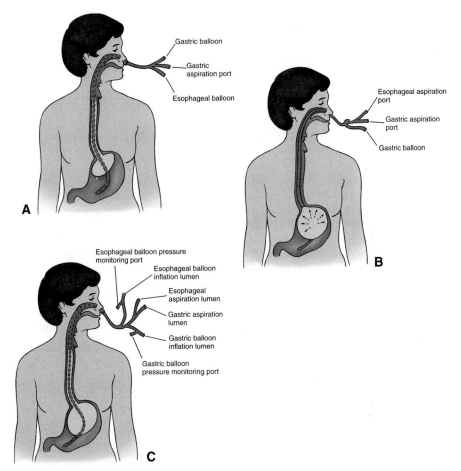

FIGURE 102-1 A, Sengstaken-Blakemore tube. **B,** Linton-Nachlas tube. **C,** Minnesota tube. (From Urden, L., Stacy, K., & Lough, M. [2006]. *Thelan's critical care nursing: Diagnosis and management* [5th ed.]. St. Louis: Mosby.)

Gastric tube (not necessary if an MN or LN is used)

Lubricating jelly (anesthetic jelly may be used if prescribed)

Local vasoconstrictor (e.g., oxymetazoline) for nasal passages (optional for nasal route only)

Topical anesthetic (viscous lidocaine, benzocaine) (optional)

Two or three 60-ml catheter-tip syringes

Bite block

Four rubber-shod clamps

One or two aneroid manometer(s) (handheld with integral bulb preferred)

Two Y-connectors or Lopez valves (a three-way stopcock that can accommodate a catheter tip syringe, manufactured by ICU Medical, San Clemente, CA)

Two intermittent suction sources

Adhesive tape

Foam rubber to pad nares

Catcher's mask or helmet with face mask (football or hockey), or commercial mask or traction setup with 1 to 3 lb weight

Normal saline solution or tap water for irrigation

Scissors

PATIENT PREPARATION

1. Intubation should be seriously considered to protect the patient's airway and help prevent aspiration, especially for patients with altered mental status (see Procedures 8 through 11).
2. Empty the stomach via lavage (see Procedure 99) and then remove the gastric tube. Failure to empty the stomach may result in vomiting and aspiration during the tube insertion.
3. Spray a topical vasoconstrictor into the nose (if prescribed).
4. *Anesthetize the conscious patient's nasopharynx (optional). Some sources discourage this practice because anesthetizing the nasopharynx may decrease the gag reflex and increase the risk of aspiration (Day, 2005). Do not exceed a 2-second spray of anesthetic. Systemic absorption of benzocaine can have serious adverse effects including death (FDA, 2006).
5. If possible, elevate the head of the bed to a 45-degree angle or higher. If the patient cannot sit upright, left lateral decubitus is acceptable. The supine position may be used with intubated patients.
6. Emergency endoscopy to diagnose the presence of esophageal varices usually precedes tube placement and may improve success rates (Attar, 2004; Pinto-Marques, Romaozinho, Ferreira, Amaro, & Freitas, 2006).

PROCEDURAL STEPS

1. Inflate both balloons with the maximum recommended amount of air and submerge them under water to check for leaks.
2. Using a Y-connector, connect each balloon inflation port to a manometer. See Figure 102-2 for assembly of the manometer and Y-connector. Alternately a Lopez valve can be used in place of the Y-connector; the three ports are attached to (1) manometer, (2) 60-ml catheter-tip syringe, and (3) one side of the gastric or esophageal balloon Y-set (Figure 102-3) (Greenwald, 2004a). The other end of each Y-set is then plugged or clamped. If clamps are used, they should be padded and applied to the thicker end of the port to prevent rupture, with resultant leaking of the balloon or crushing of the lumen, which can lead to tube impaction (Greenwald, 2004b).
3. Measure and record the pressure of the esophageal balloon when fully inflated and the pressure in the gastric balloon at 100-ml intervals up to maximal inflation; the pressures should decrease as the volume increases (Day, 2005; Greenwald, 2004b). Deflate both balloons completely and leave a manometer connected to the gastric balloon lumen for insertion.
4. *Pass the lubricated tube through the patient's mouth or nose to about the 50-cm mark (40-cm mark for 12-Fr tube) or at least 10 cm past the estimated

---

*Indicates portions of the procedure usually performed by a physician or an advanced practice nurse.

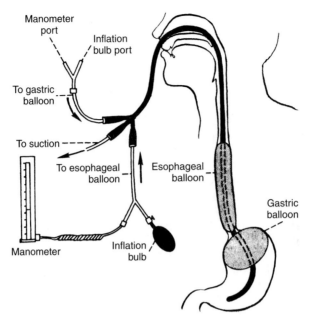

FIGURE 102-2 Measuring balloon pressure in a Sengstaken-Blakemore tube using a manometer. (From Smolen, D. [2001]. Management of clients with hepatic disorders. In J. M. Black, J. Hokanson Hawks, & A. M. Keene [Eds.], *Medical-surgical nursing: Clinical management for positive outcomes* [6th ed., p. 1242]. Philadelphia: Saunders.)

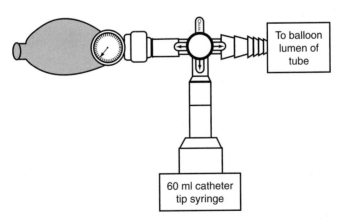

FIGURE 102-3 Assembly of Lopez valve, handheld manometer, and 60-ml catheter-tip syringe used to monitor the pressure in both gastric and esophageal balloons and to inflate the esophageal balloon.

insertion depth as measured for standard gastric tube placement (see Procedure 98) (Attar, 2004; Day, 2005). Fold the balloons around the tube to facilitate its passage. Place a bite block to prevent the patient from biting through the tube if the tube is inserted orally. Coiling of the tube during insertion is not uncommon. To prevent this, a guide wire may be inserted through the gastric aspirate port before insertion (Kaza & Rigas, 2002).

5. Attach the gastric suction port to intermittent suction (60 to 120 mm Hg) (Day, 2005; Greenwald, 2005b). Attach the esophageal suction port (MN, LN tubes only) to 120 to 200 mm Hg intermittent suction (Day, 2005; Greenwald, 2005b).

6. Assess placement via the gastric suction port per usual protocols, such as pH, appearance of aspirate, absence of end-tidal CO_2, etc. See Procedure 98 for details.

7. *Further verify tube position by instilling 50 to 100 ml of air into the gastric balloon and obtaining a chest radiograph (Chong, 2005). Other options to help ensure proper tube placement include insertion with endoscopy or fluoroscopy. Ultrasound may also confirm that the tube has traversed the lower esophageal sphincter into the stomach (Lin, Hsu, Wang, & Chong, 2006). If the patient complains of chest pain or the pressure in the gastric balloon is more than 15 mm Hg higher than baseline (indicators that the gastric tube is in the esophagus), deflate the balloon immediately and advance it another 10 cm (Attar, 2004; Day, 2005).

8. *Instill additional air in 50- to 100-ml increments into the gastric balloon per manufacturer's recommendations (a total of 250 to 300 ml in SB, 600 ml in LN, 400 ml in MN) and double-clamp the port (Attar, 2004). Monitor the patient carefully for chest pain during inflation of the gastric balloon because it may signal that the balloon is inappropriately positioned in the esophagus. In this instance, the balloon should be deflated and the tube advanced further.

9. Repeat chest radiograph to verify tube placement after full inflation (Chong, 2005).

10. *Exert gentle traction on the tube to pull up the gastric balloon and compress the varices in the upper stomach. The traction is maintained by fastening the tube to a helmet or catcher's mask placed on the patient or by using a standard traction setup with 1 to 3 lb of weight (Attar, 2004; Day, 2005).

11. Lavage the gastric suction port to clear large clots.

12. *If bleeding continues, inflate the esophageal balloon to 25 mm Hg of pressure and double-clamp the port. The bulb of the manometer can be used to inflate the esophageal balloon (Greenwald, 2004a). If the bleeding continues, add air to increase the balloon pressure in 5–mm Hg increments until the bleeding stops or to a maximum pressure of 45 mm Hg (Attar, 2004). NOTE: The LN tube does not have an esophageal balloon.

13. (SB tube only) Insert a small gastric tube through the mouth or the opposite naris to the top of the esophageal balloon and attach to 120 to 200 mm Hg

*Indicates portions of the procedure usually performed by a physician or an advanced practice nurse.

intermittent suction to remove oropharyngeal secretions and assess for proximal bleeding sites (Day, 2005).

14. Pad the nares with foam rubber to help prevent pressure necrosis as a result of the tube (for nasally inserted tubes).

15. Clearly label the ports of the tube so that the gastric balloon is not inadvertently deflated (see Complications). Consider taping both clamps closed on each (inflated) balloon port and labeling them "Do not touch or remove" (Dartmouth-Hitchcock Medical Center, 2006).

16. Lavage for gastrointestinal bleeding may continue through the gastric port as prescribed.

17. Sedate and restrain the patient as necessary to prevent the tube from becoming dislodged (see Procedure 190).

18. If possible, keep the head of the bed elevated at a 30- to 45-degree angle to help keep the stomach empty and decrease aspiration risk.

19. Place a pair of scissors in an easily visible and accessible location in case it is necessary to cut the tube and rapidly deflate the balloons to remove the tube.

20. Check balloon pressures hourly or continuously (Day, 2005). A handheld manometer with integrated bulb can be left on the port(s) continuously (Greenwald, 2004a). Pressures in the esophageal balloon will vary with respirations and may intermittantly reach 70 mm Hg (Day, 2005). The esophageal balloon may be intermittantly deflated; sources vary on this recommendation from 30 minutes every 8 to 12 hours (Day, 2005; Paskus, 2007) to 1 hour every 4 hours (Dartmouth-Hitchcock Medical Center, 2006).

21. If removal of the tube is necessary, the esophageal balloon is always deflated first except in emergencies where both balloons are deflated simultaneously by cutting the tube proximal to both inflation ports.

AGE-SPECIFIC CONSIDERATIONS

1. The SB tube is available in three sizes (Paskus, 2007):
   - Child: 12 Fr, 30 inches long with a 4.5-in esophageal balloon
   - Intermediate: 16 Fr, 39 inches long with a 6-in esophageal balloon
   - Adult: 20 Fr, 39 inches long with an 8-in esophageal balloon

2. Children usually require sedation to tolerate the tube (Paskus, 2007).

3. The recommended pressure for the esophageal balloon in children is 20 to 40 mm Hg (Paskus, 2007).

COMPLICATIONS

1. Airway obstruction as a result of dislodgement of the tube or compression of the trachea. Monitor the patient for respiratory distress, aspiration, or chest pain. Never deflate the gastric balloon with the esophageal balloon inflated or while there is traction on the tube. If the tube becomes dislodged and obstructs the airway, cut the tube below the ports and quickly remove the tube. Always keep a pair of scissors at the bedside for this purpose. A second tube, and supplies for insertion, should be readily available for reinsertion after an airway emergency is controlled.

2. Vomiting and aspiration of gastric contents or oropharyngeal secretions. This can usually be prevented by performing endotracheal intubation,

emptying the stomach before tube insertion, maintaining suction on the gastric port, and placing a proximal gastric tube to remove the secretions when an SB tube is used.

3. Esophageal erosions or rupture as a result of excess pressure in the esophageal balloon or inflation of the gastric balloon in the esophagus. Auscultation is not a reliable method of assessing tube location; radiographs should be obtained prior to full inflation of the gastric tube (Chong, 2005).

4. Atelectasis may result from increased thoracic pressure from the balloon (Simone, 2001).

5. Hiccups (Attar, 2004)

6. Cardiac arrhythmias (Attar, 2004)

7. Pulmonary edema from the pressure of the balloons on mediastinal structures (Attar, 2004)

8. Irritation or ulceration of the nares. This can be decreased by carefully padding the nares with foam rubber.

9. Impaction of the tube is uncommon but should be suspected if there is any difficulty removing it after balloon deflation. Impaction may occur with crushed balloon lumens or the introduction of particulate matter in the balloon lumen (e.g., if a syringe previously used to aspirate gastric contents is used to inflate the balloons) (Greenwald, 2004b).

10. Ruptured balloon(s) with dislodgement, airway obstruction, and/or recurrence of bleeding, depending on which balloon ruptures.

PATIENT TEACHING

1. Immediately report any chest pain, difficulty breathing, or nausea.

2. Do not pull on the tube or attempt to readjust the tube position.

3. To prevent increased bleeding or movement of the tube, it is important that you lie quietly and move only with assistance.

REFERENCES

Attar, B. M. (2004). Balloon tamponade of gastrointestinal bleeding. In E. F. Reichman, & R. R. Simon (Eds.), *Emergency medicine procedures* (pp. 448-456). New York: McGraw-Hill.

Chong, C. (2005). Esophageal rupture due to Sengstaken-Blakemore tube misplacement. *World Journal of Gastroenterology, 11*(41), 6563-6565.

Christensen, T. (2004). The treatment of oesophageal varices using a Sengstaken-Blakemore tube: Considerations for nursing practice. *Nursing in Critical Care, 9*(2), 58-63.

Dartmouth-Hitchcock Medical Center. (2006). *Minnesota four-lumen tubes (esophagogastric)*. Adult Critical Care Policy/Procedure. Lebanon, NH: Author.

Day, M. W. (2005). Esophagogastric tamponade tube. In D. J. Lynn-McHale Wiegand, & K. K. Carlson (Eds.), *AACN procedure manual of critical care* (5th ed., pp. 861-869). Philadelphia: Saunders.

Food & Drug Administration (FDA). (2006). *FDA public health advisory: Benzocaine sprays marketed under different names, including Hurricaine, Topex, and Cetacaine*. Retrieved February 17, 2007, from http://www.fda.gov/cder/drug/advisory/benzocaine.htm

Greenwald, B. (2004a). Two devices that facilitate the use of the Minnesota tube. *Gastroenterology Nursing, 27*, 268-270.

Greenwald, B. (2004b). The Minnesota tube: Its use and care in bleeding esophageal and gastric varices. *Gastroenterology Nursing, 27*, 212-217.

Kaza, C. S., & Rigas, B. (2002). Rapid placement of the Sengstaken-Blakemore tube using a guidewire (letter to the editor). *Journal of Clinical Gastroenterology, 34*, 282.

Lin, A. C., Hsu, Y. H., Wang, T. L., & Chong, C. F. (2006). Placement confirmation of Sengstaken-Blakemore tube by ultrasound. *Emergency Medicine Journal, 23*, 487.

Paskus, L. R. (2007). Esophagogastric tamponade tube: Care and management. In J. T. Verger, & R. M. Lebet (Eds.), *AACN procedure manual for acute and critical pediatric care* (pp. 701-708). Philadelphia: Saunders.

Pinto-Marques, P., Romaozinho, J. M., Ferreira, M., Amaro, P., & Freitas, D. (2006). Esophageal perforation–associated risk with balloon tamponade after endoscopic therapy. Myth or reality? *Hepatogastroenterology, 53*(70), 536-539.

Simone, S. (2001). Gastrointestinal critical care problems. In M. A. Q. Curley, & P. A. Moloney-Harmon (Eds.), *Critical Care Nursing of Infants and Children* (2nd ed., pp. 765-804). Philadelphia: Saunders.

PROCEDURE 103

Diagnostic Bladder Ultrasound

Lucinda W. Rossoll, RN, MSN, CCRN, CEN

Diagnostic bladder ultrasound is also known as *bladder scanning*. The bladder scanner is a portable ultrasound that computes bladder volume with a high degree of accuracy.

INDICATIONS

1. To check bladder volume before and after voiding
2. To diagnose and manage urinary outflow dysfunction
3. To decrease the number of bladder catheterizations necessary to check residual urine volumes, thus reducing catheter-associated urinary tract infections
4. To assess for the minimum amount of urine volume (10 ml) needed for aspiration and thereby increasing the chances for successful suprapubic aspiration with a minimum number of attempts (Munir, Barnett, & South, 2002)

CONTRAINDICATIONS AND CAUTIONS

1. This procedure is not intended for fetal use or for use on pregnant women.
2. Do not use on patients with open wounds in the suprapubic area.

3. Do not use on a patient with an indwelling catheter in the bladder.
4. Scar tissue, staples, sutures, and incision in the suprapubic area may affect the ultrasound transmission.
5. Do not use on patients with ascites.
6. Ovarian cysts, bladder diverticula, or bladder cyst may affect accuracy.

EQUIPMENT

BladderScan (Figure 103-1)
Ultrasound transmission gel or Sontac ultrasound gel pads
Isopropyl alcohol pads or soft cloth moistened with isopropyl alcohol (to clean scan head)
Washcloth (to clean gel off patient)

PATIENT PREPARATION

Position patient in a reclining or supine position.

PROCEDURAL STEPS

1. Clean scanhead with isopropyl alcohol.
2. Turn bladder scanner on.
3. Select the patient gender by pressing the MALE/FEMALE button (Figure 103-2). The female gender selection accounts for the uterus; therefore, if the patient has had a hysterectomy, select the male gender.
4. Apply a generous amount of ultrasound gel to the scan head, taking care not to incorporate air bubbles that may interfere with transmission. If the patient has excessive hair, add some gel directly onto the patient. Alternatively, the Sontac Ultrasound Gel Pad may be applied to the patient immediately superior to the symphysis pubis (Figure 103-3).
5. Orient the head icon on the scanhead toward the patient's head (Figure 103-4). Place the scanhead about 1 inch (2.5 cm) above the symphysis pubis (the bladder cannot be scanned through the pubic bone) and point it

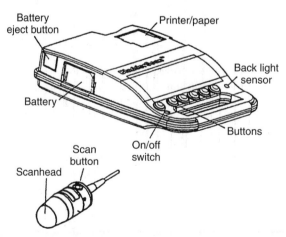

FIGURE 103-1 BladderScan. (Courtesy Diagnostic Ultrasound Corporation, Bothell, WA.)

toward the bladder. In an obese patient, more pressure may be applied to the scanhead (1 to 2 inches depression into abdomen).

6. Press the scan button on the scanhead and hold it steady until a beep is heard.
7. The volume measured will be displayed. An aiming screen with crosshairs will be displayed, with the light area on the screen representing the bladder.

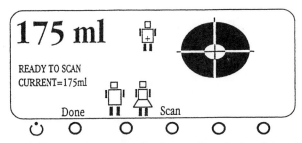

FIGURE 103-2 Bladder scanning screen showing gender selection. Select the male gender for female patients who have had a hysterectomy. (Courtesy Diagnostic Ultrasound Corporation, Bothell, WA.)

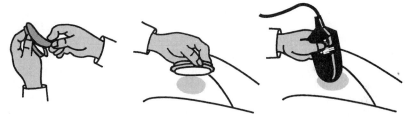

FIGURE 103-3 Application of the Sontac Gel Pad. (Courtesy Diagnostic Ultrasound Corporation, Bothell, WA.)

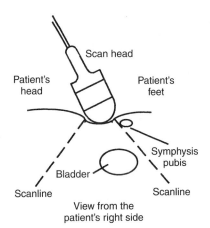

FIGURE 103-4 Positioning the scanhead. (Courtesy Diagnostic Ultrasound Corporation, Bothell, WA.)

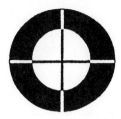

FIGURE 103-5 Aiming icon with crosshairs centered on bladder. (Courtesy Diagnostic Ultrasound Corporation, Bothell, WA.)

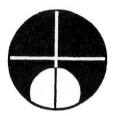

FIGURE 103-6 Aiming icon not centered on bladder indicating that the bladder was not completely scanned. (Courtesy Diagnostic Ultrasound Corporation, Bothell, WA.)

The crosshairs should be centered on the bladder (Figure 103-5). If the bladder overlaps the side of the crosshairs, the measured volume will be inaccurate (low) (Figure 103-6). Readjust the probe position and rescan until the bladder is properly centered on the aiming screen. Repeat the scan to ensure an accurate measurement.

8. Press DONE and then PRINT (if hard copy desired).
9. Turn scanner off.
10. Remove gel from patient.
11. Cleanse scanhead.

AGE-SPECIFIC CONSIDERATION

The bladder scanner may be used on patients of all ages.

COMPLICATIONS

1. To date, exposure to pulsed diagnostic ultrasound had not been shown to produce adverse effects (Diagnostic Ultrasound Corporation, 1999–2000).
2. Inacurate results that may be related to improper technique or using wrong gender selection.

REFERENCES

Diagnostic Ultrasound Corporation. (1999-2000). *BVI 3000 operator's manual*. Bothell, WA: Author.

Munir, V., Barnett, P., & South, M. (2002). Does the use of volumetric bladder ultrasound improve the success rate of suprapubic aspiration of urine? *Pediatric Emergency Care, 18*, 5.

Urinary Bladder Catheterization

Lucinda W. Rossoll, RN, MSN, CCRN, CEN

Urinary bladder catheterization is also known as *Foley catheter insertion.*

INDICATIONS

1. To obtain a sterile urine specimen for diagnostic purposes when the patient is unable to cooperate or assist in obtaining an adequate specimen.
2. To provide bladder drainage for a patient who is unable to void spontaneously (i.e., urinary tract obstruction or neurogenic bladder).
3. To ascertain the residual volume in the bladder after voiding or to facilitate bladder emptying when the patient chronically has large residual volumes after voiding. Bladder ultrasound is another alternative to ascertain residual volume (see Procedure 103).
4. To monitor urine output precisely.
5. To obtain a urine specimen for a toxicology screen from the patient who is unable or unwilling to urinate and when it is necessary that the substance ingested or injected be identified as soon as possible.
6. To fill the bladder for diagnostic radiologic procedures, such as a pelvic ultrasound or a cystogram.
7. To provide a means to deal with incontinence, only after other methods have been proved unsuccessful and when the benefits outweigh the risks.
8. To decompress the bladder before surgical procedures or peritoneal lavage.

CONTRAINDICATIONS AND CAUTIONS

1. Urinary catheterization should not be performed in a trauma patient with blood at the urinary meatus until a retrograde urethrogram is obtained. The presence of anterior pelvic fractures also requires extra caution.
2. Urinary catheterization should not be performed in a male trauma patient until a rectal examination has been performed to assess for urethral damage by palpating the prostate.
3. Strict aseptic technique should be adhered to when inserting the catheter.
4. A closed sterile drainage bag should be connected to all indwelling catheters.
5. The balloon should never be inflated until urine flow is established, thus ensuring that the catheter is in the bladder and preventing urethral rupture. Gentle pressure on the suprapubic area may help establish urine flow.
6. Institutional policy may require the presence of a chaperone when the nurse is the opposite gender of the patient.

EQUIPMENT

Antiseptic solution
Sterile gloves
Sterile fenestrated drape
Sterile towel
Sterile cotton balls
Sterile forceps
Sterile water-soluble lubricant
Sterile catheter, either straight or indwelling (6 to 22 Fr)
Sterile drainage bag
Sterile 10-ml syringe filled with sterile water
Sterile specimen container
Adhesive tape
1% lidocaine jelly (optional)
(NOTE: Prepackaged disposable kits that contain equipment for either intermittent or indwelling catheterization are available.)

PATIENT PREPARATION
Female

1. Place the patient in the supine position with her knees flexed and separated or with one knee flexed and the other leg flat on the bed.
2. If the patient is unresponsive, unstable, or combative, assistance may be necessary to keep the knees flexed and to prevent contamination of the equipment.
3. If the patient is cooperative but has decreased strength in her legs, have her flex her knees and place the bottoms of her feet together as close to her perineum as possible. This allows her knees to relax against the side rails.

Male

Place the patient in a supine position with head elevated or flat, depending on the patient's comfort, condition, and ability to cooperate.

PROCEDURAL STEPS
Female

1. Put on sterile gloves and place the sterile drape underneath the patient's buttocks, taking care that the gloves are not contaminated. Place the fenestrated drape over the perineum.
2. Open the antiseptic solution packet and pour it over the cotton balls.
3. Attach a prefilled syringe to the balloon port of the catheter (if an indwelling catheter is used). Inflate the balloon and check for leaks. Aspirate to deflate the balloon and leave the syringe attached.
4. Open the package of lubricant and dispense it onto the sterile tray surface. Lubricate 2 to 3 inches of the distal catheter.
5. If an indwelling catheter is being inserted, attach it to the drainage bag.
6. Spread the labia majora with one hand (usually the nondominant hand) to expose the urinary meatus. This hand is now considered to be contaminated and should not release the labia until the procedure is complete (Figure 104-1).

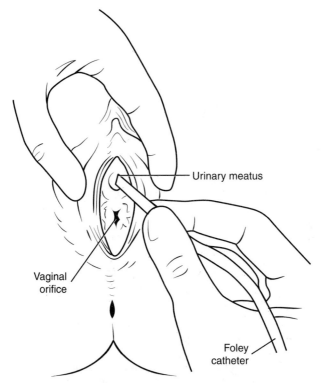

FIGURE 104-1 Exposing the urinary meatus.

7. Grasp an antiseptic-soaked cotton ball with the forceps, and wash the labia majora downward on each side with one cotton ball for each side. Spread the labia minora and repeat. Then wipe directly over the meatus with another antiseptic-soaked cotton ball.

8. Hold the lubricated catheter with the dominant hand a few inches from the tip to ease insertion and to control the direction of the catheter. Allow the distal end of the catheter to rest in the urine container if the end is not attached to a drainage bag. Gently insert the lubricated tip into the urinary meatus until urine begins to flow (about 2 to 3 inches in an adult; 1 inch in a small child). Then insert the catheter another 1 to 2 inches. This should ensure that the catheter is in the bladder, thus preventing rupture of the urethra when the balloon is inflated. Never force a catheter during insertion. If you meet resistance, stop and ask the patient to take several deep breaths or to bear down gently. This helps relax the sphincter. If you still meet resistance, seek assistance.

9. Once the catheter is inserted, hold it in place with the hand that has been separating the labia. If your first attempt to insert a catheter is unsuccessful, leave the catheter in place. This helps prevent similar misplacement on the next attempt.

10. For an indwelling catheter, inject the water or saline solution into the balloon port. Use the amount of fluid recommended by the manufacturer.

A 5-ml balloon requires about 10 ml of fluid to completely fill the balloon and the catheter lumen. Under- or overinflation may result in an asymetrical balloon, which can deflect the catheter tip to one side, causing occlusion of the drainage eyes, irritate the bladder wall, and lead to bladder spasms (Smith, 2003). When inflating the balloon, if resistance or pain is felt, aspirate the fluid back into the syringe, advance the catheter farther, and attempt to reinflate the balloon.

11. For a straight catheterization, collect the necessary amount of urine in a specimen container; then drain the rest of the urine into the collection receptacle.

12. Hang the drainage bag below the level of the bladder.

13. Attach the catheter to the upper thigh, allowing for some movement. This prevents movement of the catheter and traction on the bladder.

Female Quick Catheter Kit

A quick catheter kit is used to obtain a urine sample. It does not provide complete or continuous drainage.

1. Open the kit and place it on a flat surface. The opened package may be used as a sterile field.

2. Put on the sterile gloves (optional). Open the package of antiseptic solution–soaked swab sticks.

3. Pull the tip of the catheter out of the container until 4 to 6 inches of the catheter is free. If nonsterile gloves are used, grasp the tip of the catheter through the package to pull the catheter out without contamination. Make sure the cap is screwed on tightly. No lubricant is needed.

4. Spread the labia majora with one hand (usually the nondominant hand) to visualize the urethra. This hand is now considered to be contaminated and should not release the labia until the procedure is complete.

5. Use your other hand to cleanse the labia minora and the meatus with the antiseptic swabs, using one swab for each wipe.

6. Gently insert the catheter into the urethra until urine is seen, and fill the container. If nonsterile gloves are used, be careful to touch only the specimen tube and not the catheter. If your first attempt to insert a catheter is unsuccessful, leave the catheter in place. This helps prevent similar misplacement on the next attempt.

7. Remove the catheter from the urethra, then from the container. Close the top of the container.

Male

1. Put on sterile gloves, and place the drape over the patient's thighs. Place the fenestrated drape over the penis.

2. Open the antiseptic solution packet and pour it over the cotton balls.

3. Attach a prefilled syringe to the balloon port of the catheter (if using an indwelling catheter). Inflate the balloon, and check for leaks. Aspirate to deflate the balloon, and leave the syringe attached.

4. Open the package of lubricant and dispense it onto the sterile tray surface. Lubricate 2 to 3 inches of the catheter.

5. If an indwelling catheter is being used, attach it to the drainage bag.

6. Grasp the penis behind the glans (usually with your nondominant hand). This hand is now considered to be contaminated. If the patient is uncircumcised, retract the foreskin.

7. Grasp an antiseptic-soaked cotton ball with the forceps, and wash the meatus and then the glans using a circular motion. Repeat this step, using a new cotton ball until they all are used.

8. Filling the urethra with 1% lidocaine jelly using a syringe is optional; however, this provides more lubrication and some local anesthesia.

9. Hold the penis at a 90-degree angle (perpendicular) to the body with slight tension. This straightens the urethra and maintains a sterile field. Hold the catheter in your dominant hand about 4 to 6 inches from the tip of the catheter, and gently insert the catheter into the meatus until urine begins to flow (6 to 8 inches in an adult, 1 inch in a small child). The catheter may have to be inserted to the junction of the balloon port to obtain urine flow. When urine flow is established, insert the catheter 1 inch farther to ensure that the catheter is in the bladder and not the urethra, thus preventing urethral rupture. Never force the catheter during insertion. If you meet resistance, slightly increase your traction on the penis, ask the patient to bear down as if to pass urine to help relax the sphincter, and apply steady gentle pressure on the catheter. In a male with an enlarged prostate, a coudé catheter may be used to facilitate insertion. If this is unsuccessful, seek assistance.

10. Once the catheter is inserted, use the hand that has been holding the penis to hold the catheter in place.

11. Replace the foreskin to prevent compromised circulation and painful swelling.

12. For an indwelling catheter, inject water or saline solution into the balloon port. Use the amount of fluid recommended by the manufacturer. A 5 ml-balloon requires 9.5 to 10 ml of fluid to fill the balloon and the catheter lumen completely (Bard, 1997). When inflating the balloon, if resistance or pain is felt, aspirate the fluid back into the syringe, advance the catheter farther, and attempt to reinflate the balloon.

13. For a straight catheterization, collect the necessary amount of urine in a specimen container; then drain the rest of the urine into the collection receptacle.

14. Hang the drainage bag below the level of the bladder.

15. Attach the catheter to the upper thigh or the lower abdomen, allowing for some movement. This prevents movement of the catheter and traction on the bladder.

AGE-SPECIFIC CONSIDERATIONS

1. To insert a catheter in a young female, flex her knees and place the bottoms of her heels as near the perineum as possible, allowing the knees to relax and separate (Figure 104-2).

2. Catheter sizes for children are as listed in Table 104-1.

3. In an elderly woman who cannot abduct her legs, or in a woman who cannot lie supine, have her lie on her side with upper leg flexed at knee and hip (Figure 104-3).

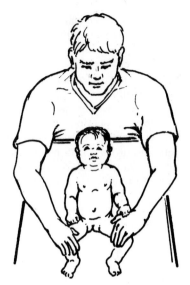

FIGURE 104-2 Position for bladder catheterization in a child. (From Gavula, D. P. [1992]. Bladder catheterization. In M. Jastremski, M. Dumas, & L. Peñalver [Eds.], *Emergency procedures* [p. 95]. Philadelphia: Saunders.)

4. If you are unable to pass the catheter in a male with prostatic hypertrophy, use a larger catheter or one with a coudé tip on the next attempt.

COMPLICATIONS

1. Urethral damage such as strictures or rupture
2. Urinary tract infection
3. Sepsis
4. Catheter obstruction with sediment, mucus, or blood clots leading to acute postobstructive renal failure

PATIENT TEACHING

If the patient is going home with an indwelling catheter, give the following instructions:

1. Wash your hands before and after you handle the catheter.

TABLE 104-1
PEDIATRIC CATHETER SIZES

Age	Size (Fr)
Neonate	5
Infant	8
1-3 yr	8-10
3-9 yr	10-12
9-14 yr	12-16

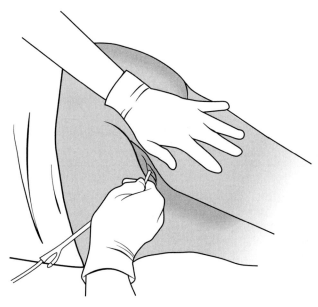

FIGURE 104-3 Side-lying position for urinary bladder catheterization in a female patient.

2. Wash the urinary meatus and the perineal area twice a day with soap and water.
3. Drink at least 8 to 12 glasses of water a day. If your urine becomes dark, increase the amount of fluid you are drinking.
4. Do not pull on the catheter.
5. Keep the drainage bag lower than your bladder.
6. Wipe all connections with alcohol when changing from leg bag to drainage bag and vice versa.
7. Report any of the following: cloudy or bloody urine, foul-smelling urine, fever, decreased urine output.

REFERENCES

Bard Urological Division. (1997). *Foley catheter inflation/deflation guidelines.* Covington, GA: Author.

Smith, J. M. (2003). Indwelling catheter management: From habit-based to evidence-based practice. *Ostomy Wound Management, 49,* 38.

Suprapubic Urine Aspiration

Lucinda W. Rossoll, RN, MSN, CCRN, CEN

Suprapubic aspiration is also known as *suprapubic "tap"* or *suprapubic bladder aspiration.*

INDICATION

To obtain a sterile urine specimen for diagnostic purposes when uncontaminated urine cannot be obtained for culture in a child who is younger than age 2, who is not toilet trained, and who has suspected sepsis or fever of unknown origin. Urethral catheterization is the preferred method for obtaining a sterile urine specimen from a child who is older than age 2. Suprapubic aspiration is rarely performed in adults but may be used when uncontaminated urine cannot be obtained for culture by other means.

CONTRAINDICATIONS AND CAUTIONS

1. Suprapubic aspiration should not be performed in a child who is older than age 2 or who is able to void on command.
2. This procedure should not be performed in a patient who has just voided. The procedure should be delayed for at least 1 hour after voiding. The bladder must be palpable or visualized on bladder scan (Stokes & Kulkarni, 2004).
3. Coagulopathy should be corrected prior to the procedure (Stokes & Kulkarni, 2004).
4. Aspiration should not be performed on patients with abdominal distention or suspected bowel obstruction (Stokes & Kulkarni, 2004).

EQUIPMENT

Antiseptic solution or antiseptic-soaked swabs
2 × 2 gauze pads
Bandage
Diaper
3- or 5-ml syringe
Topical anesthetic, i.e., EMLA (optional)
If anesthetic is to be infiltrated, add the following:
Lidocaine 1% (with or without epinephrine)
Tuberculin syringe
27-G 1-in needle
22-G 1½-in needle or 22-G 1½-in spinal needle
Sterile specimen container
Pediatric urine collection bag
Bladder scanner (optional)

PATIENT PREPARATION

1. Wait at least 1 hour after the last void before performing the procedure. This allows enough urine to collect to distend the bladder, making it easier to palpate. A bladder scanner (see Procedure 103) may be used to assess the minimum amount of urine volume (10 ml) needed for aspiration, thereby increasing the chances for successful suprapubic aspiration with a minimum number of attempts (Munir, Barnett, & South, 2002).
2. Remove the diaper. Place a sterile urine collection bag on the patient because the patient may spontaneously void during the procedure.
3. Place the patient in a supine position with the knees flexed and the bottoms of the heels as close to the perineum as possible and secure the arms. This position keeps the patient from moving during the procedure, while making it easy to observe and soothe the patient.
4. Allow the patient to use a pacifier or hold onto a security object.

PROCEDURAL STEPS

1. Use the bladder scanner (Procedure 103) to assess whether there is enough urine (10 ml) for aspiration (optional).
2. Wipe the area between the symphysis pubis and the umbilicus twice in a circular motion outward with antiseptic-soaked gauze or swabs. Allow to air dry.
3. *If the skin was not previously anesthetized with anesthetic cream, anesthetize the skin at the insertion site by infiltrating the insertion site with 1% lidocaine using the tuberculin syringe with the 27-G needle.
4. *Attach the 3- or 5-ml syringe to the 22-G, 1-in needle or the spinal needle, using sterile technique.
5. To prevent urination during the procedure, compress the infant's urethra. If the patient is a boy, squeeze the penis. If a girl, place digital pressure on the urethra.
6. *Insert the needle about 1 to 2 cm above the symphysis pubis at a 10- to 20-degree angle cephalad from the perpendicular axis in children (Figure 105-1) and angle it a little caudad in adults (Figure 105-2).
7. *Advance the needle while aspirating until urine is obtained. If urine is not obtained, pull the needle back and advance at a different angle (20 degrees cephalad or caudad). Repeat no more than three times. An ultrasound-guided aspiration may be useful, or wait another hour until more urine is present in the bladder.
8. *Withdraw the needle and the syringe.
9. Hold pressure over the site with gauze for 3 minutes and then apply a small bandage.
10. Apply a clean diaper, and give the child to the parents to comfort.
11. Place the urine in the sterile container, securing the cap tightly, and transport it to the laboratory.

---

*Indicates portions of the procedure usually performed by a physician or an advanced practice nurse.

12. Check periodically for bleeding for 1 hour after the procedure.
13. Discharge the patient after the first void, noting the time of urination and the color of the urine (pink may be expected; report frankly bloody urine to the physician).

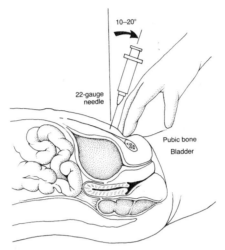

FIGURE 105-1 Proper placement of the syringe and needle for suprapubic aspiration in children. (From Roberts, J. R. & Hedges, J. R. [Eds.]. [2004]. *Clinical procedures in emergency medicine* [4th ed., p. 1099]. Philadelphia: Saunders.)

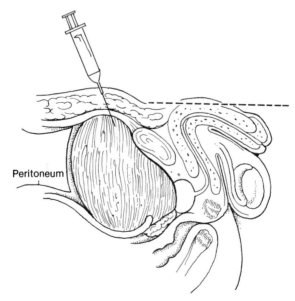

FIGURE 105-2 Proper placement of the syringe and needle for suprapubic aspiration in adults. (From Roberts, J. R. & Hedges, J. R. [Eds.]. [2004]. *Clinical procedures in emergency medicine* [4th ed., p. 1100]. Philadelphia: Saunders.)

COMPLICATIONS

1. Bowel perforation
2. Bladder or abdominal wall hemorrhage. NOTE: Microscopic hematuria is common.
3. Bleeding from the puncture site
4. Infection of the bladder or abdominal wall

PATIENT TEACHING

Report any of the following to the physician or nurse: abdominal pain, bloating, redness or drainage at the insertion site, fever, decreased urine output, bloody urine, or urine with a foul odor.

REFERENCES

Munir, V., Barnett, P., & South, M. (2002). Does the use of volumetric bladder ultrasound improve the success rate of suprapubic aspiration of urine? *Pediatric Emergency Care, 18,* 5.

Stokes, S., & Kulkarni, A. (2004). Suprapubic bladder aspiration. In E. F. Reichman, & R. R. Simon (Eds.), *Emergency medicine procedures* (pp. 1128-1133). New York: McGraw-Hill.

PROCEDURE 106

Suprapubic Catheter Insertion

Lucinda W. Rossoll, RN, MSN, CCRN, CEN

Suprapubic catheterization is also known as *suprapubic bladder drainage* or *cystostomy*. It may be performed at the bedside, in a procedure room, in the operating room, or during a cystoscopy.

INDICATIONS

To provide temporary or continuous urinary drainage in the following circumstances:

1. Instead of long-term urethral catheterization in males (may decrease the incidence of infection)
2. Patients with strictures or prostatic obstruction that makes urethral catheterization impossible

3. Patients with neurogenic bladder
4. Patients with pelvic fractures
5. In the presence of urethral injury

CONTRAINDICATIONS AND CAUTIONS

1. Caution should be exercised in the presence of coagulopathy or previous lower abdominal surgery (may use ultrasound to guide placement).
2. Contraindications include nondistended bladder, pregnancy, bladder cancer, or pelvic irradiation (Quek & Stein, 2002).
3. Gross hematuria with clots may occlude the catheter.

EQUIPMENT

†Prepackaged suprapubic catheter set (Figure 106-1)
Drainage bag (bedside bag or a leg bag)
Sterile gloves
Antiseptic solution
No. 11 scalpel
Lidocaine 1% for local anesthesia
Syringe and needles for local anesthesia
Needle holder
4-0 nylon suture
Drain sponge
Adhesive tape
Antibiotic ointment

---

†Several types of suprapubic catheters and kits are available. The method of insertion differs slightly, depending on the type of catheter being used, but the basic principles remain the same (Quek & Stein, 2002).

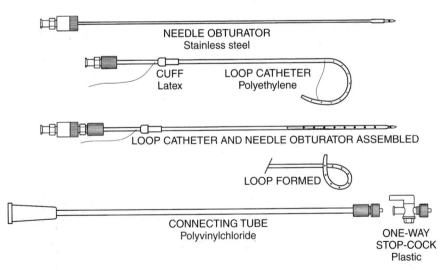

FIGURE 106-1 Contents of a Stamey percutaneous loop suprapubic catheter set. (Courtesy Cook Urological Incorporated, Spencer, IN.)

PATIENT PREPARATION

1. Fill the bladder (if not already distended) with sterile saline solution via a urethral catheter or have the patient drink fluids until the bladder is filled. This makes it easier to locate the bladder by palpation.
2. Place the patient into a supine position and expose the abdomen. A rolled towel or a blanket under the hips may be helpful.

PROCEDURAL STEPS

1. Cleanse the insertion area with an antiseptic solution.
2. *Infiltrate the insertion area with local anesthesia.
3. *Make a small midline incision about 2 to 3 cm above the symphysis pubis but below the upper edge of the bladder. No incision is needed if the catheter is inserted via a needle and guidewire set.
4. *For patients without a history of prior lower abdominal surgery, insert the catheter vertically. For patients with past lower abdominal surgery, insert the catheter at a 30-degree angle toward the symphysis pubis. Gradually advance the catheter in a caudal direction via a guide wire, needle, or cannula until urine is seen and continue 4 to 5 cm beyond that point or until the flange is against the skin. If a percutaneous loop catheter is used, pull the string to secure the retentive loop into its fully closed position (Figure 106-2). Wrap the drawstring around the catheter shaft several times and tie. Cut off the excess drawstring, and unroll the latex cuff to cover the knotted drawstring. If the catheter needs to be removed, cut the catheter and the drawstring below the latex cuff to free the catheter loop (Cook Urological Inc., 1987). If a urinary catheter is to be inserted, use a 16 to 20 Fr and inflate balloon with 10 ml of sterile water to hold the catheter in place.
5. Secure the catheter with adhesive tape or sutures. Some suprapubic catheters have a balloon to hold them in place; others are self-retaining winged catheters that have two to four wings to hold them in place.
6. Connect the catheter to a drainage bag and allow the bladder to empty.
7. Apply tincture of benzoin to the catheter shaft and the abdomen. Secure the catheter to the lateral abdomen with adhesive tape.

COMPLICATIONS

1. Bowel or peritoneal perforation
2. Infection at the insertion site or in the bladder
3. Skin breakdown around the insertion site

---

*Indicates portions of the procedure usually performed by a physician or an advanced practice nurse.

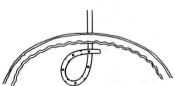

FIGURE 106-2 Retention loop of the suprapubic catheter in its fully closed position within the dome of the bladder. (Courtesy Cook Urological Incorporated, Spencer, IN.)

4. Kinking of the catheter
5. Leakage of urine around the insertion site

PATIENT TEACHING

1. Clean and dress the incision site every day. Soap and water or a swab with sterile antiseptic may be used to clean the site. Clean incision site using a circular motion, starting at the insertion site and moving outward (Perry & Potter, 2006).
2. If the catheter becomes obstructed, return to the urologist. Do not try to remove the tube yourself.
3. Call your urologist or return to the emergency department if you experience any of the following:
   a. Uncontrolled urine leakage
   b. Skin breakdown
   c. Redness or foul, purulent drainage at the insertion site
   d. Foul smelling, cloudy, or bloody urine
   e. Abdominal pain
   f. Fever
   g. Decreased urine output
4. Drink at least 2000 ml of fluids a day (if no fluid restriction) because the small-bore catheter can easily become obstructed by clots, mucus, or sediment (Perry & Potter, 2006).

REFERENCES

Cook Urological Incorporated. (1987). *Stamey percutaneous loop supracatheter set product information.* Spencer, IN: Author.

Perry, A. G., & Potter, P. A. (2006), *Clinical nursing skills & techniques* (6th ed.). St Louis: Mosby.

Quek, M. L., & Stein, J. P. (2002). Suprapubic urinary tube placement. In W. C. Shoemaker, G. C. Velamahos, & D. Demetriades (Eds.), *Procedures and monitoring for the critically ill* (pp. 139-145). Philadelphia: Saunders.

Pelvic Examination

Lucinda W. Rossoll, RN, MSN, CCRN, CEN

Pelvic examination is also known as *vaginal examination, per vaginal examination,* and *PV.*

INDICATIONS

1. To assist in the diagnosis of intraabdominal pathology in the female patient with abdominal pain.
2. To obtain specimens to diagnose vaginal and uterine infections.

CONTRAINDICATIONS AND CAUTIONS

1. Warm water should be used on the speculum instead of lubricant if cultures or other specimens are to be obtained.
2. Gloves should be changed before a rectal examination. This prevents the spread of infection from the vagina to the rectum.
3. When a multidose tube of water-soluble lubricant is used, the lubricant should be squirted onto a surface such as the speculum wrapper. This prevents cross-contamination between patients.
4. Institutional policy may require the presence of a chaperone, especially if the examiner is a male.

EQUIPMENT

Light source
Vaginal speculum (appropriate size for the patient)
Lubricating jelly (water based)
Ring forceps and gauze dressings or long swab sticks
Specimen collection supplies—any or all of the following, depending the diagnostic test requested (Papanicolaou smear, potassium hydroxide, wet mount [normal saline], specimen slide with cover slips, gonorrhea or chlamydia transport media)
Drape or sheet
Damp wash cloth and towel

PATIENT PREPARATION

1. For a woman's first pelvic examination, time should be spent explaining what will occur. Models and illustrations may be used as adjuncts to the discussion. Assess the woman's ability to cooperate with the examination.
2. Have the patient empty her bladder.
3. Assist the patient into the lithotomy position with her buttocks at the edge of the table and place a pillow under her head. Do not place the patient into this position until the examiner is ready to see her. Weak or dizzy patients may not be able to maintain this position without assistance.

PROCEDURAL STEPS

1. *To avoid startling the patient, advise her that she will feel you touching her. Touching the inner thigh first will let the woman know the examination is beginning and may place her at ease. Inspect the external genitalia for swelling, inflammation, bleeding, discharge (clear and odorless is normal), nodules, or skin changes.

2. *Insert one or two fingers into the introitus and press downward on the lower edge. Insert the appropriately sized speculum, moistened with warm water, into the introitus by passing it over your fingers. The speculum is inserted at an angle to the vaginal opening and gently rotated to avoid trauma and discomfort to the patient (Figure 107-1).

3. *Remove your fingers from the perineal body and make sure that the speculum is fully inserted into the vagina. Open the speculum and adjust it until the cervix is seen, and tighten the thumb screw to hold the blades open (Figure 107-2). If a plastic speculum is used, lock it into place by pressing down on the lever. Advise the patient that she will hear a clicking noise when the speculum is locked.

4. *If the os of the cervix is obscured, wipe the cervix with a dry gauze dressing held by a ring forceps or with a long swab stick.

5. *Inspect the cervix, noting color, lesions, bleeding, discharge (other than pale white secretions), and ulcerations, as well as the position of the uterus (see Figure 107-2).

---

*Indicates portions of the procedure usually performed by a physician or an advanced practice nurse.

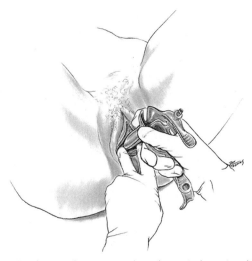

FIGURE 107-1 Inserting the speculum at an angle to the vaginal opening. (From Jarvis, C. [1996]. *Physical examination and health assessment* [2nd ed., p. 817]. Philadelphia: Saunders.)

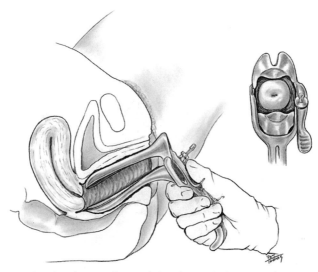

FIGURE 107-2 Opening the speculum to bring the cervix into view. (From Jarvis, C. [2000]. *Physical examination and health assessment* [3rd ed., p. 812]. Philadelphia: Saunders.)

6. *Obtain specimens as needed for the necessary diagnostic tests. These may include one or more of the following:
   a. Papanicolaou smear (if performed) should be obtained before any other specimen or lubricant is used so as not to interfere with cytology testing.
   b. Gonorrhea
   c. Chlamydia
   d. Gram's stain
   e. Potassium hydroxide slide to look for Candida (yeast) organisms
   f. Wet mount (normal saline) to look for trichomonas or clue cells for bacterial vaginosis
7. *View the vagina around the cervix by gently rotating the speculum. Gradually withdraw the speculum while rotating it to allow visualization of the vaginal walls and mucosa for color, lacerations, ulcers, discharge, or inflammation. When the cervix is cleared, release the lock on the speculum, being careful not to pinch the vagina.
8. *Perform a bimanual examination by first inserting the lubricated index and middle fingers of your dominant hand gently into the vagina. The fourth and fifth fingers are flexed on the palm, and the thumb is extended away from the perineum. Palpate the cervix, and note the position (anterior or posterior), consistency (soft or firm), mobility, and any tenderness of the cervix.
9. *Place your nondominant hand on the abdomen between the symphysis pubis and the umbilicus. Gently press down on the abdomen toward the fingers

---

*Indicates portions of the procedure usually performed by a physician or an advanced practice nurse.

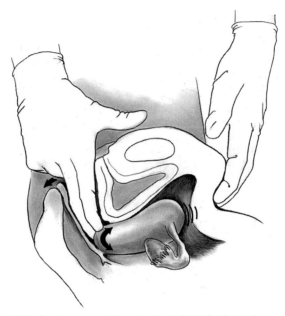

FIGURE 107-3 Palpating the uterus. (From Jarvis, C. [2000]. *Physical examination and health assessment* [3rd ed., p. 818]. Philadelphia: Saunders.)

in the vagina, and elevate the cervix and the uterus with the other hand. This allows you to feel the uterus between the two hands and palpate to identify size, shape, tenderness, and masses (Figure 107-3).

10. *Continue to palpate with the hand on the abdomen in the right lower quadrant with the fingers in the vagina to the right of the cervix and again on the left. Palpate the ovary on each side (the ovaries may be difficult to palpate 4 to 5 years after menopause) for fullness, tenderness, and any masses that might be present.

11. *Change gloves and add lubrication. Reinsert the index finger into the vagina and the middle finger into the rectum. Assess the rectovaginal wall, the posterior surface of the uterus, and the area behind the cervix.

12. Assist the patient in removing her feet from the stirrups. Offer her a damp washcloth and towel to cleanse herself after the examination.

AGE-SPECIFIC CONSIDERATIONS

1. In the well child, a gynecologic examination need only be an external examination. This may be accomplished by having the young child or infant lie in the mother's lap in the frog-leg position. The older preadolescent child may position herself with her knees to her chest. An internal examination should be performed if there is bleeding, discharge, evidence of trauma, or suspected

---

*Indicates portions of the procedure usually performed by a physician or an advanced practice nurse.

sexual abuse. This examination should be performed only by an examiner who is skilled and knowledgeable in pediatric gynecologic examination and qualified to collect forensic evidence (if applicable).

2. In virgins or those with a small introitus, the examination technique may need to be modified with the use of one finger instead of two. Use an appropriately-sized speculum, such as a pediatric speculum or a nasal speculum.

3. Allow the adolescent to choose the person she would like as a chaperone during the examination.

4. An older woman may need assistance to get into the lithotomy position. She may need to hold her knees to support her legs, because they may tire quickly in this position. If she cannot assume this position, have her lie on her side with the upper leg held up to her chest.

5. When menopause occurs or in women aged 50 or older, the decreased estrogen results in a narrowing (atrophy) of the vagina and decreased lubrication. These changes may result in some physical discomfort during the examination, and a smaller speculum may be needed.

COMPLICATIONS

1. Vaginal or labial laceration
2. Inaccurate results from an inaccurate specimen collection
3. Ruptured ovarian cyst or ectopic pregnancy from vigorous palpation
4. Spread of infection from one part of the body to another resulting from improper examination technique

PATIENT TEACHING

1. Instruct the patient on how to obtain her laboratory test results and designate the person with whom she should follow up.
2. Provide individualized instructions based on the final diagnosis.

Assessing Fetal Heart Tones

June F. Stacey, RN, BSN, CEN

Fetal heart tones (FHTs) are also known as *heart tones* or *fetal heart rate* (*FHR*).

INDICATION
To assess fetal status when the pregnant patient is ill, injured, or in labor.

CONTRAINDICATIONS AND CAUTIONS
1. To discriminate between the maternal heart rate and the FHR, the maternal pulse should be palpated simultaneously when the FHR is assessed (Doan-Wiggins, 2004).
2. A visibly pregnant patient should not remain in the supine position because hypotension may result from compression of the inferior vena cava and the aorta by the uterus, which impedes venous return. If the patient must remain supine for a prolonged period of time, a folded sheet should be placed under the right hip. If the patient requires spinal immobilization, the backboard should be tilted approximately 15 to 20 degrees to the left to decrease compression of the vena cava. If this is not possible, then the uterus should be manually displaced to the left side (Limmer, 2005).
3. FHTs may be heard with a regular stethoscope at 18 to 20 weeks' gestation and with a Doppler at 10 to 12 weeks' gestation.
4. The FHT is heard as a rapid ticking sound. A whooshing sound is the placental circulation being auscultated and is usually the same rate as the maternal pulse.
5. Anything that compromises the mother also compromises the fetus. If the condition of the mother is optimized, this helps optimize the condition of the fetus.
6. Consultation with an obstetrical nurse or physician is recommended early in the assessment of the pregnant patient to validate FHTs.
7. If continuous fetal monitoring is needed, the Emergency Nurses Association (ENA) and the Association of Women's Health, Obstetric and Neonatal Nurses (AWHONN) believe that "when a fetal monitor is being used in the emergency department, the nurse responsible for monitoring will be appropriately educated and will meet institutional standards for fetal monitoring" (ENA, 2000).

EQUIPMENT
Stethoscope
Doppler ultrasonic flowmeter (2.25-MHz frequency)
Conductive gel

PROCEDURAL STEPS

1. With the patient lying in a supine position, palpate to find the fetal position. Palpate the back of the fetus, which feels like a flat surface, and place the Doppler on the abdomen where the flat surface is palpated. The FHTs are usually located in the mother's right or left lower abdominal quadrant. The position of the fetus has an effect on where the FHTs are found (e.g., a fetus in the breech position has FHTs above the umbilicus). Before the third trimester, the fetal position is difficult to discern. During labor with a cephalic presentation, FHTs are usually best heard midway between the umbilicus and symphysis pubis (Doan-Wiggins, 2004).

2. Place the conductive gel on the abdomen or on the Doppler. If warmed gel is available, this is more comfortable for the patient.

3. Locate the heartbeat and listen at the point of maximal intensity. Changing the angle of the probe may intensify the sounds. Count the FHTs for 30 to 60 seconds between contractions (if present) to obtain a baseline rate. A normal FHT ranges between 120 and 160 beats/min. Brief accelerations may be due to fetal movement, and bradycardia often occurs during contractions, but prolonged FHT less than 110 beats/min (bradycardia) or greater than 160 beats/min (tachycardia) may indicate fetal distress and should be reported immediately (Doan-Wiggins 2004).

4. It is not unusual to have difficulty locating and auscultating the FHTs. This could be due to inexperience of the listener, excess noise from the surroundings, obesity, improper positioning of the stethoscope or Doppler, or fetal death. If the FHTs cannot be heard, reassure the mother that there are many possible reasons for this and request assistance from an obstetrical nurse or obstetrician.

5. Check the FHTs each time the mother's vital signs are checked. If the mother is in labor, FHT's should be checked at least every 15 minutes in early labor and every 5 minutes during the second stage of labor. (Doan-Wiggins, 2004)

COMPLICATION

Supine hypotension

REFERENCES

Emergency Nurses Association (ENA). (2000). *The obstetrical patient in the ED (Joint Position Statement with AWHONN)*, Des Plaines, IL: AuthorRetrieved March 7, 2007, updated September 2000, from http://www.ena.org

Doan-Wiggins, L. (2004). Emergency childbirth. In J. R. Roberts, & J. R. Hedges (Eds.), *Clinical procedures in emergency medicine* (4th ed., pp. 1117-1143). Philadelphia: Saunders.

Limmer, D. (2005). Obstetrics and gynecological emergencies. In D. Dickinson, & D. Limmer (Eds.), *Emergency care* (pp. 524-545). Upper Saddle Ridge, NJ: Pearson Prentice Hall.

Emergency Childbirth

June F. Stacey, RN, BSN, CEN, and
Jean A. Proehl, RN, MN, CEN, CCRN, FAEN

Emergency childbirth is also known as a *precipitous* (*"precip"*) *delivery* or *birth on arrival* (BOA).

INDICATIONS
To deliver an infant when birth is imminent, as evidenced by the following:
1. The woman is having contractions and is pushing.
2. The woman has the urge to defecate or bear down.
3. The woman tells you "the baby is coming."
4. The perineum is bulging (crowning), and the infant's head is seen at the vaginal opening, even between contractions. Birth is imminent if you see the infant's head at any time in a woman who has had previous vaginal deliveries.

CONTRAINDICATIONS AND CAUTIONS
1. It is important to remain calm and in control. An obstetrical nurse and an obstetrician should be contacted to come and assist, but the delivery should not be delayed.
2. Do not allow the mother to go to the bathroom, even though she may feel the urge to have a bowel movement.
3. Supine hypotension or vena cava compression syndrome is possible. When the mother is supine, the weight of the fetus, placenta, and amniotic fluid totals 20 to 24 pounds. This may compress the superior vena cava, decreasing blood return to the heart, which will decrease cardiac output causing hypotension. If this occurs, the mother should be turned to the left side-lying position.
4. Explosive delivery of the fetal head should be avoided to minimize perineal tearing, vaginal lacerations, or urethral damage to the mother.
5. If the mother is walking or in a wheelchair and there is not time to place her on a stretcher, she should be eased to the floor for the delivery.
6. The fingers should be kept out of the vagina to avoid infection. Sterility is not a priority, but sterile technique should be used when possible. The umbilical cord should not be cut until sterile equipment is available.
7. Intrapartum suctioning "on the perineum" (prior to complete delivery) is no longer recommended, even for patients with meconium-stained amniotic fluid (AHA, 2005). Suctioning is completed as indicated after delivery.
8. The infant should be stimulated to cry by suctioning, drying, rubbing the back, or flicking the soles of the feet. Do not slap the buttocks or hold the infant upside-down to stimulate respiratory effort.

9. The infant should be dried immediately and kept warm after delivery to avoid hypothermia and acidosis.

EQUIPMENT

Antiseptic solution
Gloves, preferably sterile
Basin or plastic bag
Sterile cloth towels
Baby blanket
Bulb syringe
Sterile scissors or scalpel
Two sterile cord clamps or Kelly forceps
Sterile perineal pad
(NOTE: Emergency departments should have a sterile obstetrics kit or "Precip Pack" available with all of the aforementioned items.)
Identification bands for both the mother and the infant
Resuscitation equipment should be nearby (adult and neonatal)
Heated isolette (if available)
Warm blankets (if available)

PATIENT PREPARATION

1. Obtain a brief history to determine the presence of conditions that may complicate the birth or resuscitation of the neonate. Essential questions include expected due date, number of previous pregnancies and deliveries, complications with this pregnancy, multiple birth anticipated, rupture of membranes, and color of amniotic fluid.
2. When the mother is having intense contractions lasting 60 to 90 seconds every 1½ to 2 minutes, she is not receptive to most teaching. Remain calm, and give instructions firmly and with confidence. It is important to get the mother to cooperate and assist at important times in the delivery, such as when trying to control an explosive delivery of the head.
3. The mother may need assistance or reminders to use breathing techniques to help her control the delivery. You may need to demonstrate breathing in deeply and exhaling slowly through pursed lips.

PROCEDURAL STEPS

1. Position the mother in a dorsal recumbent position with her knees bent or in a side-lying (preferably left) position with her knees bent. Raising the hips by placing the patient's buttocks on the underside of a bedpan may be helpful.
2. If time permits, cleanse the patient's perineum with soap and water or pour antiseptic solution over the area moving in an anterior to posterior direction.
3. Drape the perineal area with sterile towels.
4. If time permits, take vital signs, including fetal heart tones (see Procedure 108).
5. Place a clean towel, drape, or absorbent pad under the mother's buttocks.
6. To control the urge to push and the rate of delivery, instruct the mother to pant as the head is being delivered to help control the urge to bear down. This helps to control the rate of delivery.

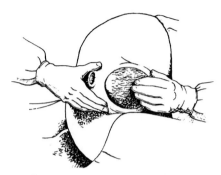

FIGURE 109-1 Placement of hands on perineum with the mother in the side-lying position. (From Roberts, J., & McGowan, N. [1985]. Emergency birth. *Journal of Emergency Nursing, 11*, p. 127.)

7. Support the perineum by applying manual pressure just above the anus with a sterile towel or sterile gauze dressing. This protects the fetus from potential fecal contamination from the anus. It also prevents excess stretching of the perineum and helps to control the rate of delivery (Figure 109-1).

8. Use gentle pressure with the palm of the other hand on the infant's head as it emerges. (Do not use the hand that is supporting the perineum.) This will control the delivery and avoid rapid expulsion of the infant (Figure 109-2). The head should never be pushed back to prevent delivery.

9. Support the head with both hands and allow it to rotate naturally. The infant turns and faces one of the mother's thighs.

10. If the membranes are still intact by the time the head is delivered, snip them at the nape of the neck and pull them away from the infant's face.

11. Use your fingers to ascertain whether the umbilical cord is around the neck. If it is, attempt to slip it over the infant's head. This is best done in between contractions. If the cord is too tight, and cannot be easily moved, immediately clamp the cord in two places and cut the cord between the clamps, before proceeding with the delivery.

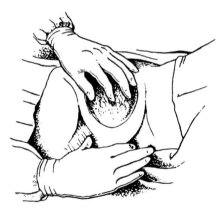

FIGURE 109-2 Placement of hands to control the emerging fetal head. (From Roberts, J., & McGowan, N. [1985]. Emergency birth. *Journal of Emergency Nursing, 11*, 128.)

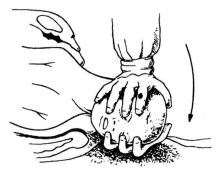

FIGURE 109-3 Delivery of the anterior shoulder. (From Roberts, J., & McGowan, N. [1985]. Emergency birth. *Journal of Emergency Nursing, 11,* 128.)

12. Deliver the shoulders by placing the palms of your hands, one on each side of the infant's head, and gently direct the head downward (Figure 109-3). This allows delivery of the anterior shoulder. If it is necessary to assist with delivery of the posterior shoulder, gently direct the infant's head upward (Figure 109-4).
13. The rest of the infant delivers rapidly. The infant is slippery, so support the body securely to prevent dropping of the infant.
14. Note the time of delivery.
15. Place one clamp approximately 4 to 5 cm from the infant's abdomen and another clamp approximately 4 to 5 cm toward the mother. Cut the cord between the two clamps with sterile scissors or a scalpel. If sterile equipment is not available, it is not necessary to cut the umbilical cord. Keep the infant at or below the level of the mother until the cord is cut.

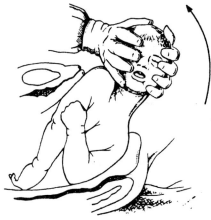

FIGURE 109-4 Delivery of the posterior shoulder. (From Roberts, J., & McGowan, N. [1985]. Emergency birth. *Journal of Emergency Nursing, 11,* 129.)

16. Rapidly assess the infant for the following: Full-term gestation? Amniotic fluid clear and without evidence of infection? Breathing or crying? Good muscle tone?

a. Full term babies who are breathing or crying, have good muscle tone, and clear amniotic fluid do not need resuscitation and should not be separated from the mother (AHA, 2005). The infant should be dried, placed directly on the mother's chest, and covered with dry blankets. Be sure the baby's head is covered. Assess Apgar scores at 1, 5, and 10 minutes (Figure 109-5).

b. If the answer to any of the above questions is "no," further resuscitation of the baby is indicated with the following sequence of resuscitative interventions (AHA, 2005). After 30 seconds at each step, reassess respirations, heart rate, and color and progress to the next step if indicated (AHA, 2005). Markers of success are a heart rate above 100, pink skin, and effective spontaneous ventilations (AHA, 2005).

i. Provide warmth, place head in sniffing position, clear airway with a bulb syringe or suction catheter, dry, stimulate breathing, and reposition. Suction the mouth first because suctioning the nose often stimulates the infant to gasp and may cause aspiration of material in the oropharynx. Endotracheal suctioning may be indicated in the presence of meconium. At this point, if the infant is breathing with an adequate heart rate but with central cyanosis, administer supplemental oxygen. If cyanosis persists, begin positive-pressure ventilation.

ii. Ventilation. If the infant is gasping or apneic, assist ventilations with a bag-mask and supplemental oxygen at a rate of 40 to 60 breaths per minute. The heart rate should promptly improve with adequate ventilation. In some instances, resuscitation is started with room air or less than 100% supplemental oxygen; oxygen should be added if there is no appreciable improvement after 90 seconds. Endotracheal intubation or the insertion of a laryngeal mask

	0	1	2
Heart rate	Absent	Less than 100	Over 100
Resp. effort	Absent	Slow, irregular	Good cry
Muscle tone	Limp	Some flexion	Active motion
Reflex irritability	No response	Grimace	Cry
Color	Pale	Body pink, extremities blue	All pink

FIGURE 109-5 Apgar score.

airway may be considered if tracheal suctioning of meconium is required, bag-mask ventilation is ineffective or prolonged, chest compressions are required, to deliver endotracheal medications, or in other special resuscitation circumstances. Continue positive-pressure ventilation until the heart rate exceeds 100 beats/min and there are spontaneous respirations.

   iii. Chest compressions. The base of the umbilical cord can be palpated to determine heart rate. However, the umbilical stump may become constricted so that the pulse cannot be palpated, so auscultate for heart sounds if in doubt. If the heart rate is less than 60 after 30 seconds of effective ventilation with supplemental oxygen, start chest compressions. Deliver chest compressions and ventilations at a 3:1 ratio at a rate that delivers 90 compressions and 30 breaths per minute. Avoid ventilating and compressing simultaneously. The two-thumb technique with both thumbs on the sternum and fingers encircling and supporting the back is preferred over the two-finger technique of chest compressions. Chest compressions are performed over the lower third of the sternum and are given with enough pressure to depress the sternum to a depth approximately one third of the anteroposterior diameter of the chest and deep enough to generate a palpable pulse. The chest should be allowed to completely re-expand between compressions but the thumbs (or fingers) should never leave the chest. Continue compressions and ventilations until the heart rate is 60 or greater.

   iv. Epinephrine and/or volume expansion. If the infant does not respond to ventilatory and circulatory support as outlined above, prepare to administer medications and IV fluid. Epinephrine is the first-line medication and IV administration is preferred over endotracheal administration. If fluid administration is indicated, the initial dose is 10 ml/kg of a crystalloid solution. Administer naloxone and glucose as indicated.

17. Withdraw 20 to 30 ml of blood from the one of the umbilical veins (Stallard & Burns, 2003). Transfer to lab tubes per institutional protocols.

18. Placing the infant to the mother's breast stimulates the release of oxytocin, causing the uterus to contract. This helps with placental separation and helps control bleeding. The placenta usually delivers spontaneously within 20 to 30 minutes after the delivery of the infant.

19. Watch for the signs of the separation and delivery of the placenta. One sign is a lengthening of the umbilical cord from the vagina. The uterus becomes firm as it contracts and changes to a globular shape. Instruct the mother to bear down to deliver the placenta. You may apply gentle traction to the umbilical cord, but do not tug the cord, because this could tear the cord or placenta or invert the uterus. Do not apply pressure to the fundus to facilitate delivery of the placenta. Deliver the placenta into the basin. Once the placenta is delivered, check for intactness. Save the placenta in a basin or plastic bag and keep it with the mother.

20. Once the placenta has been delivered, oxytocin may be administered as prescribed. Oxytocic agents should not be given prior to the delivery of the placenta due to the potential of increased complications; i.e., entrapment of placenta or undiagnosed twin.

21. Palpate the uterus. It should feel firm and about the size of a grapefruit. Massage is not necessary as long as the uterus is firm. Check the firmness of the fundus (top of the uterus) every 5 minutes to ensure that it is still firm. If the uterus does not feel firm, gently massage it by placing one hand above the symphysis pubis and the other on the top of the uterus. The palms of your hands should be facing each other. Gently massage the fundus of the uterus down toward your lower hand (Figure 109-6). This helps the uterus contract (you can feel it firm up) and prevents hemorrhage. When the uterus is firm, stop massaging. Do not overmassage the uterus.

22. Monitor the vital signs of the mother and the infant, the firmness of the uterus, and the cord stump for bleeding every 5 minutes or until the patient is stable.

23. Wash the mother's perineum and apply a sterile perineal pad.

24. Place identification bands on both the mother and the infant.

COMPLICATIONS

1. Prolapsed cord: This usually happens at the same time that membranes rupture. The umbilical cord may protrude from the vagina. Instruct the mother not to push. Elevate the hips or place the mother in the knee-chest position (kneeling with her face down and her chest to her knees) and place the bed in Trendelenberg position. Administer high-flow oxygen via nonrebreather face mask. Place a gloved hand into the vagina, and elevate the infant's head to relieve pressure on the cord. *Do not remove your hand.* Monitor the cord for pulsations. Do not try to place the cord back into

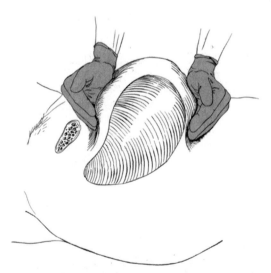

FIGURE 109-6 Uterine massage. One hand remains cupped against the uterus at the level of the symphysis pubis to support the uterus. The other hand is cupped and gently compresses the fundus toward the lower uterine segment. (From Gorrie, T., Murray, S. S., & McKinney, E. S. [2002]. *Foundations of maternal newborn nursing* [3rd ed., p. 776]. Philadelphia: Saunders.)

the vagina. If this position is to be maintained for a prolonged period of time, keep the cord moist with towel moistened with normal saline solution. Prepare for an emergency cesarean section.

2. Fetal distress (hypothermia, aspiration)

3. Shoulder dystocia: The diameter of the shoulders is too wide to pass through the pelvis. This is an emergency requiring immediate obstetrical expertise. Administer high-flow oxygen via nonrebreather facemask.

4. Breech birth: The presenting part of the infant is the buttocks or lower limbs. If one or both feet are the presenting part, this is known as a footling birth. Support the legs and the buttocks of the infant after they have delivered, and apply gentle downward traction until the axillae are visible. Gently lift the body to deliver the posterior shoulder, then gently lower the body to deliver the anterior shoulder. Place your index finger in the infant's mouth and let the infant's chin rest on the palm of your hand (this will maintain the neck in a flexed position to help with delivery). Use your other hand to grasp the neck and shoulders posteriorly. Have someone apply downward pressure over the suprapubic region to push the infant's head under the symphysis. The head should then deliver. Allow the infant to attempt to deliver spontaneously. Do not pull on the infant, or the head may become lodged in the cervix.

5. Limb presentation (one of the infant's extremities is the presenting part): Elevate the mother's hips to slow the birth and contact an obstetrician immediately. Administer high-flow oxygen via nonrebreather mask to the mother.

6. Meconium aspiration leading to respiratory distress. The infant may need endotracheal suctioning to clear the airway of meconium.

7. Fetal death

8. Retained placenta

9. Perineal tearing or vaginal lacerations

10. Postpartum hemorrhage, as evidenced by a steady flow of bright red blood, greater than 750 ml; hypotension; tachycardia; and pale, cool, clammy skin. Administer high-flow oxygen via nonrebreather mask. Place the patient in a modified Trendelenburg position. Place the infant to the breast. Start two large-bore intravenous lines. Apply manual pressure to any external lacerations. Administer intravenous oxytocin as prescribed to contract the uterus.

11. Amniotic fluid embolism. The mother has sudden onset of respiratory distress and shock. Provide treatment to support airway, breathing, and circulation. Order a blood type and crossmatch and have O-negative blood on hand, because disseminated intravascular coagulation may occur.

REFERENCES

American Heart Association (AHA). (2005). American Heart Association guidelines for cardiopulmonary resuscitation and emergency cardiovascular care. *Circulation, 112*(suppl. IV). Retrieved March 10, 2007, from http://circ.ahajournals.org/cgi/content/full/112/24_suppl/IV-188.

Stallard, T. C., & Burns, B. (2003). Emergency delivery and perimortem C-section. *Emergency Medicine Clinics of North America, 21*, 679-693.

Dilatation and Curettage

Robin A. Scott, RN, ND

Dilatation and curettage (D&C) is also known as *suction curettage.*

INDICATION

To open the cervix and empty the contents of the uterus after an incomplete or "missed" abortion and as a diagnostic tool for abnormal vaginal bleeding. The D&C procedure involves widening the cervix with a dilator and scraping the uterine cavity with a curette. Only D&Cs performed during the first trimester of pregnancy are addressed in this procedure.

CONTRAINDICATIONS AND CAUTIONS

1. The emergency department (ED) is not the best location to perform a D&C; an operating room is preferable. Only patients who have stable vital signs and are afebrile should be considered for D&C in the ED. If it is undertaken, consider consulting the anesthesiology department to manage sedation and analgesia needs.
2. In the past, D&C was the standard treatment for spontaneous abortion. However, new methods such as expectant and medical management are being explored as viable alternatives to surgical intervention. Surgical management is mostly likely to produce complete evacuation of the uterine cavity. If expectant or medical management fails, surgical intervention will ultimately be necessary (Sotiriadis, Makrydimas, Papatheodorou, & Ioannidis, 2005).
3. D&C should not be performed until ultrasound and β-hCG levels confirm the diagnosis (Puscheck & Pradhan, 2006).
4. Before the procedure, a thorough history should be taken, including last menstrual period, estimated gestational age, symptoms of pregnancy, degree of bleeding, duration of bleeding, presence of cramps, pain, or fever.
5. A D&C should always be preceded by a thorough pelvic examination to ascertain uterine position and size (see Procedure 107).
6. A single-tooth retractor can cause vascular injury (WHO, 2006).
7. Perforation of the uterus is most likely to occur when the uterine sound or dilators are inserted (Stubblefield, Carr-Ellis, & Borgatta, 2004).
8. Increased procedural difficulty may be encountered, including increased blood loss and lengthened procedure time, in patients with a body mass index (BMI) greater than 30 (Stubblefield et al., 2004).

EQUIPMENT

10-ml syringe
Spinal needle (usually 20- or 22-G)
Local anesthetic

Sterile vaginal speculum
Tenaculum (Figure 110-1)
Ring forceps
Gauze sponges
Cotton balls
Uterine sound
Curettes (Figure 110-2)
Hegar or Hank dilators (Figure 110-3)
Sterile drapes
Antiseptic solution
Pathology specimen container with preservative
Paracervical anesthesia (optional)
For suction curettage:
    Suction machine
    Sterile tubing
    Sterile plastic suction cannulas (7 to 12 mm in diameter)
    Sterile swivel handle
Oxytocin infusion (optional)

PATIENT PREPARATION

1. Insert an intravenous (IV) catheter, 16-G or larger if possible (see Procedure 60).
2. Obtain blood samples and send to laboratory for ABO and Rh typing, complete blood count, β-hCG level, and coagulation studies (White & Bouvier, 2005).
3. Review the steps in the procedure with the patient, including a review of what the patient may feel during each step.

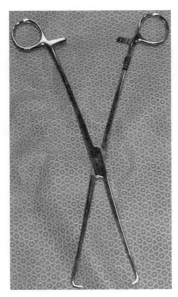

FIGURE 110-1 Tenaculum. (Photograph courtesy of R. Scott.)

4. Ask patient to empty her bladder before the procedure, or insert an indwelling catheter as needed.
5. Administer analgesia and sedation as prescribed.
6. Place the patient in dorsal lithotomy position.

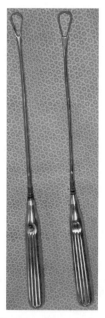

FIGURE 110-2 Currettes. (Photograph courtesy of R. Scott.)

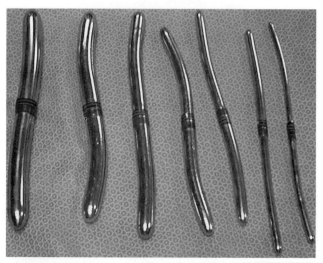

FIGURE 110-3 Hegar dilators. (Photograph courtesy of R. Scott.)

PROCEDURAL STEPS

1. *Administer anesthetic or perform a paracervical block.
2. *Cleanse the vagina and the perineum with antiseptic solution.
3. *Drape the pubic area and the inner thighs. Place a sterile towel under the buttocks.
4. *Using a speculum, visualize the cervix.
5. *Grasp the anterior lip of the cervix with the tenaculum at the 10- or 12-o'clock position (WHO, 2006).
6. *Using gentle traction, bring the cervix down toward the vaginal opening.
7. *Visualize the cervix and examine it for tears.
8. *Gently insert the uterine sound into the cervix and advance it into the uterine cavity. This is accomplished using information about the size and position of the uterus found on pelvic examination. Note the depth of the uterine cavity (WHO, 2006).
9. *Insert the largest size dilator that the cervix can accommodate and continue inserting progressively larger dilators until dilation is sufficient enough to allow evacuation of uterine contents (WHO, 2006).
10. *Evacuate the uterus using a curette and scraping the walls of the uterus until a grating sensation is felt.
11. *Inspect evacuated material for products of conception and quantity of material. Place all tissue obtained in preservative to be sent to pathology.
12. Wash antiseptic and blood from the perineal area. Place a perineal pad and lower the patient's legs gently to the table.
13. Assess the patient's vital signs in comparison to baseline findings.
14. Administer Rho(D) immune globulin (RhoGAM) if prescribed (Puscheck & Pradhan, 2006).
15. *Document estimated blood loss.

COMPLICATIONS

1. Uterine perforation (White & Bouvier, 2005)
2. Uterine hemorrhage (White & Bouvier, 2005)
3. Infection, sepsis (White & Bouvier, 2005)
4. Cervical laceration or trauma
5. Scarring of the uterine lining (Robertson, 2006)
6. Disseminated intravascular coagulation (Stubblefield et al., 2004)

PATIENT TEACHING

1. You may resume your normal daily activities as tolerated (Robertson, 2006).
2. You can expect abdominal cramping and vaginal bleeding after the procedure.
3. Do not use tampons or douche until you are reexamined by your physician.
4. Do not engage in sexual intercourse until your physician indicates that it is safe to do so, in approximately 2 weeks (Cohen, 2006).
5. Notify your physician of fever, chills, abdominal pain, severe cramping, vaginal bleeding that is heavier than a normal menstrual period or more than one pad per hour, or foul-smelling vaginal drainage or if further tissue

---

*Indicates portions of the procedure usually performed by a physician or an advanced practice nurse.

is passed. These symptoms may indicate complications such as infection and require physician evaluation.

6. Follow the instructions regarding Rho(D) immune globulin (RhoGAM) (if prescribed and administered).

7. Schedule a follow-up visit with your physician.

8. You may experience a variety of emotions, including a sense of relief, guilt, sadness, or grief for the loss of the pregnancy. Seeking a grief support group or other community resources is encouraged.

REFERENCES

Cohen, C. K. (2006). Gynecologic disorders. In S. M. Nettina (Ed.), *Lippincott manual of nursing practice* (8th ed., pp. 807-853). Philadelphia: Lippincott Williams & Wilkins.

Puscheck, E., & Pradhan, A. (2006). First trimester pregnancy loss. *eMedicine from WebMD.* Retrieved September 17, 2006, from http://www.emedicine.com/med/topic3310.htm

Robertson, A. R. (2006). D and C. *Medline Plus: A service of the U.S. National Library of Medicine and the National Institutes of Health.* Retrieved September 17, 2006, from http://www.nlm.nih.gov/medlineplus/ency/article/002914.htm

Sotiriadis, A., Makrydimas, G., Papatheodorou, S., & Ioannidis, J. P. A. (2005). Expectant, medical or surgical management of first-trimester miscarriage: A meta-analysis. *American Journal of Obstetricians and Gynecologists, 105,* 1104-1113.

Stubblefield, P. G., Carr-Ellis, S., & Borgatta, L. (2004). Methods for induced abortion. *American Journal of Obstetricians and Gynecologists, 104,* 174-185.

White, H. L., & Bouvier, D. A. (2005). Caring for a patient having a miscarriage. *Nursing, 35,* 18-19.

World Health Organization, Department of Reproductive Health and Research (WHO). (2006). *Managing complications in pregnancy and childbirth: A guide for midwives and doctors.* Retrieved September 17, 2006, from http://www.who.int/reproductive-health/impac/

Musculoskeletal Procedures

Spinal Immobilization

Kyle Madigan, RN, BSN, CEN, CFRN, CCRN

INDICATIONS

To immobilize the spine when injury is suspected. A spinal injury should be suspected in all trauma victims with impaired consciousness; complaints of neck, back, or limb pain; evidence of significant head or facial trauma; localized spinal tenderness, deformity, or paravertebral muscle spasm; signs of a focal neurologic deficit; or unexplained hypotension. The mechanism of injury should be considered in the decision to immobilize patients. A high index of suspicion should accompany the following mechanisms and patient presentations:

Motor vehicle crashes

Falls

Head, neck, or facial trauma

Distracting injury

Multiple trauma

Trauma with history of loss of consciousness, altered level of consciousness, or intoxication

Unconsciousness or confusion with potential for unwitnessed trauma

If in doubt, immobilize.

CONTRAINDICATIONS AND CAUTIONS

1. Evacuation should precede immobilization in the presence of an environmental hazard, such as fire or noxious fumes.
2. Preexisting spinal deformities secondary to conditions such as arthritis or ankylosing spondylitis may require modification of these procedures to align the head and neck in a normal position for the patient.
3. If realignment maneuvers cause additional pain or muscle spasm or compromise the airway, the maneuvers should be stopped immediately and the patient should be immobilized in the position found. If the patient holds the head rigidly angulated or is unable to move the head, realignment is contraindicated, and the patient should be immobilized in the position found.
4. Placing the patient on a backboard should be deferred until life-threatening problems (e.g., airway, breathing, circulation) are addressed and a secondary assessment is completed (see Procedures 1 and 2). Manual stabilization of the head should be used during initial resuscitative efforts.
5. Suction should be immediately available in the event that the immobilized or partially immobilized patient begins to vomit.
6. Immobilization of standing patients may be accomplished by placement of the cervical collar and backboard in a standing position before lowering

the backboard and patient as a unit to a flat position. This procedure is not addressed here. A common hospital practice is to apply a cervical collar and assist the patient to lie down on a stretcher or backboard.
7. The following immobilization technique is not intended for patients in the prehospital setting or for interfacility transport. Further immobilization may be indicated for these patients.

EQUIPMENT

Rigid cervical collar of appropriate size for the patient
Long backboard
Straps or cravats
2- to 3-in adhesive tape
Large-bore continuous oral suction
Towel rolls, foam blocks, or blankets to provide lateral head support
Four or five team members
(Vacuum mattresses are used in addition to backboards in some areas. Consult the manufacturer's instructions for use.)

PATIENT PREPARATION

1. Stabilize the head manually in the position found, and instruct the patient not to move. Large-bore oral suction should be immediately available in case the patient vomits.
2. Instruct the patient to remain as still as possible and to let the health care providers do all of the work.
3. Instruct the patient to alert you immediately if any of the maneuvers causes increased neck pain, numbness or tingling of the extremities, or difficulty breathing.
4. Assess and document neurologic status, including movement and sensation of all extremities both before and after the procedure.
5. If possible, remove the contents of the patient's back pants pockets to prevent pressure points.

PROCEDURAL STEPS

1. Return the patient's head to a neutral position unless contraindicated. A proper neutral inline position is maintained without any significant traction (Salomone & Pons, 2007). The traction pull should be just enough to support the weight of the head off the axis and cervical spine. Place your thumbs under the mandible and your index and middle fingers on the occipital ridges to avoid soft tissue compression and secure a firm hold on the patient (Figure 111-1). This manual stabilization should be maintained until the patient is securely immobilized to a spine board with a rigid cervical collar in place.
2. Apply a rigid cervical collar. Soft foam collars are inadequate for cervical spine immobilization. If possible, remove jewelry from the ears and neck before collar placement. A correctly sized collar should extend from the shoulders to the mandible. An effective cervical collar sits on the chest, posterior thoracic spine and clavicle, and trapezius muscles where the tissue movement is at a minimum (Salomone & Pons, 2007). Two commonly used rigid cervical collars are the Laerdal Stifneck Select Collar and the

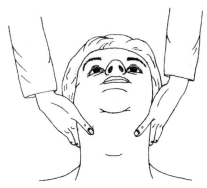

FIGURE 111-1 Manual stabilization of the head. The fingers are placed on the mandible and occipital ridges to avoid soft tissue compression and to secure a firm hold on the patient.

Ambu Perfit ACE Extrication Collar. Both of these collars are adjustable to allow for a wide variety of patient sizes.

a. *Laerdal Stifneck Select, Adult and Pediatric (Laerdal, 2005)*: With the patient in neutral alignment, use your fingers to measure the distance from the top of the shoulder to the bottom of the chin (Figure 111-2, *A*). Find the SIZING LINE on the product and match the collar size to the patient (Figure 111-2, *B*). Adjust and lock both sides of the adjustable collar by pressing the two lock tabs (Figures 111-2, *C* and *D*). Preform the collar to the appropriate shape (Figure 111-2, *E*). Apply the collar while manually maintaining neutral head alignment; ensuring the chin support is well under the chin (Figure 111-2, *F*). If a different size is needed remove, resize, and reapply the collar.

b. *Ambu Perfit ACE Collar (Ambu, 2003)*: Measure the distance between an imaginary plane drawn horizontally and immediately below the patient's chin and second horizontal plane drawn immediately on top of the patient's shoulders (Figure 111-3, *A*). Compare this distance with the distance from the collar sizing line to the lower aspect of the plastic collar body (not the foam) (Figure 111-3, *B*). The Perfit ACE collar is preset to Neckless Size 3. If a taller collar is needed, disengage the safety locks by pulling up on the safety buttons (Figure 111-3, *C*) and pull the collar apart until the distance between the sizing line and the plastic collar body equals your finger measurement (Figure 111-3, *D*). Engage the safety locks by pushing down on the safety buttons. Place an index finger on the foam side of the chin piece (on the center rivet) and the thumb on the plastic side of the chin piece (on the center rivet) and flip the chin piece from the back of the collar to the front of the collar (Figure 111-3, *E* and *F*). Apply the collar to the patient ensuring the patient's chin is securely on top of the chin piece (Figure 111-3, *G*).

3. Log roll the patient to a supine position on a long backboard. The team leader should maintain alignment of the head and coordinate the team's movements.

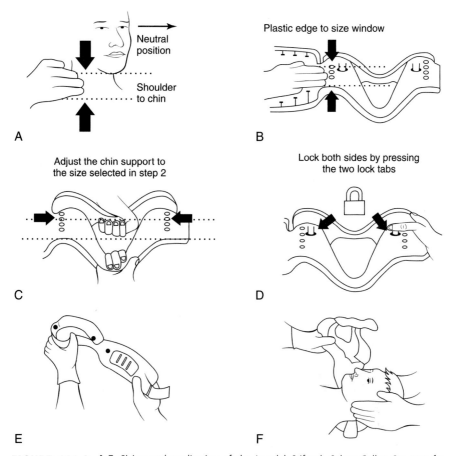

FIGURE 111-2 A-F, Sizing and application of the Laerdal Stifneck Select Collar. See text for details. (Laerdal. [2005]. *Stifneck Select directions for use* [product insert]. Wappingers Falls, NY: Author.)

A useful landmark for maintaining head position is to keep the nose aligned with the umbilicus. At least three additional people are preferred for this movement: one to roll the shoulders and hips, one to roll the hips and legs, and one to place the backboard under the patient.

4. Remove protective headgear if indicated (see Procedure 112).
5. Place padding underneath the head if necessary to prevent hyperextension when the head is lowered to the board.
6. Secure the torso and legs to the board with straps. Many different methods exist for immobilizing the torso and legs to the board. Protection against movement in any direction—up, down, left, or right—should be achieved at both the upper torso (shoulders and chest) and the lower torso (pelvis) to avoid compression and lateral movement of the vertebrae of the torso (Salomone & Pons, 2007). To use regular straps, strap under the armpits at the level of the axilla, across the upper arms, abdomen, hips, distal thighs,

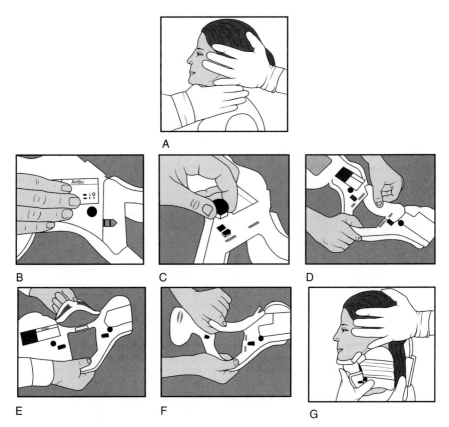

FIGURE 111-3 A-G, Sizing and application of the Ambu Perfit ACE Extrication Collar. See text for details. (Ambu. [2003]. *Ambu Perfit ACE directions for use* [product insert]. Glen Burnie, MD: Author.)

and lower legs (Figure 111-4). To use spider straps, ensure that the "Y"portion is placed over the shoulders. The remaining straps will need to be placed across the chest, pelvis, and lower extremites and secured to the hand holds on the backboard with the hook and loop closure (Figure 111-5).

7. Stabilize the head bilaterally with foam block or towel rolls, and place 2- or 3-inch adhesive tape directly on the skin across the patient's forehead and onto the board (Figure 111-6). The use of sandbags for lateral head stabilization is discouraged because the weight of the sandbags could increase head movement if the board is tipped to the side. Avoid taping across the hair or the eyebrows to prevent patient discomfort and to optimize immobilization. Place the tape directly on the skin of the forehead to improve immobilization. Chin cups or straps encircling the chin should not be used because they may impede mouth opening and lead to aspiration if the patient vomits (Salomone & Pons, 2007).

8. Discontinue manual stabilization of the head at this point.

9. Assess and document neurologic status, including movement and sensation of all extremities.

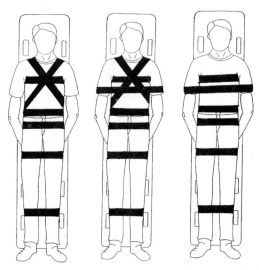

FIGURE 111-4 Acceptable strapping configurations. (From Mazolewski, P., & Manix, T. H. [1994]. The effectiveness of strapping techniques in spinal immobilization. *Annals of Emergency Medicine, 23*, 1292.)

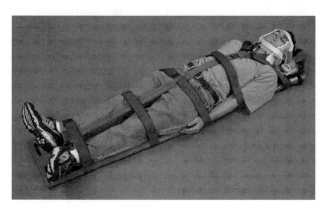

FIGURE 111-5 Proper application of spider straps. (From Sanders, M. J. [2007]. *Mosby's paramedic textbook* [3rd ed., p. 623]. St Louis: Mosby.)

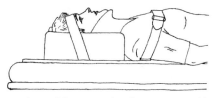

FIGURE 111-6 Head immobilization with adhesive tape and lateral head support.

10. Have suction available at all times, and be prepared to turn the patient on the board should vomiting occur.

AGE-SPECIFIC CONSIDERATIONS

1. Young children present challenges in the assessment of pain. Consider the mechanism of injury carefully to decide when to immobilize.
2. If a child is frightened and fighting, attempts at immobilization may increase movement. If possible, position a parent or caregiver at the top of the backboard in the child's direct line of vision; this can help calm the child and elicit cooperation. The parent can also assist with manual head immobilization.
3. The distinctive anatomic characteristics of infants and children up to age 8 include larger head-to-body ratio, underdeveloped cervical musculature, and incomplete vertebral ossification (Boswell et al., 2001). As a result, placement on a standard backboard may cause excess flexion. To achieve neutral alignment, padding should be placed under the trunk or shoulders, or a backboard with a "cutout" for the head may be used. Optimal position results in the external auditory meatus in line with the shoulders (Figure 111-7) (Mintz, 1994).
4. Pediatric and infant rigid collars are available. If an appropriate-sized collar is not available, a folded towel around the neck may help prevent flexion. Tape across the forehead and head blocks are crucial in this instance. Care must be taken to ensure that the towel around the neck is not too tight.
5. Standard head blocks may be too large to be effective with small children. Rolled towels or blankets can be substituted.
6. Geriatric patients may be at increased risk for skin breakdown because of thinner skin, poor peripheral circulation, loss of subcutaneous padding, and concomitant disease processes. Geriatric patients may also have kyphosis and may require 1 to 3 inches of padding under the occiput in order to avoid hyperextension of the cervical spine.
7. Spinal immobilization restricts respiration by an average of 15% (Totten & Sugarman, 1999). Geriatric patients and patients who have cardiopulmonary

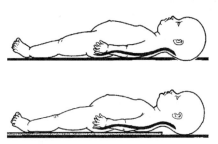

FIGURE 111-7 Immobilization of an infant with "cutout" to accommodate occiput or extra padding from shoulders down. Both techniques achieve optimal alignment (external auditory meatus in line with shoulders). (From Carruthers, G. N. [1997]. Spinal immobilization. In R. A. Dieckmann, D. H. Fiser, & S. M. Selbst [Eds.], *Pediatric emergency and critical care procedures* [p. 598]. St Louis: Mosby.)

disease may experience respiratory compromise when supine. Careful monitoring is essential to ensure that ventilatory status is adequate.

8. The main objective is to maintain neutral alignment of the cervical, thoracic, and lumbar spines throughout the immobiliztion procedure. The pediatric and geriatric population may require additional padding to be placed either under the shoulders or occiput to accomplish this.

COMPLICATIONS

1. Further damage to the spine or the spinal cord as a result of movement. Incorrectly applied straps increase this risk.
2. Respiratory compromise secondary to tight straps across the chest, aspiration of vomitus, improperly sized or placed cervical collar, or excessive neck flexion in young children.
3. Pain related to backboard and collar. Perceived comfort levels are significantly better with the vacuum mattress than with the backboard (Ahmad & Butler, 2001).
4. Tissue breakdown secondary to contact of bony prominences with the backboard or stiff cervical collar. Minimize the time spent on the backboard and pad any bony prominences to help decrease this risk.
5. Supine hypotension in pregnant patients (secondary to the pressure of the gravid uterus on the inferior vena cava). This can be minimized by tilting the backboard to the patient's left 15 to 20 degrees. Care must be taken to immobilize the patient in such a way that she does not slide to the side when the board is tilted.

PATIENT TEACHING

1. Do not move until spinal injury has been ruled out.
2. Immediately report any nausea, difficulty breathing, increased pain, numbness, or tingling.

REFERENCES

Ahmad, M., & Butler, J. (2001). Spinal boards or vacuum mattresses for immobilisation. *Emergency Medicine Journal, 18,* 379-380.

Ambu. (2003). *Ambu Perfit ACE directions for use (product insert).* Glen Burnie, MD: Author.

Boswell, H. B., Dietrich, A., Sheils, W. E., King, D., Ginn-Pease, M., Bowman, M. J., & Cotton, W. H. (2001). Accuracy of visual determination of the immobilized pediatric cervical spine. *Pediatric Emergency Care, 17,* 10-14.

Laerdal. (2005). *Stifneck Select directions for use* (product insert). Wappingers Falls, NY: Author.

Mintz, L. J. (1994). Traction. In S. L. Weinstein (Ed.), *The pediatric spine: Principles and practice* (pp. 1241-1256). New York: Raven Press.

Salomone, J. P., & Pons, P. T. (2007) *Prehospital trauma life support* (6th ed.). St Louis: Mosby.

Totten, V. Y., & Sugarman, D. S. (1999). Respiratory effects of spinal immobilization. *Prehospital Emergency Care, 3,* 347-352.

Helmet Removal

Kyle Madigan, RN, BSN, CEN, CFRN, CCRN

INDICATION

To remove protective headgear (e.g., motorcycle or athletic helmets) from patients with potential cervical spine injuries

CONTRAINDICATIONS AND CAUTIONS

1. Helmet removal may be deferred in a patient without airway compromise when cervical spine injury is strongly suspected. Leaving a helmet in place may require padding to elevate the patient's body from the shoulders down. Otherwise, flexion similar to that seen in a toddler may result with spinal immobiliztion (see Procedure 111).
2. The facemask should be removed at the earliest opportunity, before transportation and regardless of current respiratory status (Kleiner, Almquist, & Bailes, 2001).
3. The presence of football shoulder pads after the removal of a football helmet results in significant cervical extension. Therefore, football players should initially be immobilized with both helmet and shoulder pads left in place to maintain their neck in a neutral postion. The simultaneous removal of the helmet and shoulder pads is best done in a controlled atmosphere, such as the emergency department, with many trained hands (Kleiner et al., 2001).
4. Helmet removal should not be attempted without sufficient trained personnel.

EQUIPMENT

Two people skilled in this technique
NOTE: A one-person technique has been described; however, the two-person technique is the most widely endorsed procedure

PATIENT PREPARATION

1. Manually stabilize the patient's head.
2. Instruct the patient to remain as still as possible and let the health care providers do the work of removing the helmet.
3. Instruct the patient to alert you immediately if any of the maneuvers cause increased neck pain or numbness or tingling of the extremities.
4. If possible, have a second person remove the patient's glasses, necklaces, and earrings.
5. Assess and document neurologic status, including movement and sensation of all extremities both before and after helmet removal.

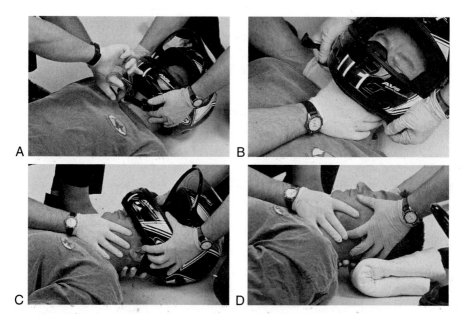

FIGURE 112-1 Helmet removal. **A,** The assistant grasps side of helmet with the palms of the hands and stabilizes the lower mandible with the fingertips. A second provider then opens or removes the face shield if needed, and undoes or cuts the chinstrap. **B,** Grasp the patient's mandible between the thumb and the first two fingers at the angle of the mandible. Then place the other hand under the patient's neck on the occiput to maintain stabilization. **C,** The provider pulls the sides of the helmet apart, then slowly and gently pulls the helmet off of the patient's head, while the assistant maintains manual stabilization. Movements need to be deliberate to minimize movement of the spinal column. **D,** Once the helmet is removed, place padding under the patient's occiput to occupy the void left from the helmet. Manual stabilization is maintained throughout entire procedure. (From McSwain, N., Jr., Frame, S., & Salomone, J. [2007]. *PHTLS: Basic and advanced prehospital trauma life support* [6th ed., pp. 268–270]. St Louis: Mosby.)

PROCEDURAL STEPS

1. *Leader:* Stand at the patient's head and apply gentle in-line stabilization by placing your thumbs on the patient's mandibles and your index fingers on the occipital ridges.

   Assistant: Cut or remove any chin strap or face guard. If the helmet has snap-out ear protectors, remove them by prying them loose with a tongue blade (Figure 112-1, *A*).

2. *Assistant:* Assume in-line stabilization from the leader by cupping the mandible with the thumb and index finger of one hand and placing the other hand on the occipital ridge (Figure 112-1, *B*).

   Leader: Spread the helmet laterally and gently remove it (Figure 112-1, *C*). As the helmet comes over the occiput, it may be necessary to rotate the helmet anteriorly over the face, taking care to avoid the patient's nose.

Assistant: Warning—the head drops as the helmet is removed unless adequate support is provided posteriorly to the occipital ridges.
3. *Leader:* Resume stabilization laterally with your fingers on the mandible and occipital ridges as described in step 1 (Figure 112-1, *D*).
   Assistant: Place a folded towel or blanket under the patient's head as necessary to maintain neutral alignment. Assemble equipment and personnel to immobilize the patient's spine (see Procedure 111).
4. Reassess and document the patient's neurologic status, including movement and sensation of all extremities.

COMPLICATION
Further damage to the spine or the spinal cord as a result of movement

PATIENT TEACHING
Instruct the patient not to move until instructed to do so by the nurse or physician.

REFERENCE
Kleiner, D. M., Almquist, J. H., & Bailes, J., et al. (2001) *Prehospital care of the spine injured athlete: A document from the Inter-Association Task Force for Appropriate Care of the Spine-Injured Athlete.* Dallas: National Athletic Trainers' Association.

PROCEDURE 113

General Principles of Splinting

Ruth L. Schaffler, RN, PhD, ARNP, CEN

INDICATIONS
1. To immobilize and stabilize suspected fractures, dislocations, or tendon ruptures as soon as possible after an injury in order to prevent further soft tissue, blood vessel, nerve, or bony damage.
2. To decrease pain from impaired neurologic function or muscle spasm.
3. To decrease swelling associated with injury by reducing blood and fluid loss into the soft tissues.

4. To immobilize injured areas after burns, bites, or stings.
5. To immobilize an area during the healing of infectious or inflammatory processes and after the surgical repair of muscles or tendons.

CONTRAINDICATIONS AND CAUTIONS

1. Injured extremities should be handled gently and movement of the affected area minimized to decrease pain and risk of complications (e.g., compartment syndrome, fat embolism, vascular or nerve damage, venous thrombosis).
2. Bony prominences should be padded to avoid undue pressure and skin breakdown.
3. The joints above and below the injury site should be immobilized.
4. Gentle longitudinal traction may be exerted while the splint is being applied, except when the injury site involves a joint, a dislocation, or an open fracture. In these cases, the injury should be splinted in the position found, unless circulatory compromise exists, in which case the injury site should be straightened only enough to restore distal pulses.
   NOTE: It is generally agreed that traction splints should be applied in cases of open femoral fractures; this is likely to cause the bone ends to slip beneath the skin. Open fractures are generally considered contaminated, and wound care becomes a high priority (ENA, 2000).
5. Align a severely deformed limb with steady gentle traction so a splint can be applied. The extremity should not be forced into the splint. The splint may have to be improvised or altered to fit the limb in the position of deformity (Buckwalter, 2005).
6. No zippers, knots, or attachments of the splinting device should be placed directly over the injury site.
7. Neurovascular status should be assessed and documented before and after splinting. If sensation and circulation are diminished after splinting, the splint must be readjusted or removed and reapplied.
8. Rigid splints should be well padded to prevent local pressure.
9. If the limb is wrapped circumferentially, the wrapping material should be expandable and nonconstricting.
10. When doubt exists, a splint should be applied.
11. All open fractures should be considered contaminated (ENA, 2000). Care should be taken to clean and cover open wounds with sterile dressings before splinting to minimize the potential for infection. Notify the physician of all open wounds and administer antibiotics promptly as prescribed.

EQUIPMENT

Splints are divided into four general categories:
- Soft (nonrigid)
- Hard (semirigid and rigid)
- Pneumatic (inflatable)
- Traction

Table 113-1 lists indications. Plaster and fiberglass splinting are not addressed in this procedure (see Procedure 124).

TABLE 113-1
DEVICES FOR INITIAL IMMOBILIZATION OF ORTHOPEDIC INJURIES

Site	Type of Splint
Clavicle	Sling and swathe
Shoulder dislocation	
Anterior	Splint to the body with elastic bandage in the position found
Posterior	Sling and swathe
Scapula	Sling and swathe
Humerus	Rigid splint with sling and swathe
Elbow	Rigid splint with sling and swathe in position found
Forearm	Rigid splint with sling, air splint
Wrist	Rigid splint with sling
Hand, fingers	Rigid splint in position of function
Spine	Backboard, stiff cervical collar, lateral head support
Pelvis	Backboard, PASG, circumferential binding
Hip	Backboard, traction splint, or secure the injured leg to the uninjured leg with cravats or bandages
Femur	Traction splint, rigid splint, or PASG
Patella	Soft or padded rigid splint placed posteriorly in position found
Tibia/fibula	Air splint, rigid splint
Ankle	Air splint or pillow
Foot	Air splint or pillow
Toes	Tape to adjacent digit on medial side, rigid splint on great toe

PASG, Pneumatic antishock garment (see Procedure 51).

Soft (Nonrigid) Splints

Bandaging material
Blanket
Cloth
Cravat
Foam rubber
Pillow
Clavicle strap
Sling and swathe
Binder

Hard (Rigid and Semirigid) Splints

Aluminum or other pliable metal
Cardboard
Fiberglass
Wire ladder splints
Leather
Molded plastic
Plaster
Vacuum
Wood, backboards
Cervical collar

Finger splint
Wrist splint
Knee immobilizer
Ankle support
Orthopedic shoe

Pneumatic (Inflatable) Splints

Air splints
Pneumatic antishock garment (PASG)

Traction (capable of maintaining longitudinal traction for lower extremity fractures)

Sager (Minto Research & Development, Redding, CA)
Hare (DynaMed, Carlsbad, CA)
Kendrick traction device (Medix Choice, El Cajon, CA)
Thomas splint
Additional equipment may include:
    Padding material
    Elastic bandage
    Roller gauze bandage
    Tape
    Safety pins

PATIENT PREPARATION

1. Cut away clothing over the injury site and remove bulky material or sharp objects from pockets that may lie under the splint after application.
2. Assess and document the neurovascular status.
3. Measure the noninjured side to determine the correct size of the splint.
4. Pad bony prominences or soft tissue areas, such as the groin.
5. Remove jewelry from injured extremities (see Procedure 114).
6. Remove boots or shoes from lower extremity injuries to assess pulses and sensation. Footwear that is difficult to remove or that is supportive to the ankle may be left on if some types of traction splints are used; however, the neurovascular status cannot be monitored.
7. Place a sterile dressing over all open wounds.
8. Pad areas of skin-to-skin contact under the splint to absorb perspiration and prevent tissue maceration.

PROCEDURAL STEPS

1. Remove clothing from the injured area to inspect for wounds, deformity, ecchymosis, and swelling.
2. Grasp the extremity with both hands, one hand below and one hand above the injury site, and exert gentle longitudinal traction to straighten any angulation. Maintain manual stabilization until the splint is secure. Fractures or dislocations of the joints should be splinted in the position found unless distal circulation is diminished or absent. In this situation, straighten the limb only enough to restore pulses. Do not attempt to realign fractures of the shoulder, elbow, wrist, or knee. Do not attempt to push protruding bone ends beneath the skin, but if bone ends slip back

into the wound, document the existence of an open fracture, and notify the physician.

3. Immobilize the joints above and below the injury site.

4. The splint should fit snugly but not be constrictive. Leave fingers and toes exposed. If possible, elevate the injured part.

5. Assess and document distal neurovascular status. If sensation or circulation is diminished, the splint must be adjusted or removed and reapplied.

6. Use traction splints for fractures of the proximal tibia or femur. Use them with caution if fractures of the pelvis or ankle are also present (see Procedure 118).

7. Leave the splint intact until definitive treatment is determined. If it is necessary to remove or readjust the splint for diagnostic procedures, reassess and document the neurovascular status after splint removal and reapplication.

AGE-SPECIFIC CONSIDERATIONS
Pediatric
1. A child's bony structure is more elastic and malleable than an adult's. It takes significant force to result in a fracture. Many injuries in children younger than 5 years are related to abuse. Nonaccidental trauma should be suspected when a child younger than age 1 year presents with a long-bone fracture. Children who are abused may have multiple fractures in various stages of healing or may have repeated fractures (Brady & Burns, 2004).

2. The epiphyses (growth plates) at the ends of long articulating bones are more susceptible to trauma in preadolescent children. Fractures that involve the epiphysis (also known as Salter fractures) may interfere with normal bone growth and result in discrepancy of limb length (Brady & Burns, 2004).

3. Children's bones have a thicker periosteal covering, which enables faster and smoother recalcification after a fracture. Nonunion is rare.

Geriatric
1. Degenerative changes that affect tendons, joints, and intervertebral discs begin in adults at about age 40. Demineralization and loss of bone mass occur over the life span but significantly increases after age 35. The bones of older adults are more brittle and susceptible to fracture, particularly postmenopausal women (Burke & Laramie, 2004). The elderly have prolonged healing times. Complete healing can take 3 to 6 months and may lead to admission into a skilled nursing facility.

2. The elderly are the fastest growing segment of the population and are at great risk for trauma. The most common orthopedic problems in the elderly are related to unsteady gait and balance problems, sensory deficits, decreased reflexes, and use of medications that increase the risk of falling (Kunkler, 2004). Nearly one-third of the elderly experience a fall every year. Half of those have repeated falls, with 1% resulting in a fracture of the hip (Buckwalter, 2005).

3. Pathologic fractures may occur as a result of chronic disease conditions such as osteoarthritis and osteoporosis (Roberts, 2004).

4. The elderly have thinner skin and less soft tissue padding; therefore, they are more prone to alterations in skin integrity.

5. Be alert to the physical and behavioral signs of abuse in all age groups, they may be covert and masked by the presenting injuries.

COMPLICATIONS

1. Decreased or absent pulses and sensation
2. Edema
3. Vascular or nerve damage
4. Compartment syndrome
5. Venous thrombosis
6. Fat embolism
7. Disruption of skin integrity and infection
8. Misalignment of bone ends
9. Increased pain

PATIENT TEACHING

1. Watch for changes in fingertips and toes—cool to touch, dusky color, swelling, altered or decreased sensation. If an elastic bandage is removed, rewrap it snugly but not too tightly.
2. Report pain that continues to increase in severity and does not respond to pain medications.
3. Elevate the limb above the level of the heart to decrease swelling and pain.
4. Use cold packs over the injured area to minimize bleeding and swelling.
5. Limit mobility and activity to allow healing of the injured site. Perform only approved activities (e.g., weightbearing, stretching, or bending of joints).
6. Do not use coat hangers or other sharp objects to scratch the skin inside the splint.
7. Review with the patient the length of time to wear the splinting or immobilization device and when to follow up with the primary health care provider or physical therapist.
8. Instruct the patient in crutch walking, if indicated, and have the patient give a return demonstration of the techniques (see Procedure 132).
9. Assess the patient's ability to continue activities of daily living and the possible need for family or professional assistance at home.
10. Discuss injury prevention strategies with patients and families.

REFERENCES

Brady, M. A., & Burns, C. E. (2004). Musculoskeletal disorders. In C. E. Burns, A. M. Dunn, M. A. Brady, N. B. Starr, & C. G. Blosser (Eds.), *Pediatric primary care: A handbook for nurse practitioners* (3rd ed., pp. 1047-1082). Philadelphia: Saunders.

Buckwalter, J. A. (2005). General orthopaedics. In L. Y. Griffin (Ed.), *Essentials of musculoskeletal care* (3rd ed., pp. 1-143). Rosemont, IL: American Academy of Orthopaedic Surgeons.

Burke, M. M., & Laramie, J. A. (2004) *Primary care of the older adult: A multidisciplinary approach* (2nd ed.). St Louis: Mosby.

Emergency Nurses Association (ENA). (2000). *Trauma nursing core course: Provider manual* (5th ed.). Des Plaines, IL: Author.

Kunkler, C. E. (2004). Nursing management: Musculoskeletal trauma and orthopedic surgery. In S. M. Lewis, M. M. Heitkemper, & S. R. Dirksen (Eds.), *Medical-surgical nursing: Assessment and management of clinical problems* (6th ed., pp. 1650-1691). St Louis: Mosby.

Roberts, D. (2004). Nursing assessment: Musculoskeletal system. In S. M. Lewis, M. M. Heitkemper, & S. R. Dirksen (Eds.), *Medical-surgical nursing: Assessment and management of clinical problems* (6th ed., pp. 1635-1649). St Louis: Mosby.

PROCEDURE 114

Ring Removal

Kyle Madigan, RN, BSN, CEN, CFRN, CCRN

INDICATION

To remove a ring when an upper extremity injury is present and when other methods, such as use of a lubricant and soap, have failed. In the presence of any extremity injury, all jewelry should be removed from the extremity as soon as possible.

CONTRAINDICATIONS AND CAUTIONS

1. If vascular compromise is present or imminent, the ring should be removed with a ring cutter as quickly as possible.
2. The string method should not be used if there are lacerations, fractures, or dislocations to the involved finger or toe; a ring cutter should be used.

PATIENT PREPARATION

1. Ring removal may not be possible without digital anesthesia if the finger (or toe) is extremely painful. A digital or metacarpal (metatarsal) block producing minimal tissue distention may be performed (see Procedure 136) (Stone & Koutouzis, 2004). Conscious sedation may also be indicated.
2. Before removal using the string method, attempt to decrease edema by using a Penrose drain wrapped distally to proximally along the finger or toe (Stone & Koutouzis, 2004). Elevate the hand or foot, apply an ice pack, and wait a few minutes.

STRING METHOD
Equipment for String Method

Penrose drain (optional)
2 to 3 feet of umbilical tape or heavy suture (1-0 or heavier silk)

Small, curved hemostat
Bar soap (optional)

Procedural Steps for String Method

1. Rub the bar soap along the length of the tape or suture. This step is optional, but it makes ring removal easier.
2. Pass the end of the string under the ring, using the hemostat if necessary.
3. Have the patient anchor the tape or suture against the palm with the thumb. Wrap the string tightly around the finger clockwise in close, concentric circles, starting next to the ring and moving toward the finger tip (Figure 114-1). Be especially careful to wrap firmly around the proximal interphalangeal joint, because this is the most difficult area of the ring removal process.
4. While pulling the proximal end of the string toward the fingertip and against the ring, unwrap the string in a clockwise direction from the finger. This moves the ring over the string-wrapped finger (see Figure 114-1).
5. Repeat the procedure until the ring is removed.
6. May also be used on a toe.

MANUAL RING CUTTER
Equipment for Manual Ring Cutter

Ring cutter
Hemostat
Pliers
Lubricant

Procedural Steps for Manual Ring Cutter

1. Insert the curved blade of the ring cutter under the narrowest part of the ring. Lubrication may be necessary (Figure 114-2).
2. Clamp the saw firmly down on the ring, and turn the blade manually until the ring is severed.

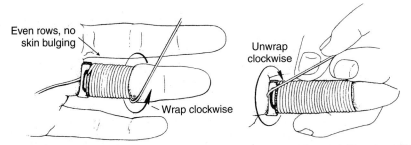

FIGURE 114-1 String method of ring removal. Wrap umbilical tape from proximal to distal in close concentric circles around the finger. Using the proximal tail of the tape, unwrap in a clockwise direction while maintaining slight traction. (Stone, D. B., & Koutouzis, T. K. (2004). Soft tissue foreign body removal. In J. R. Roberts & J. R. Hedges (Eds.), *Clinical procedures in emergency medicine* [4th ed., p. 713]. Philadelphia: Saunders.)

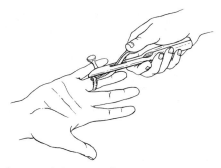

FIGURE 114-2 Use of a manual ring cutter. (From Rosen, P., & Sternbach, G. L. [1983]. *Atlas of emergency medicine* [2nd ed., p. 219]. Baltimore: William & Wilkins.)

3. Pry the ends of the ring apart and away from the finger with a hemostat, pliers, or both.
4. Remove the ring carefully to prevent injury from the severed ring ends.

BATTERY-POWERED RING CUTTER
Equipment for Battery-Powered Ring Cutter
Battery-powered ring cutter (Gem II, M. W. Mooney, Ashland, OR)
Water-soluble lubricating jelly
Hemostat or ring spreader
Pliers (optional)

Procedural Steps for Gem II Battery-Powered Ring Cutter (M. W. Mooney, 2006)

1. Check to see that the correct blade is in place. Use the blue-coated carbide disk for gold and silver. The diamond disk (red coated) is used for platinum, steel, iron, and brass.
2. Liberally cover the area to be cut with water-soluble lubricating jelly. The cutting process generates heat, and the jelly helps dissipate the heat and prevents discomfort or burns. If the warmth becomes uncomfortable, pause and apply fresh lubricant. An ice cube placed against the ring during cutting also helps decrease heat.
3. Slide the finger guard completely under the ring and the finger (or toe) (Figure 114-3).
4. Attach the cutter to the finger guard with the cutting disk on the ring.
5. Rest the blade on the surface of the ring.
6. Turn the ring cutter on by pushing the red button to activate.
7. Gently move the cutting disk backward and forward from one side of the ring to the other. The weight of the cutter head provides the necessary downward force. Do not press down on the blade. Rings made of high-tensile metal may require two cuts, one on each side of the ring. It's best to make two full-thickness cuts, separated by approximately 180 degrees (allowing for the design of any setting). This will allow the ring to be easily repaired by a jeweler. When it's not possible to make two cuts, make a single

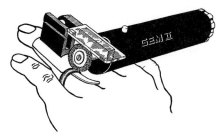

FIGURE 114-3 Gem II battery-powered ring cutter. (Courtesy M. W. Mooney & Co., Ashland, OR.)

full thickness cut and then use a ring spreading instrument or two hemostats to gently spread the ring and slip it from the finger. Spread only as far as necessary to slip the ring from the finger. To reduce the tension in the high-tensile strength metals, such as steel, first make a quarter-thickness cut and then a full-thickness cut on the opposite side of the ring. This will reduce the tension and allow the ring remover instrument to be used (M. W. Mooney, 2006).

8. A sudden increase in the rotating speed of the disk indicates that the ring is cut through.
9. Pry the ends of the ring apart and away from the finger with a ring spreader, a hemostat, or pliers.
10. Remove the ring carefully to prevent injury from the severed ring ends.

REMOVAL OF HARD METAL OR CERAMIC RINGS WITH VISE GRIP–STYLE PLIERS
Equipment for Removal of Hard Metal or Ceramic Rings
Vise grip–style locking pliers

Procedural Steps for Removal of Hard Metal or Ceramic Rings (Hajduk, 2001)
1. Place vice grip–style locking pliers over ring and adjust the jaws to clamp lightly.
2. Release and adjust tightener one-third turn and then clamp again.
3. Repeat step 2 until a crack is heard; then continue clamping in different positions on the ring until the hard material breaks away.
4. If the ring contains an inlay of gold, the exposed gold can be cut in the usual fashion.

COMPLICATIONS
1. Abrasions (from the string method)
2. Laceration of the finger from the severed ring ends (if a ring cutter is used)
3. Minor burn if inadequate lubricant is used (battery-powered ring cutter)

PATIENT TEACHING
Instruct the patient to remove rings promptly if any future injuries to the upper extremity occur.

REFERENCES

Hajduk, S. V. (2001). Emergency removal of hard metal or ceramic finger rings (letter to the editor). *Annals of Emergency Medicine, 37,* 736.

M. W. Mooney & Co. (2006). *Gem II ring cutting system operators manual.* Ashland, OR: Author.

Stone, D. B., & Koutouzis, T. K. (2004). Soft tissue foreign body removal. In J. R. Roberts, & J. R. Hedges (Eds.), *Clinical procedures in emergency medicine* (4th ed., pp. 694-716). Philadelphia: Saunders.

PROCEDURE 115

Body Jewelry Removal

Kyle Madigan, RN, BSN, CEN, CCRN, CFRN

INDICATIONS

To remove body jewelry in the presence of an injury or to facilitate diagnostic studies in which the jewelry would hinder or obstruct the ability to perform procedures or to obtain a complete examination (e.g., surgical procedure, radiographic studies, magnetic resonance imaging [MRI]). Removal of oral piercings should be attempted before intubation to decrease risk of trauma and subsequent hemorrhage, as well as aspiration of the jewelry.

NOTE: This procedure encompasses common, commercially available body jewelry inserted by professional piercers. Amateur piercings may involve other types of jewelry and materials, including homemade items. If possible, ask the patient about the nature and the material of the jewelry before attempting removal.

CONTRAINDICATIONS AND CAUTIONS

1. Health care providers may instruct patients with infected piercings to remove the jewelry; however, jewelry removal may allow healing and closure of the epidermis, while promoting abscess formation in deeper skin structures (Christiensen, Miller, Patsdaughter, & Dowd, 2000). Even momentary removal of jewelry from a healing piercing can result in amazingly rapid closure of the piercing and make reinsertion difficult or impossible (Association of Professional Piercers, 2001).

2. Electrical burns can occur if body jewelry is worn and exposed to a current, such as electrocauterization. Defibrillation during cardiac arrest could result in burns if a nipple ring is present (Christiensen et al., 2000).

3. Appropriate metal body jewelry is not magnetic and therefore does

not need to be removed for MRI procedures, unless it is located in the region being examined (Association of Professional Piercers, 2001). In emergency situations, it may be difficult to determine the type of metal used, and appropriate precautions should be taken.

4. Any jewelry that is removed should be treated as contaminated with body fluid and placed in a container with antiseptic solution (Leviton, Reilly, & Storm, 1997).

PATIENT PREPARATION

1. When possible, ask the patient to remove the piercing.
2. Ascertain type of piercing to be removed (e.g., bead ring, captive bead ring, and circular barbell/barbell) (Figure 115-1).

CAPTIVE BEAD RING/BEAD RING REMOVAL
Equipment for Captive Bead/Bead Ring Removal

Ring-expanding pliers (preferred)
Two hemostats (smooth jaw preferred to decrease damage to jewelry) (optional)
Two pairs of needle-nose pliers (optional)
External snap ring pliers (optional)

Procedural Steps for Captive Bead/Bead Ring Removal

1. When using ring-expanding pliers or external snap ring pliers, place the head of the pliers inside the captive bead ring and squeeze handle to spread jaws to remove one end from the bead, proceed to step 3 (Figure 115-2).
2. Grasp the ring on each side of the bead with hemostats or pliers, pull gently in opposite directions; one end will be removed from the bead.
3. Grasp the jewelry with hemostats and rotate away from bead, and out of the patient's tissue (Figure 115-3).

BARBELL/CIRCULAR BARBELL/LABRET REMOVAL
Equipment for Barbell/Circular Barbell/Labret Removal

Two hemostats (smooth jaw preferred) (optional)
or
Two pairs of needle-nose pliers (optional)

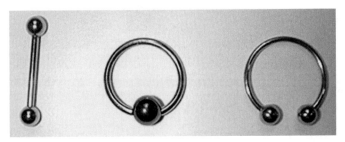

FIGURE 115-1 Barbell, captive bead ring, circular barbell. (Courtesy Association of Professional Piercers, Chamblee, GA, 2001.)

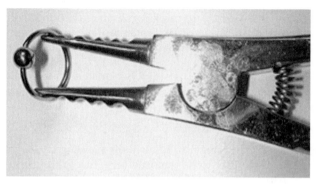

FIGURE 115-2 Ring-expanding pliers with captive bead ring. (Courtesy Association of Professional Piercers, Chamblee, GA, 2001.)

Procedural Steps for Barbell/Circular Barbell/Labret Removal

1. Using fingers or hemostats grasp both ends of the jewelry, usually in the shape of a bead (Figure 115-4).
2. Unscrew the bead in a counterclockwise rotation. One or both ends may be threaded in this type of jewelry.
3. After removal of the threaded bead, slide jewelry from tissue.

COMPLICATIONS

1. Aspiration of jewelry during oral piercing removal.
2. Additional tissue trauma during removal of tongue piercing may result in edema, further complicating airway management.
3. Use of jewelry cutting methods may have limited success because of materials used (e.g., titanium). Cutting body jewelry may produce rough, burred edges that may further damage the tissue with its removal.

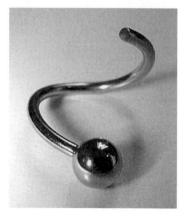

FIGURE 115-3 Captive bead ring removed with hemostats. (Courtesy Association of Professional Piercers, Chamblee, GA, 2001.)

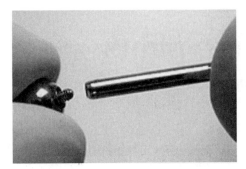

FIGURE 115-4 Removal of internally threaded barbell. (Courtesy Association of Professional Piercers, Chamblee, GA, 2001.)

4. Jewelry may be slippery secondary to blood or body fluids; be careful not to cut yourself during removal.

PATIENT TEACHING

Instruct patient that unless the piercing is well established, the track closes quickly, and it may be difficult or even impossible to reinsert (Hatfield-Law, 2001).

REFERENCES

Association of Professional Piercers. (2001). *Body piercing: Troubleshooting for you and your healthcare professional.* Available at http://www.safepiercing.org

Christiensen, M. H., Miller, K. H., Patsdaughter, C. A., & Dowd, L. J. (2000). To the point: the contemporary body piercing and tattooing renaissance. *Nursing Spectrum Online.* Retrieved December 29, 2002, from http://nsweb.nursingspectrum.com/ce/ce194.htm

Leviton, R., Reilly, J., & Storm, B. (1997). Body piercing: EMS concerns. *Emergency, 2,* 18-20.

Hatfield-Law, L. (2001). Body piercing: Issues for A&E nurses. *Accident and Emergency Nursing, 9,* 14-19.

Vacuum Splints

Ruth L. Schaffler, RN, PhD, ARNP, CEN

The information in this chapter is specific to vacuum splints and should be used in conjunction with Procedure 113.

INDICATION

To temporarily immobilize injured extremities. Vacuum splints are particularly useful for immobilizing an extremity in the position found. When ready to immobilize, the air in the splint is pumped out and the splint becomes rigid and conforms to the shape of the extremity. Once applied, the splint can be remolded if swelling or neurocompromise occurs. The splints are lightweight, radiotranslucent, and can remain in place for up to 24 hours if needed. Vacuum mattresses are also available and are useful for full-body splinting, whether the patient is lying or sitting. Full-leg vacuum splints can be used as a full-body splint for an infant or small child. In one study, the vacuum mattress was found to provide greater patient stability and comfort than a long backboard (Luscombe & Williams, 2003).

CONTRAINDICATIONS AND CAUTIONS

1. Vacuum splints are bulky and nontransparent and may not allow access to the distal limb for reassessment after splint application.
2. The splint valve should be closed tightly to prevent loss of rigidity once the splint has been applied.

EQUIPMENT

Vacuum splint
Vacuum pump
Accessory straps or tape
Talcum power or cornstarch (optional)

PATIENT PREPARATION

1. Remove clothing, jewelry, or constrictive bulky material that may lie under the splint (Procedures 114 and 115).
2. Cover open wounds with sterile dressings.
3. Apply gentle traction to align the limb, if appropriate, or prepare to splint as found (Garcia, 2002; Limmer & O'Keefe, 2005).

PROCEDURAL STEPS

1. Lay the vacuum splint flat with all straps open and the inner surface facing up. Smooth the foam beads evenly throughout the splint to ensure uniform distribution.

2. Dust the splint with talcum powder or cornstarch (optional; contraindicated in the presence of open wounds).
3. Support the bone ends above and below the injury site as the splint is placed around the limb (Figure 116-1, *A*).
4. Form or shape the splint over the sides and top of the limb.
5. Secure the splint with the attached straps or tape. Fold the distal portion of the splint outward as needed to allow inspection of fingers or toes.
6. Attach the vacuum pump to the splint and evacuate the air until the splint converts from a soft, pliable device to castlike rigidity (Figure 116-1, *B*).
7. Twist the valve clockwise until it is tight before disconnecting the pump. Some models have a spring-loaded valve that is self-sealing when the pump is removed.
8. To remove the splint, open the splint valve by turning it in a counterclockwise motion. When the splint is pliable, open the straps, and carefully support the limb while the splint is removed.

AGE-SPECIFIC CONSIDERATIONS

1. Many arm and leg vacuum splints are too large to fit on the smaller extremities of infants and children.
2. The skin of the elderly can be quite friable; a layer of padding may be needed between the skin and the splint to avoid pressure problems.

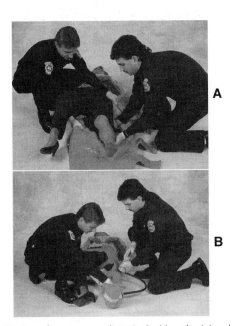

FIGURE 116-1 Application of a vacuum splint. **A,** Position the injured extremity in the center of the splint. **B,** Wrap the splint around the extremity and attach the vacuum pump. The splint forms to the extremity and becomes rigid after the air is evacuated. (From American Academy of Orthopedic Surgeons. [1993]. *Emergency care and transportation of the sick and injured* [5th ed., p. 279]. Rosemont, IL: Author.)

COMPLICATIONS

1. Accumulation of perspiration or moisture inside the splint may cause it to adhere to the skin and cause increased pain when removing or may macerate the skin. Dusting the interior of the splint with talcum powder or cornstarch before application may help decrease this.

2. The splint loses its rigidity if it is punctured or torn. Each time the splint is folded for storage it develops a corner that is susceptible to the development of cracks (Hartwell Medical, n.d.).

3. The splint may soften during significant changes in altitude and may need to be adjusted accordingly.

4. Vacuum is not maintained if the valve mechanism is not fully closed or if it is damaged.

REFERENCES

Garcia, B. (2002). Extremity trauma. In M. W. Hubble, & J. P. Hubble (Eds.), *Principles of advanced trauma care* (pp. 315-349). Albany, NY: Delmar.

Hartwell Medical. (n.d.). *Answers to frequently asked questions: Vacuum technology—EVAC-U-SPLINT products*. Retrieved August 6, 2006, from http://www.hartwellmedical.com/faqevac.html

Limmer, D., & O'Keefe, M. (2005). Musculoskeletal injuries. In D. Limmer, M. O'Keefe, E. Dickinson, H. Grant, B. Murray, & J. Bergeron (Eds.), *Emergency care* (10th ed., pp. 633-681). Upper Saddle River, NJ: Prentice-Hall.

Luscombe, M. D., & Williams, J. L. (2003). Comparison of a long spinal board and vacuum mattress for spinal immobilisation. *Emergency Medicine Journal, 20*, 476-478.

Air Splints

Ruth L. Schaffler, RN, PhD, ARNP, CEN

The information in this chapter should be used in conjunction with the information in Procedure 113.

Air splints are also known as *pneumatic splints.*

INDICATIONS

1. To temporarily immobilize injuries of the distal extremities—arm, lower leg, and ankle.
2. To decrease swelling and blood loss into the soft tissues, or to control external bleeding associated with distal extremity injuries (Griffin, 2005; Limmer & O'Keefe, 2005). A pneumatic antishock garment may also be used as an air splint for fractures of the pelvis or lower extremities (see Procedure 51).
3. Air splints are relatively "dynamic" in that pneumatic pressure can be adjusted as indicated. Air splints can align the joint and limb while decreasing the risk of secondary complications such as ischemia or pressure ulcers particularly in patients with diminished or absent sensation (Taly, Nair, Murali, & Wankade, 2002).

CONTRAINDICATIONS AND CAUTIONS

1. Air splints are not suitable for angulated fractures or fractures involving joints. The design of the splint allows immobilization only in anatomic positions.
2. Air splints should not be applied over clothing because the pressure created by buckles, buttons, or wrinkles may injure the soft tissues.
3. Air splints should not be inflated with positive-pressure devices.
4. Overinflation of an air splint may cause circulatory compromise; underinflation may not provide enough support.
5. Air splints are not effective for fractures of the humerus or femur.
6. Air pressure within a pneumatic splint is subject to fluctuations with temperature and altitude variations. The pressure increases with warmth and ascent and decreases with cold and descent. Careful monitoring is required when this type of splint is used in a changing environment.
7. Air splints may not maintain adequate immobilization because they have a tendency to leak (Taly et al, 2002).

EQUIPMENT

Air splint (appropriate size and shape for area to be immobilized)
Talcum powder or cornstarch (optional)

PATIENT PREPARATION

1. Remove any clothing or jewelry that would lie under the splint (see Procedures 114 and 115).
2. Cover open wounds with sterile dressings.

PROCEDURAL STEPS

1. Open the zipper of the air splint. If the splint has no zipper, gather the distal portion of the splint over your arm (Figure 117-1, *A*).
2. Dust the interior of the splint with talcum powder or cornstarch (optional; contraindicated in the presence of open wounds).
3. Grasp the patient's hand or foot and apply gentle longitudinal traction to straighten the limb slightly, if necessary.
4. Place the splint, free of wrinkles, on the patient's extremity (see Figure 117-1, *B*).
5. Twist the valve on the splint in a counterclockwise motion to open it.
6. Inflate the splint by mouth to a point where your finger makes a slight dent in the surface of the splint (see Figure 117-1, *C*).
7. Twist the valve clockwise to close it and prevent air loss.
8. Monitor the air pressure within the splint frequently. You should be able to indent the splint wall with your finger.

AGE-SPECIFIC CONSIDERATIONS

1. Many air splints are an inappropriate size for children's extremities.

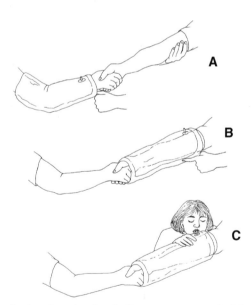

FIGURE 117-1 Application of an air splint. **A,** The rescuer supports the injured extremity with one hand and places the air splint on the other arm. **B,** An assistant slides the splint onto the patient's arm. **C,** The air splint is inflated until finger pressure makes a slight dent. (From Brabson, T. A., & Greenfield, B. S. [2004]. Prehospital splinting. In J. R. Roberts & J. R. Hedges [Eds.], *Clinical procedures in emergency medicine* [4th ed., p. 90]. Philadelphia: Saunders.)

2. The skin of the elderly can be quite friable; a thin layer of smooth padding may be necessary between the skin and the splint.

COMPLICATIONS

1. Complications of air splinting can include constriction of blood supply and compression on nerves in the extremity particularly when the splint is overinflated.
2. Excessive pressure variation within the splint may result in inadequate immobilization (decreased pressure) or compartment syndrome or soft tissue damage (increased pressure).
3. Accumulation of perspiration or moisture inside the splint may cause it to cling to the skin and can make removal difficult or cause skin maceration. Dusting the interior of the splint with talcum powder or cornstarch before application may help decrease this problem.
4. Some air splints are not transparent, and wounds under the splint cannot be visualized.

REFERENCES

In Griffin, L. Y. (Ed.). (2005). *Essentials of musculoskeletal care* (3rd ed.). Rosemont IL: American Academy of Orthopaedic Surgeons.

Limmer, D., & O'Keefe, M. (2005). Musculoskeletal injuries. In D. Limmer, M. O'Keefe, E. Dickinson, H. D. Grant, R. H. Murray, & J. D. Bergeron (Eds.), *Emergency care* (10th ed., pp. 633-681). Upper Saddle River, NJ: Prentice-Hall.

Taly, A. B., Nair, K. P., Murali, T., & Wankade, M. (2002). Pneumatic splints: Fabrication and use in neurorehabilitation. *Neurology India, 50*(1), 68-70.

PROCEDURE 118

Traction Splints

Ruth L. Schaffler, RN, PhD, ARNP, CEN

The information in this chapter is specific to traction splints and should be used in conjunction with Procedure 113.

There are four basic types of traction splints: Hare, Kendrick, Sager, or Thomas splints.

INDICATION

To align and stabilize a fracture of the femur or proximal tibia. A traction splint is the preferred splint for a femur fracture.

CONTRAINDICATIONS AND CAUTIONS

1. Traction splints are not suitable for fractures of the distal fibula, distal tibia, ankle, foot, or upper extremity (Limmer & O'Keefe, 2005; Sanders, 2005).
2. Bipolar traction splints, such as the FernoTrac, Hare, and Thomas splints, can displace the proximal third of a fractured femur because of the posterior placement of the ischial pad. To reduce this problem, the ischial pad can be placed on the lateral aspect of the extremity fracture. Unipolar traction splints, such as the Sager and Kendrick splints, do not have this risk because they are designed differently (Limmer & O'Keefe, 2005).
3. Traction splints should be used cautiously in patients who also have pelvic fractures. If pelvic pain increases after splint application, the splint should be removed.
4. Traction splints may be used with open fractures of the femur. In this case, the bone ends usually slip back beneath the skin. Known or suspected open fractures are considered surgical emergencies, are potentially contaminated, and should be reported to the physician. Do not place straps directly over an open wound.
5. Two persons are needed to apply most traction splints; however, the Sager or Kendrick splint can be applied by one person.
6. In general, clothing and footwear should be removed before applying a traction splint. If a shoe or boot is difficult to remove or if it serves as a splint for the ankle, leave it on.
7. Blood loss from a femoral fracture can be as high as 1 to 2 L (Bledsoe & Barnes, 2004; Gisness, 2005; Limmer & O'Keefe, 2005). If early signs of shock are present in a patient with a femur fracture, a pneumatic antishock garment may be a better choice than a traction splint to stabilize the fracture.

EQUIPMENT
Splint

Hare traction splint (DynaMed, Carlsbad, CA) or FernoTrac traction splint (Rancho Cordova, CA)
   Metal frame with padded ischial bar and a heel stand
   Ratchet device
   Ankle hitch
   Elastic straps
Kendrick traction device (Medix Choice, El Cajon, CA) (The Kendrick traction device collapses into a compact package for easy storage and transport.)
   Snap-out traction pole
   Thigh strap with pole receptacle
   Ankle hitch
   Elastic straps
Sager traction splint (Minto Research & Development, Redding, CA) (The Sager splint is also available in a bilateral model.)
   Ankle harness
   Thigh strap
   Elastic leg straps

Metal bar with padded arch support for groin
Attached pulley-and-cable apparatus
Thomas splint
Metal frame with padded ischial half-ring
Cravats
Padding (ABD dressings or similar material)

PATIENT PREPARATION

1. Pad the anterior groin area (not necessary with a Sager or Kendrick splint).
2. Measure against the unaffected extremity to determine the needed length of the splint (not necessary with a Sager splint).
3. Assess and document the neurovascular status.

PROCEDURAL STEPS
Hare Traction Splint or FernoTrac Traction Splint

1. Adjust the splint to a length approximately 6 to 8 inches longer than the leg.
2. Place the ankle hitch under the heel of the foot, and cross the straps over the top of the foot (Figure 118-1).
3. Have an assistant exert longitudinal traction by placing one hand behind the patient's heel and the other hand over the dorsum of the foot and then pulling firmly. The amount of traction required varies but is generally approximately 15 lbs of pulling force.
4. Support the leg while lifting it just high enough to slide the splint under the extremity, and position the padded bar against the ischial tuberosity. Seat firmly at the hip.
5. Fasten the attached ischial strap around the leg over the padding.
6. Attach the S-ring of the ratchet to the D-rings of the ankle hitch, and twist the ratchet knob to tighten traction. Be careful not to overstretch the limb. The amount of mechanical traction should equate the manual traction. Manual traction can be released only when mechanical traction is established and the splint is fully applied.
7. Secure the Velcro straps around the leg, two above and two below the knee, if possible. Do not place straps directly over the injury site.
8. Lower the heel stand into place to elevate the limb slightly. The leg should not drop but should remain stabilized in the splint.
9. Reassess distal neurovascular status.

Kendrick Traction Device (Medix Choice, 2006)

1. Adjust the plastic buckle on the thigh strap so it will be located on the anterior thigh when fastened (Figure 118-2).
2. Apply the ankle hitch slightly above the ankle and tighten the stirrup by pulling the green tab until the stirrup is snug under the patient's heel.
3. Slide the thigh strap under the leg and position it in the groin by using a see-saw motion. Ensure that male genitals are not compressed by the strap. Fasten the buckle. Cinch the strap until the traction pole receptacle rests against the belt line or the pelvic crest.

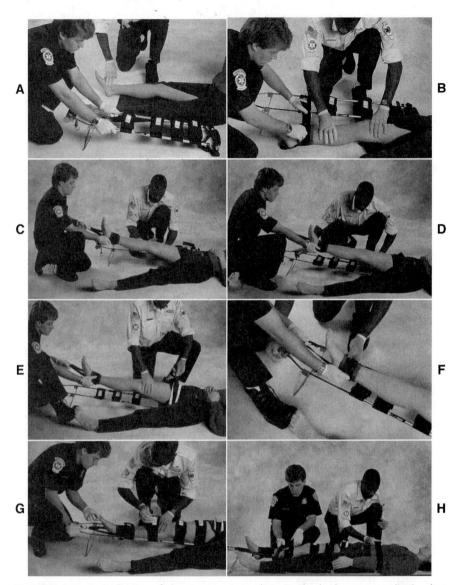

FIGURE 118-1 Application of the Hare traction splint. **A**, The leader assesses distal pulses and stabilizes the injury site while an assistant measures the splint against the unaffected side. **B**, The ankle strap is applied. **C**, Manual traction is initiated by the assistant while the leader supports the fracture site. **D**, Position the splint under the extremity. **E**, Pad the groin area and secure the ischial strap. **F**, Attach the ankle strap to the ratchet and tighten it just enough to maintain limb alignment and relieve pain. **G**, Fasten the support straps after proper mechanical traction has been applied. **H**, Secure the patient and the traction splint to a backboard. (From American Academy of Orthopedic Surgeons. [1993]. *Emergency care and transportation of the sick and injured* [5th ed., pp. 280, 281]. Rosemont, IL: Author.)

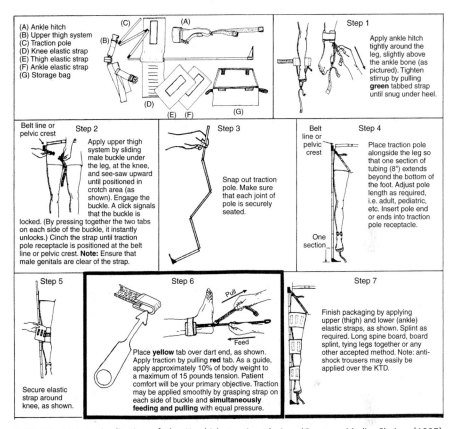

FIGURE 118-2 Application of the Kendrick traction device. (Courtesy Medix Choice. [1997]. *Instructional guide for Kendrick Traction Device.* El Cajon, CA: Author.)

4. Extend the folded traction pole, making sure that all joints are securely locked in position.
5. Place the traction pole beside the leg. Extend one end of the pole 8 inches beyond the bottom of the patient's foot. Adjust the opposite end to the patient's extremity length, and insert it into the traction pole receptacle on the groin strap.
6. Secure the elastic knee strap.
7. Place the yellow tab on the ankle strap over the dart end of the traction pole beyond the patient's heel.
8. Apply traction by simultaneously pulling and feeding the strap with both hands until 10% of the patient's body weight or a maximum of 15 lbs of tension has been reached.
9. Apply the appropriate elastic thigh and ankle straps. Avoid placing straps directly over the injury site.
10. The legs may be wrapped together as needed to provide further stability.
11. Reassess distal neurovascular status.

Sager Traction Splint (Minto, 2006)

1. Cover the cushioned arch with a shoe cover turned inside out to help keep the splint clean. Place the splint between the patient's legs (Figure 118-3). The cushioned arch should be seated against the ischial tuberosity. Tight-fitting clothing should be cut open or removed before the splint is applied.
2. Tighten the thigh strap until it fits snugly around the thigh of the injured leg.
3. Extend the shaft of the splint until the wheel of the pulley or the pulling handle is at the patient's heel level.
4. Prepare the ankle harness(es) to fit around the ankle(s) of the injured leg(s) just above the medial and lateral malleoli. Place the harness behind the ankle with one strap on either side of the ankle. Individual pads on the harness may be folded back so it fits snugly around the ankle.
5. Pull the tabs on the strap(s) to take up the slack.
6. Extend the shaft of the splint until the desired amount of traction is reached; usually 10% of the patient's body weight is adequate for a single femur fracture. More traction will be necessary if both femurs are fractured (approximately 20% of body weight).
7. Retighten the thigh strap if necessary.
8. Bind the patient's legs together with the three leg straps, the longest around the upper thighs, the middle-sized strap under the knees, and the shortest around the lower legs. This decreases movement of the legs. If you cannot bind the patient's legs together, hip rotation can be minimized with towel rolls or sandbags placed along the lateral aspect of the legs.
9. Wrap the long strap in a figure-eight method around the forefeet to prevent external rotation of the legs.
10. Reassess distal neurovascular status.
    Figure 118-4 demonstrates application of the infant Sager splint.

Thomas Splint

1. Adjust the splint to the length of the patient's leg, and allow an extension of 6 to 8 inches beyond the foot.

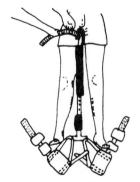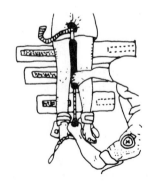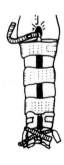

FIGURE 118-3 Application of the bilateral Sager splint. (Courtesy Minto Research & Development, Inc. [1996]. *Instructional guide.* Copyright 1992. Redding, CA: Author.)

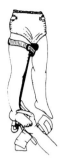

FIGURE 118-4 Application of the infant Sager Splint. (Courtesy Minto Research & Development. [1996]. *Instructional guide.* Copyright 1992. Redding, CA: Author.)

2. Apply the traction strap over the patient's foot after padding the surfaces that lie under the strap.
3. Have an assistant exert longitudinal traction on the leg by placing one hand under the patient's heel and the other over the dorsum of the foot and pulling gently. Manual traction is maintained until the splinting process is complete.
4. Place the splint under the patient's leg by lifting the leg gently and easing the padded half-ring against the ischium. Be sure that the buckle on the splint faces outside and that the half-ring is turned downward.
5. Fasten the ischial strap over the thigh and padding.
6. Bring the long free end of the foot strap over and the under the top of the notched end of the splint.
7. Pass the strap through the link at the swivel in the stirrup under the patient's foot. Apply traction by pulling the strap toward the end of the splint. If no foot strap is available, create an improvised ankle hitch and a Spanish windlass (Figure 118-5) to maintain traction as illustrated.
8. Slide the footrest on the splint until it rests against the bottom of the patient's foot.
9. Apply four or five cravats around the splint to support the leg. Make sure that no fastening device is directly over the injury site. Apply two additional cravats to support the foot and secure it to the footrest.
10. Reassess distal neurovascular status.

AGE-SPECIFIC CONSIDERATIONS

1. The pediatric/infant Sager splint should always be used in a bilateral mode to provide the best stabilization (Minto, 2006). It is appropriate for children from infancy to 6 years of age, depending on the child's height.
2. The adult Sager will fit patients over 7 feet (2 meters) tall (Fikes & Borschneck, 2004).
3. The Hare traction splint is also available in a pediatric size.
4. Frail elderly patients do not tolerate traction splints well. It may be preferable to use alternative splinting after the patient has been placed on a well-padded backboard.

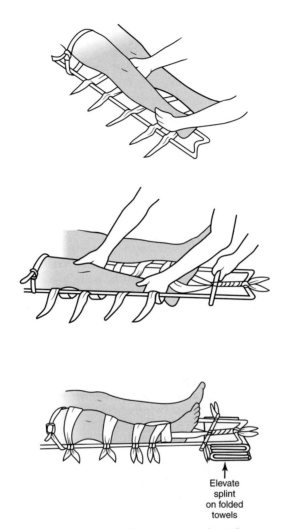

Elevate
splint
on folded
towels

FIGURE 118-5 Application of a Thomas splint using a Spanish windlass, as explained in the text.

COMPLICATIONS

1. Inappropriate use of traction splints can aggravate the existing injury or can cause damage to surrounding tissues. Many femoral injuries are accompanied by other injuries that would contraindicate the use of traction splints (Bledsoe & Barnes, 2004).
2. Compression of the sciatic nerve or perineal tissues
3. Flexion and outward rotation of the proximal femur
4. Excessive traction and overstretching of the limb
5. Compromised neurovascular status in the distal limb(s)
6. Displacement of the proximal third of the fractured femur

PATIENT TEACHING

1. Report when muscle spasm subsides and pain in the injured leg decreases during traction application.
2. Report increased pain or discomfort while in the traction splint.

REFERENCES

Bledsoe, B. E., & Barnes, D. (2004). Traction splint: An EMS relic? *Journal of Emergency Medical Services, 29*(8), 64-67.

Fikes, J. M., & Borschneck, A. G. (2004). *Sager emergency traction splints: Instructor's manual.* Redding, CA: Minto Research and Development, Inc. Retrieved October 13, 2007 from http://www.sagersplints.com/pdf/sager-manual.pdf

Gisness, C. M. (2005). Musculoskeletal emergencies. In L. Newberry, & L. Criddle (Eds.), *Sheehy's manual of emergency care* (6th ed., pp. 690-738). St Louis: Mosby.

Limmer, D., & O'Keefe, M. F. (2005). Musculoskeletal injuries. In D. Limmer, J. D. Bergeron, B. Murray, M. F. O'Keefe, & H. Grant (Eds.), *Emergency care* (10th ed., pp. 633-681). Upper Saddle River, NJ: Prentice-Hall.

Medix Choice (2006). *Instructions for application of the Kendrick Traction Device.* Retrieved July 8, 2006, from http://www.epandr.com/downloads/manuals.htm

Minto Research & Development. (2006). *Instructions for application of the Sager splint.* Retrieved July 8, 2006, from http://www.sagersplints.com/pdf/Sager-Manual.pdf

Sanders, M. (2005) *Mosby's paramedic textbook* (3rd ed.). St Louis: Mosby.

PROCEDURE 119

Pelvic Splinting

Jean A. Proehl, RN, MN, CEN, CCRN, FAEN

Pelvic splinting devices are also known as *pelvic sling, T-POD, SAM Sling, PelvicBinder, pelvic strap, pelvic harness, pelvic belt, pelvic circumferential compression device (PCCD)*, and *pelvic sheeting*.

INDICATION

To provide temporary stabilization of unstable pelvic fractures via circumferential compression. Stabilization helps realign fracture segments, decrease blood loss and pain, and prevent further injury (Bottlang & Krieg, 2002; Krieg, Mohr, Mirza, & Bottlang, 2005a; Qureshi, McGee, Cooper, & Porter, 2005). Notches may be cut in most splints to allow access to the femoral vessels for interventional radiology or for application of an external fixator.

NOTE: Pneumatic antishock garments may also be used to splint the pelvis. See Procedure 51.

CONTRAINDICATIONS AND CAUTIONS

1. Do not place the splint over an impaled object.
2. Correct positioning is important; more force is required to achieve reduction if the splint is centered higher than the level of the greater trochanters (Bottlang et al., 2002).
3. The splint is typically left in place until definitive stabilization can be achieved or unstable pelvic fracture is ruled out. However, prolonged use may lead to underlying tissue injury and necrosis. To decrease this risk (BioCybernetics, 2004; Krieg, Mohr, Mirza, & Bottlang, 2005b; Schaller, Sims, & Maxian, 2005):
   - Minimize the duration of splint use to 24 hours when possible, and monitor skin condition daily, especially with soft-tissue injury underlying the splint.
   - Release and re-tension the splint after massive fluid resuscitation, which could result in increased pressure secondary to swelling.
   - Use caution with devices that do not limit compressive forces.
   - When sheets are used, apply them over a broad area without twisting or wrinkles.
   - Document the date and time of application, preferably directly on the device.

EQUIPMENT

Commercial pelvic splint (T-POD, SAM Sling, PelvicBinder)
or
Cloth bed sheet and
Two to four large towel clamps or toothed clamps

PATIENT PREPARATION

1. Place the patient in a supine position.
2. Remove clothing from the area covered by the device. In a situation where the clothing cannot be removed, remove all objects (keys, etc.) from the pockets to prevent underlying tissue damage.
3. If possible, place a urinary bladder catheter before splint application.
4. Assess and document bilateral distal neurovascular status before and after splint application.

PROCEDURAL STEPS

Trauma-Pelvic Orthotic Device—T-POD (BioCybernetics, 2004)

1. Slide the belt under the patient and center it at the level of the greater trochanters. Trim the belt to leave a 6- to 8-inch (15- to 20-cm) gap between the belt ends at the front of the abdomen.
2. Attach the Velcro-backed pulley system to each side of the belt.
3. Slowly pull the pull-tab until the tension is tight. Elevate male genitalia out of the groin area as necessary.
4. Wrap the pulley strings around two of the plastic hooks and attach the Velcro-backed pull-tab to the opposite side of the belt (Figure 119-1).
5. The T-POD is completely radiolucent and safe for both MRI and CT scan (Julee Arbuckle, BioCybernetics, personal communication, August 25, 2006).

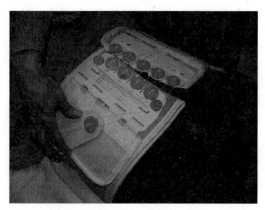

FIGURE 119-1 Securing the T-POD in place. (Photograph courtesy of John Markowitz.)

SAM Sling (Bottlang & Krieg, 2003; SAM Medical Products, 2006)

The SAM Sling has a spring loaded "autostop" buckle that indicates when the desired tension (150 Newtons or 33 lb [15 kg]) has been achieved (Bottlang et al., 2002).

1. Select the appropriate size. The SAM Sling comes in three sizes (hip circumference at the level of the greater trochanters):
   Small (28 to 46 inches [71 to 116 cm])
   Medium (33 to 50 inches [84 to 127 cm])
   Large (36 to 60 inches [91 to 152 cm])
2. Unfold the sling and place it underneath the patient with the white side up. It should be at the level of the greater trochanters and symphysis pubis.
3. Fold or cut the sling ends as needed to prevent overlapping in the front. Close the sling by placing the black Velcro on the blue surface of the sling. Try to position the buckle in the midline.
4. Pull up to release the orange handle from the flap.
5. Pull both orange handles in opposite directions to tighten the sling; this may require two people (Figure 119-2).
6. Pull until you hear a click and feel the free orange handle stop. Maintain this tension and attach the Velcro on the orange handle to the sling (blue) surface.
7. The sling can remain in place for radiographic procedures including magnetic resonance imaging (MRI) using a system operating at 3 Tesla or less. However, do not remove the sling while in the MRI room.

PelvicBinder (PelvicBinder, Inc., 2006)

1. Slide the binder under the patient and center it over the greater trochanters.
2. Cut the end of the binder to leave a 6- to 8-inch (15- to 20-cm) gap in the front of the abdomen.
3. Attach the Velcro straps and plate to the cut end of the binder.
4. Use the shoelace mechanism to tighten the binder (Figure 119-3). Close the fastener on the laces to maintain the tension.

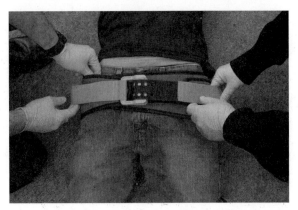

FIGURE 119-2 Tightening the SAM Sling. (Courtesy of SAM Medical Products, Newport, OR, www.pelvicsling.com.)

5. The PelvicBinder is radiolucent and MRI-compatible (Leslie White, PelvicBinder, Inc, personal communication, August 21, 2006).

Sheets (Routt et al., 2006; Schaller et al., 2005)

1. Fold the sheet lengthwise to achieve a width of 1 to 2 feet (30 to 60 cm), taking care to smooth out all wrinkles.
2. Position the sheet under the patient.
3. *Manually reduce the pelvis (optional).
4. Pull the sheet ends taut across the pelvic area.

---

*Indicates portions of the procedure usually performed by a physician or an advanced practice nurse.

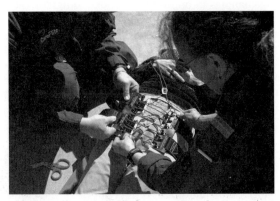

FIGURE 119-3 Tightening the PelvicBinder. (Courtesy of PelvicBinder, Inc, Dallas, TX, www.pelvicbinder.com)

5. Clamp the sheet to maintain the tension.
6. Re-assess often to make sure the clamp is maintaining appropriate tension.

AGE-SPECIFIC CONSIDERATIONS

1. The SAM Sling has not been tested on adolescents and is not recommended for use on children (Bottlang & Krieg, 2003; SAM Medical, 2006).
2. Children smaller than 50 lb (23 kg) may be too small for the T-POD if a 6-inch (15-cm) gap cannot be achieved (BioCybernetics International, 2004).
3. The T-POD is 57 inches (145 cm) long and so it will fit a patient as large as 65 inches (165 cm) around. For an obese patient, two T-POD belts may be connected. Use one power unit to link the two belts and the other as the pulley (BioCybernetics International, 2004).
4. The PelvicBinder is 60 inches (152 cm) long and will fit a patient as large as 66 inches (167 cm) around. Two PelvicBinders maybe connected for a larger patient (Leslie White, PelvicBinder, Inc, personal communication, August 21, 2006).

COMPLICATIONS

1. Soft-tissue injury and necrosis may develop under the area of the splint (Krieg et al., 2005b; Schaller et al., 2004).
2. Excessive tension could cause visceral or nerve root injury (Routt et al., 2006).
3. A pelvic splint may mask the severity of pelvic fractures both clinically and radiographically (Qureshi et al., 2005).

PATIENT TEACHING

1. The splint is a temporary device and should decrease discomfort. However, pain medication may still be needed.
2. Notify your nurse if you have any numbness or tingling in your legs or if any painful areas develop underneath the splint.

REFERENCES

BioCybernetics International. (2004). *T-POD instructions and use.* La Verne, CA: Author. Retrieved August 14, 2006, from www.tpod.com.

Bottlang, M., & Krieg, J. C. (2003). The pelvic fracture: Stabilization in the field. *Emergency Medical Services, 32*(9), 126-129.

Bottlang, M., Simpson, T., & Sigg, J., et al. (2002). Noninvasive reduction of open-book pelvic fractures by circumferential compression. *Journal of Orthopaedic Trauma, 16,* 367-373.

Krieg, J. C., Mohr, M., & Ellis, T. J., et al. (2005a). Emergent stabilization of pelvic ring injuries by controlled circumferential compression: A clinical trial. *Journal of Trauma-Injury Infection & Critical Care, 59,* 659-664.

Krieg, J. C., Mohr, M., Mirza, A. J., & Bottlang, M. (2005b). Pelvic circumferential compression in the presence of soft-tissue injuries: A case report. *Journal of Trauma-Injury Infection & Critical Care, 59,* 470-472.

PelvicBinder, Inc. (2006). *PelvicBinder fitting instructions and nursing considerations.* Dallas: Author. Retrieved July 25, 2006, from www.pelvicbinder.com.

Routt, M. L. Jr., Falicov, A., Woodhouse, E., & Schildhauer, T. A. (2006). Circumferential pelvic antishock sheeting: A temporary resuscitation aid. *Journal of Orthopaedic Trauma, 20(1 suppl)*, S3-S6.

Qureshi, A., McGee, A., Cooper, J. P., & Porter, K. M. (2005). Reduction of the posterior pelvic ring by non-invasive stabilisation: A report of two cases. *Emergency Medicine Journal, 22*, 885-886.

SAM Medical Products. (2006). *SAM Sling written instructions.* Retrieved August 14, 2006, from: http://www.sammedical.com/cgi-in/WebObjects/SamSite.woa/wa/Products/Sling #written

Schaller, T. M., Sims, S., & Maxian, T. (2005). Skin breakdown following circumferential pelvic antishock sheeting: A case report. *Journal of Orthopaedic Trauma, 19*, 661-665.

PROCEDURE 120

Sling Application

Ruth L. Schaffler, RN, PhD, ARNP, CEN

The information in this procedure should be used in conjunction with the information in Procedure 113.

INDICATION

To support an injured shoulder, clavicle, or upper extremity

EQUIPMENT

Triangular bandage measuring $40 \times 40 \times 55$ inches (can be made by folding or cutting a 40-inch square of material in half)

or

Commercially prepared sling or collar and cuff

PATIENT PREPARATION

1. Pad the axilla to absorb perspiration and prevent skin maceration if the sling is placed under the patient's clothing.
2. Splint the upper extremity as indicated before sling application.

PROCEDURAL STEPS
Sling

1. Place the longest edge of a triangular bandage vertically across the anterior chest with one tip over the uninjured shoulder. The apex of the bandage should lie under the elbow of the injured arm.

2. Place the humerus on the injured side next to the lateral chest wall, and bend the elbow so that the hand is positioned at the opposite fourth or fifth anterior rib (Figure 120-1). The weight of the arm should create an angle of slightly less than 90 degrees at the elbow while in the sling.
3. Bring the lower edge of the triangle over the injured arm, and tie a square knot to the other end of the bandage. The knot should be positioned at the side of the neck, not directly over the cervical spine. Place a pad under the knot.

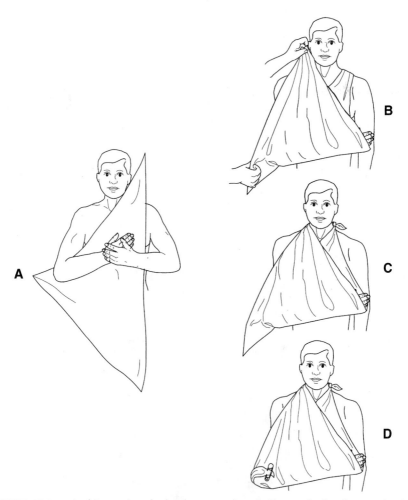

FIGURE 120-1 Applying a triangular bandage as a sling. **A,** The arm is placed across the chest and bandaged as shown. **B,** Bring the lower end of the bandage over the arm and behind the neck. **C,** Tie a square knot to the opposite end at the side of the neck. **D,** Secure the apex of the bandage with a knot or pin. The final position of the arm should create an angle of slightly less than 90 degrees at the elbow; fingers should be exposed.

4. Fold the apex of the triangle forward, and pin or tape it securely to the sling. The apex could also be twisted and knotted when it is snugly fitted against the elbow.
5. Position the edge of the sling to expose the ends of the fingers.
6. The sling should stabilize the shoulder and upper arm and maintain elevation of the lower arm and hand (Limmer & O'Keefe, 2005, Sanders, 2005).

Collar and Cuff

1. Secure the cuff to the patient's wrist.
2. Place the collar around the patient's neck, making sure that it is secure but not restrictive.
3. Loop a strap through the cuff and collar to suspend the wrist. The final position of the elbow should be at slightly less than 90 degrees flexion (Figure 120-2).

Commercial Sling

1. Place the injured arm in the fabric holder with the elbow in the seamed corner.
2. Loop the attached strap across the chest toward the uninjured side, and loop it behind the neck, and then down the chest to the D-rings at the wrist end of the holder.
3. Pass the strap upward through the rings, and secure the Velcro edges together with the elbow flexed at slightly less than 90 degrees.

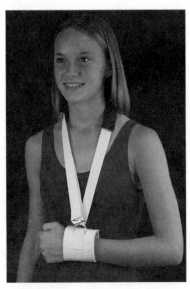

FIGURE 120-2 A collar and cuff. (Courtesy of Bird & Cronin, Inc. [2006.] Eagan, MN. www.birdcronin.com)

AGE-SPECIFIC CONSIDERATIONS

1. Slings are generally not suitable for children with fractures of the humerus or elbow. The preferred treatment is a sling and swathe, plaster casting, or surgical intervention.
2. Subluxation of the radial head in a child does not generally need immobilization after reduction, but a sling could be used (Garcia, 2002).
3. Additional padding behind the neck may be needed for an elderly patient to avoid excessive pressure over the spine from the weight of the arm in the sling.

COMPLICATIONS

1. Compression of the soft tissues in the neck
2. Increased edema of the distal limb as a result of greater than 90-degree elbow flexion in the sling

PATIENT TEACHING

1. Watch for changes in hand circulation, sensation, and motion.
2. Keep the knot positioned at the side of the neck and not directly over the spine to avoid excessive pressure on blood vessels, nerves, and spinous processes.
3. Keep the hand above elbow level, and open and close hand and wiggle fingers frequently to prevent or decrease swelling.

REFERENCES

Garcia, B. (2002). Extremity trauma. In M. W. Hubble, & J. P. Hubble (Eds.), *Principles of advanced trauma care* (pp. 315-349). Albany, NY: Delmar.

Limmer, D., & O'Keefe, M. (2005). Musculoskeletal injuries. In D. Limmer, M. O'Keefe, E. Dickinson, H. Grant, B. Murray, & J. Bergeron (Eds.), *Emergency care* (10th ed., pp. 633-681). Upper Saddle River, NJ: Prentice-Hall.

Sanders, M. (2005). *Mosby's paramedic textbook* (3rd ed.). St Louis: Mosby.

Shoulder Immobilization

Ruth L. Schaffler, RN, PhD, ARNP, CEN

The information in this procedure should be used in conjunction with the information in Procedure 113.

Shoulder immobilization is also known as *sling and swathe.* The majority of shoulder injuries result from anterior dislocations and subluxation (Hayes, Callanan, Walton, Paxinos, & Murrell, 2002). Current research and clinical trials support the use of external rotation rather than internal rotation for acute shoulder dislocations (Funk, Smith, & Carley, 2005; Murrell, 2003).

INDICATIONS

1. To immobilize the clavicle, acromioclavicular joint, shoulder, or proximal humerus. A sling and swathe is useful for anterior dislocations of the shoulder (Limmer & O'Keefe, 2005). However, new information that may change practice has shown that detachment of structures in the anterior shoulder is made worse when the shoulder is placed in internal rotation in a sling. Placing the shoulder in external rotation realigns the structures (Murrell, 2003) and reduces the rate of of dislocation recurrence (Itoi et al., 2003).
2. To immobilize unstable fractures of the proximal humerus to prevent recurrent dislocation as a result of contraction of the pectoralis major muscle.
3. To provide greater immobilization for a fractured humerus than a sling alone because the chest wall acts as a splint.
4. A sling and swathe may provide greater immobilization for a fractured humerus than a sling alone because the chest wall acts as a splint.

EQUIPMENT

Commercial sling and swathe
or
Two or three triangular bandages to create a sling and swathe
Safety pins
Axillary padding (i.e., gauze dressings, bandages, cast padding, pillows)
or
External rotation splint
   Long moldable, padded splint
   Stockinette
or
Commercial version of external rotation splint

PATIENT PREPARATION

1. Pad the axilla on the affected side, across the chest where the arm will lie, and over the opposite shoulder where the bandaging material will lie.

610

2. Flex the elbow on the injured side and place the forearm across the chest.

PROCEDURAL STEPS
Sling and Swathe
1. Apply the cloth sling to the forearm with the elbow positioned in the seamed corner, the hand extending into the open end.
2. Pass the self-fastening strap behind the neck, and secure it to the sling at the wrist.
3. Place the fabric swathe around the arm and chest to keep the extremity and shoulder immobilized (Figure 121-1).

Shoulder Immobilizer
1. Apply the elastic band around the chest, and secure with the Velcro fastener.
2. Fasten the arm strap around the humerus, and then fasten the wrist strap around the lower forearm (Figure 121-2).

External Rotation Splint
1. Curve a long moldable padded splint lengthwise at the patient's waist and bend it at the mid-point with the remaining half facing outward.
2. Insert the splint into a stockinette sleeve leaving a short tail at the arm end and a long tail at the waist end.
3. Tie a knot in the stockinette at the arm end of the splint.

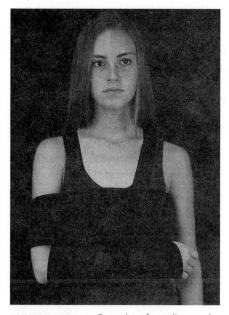

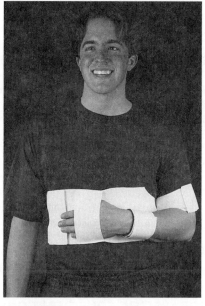

FIGURE 121-1 Example of a sling and swathe. (Courtesy of Bird & Cronin, Inc. [2006]. Eagan, MN, www.birdcronin.com)

FIGURE 121-2 Example of commercial shoulder immobilizer. (Courtesy of Bird & Cronin, Inc. [2006.] Eagan, MN, www.birdcronin.com)

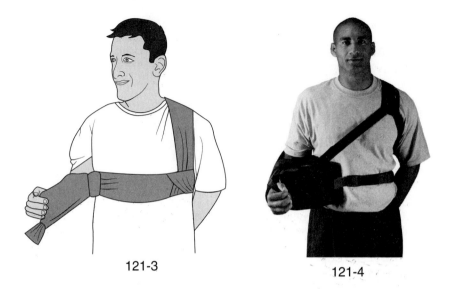

121-3

121-4

FIGURE 121-3 Example of shoulder immobilization with the arm in external rotation. (A video clip of the application of this splint can be found at http://www.ori.org.au/bonejoint/shoulder/ssfd/splint.mov)

FIGURE 121-4 Commercially available external rotation splint. When the shoulder is maintained in external rotation, the subscapularis tendon tightens and closes the joint cavity. This helps maintain proper bone position. (Courtesy of Donjoy Orthopedics, LLC, Vista, CA)

4. Cut two horizontal slits approximately the distance between the patient's elbow and wrist on the lateral side of the splint.
5. Insert the patient's arm into the stockinette through the slits on the outside of the splint.
6. Wrap the waist tail around the back of the patient, over and under the proximal forearm.
7. Tuck the tail under the wrap at the elbow, then continue wrapping the tail upward over the shoulder and behind the neck to fasten at the waist on the side opposite the injured shoulder.
8. An alternative method of wrapping is to swathe the long tail around the splint medial to the patient's elbow then upward across the patient's back, down over the opposite shoulder, and then secure at the waist (Figure 121-3).
9. Commercial devices to place the arm in external rotation are also available (Figure 121-4). The angle of rotation for splinting is determined by the physician.

AGE-SPECIFIC CONSIDERATIONS

1. Shoulder dislocation or AC joint separation is most commonly seen in patients younger than age 30. Patients older than age 50 may present with rotator cuff dysfunction due to degenerative arthritis of the AC joint.

2. Osteoporosis is common in the elderly and acute pain on emergency department presentation may indicate a humeral head fracture (Andrews, 2005).

COMPLICATIONS

1. Frozen shoulder or joint stiffness
2. Neurovascular compromise
3. Restriction of chest wall expansion
4. A sling and swathe should not be used in the bedridden because of the loss of gravity needed for alignment and union of a fracture

PATIENT TEACHING

1. Loosen the swathe and reapply if it becomes too tight or restricts breathing.
2. Report numbness, tingling, increased swelling, or pain in the distal extremity.
3. Do not lean on the elbow.

REFERENCES

Andrews, J. R. (2005). Shoulder—Overview. In L. Griffin (Ed.), *Essentials of musculoskeletal care* (3rd ed., pp. 148-149). Rosemont, IL: American Academy of Orthopaedic Surgeons.

Funk, L., Smith, M., & Carley, S. (2005). How to immobilize after shoulder dislocation. *Emergency Medicine Journal, 814*(2), 814-815.

Hayes, K., Callanan, M., Walton, J., Paxinos, A., & Murrell, G. (2002). Shoulder instability: Management and rehabilitation. *Journal of Orthopaedic & Sports Physical Therapy, 34*(10), 1-13.

Itoi, E., Hatakeyama, Y., Kido, T., Sato, T., Minagawa, H., Wakabayashi, I., & Kobayashi, M. (2003). A new method of immobilization after traumatic anterior dislocation of the shoulder: A preliminary study. *Journal of Shoulder and Elbow Surgery, 12*(5), 413-415.

Limmer, D., & O'Keefe, M. (2005). Musculoskeletal injuries. In D. Limmer, M. O'Keefe, E. Dickinson, H. Grant, B. Murray, & J. Bergeron (Eds.), *Emergency care* (10th ed., pp. 633-681). Upper Saddle River, NJ: Prentice-Hall.

Murrell, G. (2003). Treatment of shoulder dislocation: Is a sling appropriate? *Medical Journal of Australia, 179*(7), 317-370.

Knee Immobilization

Ruth L. Schaffler, RN, PhD, ARNP, CEN

The information in this procedure should be used in conjunction with the information in Procedure 113.

Knee immobilizers are also known as *knee splints* and *hinged knee braces*.

INDICATIONS

1. To immobilize a fracture, dislocation, or soft tissue injury of the knee or adjacent structures.
2. To immobilize an unstable knee joint.

CONTRAINDICATIONS AND CAUTIONS

1. The knee should be handled gently and movement of the injured area minimized to decrease pain and the risk of complications, such as damage to the popliteal artery or to the femoral and peroneal nerves (Garcia, 2002; Limmer & O'Keefe, 2005).
2. Bony prominences and body contours should be padded to avoid undue pressure or skin breakdown.
3. Not all knee injuries require an immobilizer. Unless the knee is grossly unstable (grade III sprain) or a patellar dislocation is present, consider using a hinged knee brace.
4. Realign the angulated limb into an anatomic position before splinting (Bergeron & Bizjak, 2001) if there is no concomitant injury to the hip joint (Limmer & O'Keefe, 2005). The extremity should not be forced to fit the splint. If resistance is encountered, the knee should be splinted in the position it was found if an adequate pulse is present. The splint may need to be altered to fit the deformity (Limmer & O'Keefe, 2005).
5. Neurovascular status should be assessed and documented before and after the device is applied (Garcia, 2002; Limmer & O'Keefe, 2005; McSwain, 2001). If compromise exists, a physician should be notified immediately. If deterioration occurs after splinting, the device must be readjusted or removed and reapplied.
6. Gross soft tissue swelling may make the application of an immobilizing device difficult or impossible. A plaster or fiberglass splint may need to be applied (see Procedure 124).

EQUIPMENT

Commercial knee immobilizer
or
Plaster or fiberglass splinting material
    12 to 15, 4 × 30-in or 5 × 30-in plaster strips
    Stockinette or rolled cotton padding

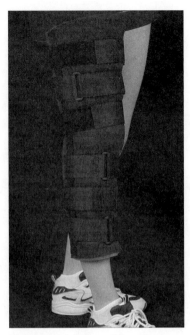

FIGURE 122-1 Example of a standard knee immobilizer (Courtesy of Bird & Cronin, Inc. [2006]. Eagan, MN. www.birdcronin.com)

Two to three rolls of 6-in elastic bandage
Bucket of lukewarm water
Absorbent pads
Pillows

PATIENT PREPARATION

1. Remove constrictive clothing that would lie under the immobilization device. If the immobilizer is to be removed occasionally and swelling is minimal, it may be applied over loose clothing.
2. Clean and dress all open wounds.
3. Measure the thigh circumference and the length of the leg to determine the correct size of the immobilizing device.
4. Assess and document neurovascular status.

PROCEDURAL STEPS
Commercial Knee Immobilizer

1. A standard knee brace holds the knee in extension (Figure 122-1). Hinged knee braces are also available and are more popular. A hinged knee brace maintains lateral support while allowing for adjustable knee flexion (Figure 122-2). Position the immobilizer under the leg while the patient is supine. If the device has a cutout in the front, place it so that the open area is over the patella. If no cutout is present, place the splint with

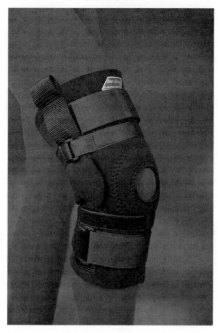

FIGURE 122-2 Example of a hinged knee immobilizer. (Courtesy of Bird & Cronin, Inc., [2006]. Eagan, MN. www.birdcronin.com)

the upper end at midthigh and the lower end at midcalf. Splints are available in various lengths.

2. Secure the device with the attached buckles or Velcro fasteners.

Plaster or Fiberglass Long Leg Posterior Splint

1. Splint fractures of the knee joint in the position found unless circulatory compromise is present. If circulatory compromise is present, gently apply longitudinal traction manually until circulation is restored.
2. If possible, place the patient in a prone position on a stretcher or examination table.
3. Measure the posterior surface of the unaffected leg from the ball of the foot to midthigh. This measurement determines the length of plaster or fiberglass splinting material needed.
4. Wrap the affected leg with rolled cotton bandage or put on a stockinette that is cut to the measured length.
5. Moisten the plaster or fiberglass material and gently pinch to remove excess water. Do not squeeze or twist (see Procedure 124).
6. Apply the plaster or fiberglass to the posterior surface of the limb from toes to midthigh. Keep the foot flexed at 90 degrees.
7. Wrap with elastic bandages to secure the splint in place.
8. Place limb on pillows for support while the splint dries. Extend the distal leg beyond the edge of the stretcher or table to allow the foot to remain in a neutral position.

9. Assess and document neurovascular status.

AGE-SPECIFIC CONSIDERATION

Commercial knee immobilizers are available in pediatric lengths (as small as 6 inches long).

COMPLICATIONS

1. Neurovascular compromise
2. Increased edema
3. Increased pain
4. Joint stiffness resulting from prolonged immobilization
5. Joint effusion
6. Compartment syndrome

PATIENT TEACHING

1. Keep the splint clean and dry.
2. Apply ice packs to the affected area to minimize swelling and pain.
3. Elevate the lower extremity above the level of the heart to reduce swelling.
4. Follow crutch walking and weight-bearing limitations if indicated (see Procedure 132).
5. Notify your primary health care provider or return to the emergency department for any symptoms of numbness, tingling, increased swelling, increased pain, or discoloration of the foot.
6. Wear the immobilization device for the recommended length of time and keep your appointments with your primary health care provider or physical therapist. (Patients who have sustained a knee injury should be referred to an orthopedic specialist.)

REFERENCES

Bergeron, J. D., & Bizjak, G. (2001) *First responder* (6th ed.). Upper Saddle River. NJ: Prentice-Hall.

Garcia, B. (2002). Extremity trauma. In M. W. Hubble, & J. P. Hubble (Eds.), *Principles of advanced trauma care* (pp. 315-349). Albany, NY: Delmar.

Limmer, D., & O'Keefe, M. (2005). Musculoskeletal injuries. In D. Limmer, M. O'Keefe, E. Dickinson, H. Grant, B. Murray, & J. D. Bergeron (Eds.), *Emergency care* (10th ed., pp. 633-681). Upper Saddle River, NJ: Prentice Hall.

Finger Immobilization

Jean A. Proehl, RN, MN, CEN, CCRN, FAEN

The information in this procedure should be used in conjunction with the information in Procedure 113.

INDICATIONS

1. To relieve pain, provide stability, promote healing, and prevent functional disability in the presence of finger fractures.
2. To protect a repaired tendon, nerve, or vessel from tension.
3. To protect soft tissue injuries from further trauma.
4. Specific splinting recommendations are based on fracture location and type.
   - *Dorsal splint:* Distal phalanx only for mallet-type injury of the distal phalanx involving less than 25% of the articular surface or for avulsion of the profundus tendon at the attachment; hyperextension of the distal interphalangeal joint may be indicated in some instances (Simon, Sherman, & Koenigsknecht, 2007). Dorsal splints may also be applied to the length of the digit for sprains, soft tissue injuries, or stable distal or middle phalangeal fractures.
   - *Plaster or fiberglass gutter splint:* For stable fractures of the middle and proximal phalanx that do not involve articular surfaces (see Procedure 124).
   - *Volar splint (plaster, fiberglass, or aluminum splint):* For uncomplicated extraarticular fractures, sprains, and dislocations and for temporary immobilization until operative reduction can be accomplished (see Procedure 124).
   - *Buddy taping (also known as dynamic splinting):* For middle and proximal phalanx extraarticular fractures that are stable and nondisplaced.
   - *Prong, hairpin, or cage splints:* For protection of distal finger injuries such as tuft fractures, fingernail avulsions, or tip amputations.
   - *Internal fixation (Kirschner wire or pin or K-wire, smooth wire, Riordan pin):* For precise reduction with unstable or intraarticular fractures.

CONTRAINDICATIONS AND CAUTIONS

1. The fingers should not be immobilized in full extension; fingers should be immobilized in the position of function. Position of function for the hand is 15-degree wrist extension with the thumb in palmar abduction, 50- to 90-degree flexion of the metacarpophalangeal joints, and 15- to 20-degree flexion of the interphalangeal joints. The thumb is immobilized slightly abducted, neither flexed nor extended (Simon et al., 2007).

2. *Rotational malalignment and angulation should be assessed. With the fingers flexed, lines drawn through the fingernails meet at the scaphoid in the normal hand (Figure 123-1, *A*). Rotational malalignment is not acceptable in metacarpal and phalangeal fractures (Figure 123-1, *B*) (Simon et al., 2007).
3. The hand performs many intricate maneuvers, and even small deficits may cause significant functional limitations. The history should include hand dominance and vocations and avocations that involve use of the injured hand (e.g., musical instruments, sports, crafts).
4. Open fractures require antibiotic administration. Clean, distal phalangeal fractures without significant soft tissue damage or crushing may be managed in the emergency department; all other open fractures of the hand are generally managed in the operating room (Simon et al., 2007).

PATIENT PREPARATION
1. Remove all rings on the injured hand (see Procedure 114).
2. Assess and document neurovascular status.

DORSAL SPLINT
Equipment
½- to 1-in tape
Dorsal splint (metal, plastic)

---

*Indicates portions of the procedure usually performed by a physician or an advanced practice nurse.

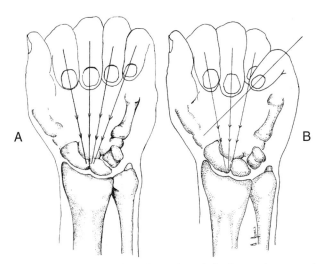

FIGURE 123-1 A, In a normal hand, lines drawn through the fingernails meet at the scaphoid. **B,** In the presence of a finger fracture with rotational malalignment, the fingernail of the fractured finger does not point to the scaphoid. (From Simon, R. R., Sherman, S. C., & Koenigsknecht, S. J. [2007]. *Emergency orthopedics: The extremities* [5th ed., p. 124]. New York: McGraw-Hill.)

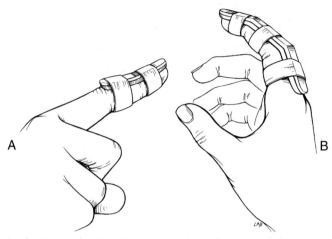

FIGURE 123-2 A, Dorsal splint of distal interphalangeal joint. **B,** Dorsal splint of finger. (From Chudnofsky, C. R., & Byers, S. [2004]. Splinting techniques. In J. R. Roberts & J. R. Hedges [Eds.], *Clinical procedures in emergency medicine* [4th ed., pp.1000-1001]. Philadelphia: Saunders.)

Procedural Steps

1. Extend the distal joint fully for a mallet finger; for other injuries, bend each interphalangeal joint 15 degrees.
2. Size the splint, apply it to the dorsum of the finger, and tape it to the middle phalanx. Place the splint over any necessary dressings or padding (Figures 123-2, *A-B*).

BUDDY TAPING
Equipment
½- to 1-in tape
Cast padding or felt

Procedural Steps

1. Place a single layer of cast padding or felt between the injured finger and the adjacent finger. Use the adjacent finger that is longer than the injured finger. If the middle finger is the injured finger, use the adjacent ring finger.
2. Tape circumferentially around both fingers at the level of the proximal phalanx and the distal phalanx (Figure 123-3).

PRONG OR CAGE SPLINT
Equipment
Prong or cage splint
½- to 1-in tape

Procedural Steps

1. Size splint and mold to fit over finger or dressing.

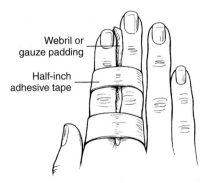

Webril or
gauze padding

Half-inch
adhesive tape

FIGURE 123-3 Buddy taping or dynamic splinting. (From Chudnofsky, C. R., & Byers, S. [2004]. Splinting techniques. In J. R. Roberts & J. R. Hedges [Eds.], *Clinical procedures in emergency medicine* [4th ed., p. 1000]. Philadelphia: Saunders.)

2. Leave a small gap between the distal end of the digit and the splint to prevent transfer of force if the splint is hit.

K-WIRE/RIORDAN FIXATION PIN
Equipment
Antiseptic solution
Pin and drill
Dressing supplies

Procedural Steps
1. *Anesthetize the finger with a digital block before manipulation or reduction of the fracture (see Procedure 136). A regional block at the wrist or a Bier block may also be used (see Procedure 137).
2. Cleanse the affected hand with particular attention to the skin overlying the insertion site with antiseptic solution.
3. *Drill the wire through skin and into the bone.
4. *Test fracture site for stability.
5. Obtain an x-ray study to confirm reduction and pin placement.
6. *Cut the pin off below the skin line.
7. Apply a dressing.
8. Apply an external splint if indicated.

COMPLICATIONS
1. Fracture deformity or nonunion
2. Infection of soft tissue or bone if the skin was broken
3. Loss of mobility, function, or both if the fracture is inadequately reduced, splinted improperly, or the patient does not receive appropriate rehabilitation

---

*Indicates portions of the procedure usually performed by a physician or an advanced practice nurse.

PATIENT TEACHING

1. Elevate your arm with your hand above the level of the elbow and the heart.
2. Apply cold packs to fracture site.
3. Report signs of infection, such as redness, swelling, and draining pus (for open fractures or pin insertions).
4. Report increasing pain, numbness, or swelling.
5. Wear splint until directed to remove it.

REFERENCE

Simon, R. R., Sherman, S. C., & Koenigsknecht, S. J. (2007). *Emergency orthopedics: The extremities* (5th ed). New York: McGraw-Hill.

PROCEDURE 124

Plaster and Fiberglass Splinting

Karen Sue Hoyt, RN, PhD, FNP, APRN-BC, CEN, FAEN

The information in this chapter is specific to plaster and fiberglass splints and should be used in conjunction with Procedure 113.

INDICATIONS

1. To immobilize extremities in order to:
   a. Maintain bony alignment
   b. Rest ligamentous injuries
   c. Decrease pain
   d. Prevent further soft tissue injury from movement of fracture fragments
   e. Decrease risk of clinically significant fat embolism
2. To allow soft tissue swelling to occur without circulatory compromise, in contrast to circumferential plaster or fiberglass casts

The author would like to thank Deborah Palmer, RN, NP, ONP-C, for her expert review of this procedure.

CONTRAINDICATIONS AND CAUTIONS

1. Bony prominences should be protected by using the appropriate size of splint and shaping it carefully. Patients with diabetes or who are long-term steroid users are also at high risk. Additional padding over bony prominences is recommended.
2. Hot water should never be used to wet the plaster or fiberglass (BSN Medical, 2006). The chemical reaction that sets the agents into an active state is exo-thermic (heat producing). This heat, in combination with the heat of the water, may burn the patient. Hot water also accelerates hardening and makes the splint difficult to mold.
3. When using plaster splinting material, the desired position of the extremity should be maintained from the time the first layer of padding or splinting material is applied. Any movement during the splinting process may weaken the splint and may move the extremity out of acceptable alignment.
4. A plaster or fiberglass splint should never completely encircle an extremity because this does not allow for postinjury swelling.
5. Wear gloves to protect your skin when working with exposed fiberglass or plaster.
6. Fiberglass edges can be sharp and cause lacerations and abrasions; be sure to cover all exposed edges.

EQUIPMENT

Cotton or synthetic cast padding (SoftRoll, Webril)
Plaster or fiberglass splints or roll
Scissors or knife (to cut plaster or fiberglass)
Measuring tape
Spray bottle (for fiberglass) or soaking bucket (for plaster)
Elastic bandages
Towels
(Preassembled plaster and fiberglass splinting material with incorporated padding is available in 1- [fiberglass only], 2-, 3-, 4-, 5-, and 6-inch widths in rolls or packaged lengths. Padding such as stockinette or sheet wadding [SoftRoll or Webril] is used with plain plaster splinting material to provide protection for friable skin or over bony prominences.)

PATIENT PREPARATION

1. Assess and document neurovascular status and skin integrity before splint application. If there is a break in the skin at or near a fracture site, an open fracture must be considered. Notify the physician before applying the splint.
2. Dress all wounds before splint application.
3. Cleanse and dry the extremity before splint application.
4. Remove all jewelry from the injured extremity (see Procedure 114).

PROCEDURAL STEPS

1. Place the patient in a position of comfort. If the injury is an upper extremity, the position may be upright; if a lower extremity, the patient may be flat on the abdomen (for short leg posterior splint) or supine (for long leg splint). The prone (inverted) position should be avoided with unstable ankle fractures and obese patients who have trouble breathing when they

lie on their abdomen. Also, in this position, the calf is flexed, and the splint may not fit as well when the patient returns to a supine or upright position.

2. For plaster, prepare bucket of tepid water, 21° to 29° C (70° to 84° F). For fiberglass splints, only a small amount of water is used, and a water bottle or spray bottle is adequate.

3. If possible, measure for the splint on the unaffected extremity. Accuracy is increased and discomfort decreased by avoiding movement of the injured extremity.

4. Cut prepared splints, rolls, or loose sheets to measured length. Width is determined by the largest surface to be supported.

5. With loose plaster splint sheets, the number of layers required depends on the size of the extremity to be supported, with variance between 8 and 20 sheets. When using loose sheets or plain plaster, pad the entire area to be splinted. One or two layers (some prefer three to four layers) of cast padding are sufficient, unless there is marked edema, friable skin, or bony prominences. These conditions require extra padding. Padding is wrapped in circular motion from distal to proximal, seeking conformity and uniform pressure. If padding is too loose, it wrinkles, and pressure sores can develop. If it is too tight, swelling causes constriction. Alternatively, the padding may be folded and placed directly under the splint. This avoids circumferential wrapping of the extremity.

6. When incorporating digits in splints (e.g., gutter splints), place a single layer of padding between them to prevent tissue maceration.

7. Activate the splint.

   Preassembled fiberglass splint rolls: Use a minimum amount of water, a single line of water down the middle of splints 3 inches wide or less, and a zigzag line of water down wider splints (Figure 124-1, *A*). Roll the moistened splint up inside a towel, and press it smooth to remove excess moisture (do not squeeze); repeat on the dry side of the towel (Figure 124-1, *B*).

   Plaster splints: Immerse and maintain plaster splints in the soaking bucket until bubbling stops, take from the bucket, and gently squeeze to remove excess moisture, then smooth together to meld the layers (Figure 124-2).

8. Apply the now activated and smoothed splinting material and form and shape using the palmar surface of the hand and an elastic bandage (Figure 124-3). Apply the elastic bandage in a circular motion, wrapping from the distal to the proximal, seeking uniform pressure and conformity.

9. Assess and document the neurovascular status after splint application.

10. Elevate on a smooth surface, and allow 15 minutes drying time before dismissal. Do not place the splint on a plastic surface for drying, because plastic reflects the heat produced by the curing process of the plaster or fiberglass, and the splint may get too hot.

11. In the case of upper extremity injury, if a sling is appropriate, apply it after the splint has been cured to firmness (Chudnofsky & Byers, 2004).

    NOTE: See Figures 124-4 through 124-10 for information about specific types of splints.

AGE-SPECIFIC CONSIDERATIONS

1. In pediatric or geriatric populations, splints and elastic bandage size should be in accordance with the width of the extremity to be splinted.
2. In both the pediatric and the geriatric population, the skin tends to be thinner and thereby at higher risk for maceration, pressure sores, and exothermic burns. Attention to the cautions and the procedural steps assists in minimizing the risks.

COMPLICATIONS

1. Pressure sores may develop because of wrinkling of the cotton padding or indentations of the plaster. When this pressure continues, compression of the skin and underlying fat can result in tissue necrosis.
2. Plaster burns can occur because of the chemical accelerators, the temperature of the water bath, the amount of water in the splinting material, the thickness of the splint, and sensitivity to the product. To aid in prevention of burns, use cool to tepid water to activate the material, follow the manufacturer's suggestions for padding and protection of the skin, and allow adequate air circulation to aid in the drying process. If the patient complains that the splint is burning, remove it immediately.
3. Improper positioning of the splinted extremity can result in misalignment, neurovascular compromise, or both. Verify the desired position before splint application, and check pulses, sensation, and capillary refill before and after application of the splint.
4. Although it is less common with splint application than with full casts, compartmental syndrome can develop in conjunction with injury or as a result of splint application.

PATIENT TEACHING

1. Fiberglass activates in minutes and is cured when it is no longer warm. Plaster requires at least 12 to 24 hours of drying time. For both products, care should be taken to prevent impression during the first 12 to 24 hours, which could result in misalignment or pressure sores.
2. Elevate and ice the injured extremity to minimize edema and increase comfort (see Procedure 129).
3. Watch for swelling, increasing pain, numbness, pale or blue fingers or toes, or tingling in the extremity. If any of these occur, loosen the elastic wrap and elevate the extremity above the level of the heart. If symptoms persist, contact your physician or return to the emergency department.
4. Splints should be kept dry. If a plaster splint gets wet, it crumbles, and it will not harden again. If the fiberglass product gets wet, it should be blotted with a towel, then fully dried with blow dryer (hair dryer). Do not wear a wet splint, because skin breakdown may occur.
5. Do not stick anything into the splint. If itching is a problem, use an ice pack over the area, or rearrange the splint and elastic bandage.
6. Do not use or walk on the injured extremity. Splints are not strong enough to support the body weight (see Procedures 131 and 132).

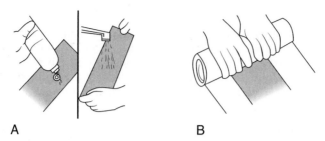

FIGURE 124-1 A, Activate preassembled fiberglass splints with a minimum amount of cool water. Then roll or fold to squeeze out any excess water. **B,** Roll the splint in a towel and squeeze to further remove water. Repeat on the dry side of the towel. (BSN Medical. [2006]. *Ortho-Glass splinting course manual* [6th ed., p. 4]. Charlotte, NC: Author.)

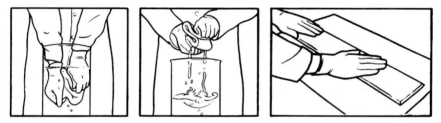

FIGURE 124-2 Submersion, water removal, and smoothing of plaster or fiberglass splint. (Courtesy Johnson & Johnson, Inc. Orthopedics. *Specialists J Splints.* New Brunswick, NJ.)

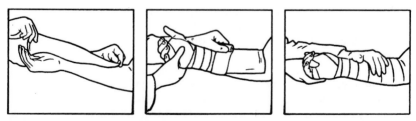

FIGURE 124-3 Application of a splint and an elastic bandage, and molding of the splint to the extremity. (Courtesy Johnson & Johnson, Inc., Orthopedics. *Specialists J Splints.* New Brunswick, NJ.)

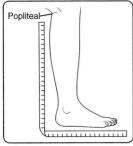

1 Measure from 2 inches below the popliteal to 2 inches beyond the toes. Prepare the splint as directed. Roll twice in a towel.

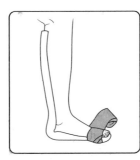

2 Fold the splint under 1 inch at the toes to make a reinforcing toe plate. Place the splint under the foot, extending slightly beyond the toes and wrap as follows: start at the toes, work up the foot, skip the ankle and wrap behind the achilles.

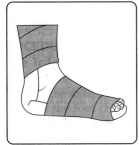

3 Below the malleolus, overlap corners of the splint. Take care not to push in and cause a pressure point.

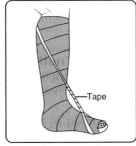

4 Wrap the heel and continue wrapping the rest of the leg. Mold and position as prescribed by physician. Tip: To hold position, wrap splint with figure-8 taping technique.

FIGURE 124-4 Posterior short leg splint. (BSN Medical. [2006]. *Ortho-Glass splinting course manual* [6th ed., p. 25]. Charlotte, NC: Author.)

Also known as: Posterior boot, posterior slab.

Indications: Fracture or soft tissue injuries of the foot or ankle.

Equipment: 4- to 5-in cast padding.

4- to 6-in plaster (10–15 layers) or fiberglass.

4- to 6-in elastic bandage.

Measure: From the metatarsal 2 in below the popliteal area to 2 in beyond the toes.

Extremity position: Foot should be at a 90-degree angle to the leg. The splint should not impede knee flexion. Fold the splint under 1-inch at the toes to provide reinforcement.

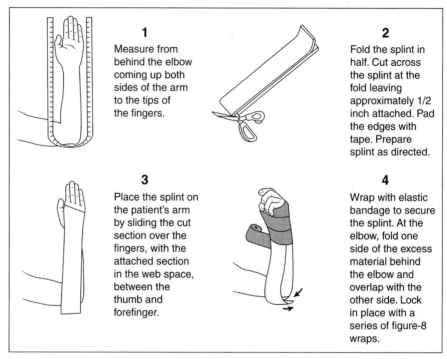

1
Measure from behind the elbow coming up both sides of the arm to the tips of the fingers.

2
Fold the splint in half. Cut across the splint at the fold leaving approximately 1/2 inch attached. Pad the edges with tape. Prepare splint as directed.

3
Place the splint on the patient's arm by sliding the cut section over the fingers, with the attached section in the web space, between the thumb and forefinger.

4
Wrap with elastic bandage to secure the splint. At the elbow, fold one side of the excess material behind the elbow and overlap with the other side. Lock in place with a series of figure-8 wraps.

FIGURE 124-5 Forearm sugar tong splint. (BSN Medical. [2006]. *Ortho-Glass splinting course manual* [6th ed., p. 18].Charlotte, NC: Author.)

     Also known as: Anterior posterior splints, sandwich splints, reverse sugar tong.

     Indications: Fractures or soft tissue injuries of the forearm/wrist.

     Equipment: 3- to 4-in cast padding.

             3- to 4-in fiberglass or plaster splints (8–10 layers).

             3- to 4-in elastic bandage.

     Measure: From the fingertips, over the dorsum of the hand, over the flexed elbow, and on over the volar aspect of the forearm to the fingertips. Fold the splint in half and cut across the fold, leaving approximately ½-inch attached. Slide the splint over the patient's arm with the attached section in the web space between the thumb and index finger. Wrap with elastic bandage and fold excess splint around the elbow and overlap with the other side.

Extremity position: Forearm with thumb up and 90-degree flexion of the elbow (consult with physician for prescribed position as other positions may be indicated).

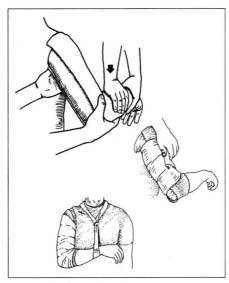

FIGURE 124-6   Humerus sugar tong. (From Simon, R., & Brenner, B. [2002]. *Emergency procedures and techniques* [4th ed., p. 269]. Baltimore: Williams & Wilkins.)

    Also known as: Hanging humeral splint

      Indications: Immobilization of a humeral shalt fracture

       Equipment: 4- to 5-in. cast padding

               4- to 5-in. fiberglass or plaster (8–15 layers)

               4- to 5-in. elastic bandage

        Measure: From the acromicoclavicular (AC) joint, over the humerus, around the albow, and up the axillary crease.

Extremity position: Forearm is either pronated or supinated with a 90-degree flexion of the elbow (consult with physican for prescribed position).

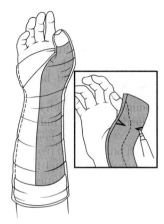

FIGURE 124-7 Thumb spica splint. (From Chudnofsky, C. R., & Byers, S. [2004]. Splinting techniques. In J. R. Roberts & J. R. Hedges [Eds.], *Clinical procedures in emergency medicine* [4th ed., p. 998]. Philadelphia: Saunders.)

Also known as: Wrist gauntlet.

Indications: Soft tissue injury, metacarpal fracture of the thumb, or fracture of the navicular or scaphoid bone.

Equipment: 2- to 3-in cast padding.

2- to 3-in fiberglass or plaster splints (8–10 layers).

2- to 3-in elastic bandage.

Measure: From the distal tip of the thumb to approximately two-thirds of the way up the forearm or it may include the elbow. The fingers should be free, allowing full motion of the metacarpophalangeal joints.

Extremity position: Position the hand as if holding a wineglass, with the thumb curved toward the fingers and the wrist dorsiflexed approximately 20 degrees (Chudnofsky & Byers, 2004).

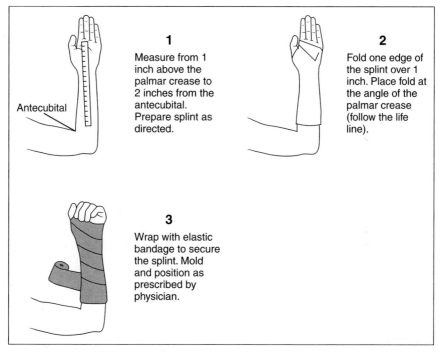

1

Measure from 1 inch above the palmar crease to 2 inches from the antecubital. Prepare splint as directed.

Antecubital

2

Fold one edge of the splint over 1 inch. Place fold at the angle of the palmar crease (follow the life line).

3

Wrap with elastic bandage to secure the splint. Mold and position as prescribed by physician.

FIGURE 124-8   Volar forearm splint. (BSN Medical. [2006]. *Ortho-Glass splinting course manual* [6th ed., p. 13]. Charlotte, NC: Author.)

Also known as: Anterior splint or radial slab.

Indications: Fracture or soft tissue injury to the wrist or carpal bones.

Equipment: 3- to 4-in cast padding.

3- to 4-in fiberglass or plaster splint (8–10 layers).

3- to 4-in elastic bandage.

Measure: From palmar crease to approximately 3 cm proximal to the antecubital fossa.

Extremity position: Wrist in a neutral position, slightly extended, with the fingers at 10–20 degrees of flexion, with the thumb pointing up. Fold the splint at an angle across the palmar crease.

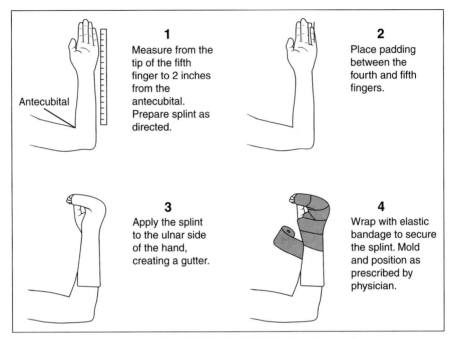

FIGURE 124-9 Ulnar gutter splint. (BSN Medical. [2006]. *Ortho-Glass splinting course manual* [6th ed., p. 17]. Charlotte, NC: Author.)

Also known as: Phalangeal or metacarpal gutter splint, boxer splint.

Indications: Fracture or soft tissue injury of the fourth and fifth metacarpals.

Equipment: 2- to 3-in. cast padding.
2- to 3-in fiberglass or plaster splints (6–8 layers).
2- to 3-in elastic bandage.

Measure: From the fingertips and up two thirds of the forearm.

Extremity position: Position the hand with the fingers held at 60–70 degrees of flexion at the metacarpophalangeal joint, the wrist dorsiflexed 20 degrees, and the interphalangeal (IP) joints extended or slightly flexed at 10 degrees (Chudnofsky & Byers, 2004). The wrist should be slightly extended. Place padding between the fourth and fifth fingers.

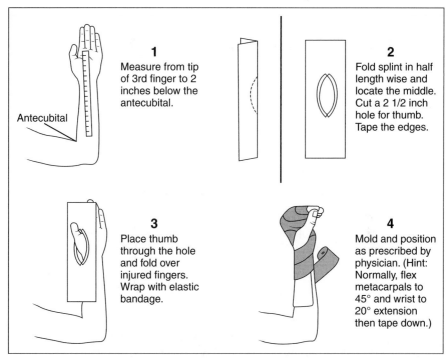

1
Measure from tip of 3rd finger to 2 inches below the antecubital.

Antecubital

2
Fold splint in half length wise and locate the middle. Cut a 2 1/2 inch hole for thumb. Tape the edges.

3
Place thumb through the hole and fold over injured fingers. Wrap with elastic bandage.

4
Mold and position as prescribed by physician. (Hint: Normally, flex metacarpals to 45° and wrist to 20° extension then tape down.)

FIGURE 124-10   Radial gutter splint. (BSN Medical. [2006]. *Ortho-Glass splinting course manual* [6th ed., p. 16]. Charlotte, NC: Author.)

    Also known as: Teardrop, phalangeal, or metacarpal gutter splint.
      Indications: Fractures or soft tissue injuries of the first through third metacarpals.
       Equipment: 2- to 3-in cast padding.
                  2- to 3-in fiberglass or plaster splints (6–8 layers).
                  2- to 3-in elastic bandage.
         Measure: From the pulp of the distal finger up to the proximal forearm (Chudnofsky & Byers, 2004). Cut a 2½-inch hole for the thumb and tape the edges.
Extremity position: Position the hand with the fingers held at 60–90 degrees of flexion at the metacarpophalangeal joint and the interphalangeal joints extended or slightly flexed to 10 degrees. The wrist should be slightly dorsiflexed to 20 degrees (Chudnofsky & Byers, 2004).

REFERENCES

BSN Medical. (2006). *Ortho-glass splinting course manual* (6th ed.). Charlotte NC: Author.

Chudnofsky, C. R., & Byers, S. (2004). Splinting techniques. In J. R. Roberts, & J. R. Hedges (Eds.), *Clinical procedures in emergency medicine* (4th ed., pp. 989-1009). Philadelphia: Saunders.

Removal and Bivalving of Casts

Margo E. Layman, MSN, RN, RNC, CN-A

Bivalving is also known as a *bilateral split* or *splitting a cast.*

INDICATIONS

1. To relieve neurovascular impairment caused by pressure from the cast
2. To facilitate care and access when the circumferential strength is no longer required
3. To remove a cast when it is no longer required or when a new cast is indicated

CONTRAINDICATIONS AND CAUTIONS

1. Cutting directly over a bony prominence should be avoided.
2. Cast cutter blades vibrate instead of rotate. Therefore, skin injury is unlikely. If excessive pressure is used when the plaster or fiberglass is cut, however, lacerations or abrasions may occur.
3. When bivalving to relieve pressure, the inner wadding needs to be split all the way to the skin.
4. Fiberglass is significantly more difficult to cut than is plaster.

EQUIPMENT

Cover sheet
Cast cutter or saw
Cast spreader
Protective eyewear
Elastic bandages (for bivalving)
Scissors

PATIENT PREPARATION

1. Arrange a nonverbal signal so that the patient can communicate despite the noise when excessive heat or pressure is felt. Heat is generated with the movement of the cast blade. A brief pause relieves the sensation.
2. Demonstrate the safety of the cutter by touching the blade to your thumb or the stretcher mattress, which stops the motion of the blade.

PROCEDURAL STEPS
Bivalving

1. Place a sheet under the cast to collect plaster material and cover the patient's clothing.

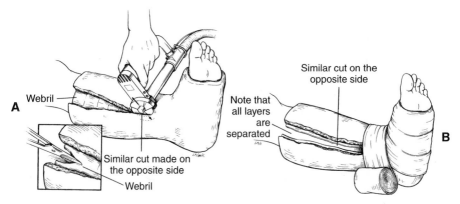

FIGURE 125-1 Bivalving a cast. See text for explanation. (From Chudnofsky, C. R., & Byers, S. [2004]. Splinting techniques. In J. R. Roberts & J. R. Hedges (Eds.), *Clinical procedures in emergency medicine* [4th ed., p. 1008]. Philadelphia: Saunders.)

2. Mark the cast lengthwise into two equal parts, avoiding bony prominences. Univalving the cast may be sufficient if neurovascular impairment resolves after one side of the cast is cut. Wedges are commercially manufactured to hold the cast open so that it does not have to be bivalved in all cases.
3. Cut with an even up-and-down motion, releasing when you feel the cutter break through the plaster or fiberglass material (Figure 125-1, *A*).
4. Separate the cast with the cast spreader, and cut the cotton wadding with scissors (see Figure 125-1, *A*).
5. Reassess neurovascular status, and notify the physician of residual deficits.
6. Wrap the cast with an elastic bandage to secure it in place (see Figure 125-1, *B*).

Removal of Cast
1. Bivalve cast as directed previously.
2. Once the cast is split through to the skin surface, remove the anterior portion of the cast.
3. With support to the extremity, remove the posterior portion. Clean and dry the skin gently.
4. Apply splints or other orthopedic adjuncts as prescribed.

AGE-SPECIFIC CONSIDERATIONS
1. The noise of the cast saw is intense and can be disturbing. Pediatric patients should be warned about the sounds and the process before the saw is turned on.
2. Elderly patients have thinner, more friable skin and are at increased risk for abrasions or lacerations.

COMPLICATIONS
1. Laceration or abrasion of the skin with the cast cutter
2. Displacement of an unhealed fracture

PATIENT TEACHING

1. Exercise and weight bearing are specified by the physician on the basis of the injury and the healing process.
2. It is normal to have peeling, dry skin where the cast had been; this resolves within a few days. Moisturizing lotions may be applied.
3. If the extremity has atrophied because of lack of muscle activity, reassure the patient that with exercise the limb will eventually strengthen and normalize.

Elastic Bandage Application

Margo E. Layman, MSN, RN, RNC, CN-A

Elastic bandages are also known as *Ace wraps* and *crepe bandages*.

INDICATIONS

1. To immobilize a fracture in conjunction with a splint
2. To provide a hemostatic dressing
3. To anchor dressings and decrease tension on sutures
4. To provide support, minimize swelling, and prevent further injury in the presence of soft tissue trauma

CONTRAINDICATIONS AND CAUTIONS

1. The patient may have an allergy to the sizing material in new fabrics or latex allergy (may use flannel or muslin bandage instead). Latex-free elastic bandages are available.
2. Elastic bandages may decrease peripheral circulation and should be used with caution in the presence of peripheral vascular disease or diabetes.

EQUIPMENT

Elastic bandage (for legs and knees, 3- to 4-in wide; for hands, wrist, and elbows, 2- to 3-in wide)
Tape or safety pins or clips
Dressings as indicated
Cast padding (optional)

PATIENT PREPARATION

1. Place extremity in the position of function. See Procedure 124 for information on positioning.

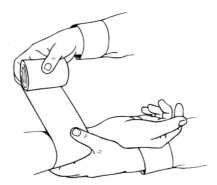

FIGURE 126-1 Elastic bandage application: anchor the bandage by circling twice around the extremity. (From Proehl, J. A., & Jones, L. M. [1998]. *Mosby's emergency department teaching guides* [pp. I-2]. St Louis: Mosby.)

2. If possible, before application, elevate the extremity for 15 to 30 minutes to facilitate venous return and help decrease edema.
3. Optional: Apply three or four layers of cast padding under the area to be wrapped. The wrapping configuration is the same as that used for the overlying elastic bandage. Be careful not to stretch the padding during application or it may become too tight.

PROCEDURAL STEPS

1. Unroll 3 to 4 inches and hold the bandage with the roll facing up, and anchor the bandage by circling twice around the distal extremity (Figure 126-1).
2. To ensure uniform pressure, unroll the bandage as you wrap the body part. Stretch the bandage only slightly while wrapping.
3. Overlap each layer of the bandage by half to two thirds the width of the bandage.
4. Wrap firmly but not tightly. You should be able to insert a finger easily under the bandage.
5. Include the wrist when wrapping the hand and the foot when wrapping the ankle.
6. Use a figure-eight wrap on joints (Figure 126-2). A spiral wrap is used if a joint is not involved. Toes and fingers should be visible for follow-up circulation assessment.
7. Secure the bandage with tape or pins or clips. Do not place pins or clips on posterior or medial surfaces because they may cause soft tissue injury if pressure is applied to them.

AGE-SPECIFIC CONSIDERATIONS

1. Young children may not be able to complain of pain or tingling. Instruct caregivers to check the bandage frequently. They should be able to easily place one finger under bandage—otherwise, it is too tight (Roe, 2003).
2. Older patients may need assistance removing the bandage and inspecting their skin for tissue damage.

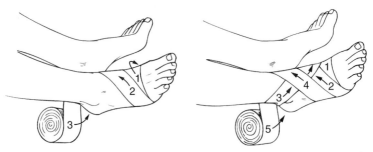

FIGURE 126-2 Figure-eight wrap around joint. (From Proehl, J. A., & Jones, L. M. [1998]. *Mosby's emergency department teaching guides* [pp. I-2]. St Louis, Mosby.)

COMPLICATIONS

1. Neurovascular impairment or skin irritation may be caused by bandages that are too tight. Assess and document neurovascular status before and after bandage application.
2. Distal edema as a result of obstruction of venous return can occur. This edema can be decreased by including the hand or foot in distal extremity wraps and by elevating the wrapped extremity.

PATIENT TEACHING

1. Reapply the bandage if it loosens unless otherwise instructed.
2. Launder the bandage in cold water as needed; either by hand or by placing it in a mesh bag in a washing machine.
3. Watch for numbness, tingling, coldness, swelling, or discoloration of the hand or foot. Loosen the bandage and elevate the extremity if any of these signs or symptoms occur. Report any symptoms not relieved by loosening the bandage or elevating the extremity.
4. Elevate the extremity and apply ice as directed to help prevent and decrease swelling.

REFERENCE

Roe, S. (2003). Applying an elastic bandage. In S. Roe (Ed.), *Delmar's clinical skills and concepts* (pp. 672-677). Clifton Park, NY: Thomson Learning.

Skeletal Traction

Jean A. Proehl, RN, MN, CEN, CCRN, FAEN

Skeletal traction is also known as *Steinmann pin, Kirschner wire,* and *K-wire.*

INDICATIONS

To maintain alignment of fractured bone ends via continuous traction on a pin or wire through bone. Traction helps decrease muscle spasm and movement of bone ends. Skeletal traction may be used when heavier weights and longer periods of immobilization are required than are permitted by skin traction. It is most frequently used with fractures of the femur but is also used for fractures of the tibia and humerus. The cervical spine may also be immobilized with traction (see Procedure 94).

CONTRAINDICATIONS AND CAUTIONS

1. Aseptic technique must be maintained to prevent contamination of the pin sites during insertion.
2. Pins are not inserted through infected or abraded soft tissue.

EQUIPMENT

Antiseptic solution
Local anesthetic
Syringes and needles for local anesthesia administration
No. 11 or 15 scalpel
Steinmann pin or Kirschner wire set (assorted sizes) (NOTE: Kirschner wires [K-wires] are generally smaller in diameter than Steinmann pins. Either may be smooth or threaded.)
Drill to drive pin
Pin cutter
Cork, tape, or rubber stoppers (e.g., those from blood tubes) to place over the cut pin ends
Gauze dressings
Antibiotic ointment (optional)
Traction bow or caliper (Bohler-Steinmann pin holder or Kirschner wire tractor)
Hospital bed with traction setup as indicated
Rope

The author would like to thank Gary Smith, Orthopedic Technician, for his expert review of this procedure.

Weights, usually 7 to 12 kg (15 to 25 lbs) for longitudinal traction on extremity fractures (Additional weight may be needed for other parts of the traction setup.)

PATIENT PREPARATION

1. Move the patient onto the hospital bed before removal of the temporary splint.
2. Assess and document neurovascular status distal to the injury.

PROCEDURAL STEPS

1. Cleanse the skin at the pin insertion site with antiseptic solution.
2. *Anesthetize the skin, tissue, and periosteum along the intended tract of the pin on both sides (see Procedure 135).
3. *Make a small incision in the skin at the insertion site in the direction of the pull of traction.
4. *Attach the pin to the drill.
5. *Drive the pin through the bone perpendicular to the long axis of the bone. Drilling too quickly can generate heat and should be avoided for secure pin placement.
6. *Incise the skin over the exit site as it is tented by the exiting pin.
7. *Remove the drill when the pin is sufficiently through the bone to attach the traction bow.
8. *Apply the traction bow, and cut off the excess pin.
9. Place cork, tape, or rubber stoppers over the cut pin ends.
10. *Attach the rope to the traction bow, run it through the pulley, and attach the weights.
11. *Suspend the extremity as indicated. The most common and most versatile traction setup for femur fractures is balanced suspension with a Thomas splint and a Pearson attachment. The patient is able to move about in bed while the leg remains supported and traction is constant (Figure 127-1).
12. Assess and document neurovascular status.
13. Perform pin care per institutional protocol. There is insufficient evidence to make strong recommendations about specific pin care techniques (Holmes & Brown, 2005). Options include:
    a. Chlorhexidine solution may be the most effective agent for cleaning the site (Holmes & Brown, 2005).
    b. Gauze dressing around the pin
    c. Antibiotic ointment around the pin entrance and exit
    d. No dressing or ointment to sites
14. Obtain postreduction x-ray studies.
15. Secure all rope knots with tape.

COMPLICATIONS

1. Osteomyelitis at the pin insertion site
2. Skin necrosis at the pin site

---

*Indicates portions of the procedure usually performed by a physician or an advanced practice nurse.

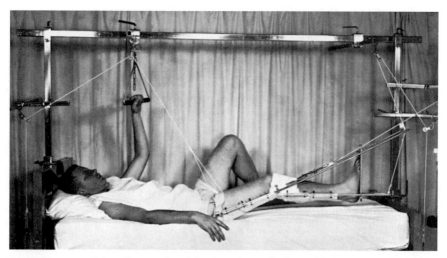

FIGURE 127-1 Balanced suspension skeletal traction to the femur. (Thompson, J. M., McFarland, G. K., Hirsch, J. E., & Tucker, S. M. [Eds.]. [2002]. *Mosby's clinical nursing* [5th ed., Fig. 6-37]. St Louis: Mosby.

3. Sudden loss of traction and motion of fractured bone ends caused by equipment failure. Be sure that traction weights hang freely at all times and that knots in the traction rope are not caught in the pulleys. Traction should not be interrupted.

4. Wire or pin migration during insertion or slips after insertion. Both are more common with smooth wires or pins.

5. Compartmental syndrome as a result of excessive traction.

PATIENT TEACHING

1. Do not attempt to adjust traction device. Request help to reposition yourself in bed.

2. Report any signs of infection immediately, including redness, swelling, increased pain, or pus.

3. Report any signs of compartmental syndrome immediately, including pain, swelling, numbness, or tingling.

4. Report any problems with the pin or traction.

REFERENCE

Holmes, S. B., & Brown, S. J., Pin Site Care Expert Panel. (2005). Skeletal pin site care: National Association of Orthopedic Nurses guidelines for orthopedic nursing. *Orthopedic Nursing,* *24*(2), 99-107.

Heat Therapy

Daun A. Smith, RN, MSN

Heat therapy is also known as *hot compress, hot pack,* and *warm moist pack.*

INDICATIONS

1. To decrease the pain and stiffness associated with subacute and chronic injuries of soft tissues and joints. Heat increases blood flow, producing an inflammatory response that may be beneficial at some stages of a disease or injury process.
2. To assist in the treatment of dermatologic or infectious conditions and pain associated with muscle spasm in the patient with degenerative joint disease.

CONTRAINDICATIONS AND CAUTIONS

1. To avoid burns, heat therapy should be avoided in the presence of severe peripheral vascular disease, venous insufficiency, vasculitis, thromboangiitis obliterans, thrombophlebitis, vasospastic disorders (e.g., Raynaud's phenomenon), immature scar tissue, infected wounds, bleeding tendencies, and known sensitivity to heat. Use extreme caution with paralyzed or insensate areas.
2. Heat treatments should be instituted after the 48-hour acute phase of injury. When the treatments are started prematurely, increased bleeding and swelling may result and prolong the inflammatory process.

EQUIPMENT

Dry towel or cloth
Hot moist pack
or
Heat lamp or commercial hot pack
(Commercial products are available that offer temperature control and delivery of moist heat.)

PROCEDURAL STEPS

1. Place a towel in warm water: 36° to 39° C (96° to 103° F).
2. Express excess water, place in a dry towel, and apply to the injured area. You may also use a thin plastic wrap to contain the heat and excess moisture.
3. For appropriate penetration and to prevent burns and rebound phenomena, the application must be left in place for no longer than 15 to 20 minutes (Wimberley, 2007).
4. Heat lamps can also be used in conjunction with wet packs (see Procedure 149).

AGE-SPECIFIC CONSIDERATIONS

1. Infants and young children have thinner skin and are easily burned with temperatures that would not affect adult skin. Warm—not hot—water is recommended.
2. Aging skin is less vascular, thinner, and therefore more easily injured. Care should be taken to ensure that water temperature or heat is within the stated parameters and that the duration of the therapy is 20 minutes or less in the elderly patient

COMPLICATIONS

1. If applied acutely in the injured patient, heat increases tissue edema.
2. Excessive or prolonged heat can burn the skin.
3. Prolonged contact with a moist pack can result in skin maceration.

PATIENT TEACHING

1. Heat treatments applied for 20- to 30-minute intervals two to four times daily assist with healing and resumption of normal function.
2. Full trunk and extremity immersion may be used. Use caution to avoid prolonged direct pressure from air jets on the injured area because this may cause increased damage to the tissues.

REFERENCE

Wimberley, T. (2007). Skin integrity & wound healing. In J. M. Wilkinson, & K. Van Leuven (Eds.), *Fundamentals of nursing: Theory, concepts, & applications* (pp. 842-843). Philadelphia: F. A. Davis.

PROCEDURE 129

Cold Therapy

Daun A. Smith, RN, MS, CEN

Cold therapy is also known as *cryotherapy, cold pack,* and *ice pack.*

INDICATIONS

To control soft-tissue pain and edema in the presence of fractures, soft tissue injuries, sprains, and strains. The initial physiologic response is constriction of the local cutaneous and subcutaneous vessels, which results in reduced blood volume to the affected site, which decreases edema.

CONTRAINDICATIONS AND CAUTIONS

1. Cold therapy should be avoided in patients with a history of severe peripheral vascular disease, venous insufficiency, vasculitis, thromboangiitis obliterans, thrombophlebitis, vasospastic disorders (e.g., Raynaud's phenomenon, Buerger's disease), anesthetized extremities, or known sensitivity to cold. Use extreme caution with paralyzed or insensate areas. In these conditions, the vasoconstriction caused by cold therapy may exacerbate underlying tissue perfusion problems.
2. Excessive or prolonged cold treatments can freeze the skin, resulting in frostnip, superficial frostbite, or deep frostbite and vascular damage. Ice bags should have a dry interface with the skin to decrease the risk of damage to the skin.
3. Cold should be discontinued if the skin blanches and then turns red after application (Titler & Rakel, 2001). This is an indication of reflex vasodilation, which may increase blood flow to the area, potentially increasing edema (Fujise, 2006).

EQUIPMENT

Ice in waterproof bag
or
Commercial cold or gel pack
Small cloth or towel
(NOTE: Chemical cold packs should not be used on the face because puncture of the bag may result in chemical injury to the eyes.)

PROCEDURAL STEPS

1. Place cubed or crushed ice in a waterproof bag.
2. Wrap the bag in a dry cloth or towel before application to the skin.
3. If a commercial product is used, follow the instructions regarding insulation and application to the skin surface.
4. Complete extremity immersion can be performed for irregularly shaped areas. The mixture of water and ice should be at 55° to 60° F (13° to 16° C). Reassess distal circulation after 10 to 15 minutes.
5. Cold packs or ice water immersion is applied for a period of 20 to 30 minutes per exposure. To avoid skin and tissue damage, longer application is not recommended (Titler & Rakel, 2001).
6. Reapply cold every 1 to 2 hours for 24 to 72 hours after injury.

AGE-SPECIFIC CONSIDERATIONS

1. Cold therapy is recommended for all populations after acute injury or after orthopedic surgery. The application time should be shortened to 15 to 20 minutes on a 3- to 4-hour reapplication cycle in pediatric and geriatric patients who have thinner, more easily injured skin.
2. Monitoring for signs of frostnip or frostbite must be stressed during patient and family teaching for these populations.

COMPLICATIONS

Frostnip, superficial frostbite, or deep frostbite and vascular damage from excessive or prolonged cold treatment.

PATIENT TEACHING

1. Always put a dry cloth between the cold pack and the skin.
2. Apply cold for 20 to 30 minutes every 1 to 2 hours in conjunction with rest and elevation of the affected site to assist with lessening pain and edema. Small children and elderly patients have thinner skin. To prevent injury in the very young or very old, apply cold for 15 to 20 minutes every 3 to 4 hours.
3. The effective cycling period for this treatment in the acute phase is 24 to 72 hours.
4. Complete extremity immersion can be performed with caution, limiting the exposure time to 20 to 30 minutes and elevating the injury site after therapy.
5. Discontinue cold therapy if the skin blanches and turns red or if the area becomes completely numb.

REFERENCES

Fujise, N. (2006). Skin integrity and wound healing. In S. C. DeLaune, & P. K. Ladner (Eds.), *Fundamentals of nursing: Standards and practice.* (3rd ed., pp. 1224-1227). New York: Thompson Delmar Learning.

Titler, M. G., & Rakel, B. A. (2001). Nonpharmacological treatment of pain. *Critical Care Clinics of North America, 13,* 221-232.

PROCEDURE 130

Measuring Compartmental Pressure

Jean A. Proehl, RN, MN, CEN, CCRN, FAEN

Compartmental pressure is also known as *compartment pressure, intracompartmental pressure,* and *tissue pressure.*

INDICATION

To measure tissue pressure when compartmental syndrome is suspected. Causes of compartmental syndrome include, but are not limited to, fractures, soft tissue or vascular trauma, crush injuries, exercise, envenomation, tight casts or circumferential dressings, pneumatic antishock garments, automatic blood pressure devices, massive fluid resuscitation, and burns.

Tissue pressure is normally 10 mm Hg or less. Follow-up monitoring is indicated if tissue pressures are between 20 and 30 mm Hg. Pressures in excess of 30 to 40 mm Hg in the presence of positive clinical findings suggest the need for decompression of the compartment via fasciotomy. Metabolically, the differential pressure between diastolic blood pressure and compartment pressure may be more important than absolute compartment pressure. A differential pressure of less than 30 mm Hg (diastolic blood pressure – compartmental pressure) was a safe indicator for fasciotomy in one study (McQueen & Court-Brown, 1996). Recent research has suggested that the pressure differential diagnostic for compartmental syndrome may actually be much lower, approximately 20 mm Hg (Kosir et al., 2007).

CONTRAINDICATIONS AND CAUTIONS

1. When compartmental syndrome is clinically evident, there is no need to measure compartmental pressures, and the patient should be taken immediately to the operating room for decompression via fasciotomy.
2. Avoid inserting the needle or catheter through infected or contaminated tissue.
3. The needle or catheter should be inserted as far away from fractured bone ends as possible to prevent conversion of a closed fracture to an open fracture. An open fracture does not rule out the possibility of a compartmental syndrome (McQueen & Court-Brown, 1996).
4. Application of cold packs to suspect extremities is controversial because further vasoconstriction may exacerbate the already decreased tissue perfusion. Consult with the physician before applying cold packs.
5. The Whitesides technique is the least precise of methods and produced unacceptable results in one study (Boody & Wongworawat, 2005). In addition, the Whitesides technique uses mercury manometers, which are no longer commonly available. Therefore, that technique is not addressed in this procedure.
6. Side port needles and slit catheters are more accurate than straight needles (Boody & Wongworawat, 2005).

PATIENT PREPARATION

1. Remove circumferential dressings or casts (see Procedure 125).
2. Keep the extremity at the level of the heart (not elevated) to optimize blood flow to the tissues until compartmental syndrome has been ruled out.
3. Treat systemic hypotension with fluids, medications, or both to sustain tissue perfusion.
4. Cleanse the skin overlying the insertion site with antiseptic solution. Multiple insertion sites may be used to measure pressures in different compartments of the same extremity (Figure 130-1).
5. *Infiltrate the insertion site with local anesthetic (optional). If local anesthetic is used, care should be taken to infiltrate only the skin because

---

*Indicates portions of the procedure usually performed by a physician or an advanced practice nurse.

Four compartments of the leg: the anterior compartment (AC), the lateral compartment (LC), the superficial posterior compartment (SPC), and the deep posterior compartment (DPC).

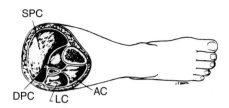

Two compartments of the forearm: the volar compartment (VC) and the dorsal compartment (DC).

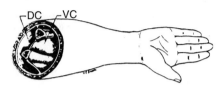

Five interosseous compartments of the hand.

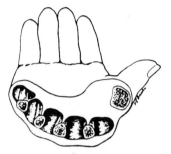

FIGURE 130-1 Compartments of the lower leg, forearm, and hand. (From Matsen, F. A., III. [1980]. Compartmental syndromes [p. 82]. New York: Grune & Stratton, with permission.)

injection of additional fluid into the compartment could increase the tissue pressure.

6. Instruct the patient to keep the extremity relaxed during pressure measurements because movement causes the pressure to change.

STRYKER INTRACOMPARTMENTAL PRESSURE MONITOR
Equipment
Antiseptic solution
Gauze dressings
Local anesthetic with needles and syringe (optional)
Intracompartmental pressure monitor (Stryker, Kalamazoo, MI)
Side-port needle, transducer, and syringe assembly supplied by manufacturer
(Through-the-needle slit catheters are also available for continuous pressure monitoring with this unit.)

Procedural Steps (Stryker, 2006)
1. Turn the pressure monitor on. "_ _" is displayed for 5 seconds and then disappears.

2. Assemble the needle, transducer, and syringe and place into the pressure monitor with the black side of the transducer down (Figure 130-2).
3. Close the cover of the pressure monitor until the latch snaps.
4. Remove the clear end cap of the syringe, and attach the plunger to the syringe.
5. Hold the monitor at a 45-degree angle with the needle upright, and push on the plunger to purge the unit of air. Do not allow fluid to flow back into the transducer well.
6. *Hold the monitor at the intended angle of insertion into the skin, and press the zero button (Figure 130-3). The digital display should read "00" after a few seconds. The display *must* read "00" before continuing.
7. *Insert the needle into the compartment. Slowly inject less than 0.3 ml of saline into the compartment to equilibrate the monitor with the interstitial fluids.
8. Wait for the digital display to equilibrate, and note the pressure. For additional measurements, repeat steps 5 through 8. Make sure unit is reset to zero.

INTRAVENOUS PUMP WITH PRESSURE SENSING CAPABILITY
(Uliazsz, Isheida, Fleming, & Yamamoto, 2003)
Equipment
Intravenous (IV) pump with pressure sensing capability and "micro" capability (able to administer at rates in tenths of an ml)
Normal saline IV fluid, 50- to 100-ml bag
Pump tubing
Needle (side port preferred), slit or wick catheter
Antiseptic solution
Local anesthetic with needles and syringe (optional)

---

*Indicates portions of the procedure usually performed by a physician or an advanced practice nurse.

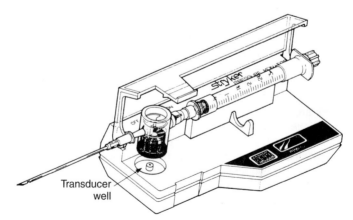

Transducer well

FIGURE 130-2 Assemble the needle, the transducer, and the syringe. Place in the pressure monitor with the black side of the transducer down. (Courtesy Stryker Surgical. [2006]. *Intra-compartmental pressure monitor system: Maintenance manual and operating instructions.* Kalamazoo, MI.)

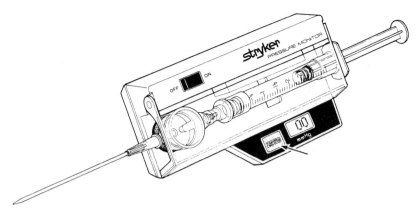

FIGURE 130-3 Hold the monitor at the intended angle of insertion and press the "zero" button. (Courtesy Stryker Surgical. [2006]. *Intra-compartmental pressure monitor system: Maintenance manual and operating instructions.* Kalamazoo, MI.)

Procedural Steps

1. Set the IV pump to manometry mode per manufacturer's instructions.
2. Attach the needle to the pump tubing and prime the tubing and needle with fluid.
3. Zero the pressure on the IV pump.
4. *Insert the needle into the compartment.
5. Infuse 0.3 ml of saline at a slow rate.
6. Read the pressure.

HEMODYNAMIC MONITOR
Equipment
Invasive pressure monitor
Transducer and pressure tubing set-up
30-ml syringe
50-ml normal saline
Needle (side port preferred), slit, or wick catheter
Antiseptic solution
Local anesthetic with needles and syringe (optional)

Procedural Steps

1. Assemble the pressure tubing and transducer. Remove the proximal part of the tubing (drip chamber and spike assembly) and replace it with a 30 ml syringe of saline. Prime the tubing as described in Procedure 88.
2. Turn on the monitor and select 30 or 60 mm Hg pressure scale. Connect the monitor to the transducer system.

---

*Indicates portions of the procedure usually performed by a physician or an advanced practice nurse.

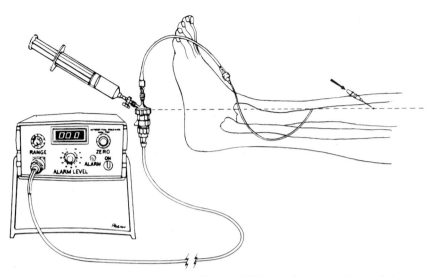

FIGURE 130-4 Zeroing the transducer with the air-fluid interface at the level of the tip of the needle or catheter. (From Gallagher, J. J. [2005]. Intracompartmental pressure monitoring. In D. J. Lynn-McHale Wiegand & K. K. Carlson [Eds.], *AACN procedure manual for critical care* [5th ed., Fig. 132-5]. Philadelphia: Saunders.)

3. Remove the cap from the side port of the distal stopcock (next to the transducer) and position it so it is open to air and to the syringe. Position the air-fluid interface (zeroing stopcock) level with the intended insertion site of the needle (Figure 130-4) (Gallagher, 2005). Zero the system.
4. Connect the needle or slit catheter to the distal end of the tubing and flush it with saline.
5. *Insert the needle or slit catheter into the compartment.
6. Read the pressure.
7. Squeeze the compartment to verify that the reading is accurate. A rapid increase in compartment pressure should be noted with pressure or muscle contraction. In a normal compartment, the pressure will fall back to baseline quickly. Patients with compartment syndrome will have a slow return to baseline (Gallagher, 2005).

AGE-SPECIFIC CONSIDERATIONS

1. Needles as small as 25-G (without a sideport) can be used to measure compartmental pressure accurately (Mars, Tufts, & Hadley, 1997).
2. Compartmental syndrome may develop more rapidly in children because the size of the compartment is relatively smaller and the fascial tissue is tighter.

---

*Indicates portions of the procedure usually performed by a physician or an advanced practice nurse.

COMPLICATIONS

1. Inaccurate pressures if the needle is inserted into a tendon or occluded with tissue. Needle function can be tested by squeezing the extremity; immediate pressure fluctuations should be noted if the needle is patent.
2. Infection (late)

PATIENT TEACHING

1. Report the following symptoms immediately: pain of increasing severity; pain that does not respond to prescribed pain medications; pain on passive movement; numbness or tingling; weakness; tenseness of the injured extremity in comparison to the noninjured extremity; pallor, mottling, cyanosis, or coldness of the extremity.
2. Position the injured extremity as instructed. (Note: If an early compartmental syndrome is suspected, the patient is instructed to keep the extremity at the level of the heart to optimize blood flow to the tissue.)

REFERENCES

Boody, A. R., & Wongworawat, M. D. (2005). Accuracy in the measurement of compartment pressures: A comparison of three commonly used devices. *Journal of Bone and Joint Surgery, 87-A*, 2415-2422.

Gallagher, J. J. (2005). Intracompartmental pressure monitoring. In D. J. Lynn-McHale Wiegand, & K. K. Carlson (Eds.), *AACN procedure manual for critical care* (5th ed.). Philadelphia: Saunders.

Kosir, R., Moore, F. A., Selby, J. H., Cocanour, C. S., Kozar, R. A., Gonzalez, E. A., & Todd, S. R. (2007). Acute lower extremity compartment syndrome (ALECS) screening protocol in critically ill trauma patients. *Journal of Trauma, 63*, 268-275.

Mars, M., Tufts, M. A., & Hadley, G. P. (1997). Towards reducing the trauma of direct intracompartmental pressure measurement for children: An in vitro assessment of small diameter needles. *Pediatric Surgery International, 12*, 172-176.

McQueen, M. M., & Court-Brown, C. M. (1996). Compartment monitoring in tibial fractures: The pressure threshold for decompression. *Journal of Bone and Joint Surgery, 78-B*, 99-104.

Stryker Instruments. (2006). *Intra-compartmental pressure monitor system.* Kalamazoo, MI: Author.

Uliazsz, A., Isheida, J. T., Fleming, J. K., & Yamamoto, L. G. (2003). Comparing the methods of measuring compartment pressures in acute compartment syndrome. *American Journal of Emergency Medicine, 21*, 143-145.

Measuring and Fitting for Ambulation Aids

Margo E. Layman, MSN, RN, RNC, CN-A

Ambulation aids include crutches, canes, and walkers.

INDICATIONS

1. To provide support or stability when walking
2. To compensate for impaired balance, decreased strength, pain during weight bearing, or injury of a lower extremity

CONTRAINDICATIONS AND CAUTIONS

1. If initial measurement is performed with the patient in a position other than standing, the fit of the aid must be evaluated and adjusted accordingly when the patient is upright.
2. An improperly fitted aid adversely affects the patient's gait pattern and may result in unstable or unsafe ambulation, decreased function, and decreased safety for the patient. Improperly fitted crutches may cause pain, nerve damage, or paralysis if excessive pressure is exerted on the axillae.
3. The energy consumption associated with non–weight bearing is substantial. Elderly, debilitated, or sedentary patients could be at risk for severe exercise challenge and pronounced fatigue. These patients may need a walker or wheelchair.
4. The patient should be instructed that the fit may need to be revised as she or he becomes stronger and more proficient with the ambulation aid.

EQUIPMENT

Measuring tape
Prescribed ambulation aid (crutches, cane, or walker)

PATIENT PREPARATION

1. Assess the patient's limitations and capabilities to determine which ambulation device is appropriate. Assessment should include strength, mobility, range of motion, visual acuity, perceptual difficulties, and balance.
2. If at all possible, the patient should be fitted wearing the shoes he or she intends to wear when using the ambulation aid.

PROCEDURAL STEPS
Cane

1. Determine the length of the cane with the patient standing or supine.

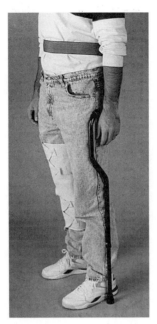

FIGURE 131-1 Confirming the fit of a cane. (From Pierson, F. M., & Fairchild, S. L. [2002]. *Principles and techniques of patient care* [3rd ed., p. 219]. Philadelphia: Saunders.)

2. The handgrip of the cane should be level with the greater trochanter or the ulnar crease of the wrist when the arm is straight down at the side.
3. With the cane parallel to the femur and tibia, the foot (tip) of the cane should be on the floor or at the bottom of the heel of the shoe (Figure 131-1).
4. Confirm the fit with the patient standing. There should be approximately 20 to 30 degrees of elbow flexion when the patient grasps the hand piece and positions the aid for ambulation. To position for ambulation, the tip of the cane is placed forward approximately 4 to 5 inches and laterally to the forefoot approximately 2 to 4 inches with cane on stronger side of body.

Crutches
1. If the patient's height is known, subtract 16 inches from the height; the resulting value approximates the length from the axillary pad to the crutch tip.
2. If height is uncertain or unknown, measure the supine patient from the anterior axillary fold (crease of armpit) to a point approximately 6 to 8 inches lateral to the patient's heel. This value represents the overall crutch length.
3. To determine the hand piece height, with the patient's arm held close to his or her side, measure from the anterior axillary fold to the trochanter or ulnar wrist crease (Figure 131-2). Use this value to position the hand piece by measuring down from the center of the axillary pad 1.5 to 2 inches or three finger widths.

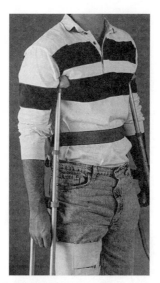

FIGURE 131-2 Determining hand piece height. (From Pierson, F. M., & Fairchild, S. L. [2002]. *Principles and techniques of patient care* [3rd ed., p. 222]. Philadelphia: Saunders.)

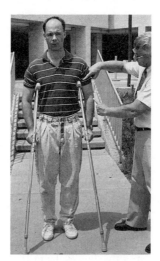

FIGURE 131-3 Confirming the fit of crutches. (From Pierson, F. M., & Fairchild, S. L. [2002]. *Principles and techniques of patient care* [3rd ed., p. 222]. Philadelphia: Saunders.)

4. Confirm the fit with the patient standing with head and trunk erect, shoulders relaxed and level, feet flat on the floor, and knees slightly flexed. The crutch tips should be 2 to 4 inches lateral and 4 to 6 inches anterior to the toes of the forefoot. The elbows should be flexed approximately 15 to 25 degrees when the hand piece is grasped with the wrist in a neutral position (Figure 131-3).

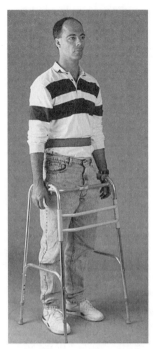

FIGURE 131-4 Confirming the fit of a walker. (From Pierson, F. M., & Fairchild, S. L. [2002]. *Principles and techniques of patient care* [3rd ed., p. 221]. Philadelphia: Saunders.)

Walker

1. Measurement can be accomplished with the patient either standing or supine.
2. The handgrip of the walker should be level with the ulnar wrist crease or greater trochanter with the walker in front of and along the patient's sides.
3. The feet of the walker should rest on the floor or be even with the heels of the shoes with the hips and knees straight (Figure 131-4).
4. Confirm the fit with the patient standing. There should be approximately 15 to 25 degrees of elbow flexion when the patient grasps the hand piece and positions the aid for ambulation. To position for ambulation, the tips of the aid are placed forward approximately 4 to 5 inches and laterally to the forefoot approximately 2 to 4 inches.

PATIENT TEACHING

See Procedure 132.

Patient Teaching for Ambulation Aids

Margo E. Layman, MSN, RN, RNC, CN-A

INDICATION

To teach a patient how to walk with crutches, a cane, or a walker. The patient may need an ambulation aid to compensate for impaired balance, decreased strength, pain during weight bearing, or injury of a leg.

CONTRAINDICATIONS AND CAUTIONS

1. The energy consumption associated with non–weight-bearing crutch walking is considerable. Elderly, debilitated, or sedentary patients could be at risk for severe exercise challenge and pronounced fatigue. The three-point gait requires the most strength and balance. These patients may do better with a walker or wheelchair.
2. Selection of the proper ambulation device and gait pattern is essential for the patient's safety and well-being.
3. Before discharge, the patient must be able to demonstrate use of the ambulation aid safely.

PATIENT PREPARATION

1. Measure and adjust the ambulation aid (see Procedure 131).
2. Ensure that the patient is wearing shoes with nonslip soles. Free the area of potential hazards (equipment or furniture in the path or a wet floor surface).
3. Assess the patient for strength, mobility, range of motion, visual accuity, perceptual difficulties, and balance.

PROCEDURAL STEPS
Three-Point Pattern (Two Crutches or a Walker)

1. This pattern is referred to as a step-to or step-through pattern and is used when the patient is able to bear weight fully on one leg but cannot bear weight on the opposite leg. This is the least stable pattern and requires balance, coordination, and good strength in the arms, trunk, and the unaffected leg. This pattern requires considerable energy expenditure while allowing for rapid ambulation.
2. The walker or crutches and the injured leg are advanced, and the patient steps up to the walker or slightly ahead of the crutches (Figure 132-1).

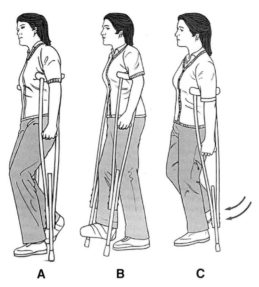

FIGURE 132-1 Three-point gait with crutches. **A,** Standing with crutches, all weight is on the good leg. **B,** Move crutches and injured leg forward simultaneously. **C,** Bearing weight on the palms of the hands, step forward onto the good leg. (From Proehl, J. A., & Jones, L. M. [1998]. *Mosby's emergency department patient teaching guides* [pp. I-7]. St Louis: Mosby.)

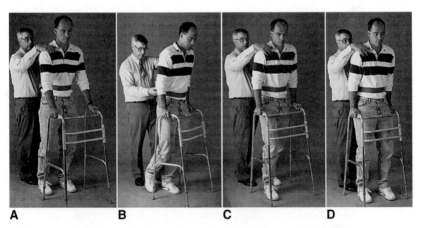

FIGURE 132-2 Modified three-point gait pattern. (From Pierson, F. M., & Fairchild, S. L. [2002]. *Principles and techniques of patient care* [3rd ed., p. 234]. Philadelphia: Saunders.)

Modified Three-Point Pattern (Two Crutches or a Walker)

1. This pattern is used when the patient is permitted full weight bearing on one leg and partial weight bearing on the other. This is a more stable pattern than the three-point pattern and requires less strength and less energy expenditure.
2. The walker or crutches are advanced simultaneously with the partial weight-bearing leg (Figure 132-2, *A* and *B*).
3. The full weight-bearing leg is then advanced (Figure 132-2, *C* and *D*).

Modified Two-Point Pattern (One Cane or Crutch)

1. This pattern requires one ambulation aid and is used when additional support, protection, or improved gait stability is needed.
2. Hold the ambulation aid in the arm opposite to the leg that requires protection or support (Figure 132-3, *A*).
3. From a stationary position, the ambulation aid comes forward simultaneously with the leg to be protected. This broadens the base of support and stabilizes the gait pattern (Figure 132-3, *B*).
4. The ambulation aid and protected leg maintain position while the unaffected leg steps forward (Figure 132-3, *C*).

Four-Point Pattern (Two Crutches or Canes)

1. This gait approximates a normal step pattern, is stable, and requires low energy expenditure. It uses alternate and reciprocal forward movement. The patient must be able to bear weight on both legs.
2. The right crutch or cane comes forward, then the left leg (Figure 132-4, *A*).
3. The left crutch or cane comes forward, then the right leg (Figure 132-4, *B*).

Sitting Down or Standing Up From a Chair

1. To sit down in a chair:
    a. Hold both crutches in one hand on the affected leg side.
    b. Place the unaffected leg close to the chair edge.

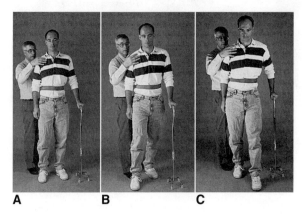

FIGURE 132-3 Modified two-point pattern. (From Pierson, F. M., & Fairchild, S. L. [2002]. *Principles and techniques of patient care* [3rd ed., p. 222]. Philadelphia: Saunders.)

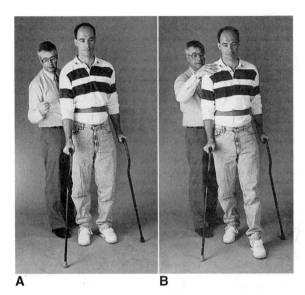

FIGURE 132-4 Four-point pattern. (From Pierson, F. M., & Fairchild, S. L. [2002]. *Principles and techniques of patient care* [3rd ed., p. 228]. Philadelphia: Saunders.)

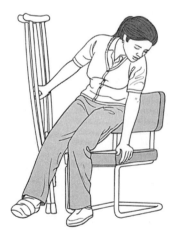

FIGURE 132-5 Sitting down or standing up from a chair. (From Proehl, J. A., & Jones, L. M. [1998]. *Mosby's emergency department patient teaching guides* [pp. I-7]. St Louis: Mosby.)

    c. Put the free hand on the seat bottom and lower to chair using crutches, the unaffected leg, and the free hand for balance and support (Figure 132-5).

2. To stand:

    a. Hold both crutches in one hand on the affected leg side.

    b. Push up using the free hand, the unaffected leg, and the hand that is holding the crutches.

Ascending and Descending Stairs

1. Going up and down stairs with crutches can be difficult and dangerous. A safer alternative may be to sit down and scoot up and down the stairs. An assistant may be necessary to help support an injured leg and carry the crutches.
2. Remember "up with the good, down with the bad" (Ogle, 2000).

With a Handrail

1. To go up stairs with a handrail:
   a. Hold both crutches in the hand opposite the handrail.
   b. Push down on the crutches and the handrail while stepping up with the good leg.
   c. Straighten the back, and lift the crutches and injured leg up to the same step (Figure 132-6).
2. To go down stairs with a handrail:
   a. Hold both crutches in the hand opposite the handrail.
   b. Bend the good leg (to assist with balance), and lower both crutches and the injured leg one step.
   c. Leaning on the crutches and the handrail, step down to the same step with the good leg (Figure 132-7).

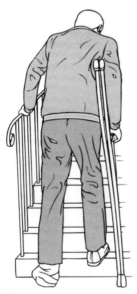 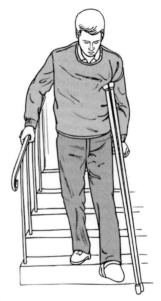

FIGURE 132-6 Ascending stairs with a handrail.

FIGURE 132-7 Descending stairs with a handrail.

(From Proehl, J. A., & Jones, L. M. [1998]. *Mosby's emergency department patient teaching guides* [pp. I-8]. St Louis: Mosby.)

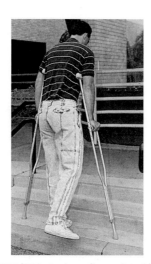

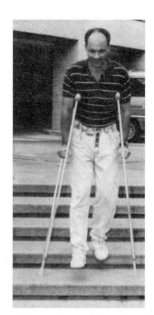

FIGURE 132-8 Ascending stairs without a handrail.   **FIGURE 132-9** Descending stairs without a handrail.

(From Pierson, F. M., & Fairchild, S. L. [2002]. *Principles and techniques of patient care* [3rd ed., p. 263]. Philadelphia: Saunders.)

Without a Handrail

1. To go up stairs without a handrail:
   a. Use the three-point gait pattern.
   b. Advance the crutches and good leg, then step up.
   c. Extend the hip and flex the knee on the injured side to 90 degrees to assist with safely clearing the stair (Figure 132-8).
2. To go down stairs without a handrail:
   a. Bend the good leg (to assist with balance), and lower both of the crutches and the injured leg to the step.
   b. Lean on the crutches, and step down with the good leg (Figure 132-9).

AGE-SPECIFIC CONSIDERATIONS

1. By age 4 to 6, children should be able to use ambulation aids. Their ability to do so depends on their growth, development, strength, and coordination.
2. The elderly patient may have difficulty using gaits such as the three-point pattern, which requires considerable energy expenditure, good balance, and arm strength. A walker, rather than crutches, and modified gait patterns may be needed.

COMPLICATIONS

1. If weight bearing is inappropriately placed with pressure to the axilla, damage to the brachial plexus and radial nerve can occur, causing pain, triceps weakness, and paralysis.

2. Falls, with the potential for additional injury

PATIENT TEACHING

1. Wear sturdy, low-heeled nonslip shoes.
2. Remove trip hazards, such as throw rugs and toys, from the walking environment. Be careful around pets and small children.
3. Be extremely careful when taking medications or alcohol because perception and judgment are affected.
4. Use caution on wet, icy, or snow-covered surfaces. Attachments are available to help prevent crutches from slipping on icy or snow-covered surfaces.
5. Do not rest on your armpits when using crutches; nerve damage may occur.
6. A backpack may be used to carry items, but be careful because it shifts the center of gravity and may alter your gait.

REFERENCE

Ogle, A. (2000). Canes, crutches, walkers, and other ambulation aids. *Physical Medicine and Rehabilitation: State of the Art Reviews, 14,* 485-492.

PROCEDURE 133

Arthrocentesis and Intraarticular Injection

Andrew A. Galvin, APRN,BC, CEN

Arthrocentesis is also known as *joint aspiration* and *joint tap.*

INDICATIONS

1. To relieve the pain and distention associated with intraarticular fluid accumulation. Joint drainage can decompress the joint, improve blood flow as well as remove bacteria and toxins (Ross, 2005).
2. To determine the cause of acute joint swelling. Joint swelling may be due to trauma, gout, infection, or rheumatoid arthritis.
3. To inject medications, usually steroids, into the joint space.

CONTRAINDICATIONS AND CAUTIONS

1. Infection of the joint space tissue at the puncture site; arthocentesis should not be attempted if the skin or tissue overlying the joint is infected (Parrillo & Fisher, 2004; Wise, 2005).

2. Bleeding disorders are a *relative* contraindication. There are relatively few data to suggest danger in an anticoagulated patient. However, care should be exercised with patients who have bleeding disorders or who are anticoagulated (Parrillo & Fisher, 2004).
3. An orthopedic surgeon should be consulted for prosthetic joints (Milne, 2001).
4. Repeated steroid injections can cause tissue damage.

EQUIPMENT
Antiseptic solution
Gauze dressings
Elastic bandage (optional)
Local or topical anesthetic (1% or 2% lidocaine)
Syringes and needles for infiltration of local anesthetic
Sample tubes for laboratory specimens (One tube should contain anticoagulant such as EDTA)
10- to 20-ml syringe (for knee aspiration, a 30- to 60-ml syringe may be necessary)
18- to 23-G 1½-in needles
Three-way stopcock (optional)
One pair hemostats
Medications for intraarticular injection
Sterile towels or drapes and gloves

PATIENT PREPARATION
The joint may be wrapped with an elastic bandage, leaving the puncture site exposed, to help compress the fluid into the puncture area (Reichman & Waddell, 2004).

PROCEDURAL STEPS
1. Cleanse the skin at the puncture site with an antiseptic solution for 5 minutes and allow to dry. If iodine is used, the puncture site is then cleansed with alcohol in order to prevent the transference of iodine into the joint space (Parillo & Fisher, 2004). The needle is usually introduced on the extensor surface of the joint to decrease the risk of neurovascular injury. Also, the synovial pouch is closer to the skin on the extensor surface (Reichman & Waddell, 2004).
2. *Anesthetize the skin and soft tissue down to the level of the joint capsule. Topical application of ethyl chloride or ice may also be used (Reichman & Waddell, 2004).
3. Position the joint in either full extension or 15 to 20 degrees flexion in order to open the joint space (Parrillo & Fisher, 2004).
4. *Insert the needle into the joint space while aspirating, and advance until synovial fluid is obtained (Figure 133-1).

---

*Indicates portions of the procedure usually performed by a physician or an advanced practice nurse.

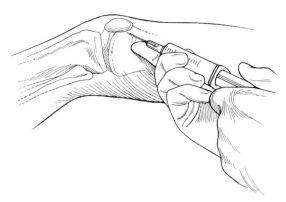

FIGURE 133-1 Arthrocentesis of the knee. (From Milne, L. W. [2001]. Arthrocentesis of the knee. In P. Rosen, T. C. Chan, G. M. Vilke, & G. Sternbach (Eds.), *Atlas of emergency procedures* [p. 233]. St Louis: Mosby.)

5. Removal of synovial fluid:
   a. Apply manual pressure to the opposite side of the joint to help force fluid over to the needle.
   b. *Aspirate all readily accessible fluid. A three-way stopcock placed between the needle and the syringe may be used for draining large effusions.
   c. Place fluid in appropriate specimen containers to send to the laboratory. Commonly performed laboratory tests include viscosity, cell count, protein, glucose, culture, and Gram's stain. Synovial fluid requires special handling; package it per laboratory protocol.
6. Injection of medications:
   a. *Taking care not to displace the needle, remove the syringe from the needle, and attach the syringe containing the medication.
   b. *Inject the medication into the joint space.
7. *Remove the needle.
8. Apply direct pressure to the puncture site for 2 minutes; then apply a sterile dressing.
9. Apply an elastic bandage to help stabilize the joint if a large amount of fluid was aspirated (see Procedure 126).

AGE-SPECIFIC CONSIDERATION

Lidocaine infiltration for anesthesia is usually avoided in children because it increases the number of skin punctures necessary. Eutectic mixture of local anesthesia (EMLA) cream may be used instead (Hostetler & Weisman, 2001).

---

*Indicates portions of the procedure usually performed by a physician or an advanced practice nurse.

COMPLICATIONS

1. Joint infection; a rare complication if proper attention is paid to aseptic technique (Parrillo & Fisher, 2004)
2. Hemarthrosis (Milne, 2001)
3. Dry tap
4. Trauma to intraarticular or neurovascular structures (Milne, 2001)

PATIENT TEACHING

1. Report any fever, increased pain, redness, or recurrent swelling, which could indicate infection.
2. Avoid excessive use of the joint for the next few days. If the injection/aspiration was in the knee, ankle, or foot, crutches may be prescribed to prevent weight bearing.
3. Apply ice to the joint and elevate it above the level of the heart to help prevent recurrent swelling.
4. Change dressings as indicated if the joint is draining.
5. Wear the elastic bandage as instructed to help stabilize the joint.
6. If steroids were injected, skin lightening and sun sensitivity may occur in the area (Hostetler & Weisman, 2001).

REFERENCES

Hostetler, M. A., & Weisman, D. S. (2001). Orthopedic procedures. In J. G. Goepp, & M. A. Hostetler (Eds.), *Procedures for primary care pediatricians* (pp. 152-184). St Louis: Mosby.

Milne, L. W. (2001). Arthrocentesis of the knee. In P. Rosen, T. C. Chan, G. M. Vilke, & G. Sternbach (Eds.), *Atlas of emergency procedures* (pp. 232-233). St Louis: Mosby.

Parrillo, S. J., & Fisher, J. (2004). Arthrocentesis. In J. R. Roberts, & J. R. Hedges (Eds.), *Clinical procedures in emergency medicine* (4th ed., pp. 1042-1056). Philadelphia: Saunders.

Ross, J. J. (2005). Septic arthritis. *Infectious Disease Clinics of North America, 19*(4), 799-817.

Reichman, E. F., & Waddell, R. (2004). Arthrocentesis. In E. F. Reichman, & R. R. Simon (Eds.), *Emergency medicine procedures* (pp. 559-584). New York: McGraw-Hill.

Wise, C. (2005). Arthrocentesis and injection of joints and soft tissues. In E. D. Harris, R. C. Budd, G. S. Firestein, M. C. Genovese, J. S. Sergent, S. Ruggy, & C. B. Sledge (Eds.), *Kelley's textbook of rheumatology* (7th ed., pp. 692-698). Philadelphia: Saunders.

Integumentary Procedures

Wound Cleansing and Irrigation

Joni Hentzen Daniels, MSN, RN, CEN, CCRN

Wound cleansing and irrigation is also known as *wound preparation* or *scrub*.

Cleansing and irrigation are the fundamentals of good wound care. Although these steps can be the most tedious and time consuming, it is essential that all contaminants and devitalized tissue be removed before wound closure. The risk of infection depends on the location, mechanism, host, and care—the risk in a clean facial wound produced by an incision is less than 1%, whereas a dirty crush injury to the foot may have a greater than 20% risk (Simon & Hern, 2006). Factors contributing to the greatest risk of wound morbidity are prolonged time since injury; crush mechanism; deep, penetrating wounds; high-velocity missiles; and contamination with saliva, feces, soil, or other foreign matter (Simon & Hern, 2006).

INDICATIONS

1. To cleanse any disruption in skin integrity.
2. To cleanse the skin before suturing, incision and drainage, invasive procedures, and removal of foreign bodies.
3. To promote healing without infection.
4. To provide the best possible function and appearance for the patient.

CONTRAINDICATIONS AND CAUTIONS

1. Injuries that require special care include:
   a. Eyelids: The eye itself should be assessed for trauma and visual acuity checked (see Procedure 153). Suturing of the eyelid may require specialist consultation.
   b. Neck: Wounds of the neck can appear superficial. Care should be taken not to underestimate a penetrating injury that could quickly compromise the patient's airway.
   c. Spray gun injuries: Extensive tissue destruction may be present despite a benign-appearing entrance wound. Injected chemicals or embedded foreign bodies frequently require surgical exploration.
   d. Scalp: Lacerations may disguise skull fractures, and the patient may lose a significant amount of blood because of the scalp's extensive vascularity. The extent of a scalp laceration can be easily overlooked because of hair matting or the patient lying supine on a backboard.
   e. Crush or avulsion injuries: Wounds with extensive tissue damage or loss of tissue are at increased risk for infection and delayed healing.
   f. Facial: Meticulous care of facial wounds is required for optimal cosmetic results.

g. Hand: Impairment of hand function, especially the dominant hand, may result in permanent disability.

h. Associated fractures: Open fractures are at high risk for infection. Specialty consultation is indicated.

i. Puncture wounds: The type and condition (e.g., rusty or dirty) of the penetrating object are important. If the puncture occurred through clothing or a shoe, the wound should be evaluated for the presence of a foreign body. Puncture wounds are at increased risk for infection.

j. Bite wounds: The risk of rabies should be evaluated. Patients are frequently discharged with antibiotics and instructions to return in 24 to 48 hours for follow-up care. Obtaining skull films in bite wounds to the cranium in children should be considered because of possible penetration of the skull. Bites wounds, especially wounds from cat bites, are at increased risk for infection.

2. Soaking macerates the skin, and povidone-iodine causes tissue destruction. There is no evidence that soaking wounds in saline and povidone-iodine is of any benefit (Simon & Hern, 2006).

3. Excessive scrubbing and powerful irrigation can damage healthy tissue.

4. Wound cleansing agents:

a. Hydrogen peroxide should be used with caution. It is a weak disinfectant and is ineffective against anaerobes, it absorbs oxygen in the wound, and it destroys cells. It is toxic to tissue in open wounds (Simon & Hern, 2006).

b. Povidone-iodine solutions provide good antimicrobial activity and effectively kills gram-positive and gram-negative rods, fungi, and viruses with little toxicity or damage. Iodine compounds are less irritating to tissue than is tincture of iodine but may still cause cellular damage and allergic reactions (Simon & Hern, 2006).

c. Nontoxic agents such as poloxamer 188 (Shur-Clens) are nontoxic to open wounds and eyes. Although they have no antimicrobial activity, they appear to be safe and effective and cause minimal cellular damage (Simon & Hern, 2006).

d. Baby shampoo provides gentle cleaning of fragile tissue but is nonsterile and is not antimicrobial. It is used for facial lacerations in some institutions.

EQUIPMENT

Wound cleansing agent (see discussion under Contraindications and Cautions)

Sterile sponges or gauze dressings

Cotton swabs

Sterile drapes or towels

Wound irrigation supplies:

16- or 18-G blunt needle or plastic cannula

30- to 35-ml syringe

Splash shield (optional)

Sterile basin

Normal saline solution

(Preassembled irrigation kits with splash shields are also available.)

For contaminated wounds and wounds embedded with foreign bodies:
    Sterile toothbrush or surgical brush
    No. 11 scalpel blade
For tar wounds:
    Petroleum jelly, topical antibiotic ointment, or mineral oil

PATIENT PREPARATION

1. Obtain a history, including time of injury, mechanism of injury, location and extent of injury, other injuries, and potential for the wound to be contaminated with soil or dirt. Assess the wound for foreign objects, such as clothing, grass, and glass. Also assess tetanus immunization status and potential for rabies (bite wounds).
2. Assess and document neurovascular status. Assess for adjacent bony injury or open fractures. Suspect damage to muscle and tendons if deep fascia is involved.
3. Obtain radiology studies as indicated to rule out the presence of foreign bodies, fractures, and air in joint spaces.
4. Anesthetize the area as indicated (see Procedures 135, 136, and 137).
5. Drape or undress the patient to protect clothing if extensive wound preparation and irrigation is planned.

PROCEDURAL STEPS

1. Maintain hemostasis by direct pressure. *Clamp and ligate vessels if necessary. Use a pneumatic tourniquet or a blood pressure cuff to help control bleeding during wound cleansing and repair, if prescribed by a physician.
2. Shaving is seldom indicated. Shaving causes many small wounds and skin nicks and increases the chance of infection. If hair removal is necessary, clip the hair close to the wound edge or smooth hair out of the way with lubricant or antibiotic ointment. Never shave eyebrows because realignment is difficult to achieve without the landmark hair, and the hair may not grow back completely.
3. Begin wound cleansing using sponges or brushes and a cleansing agent. Preparation should begin at the wound site and should move distally, encompassing a large area of skin surrounding the wound. For example, with hand lacerations, clean the hand and arm to the elbow. Continue until the wound is clean.
4. Irrigate wounds that are contaminated or those containing foreign bodies. Wound irrigation helps remove foreign bodies and dilutes bacteria. Irrigation is particularly important in bite wounds. Eight to 12 pounds per square inch of pressure is recommended to irrigate most wounds and can be achieved with an 19-G needle or plastic cannula and a 35-ml syringe held 2 inches from the wound (Figure 134-1) (Flippin, 2004). Mask, goggles, and gown are recommended in addition to a splash shield to prevent exposure to blood. Other options include a needle attached to a pressurized intravenous bag or tubing or a commercially available irrigation setup. Normal saline solution

---

*Indicates portions of the procedure usually performed by a physician or an advanced practice nurse.

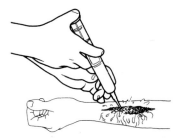

FIGURE 134-1 Irrigation of a wound. An 18-G needle or plastic cannula attached to a 35-ml syringe is ideal for providing proper irrigation pressure. (From Simon, R., & Brenner, B. [2002]. *Emergency procedures and techniques* [4th ed., p. 363]. Baltimore: Williams & Wilkins.)

is most commonly used. Low-pressure irrigation (e.g., bulb syringe) is not effective.

The following formula for determining volume of irrigant has been associated with less than 0.01% wound infection (Daniels, 2003):

100 ml/inch of length of laceration/hours since injury

Thus, a 3-in laceration that was 6 hours old would be irrigated with 1800 ml $(100 \times 3 \times 6 = 1800 \text{ ml})$.

5. Abrasions with embedded foreign bodies (except glass) require careful wound preparation to remove the foreign bodies and prevent traumatic tattooing. Use surgical scrub brushes, sterile toothbrushes, and the point of a No. 11 or 15 blade for foreign body removal (Figure 134-2) (Flippin, 2004). Wounds with glass embedded require special evaluation and management; radiographic imaging may be needed. *Wound débridement may be necessary after anesthesia is completed.

6. Use petroleum jelly, antibiotic ointment, or mineral oil to facilitate tar removal. After application, allow tar to dissolve for 10 to 15 minutes before attempting removal. Repeat applications may be necessary.

---

*Indicates portions of the procedure usually performed by a physician or an advanced practice nurse.

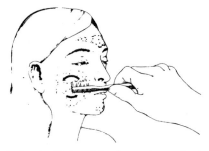

FIGURE 134-2 Removal of embedded particles from a traumatic abrasion with a sterile toothbrush. The tip of a No. 11 blade can be used to remove deeply embedded or larger particles. (From Simon, R., & Brenner, B. [2002]. *Emergency procedures and techniques* [4th ed., p. 363]. Baltimore: Williams & Wilkins.)

AGE-SPECIFIC CONSIDERATIONS

1. Parents may not know the full details of the mechanism of injury; careful wound assessment is necessary in young children.
2. Patient age is an important factor in host resistance to infection; those individuals at extremes of age—young children and the elderly—are at greatest risk.

COMPLICATIONS

1. The chance of infection, including cellulitis, soft tissue abscess, and osteomyelitis, increases in wounds to the hands and feet because of poor circulation in the extremities. Infection is also more common in dirty or old wounds. Bacterial growth begins in wounds after 3 hours.
2. Medications such as steroids and hormones may impair wound healing.
3. Other medical conditions may impair wound healing. Patients with diabetes, immune diseases, associated trauma, hypoxia, uremia, circulatory impairment, and infection, as well as the elderly, are all at increased risk for infection and delayed healing.

PATIENT TEACHING

1. High-risk patients should return for wound evaluation and dressing change within 24 to 48 hours.
2. The wound should be kept dry for the first 24 hours. The patient may then shower but should not soak in a tub. Wet dressings should be changed as soon as possible.
3. The wound should be cleaned four times a day with water and/or mild soap water. Crusted material should be gently removed with cotton swabs. Keeping crusted material off allows for quicker epithelialization.
4. Apply a light layer of topical antibiotic ointment after wound cleansing. A gauze dressing may be applied, depending on the wound location, especially for the first 48 hours.
5. Watch for bleeding, a wound that reopens, signs of circulatory compromise, or signs of infection (wound tenderness, redness, swelling, draining pus, fever). A minor amount of wound redness is normal.
6. Elevate the injured area as much as possible.
7. New wounds should not be exposed to the sun for 6 months. Permanent hyperpigmentation may result. Sun block is advisable, especially for facial wounds.
8. Complete wound healing and scar reduction may not be evident for 1 year.

REFERENCES

Daniels, J. H. (2003). Unpublished data. Sugarland, TX.
Flippin, A. L. (2004). General principles of wound management. In E. F. Reichman, & R. R. Simon (Eds.), *Emergency medicine procedures* (pp. 693-709). New York: McGraw-Hill.
Simon, B., & Hern, H. G. (2006). Wound management principles. In J. A. Marx, R. S. Hockberger, & R. M. Walls, et al. (Eds.), *Rosen's emergency medicine: Concepts and clinical practice* (6th ed., pp. 842-858). St Louis: Mosby.

Wound Anesthesia: Local Infiltration and Topical Agents

Maureen T. Quigley, MS, ARNP

INDICATIONS

To provide local and topical anesthesia before:
- Suturing of a laceration
- Removal of an embedded foreign body
- Incision and drainage of an abscess
- Invasive procedures, such as lumbar puncture or chest tube insertion
- Wound débridement and cleansing
- Insertion of nasal packing or nasal tubes
- Venous cannulation, venipuncture, or any needle insertion, including preinfiltration anesthesia

CONTRAINDICATIONS AND CAUTIONS

1. A known sensitivity or history of allergic reaction to a local anesthetic is a contraindication to its use. Patient-reported allergic reactions to amide preparations are rare (see Background Information).
2. The use of agents containing epinephrine may be contraindicated in patients with known peripheral vascular disease. Because of epinephrine's vasoconstrictive action, it may delay healing and increase the risk of infection.
3. The use of epinephrine may be helpful in vascular areas, such as the face and scalp, to slow absorption and lower peak blood levels of anesthesia. Epinephrine also decreases bleeding at the site.
4. The use of epinephrine preparations is contraindicated in cartilaginous areas of the ear and nares and in areas served by end arteries (fingers, toes, and penis). Epinephrine also distorts and discolors the vermilion border of the lip and is contraindicated in lip lacerations that extend through the lip border.
5. Injection of anesthetic agents can distort wound margins, which may increase the complexity of plastics repair. Care should be used in flap-type lacerations to preserve vascularity of the flap by not injecting directly into the flap and avoiding the use of epinephrine-containing preparations.
6. Avoid rapid infiltration of the wound to decrease pain.
7. Amide preparations should be used cautiously in patients with liver disease (see Background Information).

673

8. The use of topical anesthetics containing cocaine (such as TAC) is not recommended because of potential adverse side effects and cost (Eidelman, Weiss, Enu, Lau, & Carr, 2005). Lidocaine (5%), epinephrine (1:2000), and tetracaine (1%) (LET) is a safe and effective alternative to TAC for topical use. LET can be used as a liquid or mixed with methylcellulose to form a gel. LET should be not used on mucous membranes, noses, pinna of the ear, fingers, toes, and penis.

9. Benzocaine is found in a wide variety of over-the-counter preparations for sunburn and abrasions. Toxic and allergic reactions are common. It may cause life-threatening methemoglobinemia.

10. Cetacaine spray has two principal ingredients: benzocaine and tetracaine. Tetracaine is rapidly absorbed by the pharynx and tracheobronchial tree and is long acting. Spray application greater than 2 seconds is contraindicated because of rapid mucosal absorption and potential toxicity of benzocaine and tetracaine.

11. Eutectic mixture of local anesthesia (EMLA) is an effective topic anesthetic for intact skin in the pediatric population. Local skin reactions are relatively common but are generally mild and transient, resolving after cream is removed. Methemoglobinemia may be caused by EMLA because of the metabolites of prilocaine, but this is rare when the preparation is used properly. EMLA should not be used in any infant younger than 3 months and in infants between ages 3 and 12 months old who are being treated with methemoglobinemia-inducing drugs, such as acetaminophen, phenobarbital, nitrites, sulfonamides, and antimalarial agents (McGee, 2004). Patients with anemia, respiratory or cardiovascular disease, or glucose-6-phosphate dehydrogenase (G-6-PD) or methemoglobin reductase deficiency are at higher risk for untoward effects (McGee, 2004).

12. When blood or central nervous system concentrations exceed safe limits of local anesthetics, systemic toxicity can occur (see Table 135-1). Epinephrine potentiates cardiac toxicity when added to a local anesthetic (Paris & Yealy, 2006).

TABLE 135-1
GUIDELINES FOR MAXIMUM DOSES OF COMMONLY USED AGENTS[1]

Agent	Without Epinephrine	With Epinephrine
Lidocaine HCl[2]	3–5 mg/kg	7 mg/kg
Mepivacaine HCl	8 mg/kg	7 mg/kg[3]
Bupivacaine HCl[4]	1.5 mg/kg	3 mg/kg

[1]All maximum doses should be reduced 20% to 25% in very young, old, and very sick patients.
[2]A lidocaine level of 0.5 to 2 mg/ml may be reached for every 100 mg of lidocaine infiltrated for blocks.
[3]Epinephrine adds to the potential cardiac toxicity of this drug.
[4]Not to be used for pudendal blocks or intravenous regional anesthesia. Not recommended for children younger than age 12.
(From Marx, J. A., Hockberger, R. S., Walls, R. M., et al. (Eds.) (2006). *Rosen's emergency medicine: Concepts and clinical practice* [6th ed., p. 2932]. St Louis: Mosby; adapted from Stewart, R. D. [1988]. Local anesthesia. In P. M. Paris & R. D. Stewart [Eds.], *Pain management in emergency medicine.* Norwalk, CT: Appleton & Lange.)

EQUIPMENT

Antiseptic wipes
3-, 5-, and 10-ml syringes (for infiltration)
18-, 25-, and 27-G needles (for infiltration)
Local or topical anesthetic as prescribed:
   1% Lidocaine without epinephrine
   1% Lidocaine with epinephrine
   2% Lidocaine without epinephrine
   2% Lidocaine with epinephrine
   0.25% to 0.5% bupivacaine
   LET solution or gel
   EMLA (2.5% lidocaine and 2.5% prilocaine)
Clear bio-occlusive dressing (optional)
Elastic bandage (optional)

BACKGROUND INFORMATION

1. There are two general types of local anesthetics: ester compounds (procaine, cocaine, and tetracaine) and amide compounds (bupivacaine, lidocaine, and mepivacaine).
2. Amide compounds are metabolized in the liver. Ester compounds are hydrolyzed by the pseudocholinesterase in the serum. The lone exception is cocaine, which is excreted unchanged in the urine. All ester agents except cocaine share a common degradation pathway via serum to *para*-aminobenzoic acid, which can produce allergic or sensitizing reactions. Amide-type agents are believed to be incapable of stimulating antibody formation and so are noteworthy for their low evidence of sensitivity reactions. Reactions probably are toxic rather than allergic. Patients may be allergic, however, to the preservatives found in multiple-dose vials. Care must be taken to administer safe doses to avoid systemic toxicity.
3. The mechanism of local anesthesia is to decrease the rate and degree of depolarization and repolarization, decrease the conduction velocity, and prolong the refractory period of the neural action potential.
4. Nerve fibers are classified by their conduction velocity. Smaller fibers responsible for pain, temperature, and autonomic activity are affected rapidly by anesthetic. Local infiltration provides pain reduction without blockage of motor function.
5. All local anesthetic agents are vasodilators because of the relaxant effect on smooth muscles, with the exception of cocaine, which causes vasoconstriction.
6. Epinephrine added to the anesthetic solution helps with wound hemostasis and slows systemic absorption.
7. Similar to reactions to infiltration anesthesia, toxic reactions to topically applied anesthetics correlate with the peak blood levels that were achieved and not necessarily with the dose that was administered. Systemic absorption of a topical agent is more rapid and therefore achieves a higher peak blood level than the same dose given by infiltration.

PATIENT PREPARATION

Carefully question the patient about medication allergies. Patients may confuse vagal response with allergy history. True allergy is rare but does occur and may include urticaria, bronchospasm, changes in neurologic status, and fatal cardiac collapse. Allergic reaction is more common with ester preparations such as cocaine, benzocaine, tetracaine, and procaine.

PROCEDURAL STEPS
Topical Agents—Options

1. Apply a thick layer (1 to 2 grams [g]/10 cm^2) of EMLA to intact skin under an occlusive dressing for approximately 30 minutes to 1 hour before a procedure. For minor procedures such as needle insertions, apply 2.5 g of EMLA over 20 to 25 cm^2 for at least 1 hour. Preparation of two potential sites is recommended when an intravenous line is started, in the event of technical difficulties at the initial site. When a more painful procedure is anticipated, 2 g of EMLA/10 cm^2 should be applied for at least 2 hours (McGee, 2004).
2. Apply lidocaine topically as a liquid, ointment, jelly, or viscous fluid (2% to 10%). Absorption is rapid. Do not exceed recommended dosage (maximum safe dosage is 250 to 300 mg) because total absorption cannot be calculated (McGee, 2004).
3. Use sprays containing benzocaine and tetracaine (e.g., Cetacaine, Hurricaine) primarily for oral procedures. Spray application should not exceed 2 seconds because toxicity including methemoglobinemia may result from excessive doses.
4. Anesthetic solutions: Use LET primarily for minor facial and scalp lacerations in lieu of injectable anesthetic, especially in children.
   a. Clean the wound to remove debris and clots before using LET to increase its efficacy. Apply LET solution by saturating sterile gauze and applying it to the wound with firm pressure for 15 to 20 minutes with gloved hands to prevent skin absorption for the caregiver. LET solution may also be applied by dripping into a wound with a syringe or by applying to a wound with sterile cotton swabs. LET gel is spread directly in the wound. The gel or solution-soaked gauze may be held in place with a clear bio-occlusive dressing or elastic bandage.
   b. Take care to ensure that LET does not run or drip into the eyes, nasal passages, or mouth. Observe the patient carefully during and after administration. If the first dose of LET is not effective, infiltrate the laceration with local anesthesia; do *not* apply another dose of LET.
5. Assess adequacy of anesthesia by testing sharp-dull sensation and observing blanching before beginning the procedure.

Wound Infiltration

1. Several techniques can be used during wound infiltration to decrease pain. Slow administration of anesthetic intradermally through the inside margins of wound edges with small-gauge needles causes less pain.
2. Buffering lidocaine may reduce pain with injection. Lidocaine is buffered by adding 1 ml of sodium bicarbonate (8.4%) to every 10 ml of lidocaine solution. It remains effective after mixing for 1 week (Paris & Yealy, 2006).

3. Consider the anesthetic agent that most fits the patient's need. A longer-acting local anesthetic (bupivacaine) may prevent the wound from having to be reinfiltrated, especially in a busy emergency department. Lidocaine has a more rapid onset, but it has a short duration of action. Attempt to avoid reinfiltration, especially in children or in wounds in which tissue viability is already a problem, such as in the face. If prolonged postanesthesia pain is anticipated, bupivacaine is useful.

4. Use the smallest possible needle for infiltration. A 27-G needle is usually adequate except for digital blocks, the scalp, or callused areas; in these situations, a 25-G needle may be required.

5. *Infiltrate wound edges through the dermis and not through the skin. Approaching the dermal layer directly from the inside edges of the cut margin of the wound is less painful. Continue to infiltrate as the needle passes through the dermis, injecting as you go. Some clinicians recommend injection through surrounding intact skin if the wound is grossly contaminated (Figure 135-1).

6. *As additional needle entry is needed, reenter through areas already infiltrated with anesthetic to lessen the pain of infiltration.

7. Assess sharp-dull sensation to ensure adequate anesthesia before beginning the procedure. If epinephrine has been used, observe the wound edges for blanching.

---

*Indicates portions of the procedure usually performed by a physician or an advanced practice nurse.

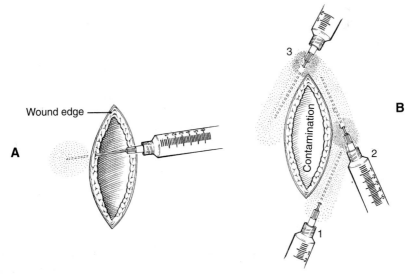

FIGURE 135-1 **A**, Injection of local anesthetic into the dermal layer of a wound margin. **B**, In the event of gross contamination, injection may be via surrounding intact skin. (From McGee, D. [2004]. Local and topical anesthesia. In J. R. Roberts & J. R. Hedges (Eds.), *Clinical procedures in emergency medicine* [4th ed., p. 543]. Philadelphia: Saunders.)

AGE-SPECIFIC CONSIDERATIONS

1. Calculate dosages carefully when administering local and topical anesthesia with children. Incorrect dosage calculations can cause significant side effects.
2. For extensive wound repair in children, consider the use of sedation (see Procedure 177) in conjunction with local anesthesia. If necessary, consider repair in a surgery or minor procedure area.
3. Viscous lidocaine should not be used for infants who are teething or have oral irritation, because they cannot expectorate well.
4. The use of distraction may be helpful in reducing pain associated with administration of local anesthesia.

COMPLICATIONS

1. Local reactions may include irritation, burning, erythema, and skin sloughing.
2. The major cause of systemic reactions is high serum levels. This is most common after topical applications to the trachea and upper airway passages because of rapid bronchial tree absorption.
3. Topical anesthesia of the nose, mouth, and pharynx may create an inadvertent suppression of the gag reflex, which may cause aspiration when combined with difficulty swallowing.
4. Resistance to injection or patient complaint of paresthesia may indicate intraneural injection. Withdraw the needle 1 to 2 mm and reinject to avoid disrupting nerve fibers.
5. Signs of central nervous system toxicity include apprehension, nausea, vomiting, tremor, light-headedness, muscle twitching, incoherent speech, and seizures. As toxicity increases, the anesthesia may interfere with electrical and mechanical function of the myocardium. Symptoms include a prolonged PR and QRS interval, bradycardia, hypotension, and asystole. Factors influencing toxicity include quantity and concentration of solution, presence or absence of epinephrine, vascularity of injection site, rate of absorption of drug, rate of destruction of drug, hypersensitivity of patient, and patient age, physical status, and weight.
6. Methemoglobinemia can occur related to the use of prilocaine or benzocaine. Signs of toxicity include dyspnea, lethargy, cyanosis, and coma.
7. True allergic reactions are rare and may occur in response to the preservatives found in multiple-dose vials. Symptoms include bronchospasm and urticaria. If epinephrine has been used, the patient may experience pallor, anxiety, palpitations, tachycardia, hypertension, and tachypnea.

PATIENT TEACHING

1. Instruct the patient when to expect the return of sensation.
2. Protect the area until sensation returns.
3. Provide analgesia when local anesthesia wears off.
4. Use of oral topical anesthetic agents, such as viscous lidocaine and benzocaine (including over-the-counter preparations), can cause difficulty swallowing. The medication should be used at the appropriate interval, and patients should be cautioned to avoid using it more frequently. It should be swished and expectorated within 1 to 2 minutes, not swallowed. Food and drink should be avoided for 1 hour after application to prevent aspiration.

REFERENCES

Eidelman, A., Weiss, J, Enu, I., Lau, J., & Carr, D. (2005). Comparative efficacy and costs of various topical anesthetics for repair of dermal lacerations: A systematic review of randomized, controlled trials. *Journal of Clinical Anesthesia, 17*, 106-116.

McGee, D. (2004). Local and topical anesthesia. In J. R. Roberts, & J. R. Hedges (Eds.), *Clinical procedures in emergency medicine* (4th ed., pp. 533-551). Philadelphia: Saunders.

Paris, P., & Yealy, D. (2006). Pain management. In J. A. Marx, R. S. Hockberger, & R. M. Walls, et al. (Eds.), *Rosen's emergency medicine: Concepts and clinical practice* (6th ed., pp. 2913-2935). St Louis: Mosby.

PROCEDURE 136

Digital Block

Joni Hentzen Daniels, MSN, RN, CEN, CCRN

The digital nerve block is one of the most useful and commonly performed blocks in the emergency department and is considered superior to local infiltration in most circumstances (Kelly & Spektor, 2004). Wound infiltration may be difficult in the digit that has tight skin and can accept only a limited volume of anesthesia. Distortion of the anatomic landmarks or reduced capability for good wound approximation is also associated with local infiltration of a digit.

INDICATIONS

To provide digital anesthesia for patients:
1. With isolated finger/toe lacerations or fingertip amputations
2. Requiring removal of a fingernail or repair of a nailbed
3. Requiring reduction of interphalangeal joint dislocation
4. To obtain a satisfactory examination of the digit if pain prevents patient cooperation

CONTRAINDICATIONS AND CAUTIONS

1. Known sensitivity or history of allergic reaction to local anesthetics is a contraindication.
2. Digital blocks should not be performed on the stump of digits under consideration for replantation.
3. The vascular status of the finger should be monitored during and after injection.
4. Preparations containing epinephrine have historically not been used for digital blocks although there have been several studies demonstrating

epinephrine can be used as an adjunct for digital block anesthesia (Wilhelmi, Blackwell, & Miller, 2001).

5. Circumferential ring block (placing a ring of anesthesia in a circle around a finger) is generally contraindicated because of the risk of vasospasm and ischemia, except in the thumb and great toe.

EQUIPMENT

Local anesthetic without epinephrine (usually, lidocaine 1% to 2% or bupivacaine 0.25% to 0.5%)
5-ml syringe
18-G and 25- or 27-G needles
Povidone-iodine or alcohol wipe

BACKGROUND INFORMATION

Before using local anesthetic agents, the practitioner must understand the principal agents and the mechanisms of their actions (see Procedure 135). Knowledge of the anatomy of the hand and foot is essential for successful digital blocks.

1. Hand and fingers (Figure 136-1):
    a. The primary nerve supply of the hand is received from the radial, ulnar, and median nerves (Figure 136-2). Anatomic variation of the radial nerve can be significant, making the thumb difficult to block.
    b. Each digit is supplied by four nerve branches that are the terminal branches of the radial, ulnar, and median nerves (two dorsal and two palmar). Thus, the digital nerves lie in pairs on either side of the phalanges.

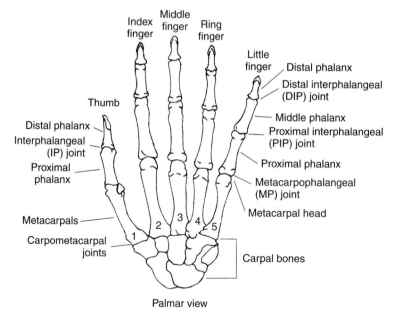

FIGURE 136-1 Bony anatomy of the hand.

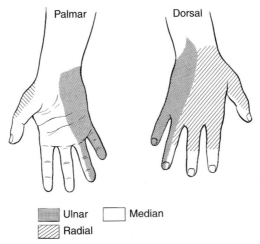

FIGURE 136-2 Sensory distribution in the hand. (From Dunmire, S. M., & Paris, P. M. [1994]. *Atlas of emergency procedures* [p. 47]. Philadelphia: Saunders.)

2. Foot and toes:
   a. Two dorsal and two volar nerves supply each toe. These nerves are branches of the major nerves of the ankle. In the toes, the nerves lie at the 2, 4, 8, and 10 o'clock positions in close relationship to the bone.
   b. The digital nerves can be blocked at the metatarsals, interdigital web spaces, or toes.

PATIENT PREPARATION

1. Place the patient in a supine position with the hand or foot extended on a firm surface.
2. Assess and document sensation, circulation, and mobility distal to the wound. Mobility can be tested by testing grip, opposition of thumb and finger, and function of the interphalangeal and metacarpophalangeal joints. Sensation can be effectively evaluated by the use of two-point discrimination using two blunt ends of a paper clip. Assess for tendon damage by having the patient flex and extend the finger or toe against pressure.
3. Suspect nerve injury if a digital artery laceration is present because of the nerve's proximity to the artery. Do not attempt to clamp a digital artery because of the risk of damaging a digital nerve. Digital nerve laceration causes hemisensory loss to the finger.

PROCEDURAL STEPS
General Remarks for Any Technique

1. *Determine anesthetic of choice. Patients almost always benefit from the use of a longer-acting anesthetic, such as bupivacaine, especially if a lengthy repair is anticipated or the patient is expected to have pain after a

---

*Indicates portions of the procedure usually performed by a physician or an advanced practice nurse.

shorter-acting anesthetic wears off. Consider using buffered lidocaine if a less lengthy repair is required. Digital blocks are less painful when buffered lidocaine is used.

2. *After infiltration of local anesthesia, gently massage the tissue to facilitate spread of anesthetic and increase absorption.

3. *Anesthesia is not effective if the periosteum has not been anesthetized. Introduce the needle down to the periosteum, and infiltrate closely to the bone.

4. *It is difficult to reach the nerves on both sides of a finger with a single injection. Separate injections on either side of the digit are usually needed.

5. Several approaches may be used to block the common digital nerves. The metacarpal and dorsal approaches are described here.

Fingers: Metacarpal Approach

1. *Palpate the metacarpal head approximately at the level of the distal palmar crease.

2. *Cleanse the palmar surface at the injection site with an antiseptic wipe.

3. *On the palmar surface of the hand, insert a 25-G needle perpendicular to the skin just medial or lateral to the metacarpal head into the web space (Figure 136-3).

4. *After aspirating to ensure vascular penetration has not occurred, inject 1 to 2 ml (depending on size of the finger) as the needle is advanced to the periosteum.

---

*Indicates portions of the procedure usually performed by a physician or an advanced practice nurse.

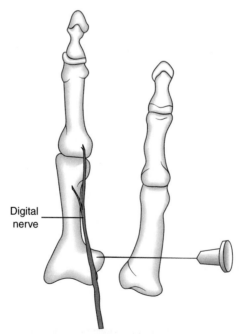

Digital nerve

FIGURE 136-3 Digital nerve block.

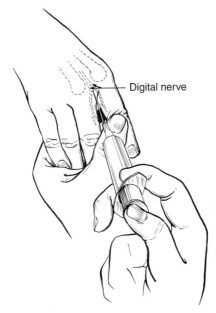

Digital nerve

FIGURE 136-4 Dorsal approach for digital nerve block in the web space. (From Dunmire, S. M., & Paris, P. M. [1994]. *Atlas of emergency procedures* [p. 48]. Philadelphia: Saunders.)

5. *Repeat step 4 on the opposite side of the metacarpal head. In total, 3 to 4 ml of anesthetic is required for effective anesthesia for both sides of the digit.
6. *The radial nerve innervates the dorsal surface of the index and middle finger (see Figure 136-2). It may also be necessary to infiltrate locally the dorsal side of the finger at the metacarpal head if injury is present to either of these fingers on the dorsal side of the hand.

Fingers: Dorsal Approach

1. *Cleanse dorsal surface with an antiseptic wipe.
2. *Inject anesthetic with a 25-G needle to raise a wheal of anesthesia on the dorsum of the finger near the base (Figure 136-4).
3. *Inject a total of 3 to 5 ml of anesthetic through the wheal by passing the needle downward until the needle is felt on the palmar surface (do not pierce the palmar skin).
4. *Subcutaneous infiltration is now accomplished at the base of the finger into the intraosseous spaces.
5. *For the index and little finger, the appropriate digital nerve is located in subcutaneous fatty tissue just anterior to the metacarpal head. Injection of anesthesia produces a half-ring wheal on the radial border of the index finger and on the ulnar border of the little finger.

---

*Indicates portions of the procedure usually performed by a physician or an advanced practice nurse.

Thumb

1. *Circumferential block is completed by placing a ring of anesthetic around the thumb. Block of the thumb is more difficult to attain because it is supplied by multiple branches of the radial and medial nerves.
2. *Insert the needle at the base of the thumb on the dorsal surface, and angle it toward the web space while injecting the anesthetic. Then reverse the needle direction and inject toward the opposite side of the thumb. Inject close to the periosteum, as noted earlier.
3. *Next, inject on the palmar side at the base of the thumb while angling the needle toward the web space. Then reverse the needle direction while injecting toward the opposite side of the thumb, thus completing the ring.
4. Effective anesthesia can usually be accomplished by injecting a total of 4 to 5 ml of anesthetic.

Toes

1. *Anesthesia of the great toe requires a band of anesthesia introduced via three separate injections (Figures 136-5 and 136-6). This block usually takes 5 to 10 minutes to take effect.
2. *To perform digital nerve blocks of other toes, introduce the needle at the dorsal side at the base of the midpoint of the involved toe (Figure 136-7).
3. *Angle the needle toward the bone, while slowly injecting anesthetic.

---

*Indicates portions of the procedure usually performed by a physician or an advanced practice nurse.

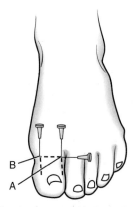

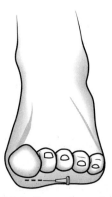

FIGURE 136-5 Digital block of the great toe. The needle is first inserted at point A and directly medially while injecting. Then, the needle is redirected posteriorly through the same puncture and anesthetic is injected in this direction. Then insert the needle at point B along the medial portion of the great toe and inject anesthetic posteriorly.

FIGURE 136-6 To complete a digital block of the great toe, the needle is inserted at the lateral, posterior aspect of the toe and directed medially while injecting anesthesia.

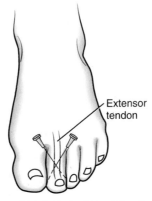

FIGURE 136-7 Digital block of toes other than the great toe.

4. *Before withdrawing the needle, redirect the needle toward the opposite side of the toe, and infiltrate the second side of the toe.
5. Effective anesthesia can be achieved by injecting a total of 3 ml in the small toes and a total of 4 to 6 ml in the great toe.

AGE-SPECIFIC CONSIDERATIONS

1. Calculate anesthetic dosages and total anesthetic volume for the pediatric patient to avoid circulatory compromise of the digit.
2. The pediatric patient is not able to monitor return of sensation after digital block. Instruct the parents to assess circulation and limit activity until the return of expected normal sensation.

COMPLICATIONS

1. Avoid repeated jabbing while injecting to minimize hematoma formation and decrease postanesthesia neuritis.
2. Position the needle adjacent to the nerve. Intraneural infiltration should be suspected if excessive injection force is required. The patient may also complain of tingling or feeling a shock if the nerve is touched. Reposition the needle to avoid nerve injury.
3. Frequent aspiration helps avoid intravascular infiltration.
4. Vascular compromise may result if too large a volume of anesthesia is used. The amount required varies with each patient. An effective block can usually be accomplished with 3 to 4 ml in the digits, 4 to 5 ml in the thumb, and 4 to 6 ml in the great toe.
5. Digital block is used with finger injuries or infections. Local wound infiltration of the finger is contraindicated because of the risk of circulatory impairment.
6. Consider regional or general anesthesia if finger injury is severe or more than two fingers need digital blocks.

---

*Indicates portions of the procedure usually performed by a physician or an advanced practice nurse.

PATIENT TEACHING

1. Teach the patient how to assess circulatory compromise and motor or nerve impairment. Instruct the patient to return to the emergency department if compromise or impairment is suspected.
2. Adjacent fingers may also be numb because of the nerve pathways. While applying dressings to the digit, consider immobilizing the adjoining digit(s) depending on the severity of the injury.
3. Begin analgesia when anesthesia wears off, if needed. Instruct the patient when to expect return of sensation if lidocaine (1 to 2 hours) or bupivacaine (4 to 8 hours) is used. If numbness persists longer than 24 hours, instruct the patient to contact a physician or return to the emergency department.
4. Provide wound or fracture care instructions as indicated.

REFERENCES

Kelly, J. J., & Spektor, M. (2004). Nerve blocks of the thorax and extremities. In J. R. Roberts, & J. R. Hedges (Eds.), *Clinical procedures in emergency medicine* (4th ed., pp. 567-590). Philadelphia: Saunders.

Wilhelmi, B. J, Blackwell, S. J., & Miller, J., et al. (2001). Do not use epinephrine in digital blocks: Myth or truth? *Plastic Reconstructive Surgery, 107*(2), 393-397.

PROCEDURE 137

Intravenous Regional Anesthesia

Joni Hentzen Daniels, MSN, RN, CEN, CCRN, and
Jean A. Proehl, RN, MN, CEN, CCRN, FAEN

Intravenous regional anesthesia (IVRA), commonly known as a *Bier block*, was invented in 1908 by August Bier and is a regional block that uses local anesthesia to temporarily block nerve conduction. Venous blood of the injured extremity (usually upper extremity) is drained by gravity or bandaging and filled with local anesthetic held in place by a tourniquet. This type of regional anesthesia provides a bloodless field and anesthesia for fracture reduction or repair of extensive wounds. The method involves the IV injection of a local anesthetic agent into the previously exsanguinated limb. Lidocaine is the only anesthetic approved by the U.S. Food and Drug Administration for IVRA (Wilhelmi, 2006). However, other local anesthetics may be used at the discretion of the physician.

INDICATIONS

1. To provide regional anesthesia for patients who require evaluation of soft-tissue injuries, for fracture reduction, for repair of nerves and tendons, and for complex suturing in an extremity.
2. This technique is best used for minor procedures up to 1 hour in duration (Candido, Pedicini, & Winnie, 2004).
3. To permit patient cooperation when constant evaluation of nerve and motor function is required. IVRA decreases the patient's pain and anxiety.
4. To provide regional anesthesia for extremities when systemic anesthesia is not an option because a patient has recently eaten or is compromised by alcohol or drug ingestion.
5. To provide regional anesthesia in anticoagulated patients (Candido et al., 2004).

CONTRAINDICATIONS AND CAUTIONS

1. Sensitivity or history of allergic reaction to local anesthetics is a contraindication.
2. IVRA should not be used in patients with peripheral vascular disease, open fractures, local skin infections, or cellulitis; when peripheral IV access cannot be achieved in the injured limb; or when tourniquet application is contra-indicated (Candido et al., 2004).
3. Caution is advised with extensive crush injury of the affected limb where tissue perfusion may already be compromised.
4. If the patient exhibits excessive fear or anxiety that prevents cooperation, IVRA could still potentially be used with appropriate sedation and analgesia (see Procedure 177).
5. Close attention must be paid to proper maintenance of the pneumatic tour-niquet with detailed check of equipment before use. Standard blood pressure cuffs should not be used.
6. IVRA can be used only when adequate personnel and monitoring and resus-citation equipment are available.
7. There are more safety issues and problems with tourniquets when IVRA is used in the lower extremity (Candido et al., 2004).
8. Do not release the tourniquet for at least 30 minutes after the last injection of anesthetic, fatal systemic toxicity may result (Candido et al., 2004).

EQUIPMENT

Local anesthetic without preservative
Antiseptic wipes
60-ml syringe
18- and 21-G needles for anesthesia
Equipment to obtain IV access
Cardiac monitor/defibrillator
Resuscitation equipment
3- to 4-in elastic bandage
Cast padding

Cast or splinting material

Pneumatic tourniquet with double cuffs (The use of a standard blood pressure cuff is not acceptable because of the risk of air leakage and systemic release of anesthesia.)

PATIENT PREPARATION

1. Establish IV access distal to site of injury (see Procedure 60).
2. Establish a second IV site in an uninjured extremity for emergency access, if needed.
3. Initiate pulse oximetry and cardiac monitoring (see Procedures 21 and 55).
4. Apply two or three layers of cast padding at the tourniquet site to protect the skin.
5. Assess and document vital signs.
6. Place the patient in a supine position.
7. Consider IV administration of a sedative to decrease patient anxiety and an analgesic to decrease cuff discomfort during the procedure (see Procedure 177).

PROCEDURAL STEPS

1. Test the pneumatic tourniquet cuffs by inflating them to 250 mm Hg, and ensure that there is no air leakage.
2. *Place both pneumatic tourniquets around the extremity proximal to the injury (Figure 137-1).
3. *Exsanguinate the extremity by elevating the extremity and wrapping it with a tight elastic bandage applied distally to proximally. Proper exsanguination allows even distribution of anesthesia, ensures a bloodless field, and decreases early tourniquet pain (Figure 137-2). If the patient's injury precludes the application of an elastic bandage, exsanguinate the extremity by elevating it and occluding the artery for 5 minutes.

---

*Indicates portions of the procedure usually performed by a physician or an advanced practice nurse.

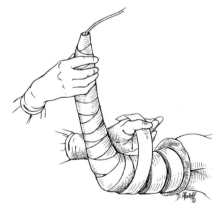

FIGURE 137-1 Exsanguinate the extremity by wrapping with an elastic bandage and/or elevating the extremity. (Courtesy of P. Rosen, M.D.)

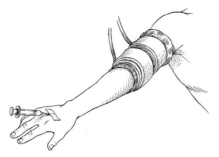

FIGURE 137-2 A double-tourniquet system. (Courtesy of P. Rosen, M.D.)

4. *Apply digital pressure to occlude the axillary artery (for the arm) or the femoral artery (for the leg) and maintain this pressure during cuff inflation. Inflate the proximal cuff to 50 to 100 mm Hg higher than the patient's systolic blood pressure (Candido et al., 2004).

5. *With the tourniquet inflated, inject the anesthesia into the IV line of the injured extremity. The anesthetic agent of choice depends on physician preference, rapidity of onset, duration and degree of motor block needed, relative toxicity of agent, and spreading power of agent. Dosage should be individualized by patient weight. (See Procedure 135, Table 135-1, for maximum doses.) Do not use anesthetic agents that contain preservatives. Lidocaine 3 mg/kg without preservative is a commonly used anesthetic. Opioids, neuromuscular blocker, and nonsteroidal antiinflammatory drugs may also be included to decrease the amount of local anesthetic required. Consultation with anesthesiology should be considered in this event.

6. Approximately 25 to 30 minutes after the onset of anesthesia or when the patient begins to develop tourniquet pain, inflate the distal cuff 50 to 100 mm Hg higher than the patient's systolic blood pressure. Slowly deflate the proximal cuff so that the local anesthetic does not rush back into the systemic circulation. The area under the distal cuff is already anesthetized and the patient does not experience tourniquet pain.

7. Monitor vital signs, cardiac rhythm, SpO_2, and level of consciousness continuously during the procedure. Monitor the pressure in the pneumatic cuffs.

8. If the patient has a fracture or dislocation, postreduction films are performed before the tourniquet is released.

9. *At completion of the procedure, tourniquet release is begun. Do not release the tourniquet for at least 30 minutes after the last injection of anesthetic (Candido et al., 2004).
   a. Deflate the tourniquet totally and immediately reinflate it for 1 minute.
   b. Assess the patient for symptoms of local anesthetic toxicity such as lightheadedness, tinnitus, or a metallic taste.

---

*Indicates portions of the procedure usually performed by a physician or an advanced practice nurse.

    c. If there are no symptoms of systemic toxicity, deflate the tourniquet totally and immediately reinflate it. Assess the patient for systemic local anesthetic toxicity.

    d. If there are no symptoms of systemic toxicity after 1 to 2 minutes, deflate the cuff and remove it.

10. During and after release of the tourniquet, continue to monitor vital signs, cardiac rhythm, SpO_2, level of consciousness, and symptoms of anesthetic toxicity. After the tourniquet release, the patient should be monitored for a minimum of 30 to 60 minutes. Circulation, sensation, and movement of the injured extremity should also be monitored during this time.

11. A large amount of anesthetic remains within the tissues of the extremity even after tourniquet release. To prevent rapid mobilization into the systemic circulation, the extremity should remain at rest for some time after the procedure (Candido et al., 2004).

AGE-SPECIFIC CONSIDERATION

Children may require additional sedation before the procedure.

COMPLICATIONS

1. Severe toxicity is rare and is usually due to a faulty tourniquet. High blood concentrations of anesthetic as a result of rapid release into the systemic circulation may be life-threatening. Systemic toxicity is dose dependent and is related to the effects of anesthesia on the cardiovascular or central nervous systems. Cardiovascular effects may include hypotension and arrhythmias, such as conduction disturbances, bradycardia, tachycardia, and asystole. Central nervous system effects are more common and include perioral numbness, dizziness, visual disturbances (blurred vision), light-headedness, near-syncope, seizure, and coma (Cox, Duriex, & Marcus, 2003).

2. Central nervous system symptoms may be masked in patients premedicated with anticonvulsants such as benzodiazepines or barbiturates. The first sign of toxicity in these premedicated patients may be cardiovascular depression (Cox et al., 2003).

3. Reactions are more common if the tourniquet is released within less than 30 minutes, if the tourniquet is released too rapidly, or if the anesthetic dosage is too high.

4. True allergic reactions are rare and are usually caused by ester-derivative anesthetics not used in IVRA (see Procedure 135).

5. Compartmental syndrome

PATIENT TEACHING

1. Keep the injured extremity still with limited active movement for at least an hour after the procedure.

2. Teach the patient symptoms of circulatory compromise and nerve and motor impairment, and ask the patient to contact a physician or return to the emergency department if problems are suspected.

3. Instruct the patient when to expect return of sensation and to begin analgesia promptly.

REFERENCES

Candido, K. D., Pedicini, E. L., & Winnie, A. P. (2004). Intravenous regional anesthesia. In E. F. Reichman, & R. R. Simon (Eds.), *Emergency medicine procedures* (pp. 984-994). New York: McGraw-Hill.

Cox, B., Duriex, M. E., & Marcus, M. A. (2003). Toxicity of local anesthetics. *Best Practice and Research Clinical Anesthesiology, 17*, 111-136.

Wilhelmi, B. J. (2006). *Hand anesthesia: Blocks.* Retrieved August 31, 2006, from http://www.emedicine.com/plastic/topic297.htm

---

PROCEDURE 138

Fishhook Removal

Daun A. Smith, RN, MSN

INDICATION

To remove fishhooks embedded in soft tissue

CONTRAINDICATIONS AND CAUTIONS

1. There are two types of fishhooks; both are curved with an extremely sharp tip. One has a barbed shaft, with the barb just distal to and on the inside of the curve, and the other has an unbarbed shaft.
2. Fishhooks embedded in or near the eye may need to be removed by an ophthalmologist. Emergency or field treatment should consist of covering the affected eye with a shield or cup (see Procedure 161). Patching the unaffected eye decreases movement in the injured eye (see Procedure 159).
3. Fishhooks embedded in bone or cartilage; in the oropharynx, nose, ear, or other orifice; or associated with neurovascular dysfunction distally may need to be removed surgically.

EQUIPMENT

Wound cleaning supplies
Local anesthetic
Other specific supplies depend on the removal method and may include the following:
    Heavy silk suture material (00 or 1-0) or umbilical tape
    Forceps (curved or straight) or needle holder
    Wire cutters
    Scalpel with No. 11 blade
    19-G needle

PATIENT PREPARATION

1. Cleanse the wound (see Procedure 134).
2. Consider local anesthesia (see Procedures 135 and 136).
3. Consider radiographic studies to locate tip of fishhook and visualize barbs.
4. Administer tetanus immunization as indicated.
5. *Perform a neurovascular assessment of distal structures before attempting to manipulate the fishhook.
6. Remove unnecessary fish line and lure; remove extra hook tips on fishhooks with multiple hooks (Thommasen & Thommasen, 2005).

PROCEDURAL STEPS

Numerous methods exist for the removal of fishhooks, depending on the depth of hook penetration, the location of the fishhook, and the remover's preference.

Simple Retrograde Removal

This method works best with superficially embedded or unbarbed hooks (Thommasen & Thommasen, 2005).
1. *Gently press down on the shank of the fishhook (this releases the barb at the tip) (Figure 138-1).
2. *Remove the fishhook by backing it out, following the pathway of entry.

String Method

This method works best for small- and medium-sized hooks (Thommasen & Thommasen, 2005).
1. For this technique, wear eye protection (both operator and patient) because the fishhook exits from the skin in an uncontrolled manner.
2. *Wrap the middle of a piece of umbilical tape or heavy silk suture material (at least 10 inches long) around the bend of the fishhook, grasping both free ends in your dominant hand, holding the ends in the opposite direction from the direction of the fishhook entry (Figure 138-2).
3. *Gently press down on the shank of the fishhook, disengaging the barb.
4. *Tug or snap the ends of the tape or suture material in the direction away

---

*Indicates portions of the procedure usually performed by a physician or an advanced practice nurse.

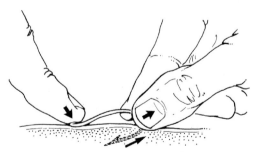

FIGURE 138-1 Simple retrograde removal. (From Jastremski, M. S. [1992]. Fishhook removal. In M. S. Jastremski, M. Dumas, & L. Peñalaver [Eds.], *Emergency procedures* [p. 129]. Philadelphia: Saunders.)

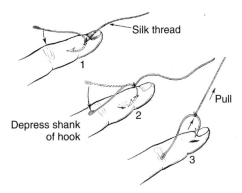

Silk thread

Depress shank
of hook

Pull

FIGURE 138-2 String removal method. (From Jastremski, M. S. [1992]. Fishhook removal. In M. S. Jastremski, M. Dumas, & L. Peñalaver [Eds.], *Emergency procedures* [p. 129]. Philadelphia: Saunders.)

from the fishhook entry and parallel to the skin. This action removes the fishhook in a retrograde fashion.

Advance and Cut

This method is used for deeper fishhook penetrations, when multiple barbs are embedded, or when other methods have failed.

1. *Advance the tip of the fishhook through the skin using the forceps or the needle holder (Figure 138-3).
2. *Cut the tip and barb from the fishhook with wire cutters.
3. *Remove the remainder of the fishhook in a retrograde manner.
4. *If the fishhook shaft is barbed, the eye of the fishhook is cut off with wire cutters and the fishhook is removed in an antegrade fashion.
5. Reassess the distal neurovascular function, and clean the wound according to institutional guidelines.

Needling Technique

This technique is more successful, less painful, and less traumatic than other techniques (Ainsworth-Smith, 2005).

1. Insert a large-gauge needle through the puncture wound on the inside of the hook and slide it over the barb (Figure 138-4).
2. Hold the needle and the hook together firmly and remove as a unit.

COMPLICATIONS

1. Infection
2. Distal neurovascular compromise

PATIENT TEACHING

1. Monitor for signs and symptoms of infection, including pain, swelling, drainage, tenderness, and redness.
2. Report any signs of infection to your primary care provider.

---

*Indicates portions of the procedure usually performed by a physician or an advanced practice nurse.

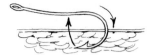

Advance hook through skin

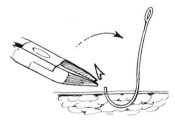

Cut off barb

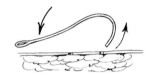

Reverse direction and extract hook

FIGURE 138-3 Advance and cut method. (From Dunmire, S. M., & Paris, P. M. [1994]. *Atlas of emergency procedures* [p. 111]. Philadelphia, Saunders.)

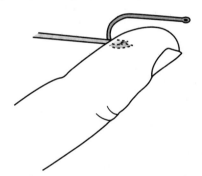

FIGURE 138-4 Removal with a large-gauge needle.

REFERENCES

Ainsworth-Smith, M. (2005). Fishing hook removal. *Emergency Nurse, 13*(6), 12.

Thommasen, H. V., & Thommasen, A. (2005). The occasional removal of an embedded fishhook. *Canadian Journal of Rural Medicine, 10*(4), 254-259.

Wound Care for Amputations

Jean A. Proehl, RN, MN, CEN, CCRN, FAEN

INDICATION

To preserve amputated or avulsed tissue or appendages for possible replantation or revascularization. *Replantation* is the correct term for "complete amputations;" partial amputations are revascularized. For simplicity, the term *replantation* is used for both situations in this procedure.

CONTRAINDICATIONS AND CAUTIONS

1. Replantation is attempted only after life-threatening problems are resolved.
2. The decision to attempt replantation is made by the surgeon after consideration of technical, esthetic, medical, and psychosocial factors. A promise should not be made to the patient that replantation will be attempted. The replantation team should be consulted as soon as possible to determine whether a replantation attempt is indicated.
3. Time is of the essence for successful replantation. Cooling the tissue prolongs its viability. The more muscle, the higher are the metabolic needs, and the shorter is the acceptable ischemic time frame. Fingers have relatively little muscle in comparison to extremities.
4. The amputated tissue should not be allowed to freeze. Freezing causes cell membrane rupture and irreversibly damages the tissue. A temperature of $4°$ C is optimal (Dalsey & Luk, 2004). Dry ice should not be used because it results in temperatures that are too cold.
5. No tissue bridge should be severed, no matter how thin. It should be treated as a partial amputation and splinted to preserve the integrity of the skin bridge.
6. Tourniquets, tying, or clamping vessels in the stump should be avoided, because these maneuvers may damage the structures that will be reanastomosed during replantation. Bleeding should be controlled with direct pressure if possible. A blood pressure cuff on the proximal extremity inflated to 30 mm Hg above systolic blood pressure can be used to help control bleeding if necessary (Dalsey & Luk, 2004).
7. Digital block anesthesia of the stump should be avoided (O'Hara-Speert & Mullaly, 1996).
8. All avulsed or amputated tissue should be preserved; even if replantation is not attempted, the tissue may be used for grafting.

EQUIPMENT

Gauze dressings

Insulated container (for prolonged storage or transport to another facility)

Plastic bag or waterproof container

Ice

Sterile normal saline solution or lactated Ringer's solution

Antibiotic, if prescribed, for tissue preservation solution

PATIENT PREPARATION

1. Consult with your referral replantation team as soon as possible to determine the feasibility of replantation and to receive specific instructions regarding care of the amputated part and the patient.
2. Remove all jewelry from the injured area (see Procedures 114 and 115).
3. Obtain wound cultures before antibiotic administration. Send laboratory specimens for type and crossmatch as indicated.
4. Administer parenteral antibiotics, analgesia, and sedation as prescribed.
5. Administer tetanus prophylaxis as indicated.
6. Administer aspirin or low-molecular-weight dextran if prescribed by the replantation surgeon.
7. Obtain x-ray studies of the stump and the amputated part.
8. Keep the patient warm to prevent vasoconstriction (Wilhelmi, Weiner, Pagenstert, & Ma, 2006).
9. Prepare the patient for transport if indicated (see Procedure 193).

PROCEDURAL STEPS
Complete Amputation

1. Cleanse the stump and the amputated part by gently rinsing with normal saline solution to remove gross contamination. Do not scrub or use antiseptic solution.
2. Apply a soft-pressure dressing and elevate the stump. Splint the stump as indicated.
3. Wrap the amputated part in gauze moistened with saline solution and seal it in a plastic bag; do not immerse the part in water (Wilhelmi et al., 2006). Be sure to wrap the part well so that it is protected from freezing.
4. Place the plastic bag or container on ice in an insulated container.
5. Label the bag or container containing the amputated part so that it is not inadvertently discarded.

Partial Amputation

1. Wrap the entire extremity in moist dressings per replantation team orders.
2. Splint and elevate the extremity.
3. Cooling the extremity may not be possible because it can be painful. If there is evidence of arterial insufficiency, attempt to cool the distal part with ice packs.

AGE-SPECIFIC CONSIDERATION

Children have better nerve regeneration capability and usually have better functional outcomes than adults. Replantation attempts are often considered in children, even in the presence of relative contraindications (Yoshida, 1997).

COMPLICATIONS

1. Cellular damage or death as a result of freezing or inadequate cooling.
2. Cellular damage or death as a result of excess time between injury and replantation. Time limits vary with the type of injury, the body part involved, and how the part is stored. Every effort should be made to replant the part as soon as possible.

PATIENT TEACHING

1. Do not smoke, eat, or drink until after surgery. Caffeine and nicotine are not allowed for several months if replantation is attempted.
2. Keep the injured part elevated.
3. The replantation surgeon is the most qualified person to discuss your prognosis with you.

REFERENCES

Dalsey, W. C., & Luk, J. (2004). Management of amputations. In J. R. Roberts, & J. R. Hedges (Eds.), *Clinical procedures in emergency medicine* (4th ed., pp. 919-926). Philadelphia: Saunders.

O'Hara-Speert, M., & Mullaly, S. G. (1996). Nursing care of the patient with a complete scalp avulsion. *Journal of Emergency Nursing, 22*, 552-558.

Wilhelmi, B. J., Weiner, L., Pagenstert, G. I. B., & Ma, J. W. (2006). Hand amputations and replantation. *E-Medicine*, updated June 28, 2006. Retrieved March 11, 2007, from http://www.emedicine.com/plastic/topic536.htm

Yoshida, D. (1997). Amputations. In R. A. Dieckmann, D. H. Fiser, & S. M. Selbst (Eds.), *Illustrated textbook of pediatric emergency and critical care procedures* (pp. 645-649). St Louis: Mosby.

Surgical Tape Closures

Jean A. Proehl, RN, MN, CEN, CCRN, FAEN

Surgical tape closures are also known as *tape closures, skin tapes, butterfly closures, Steri-Strips, Cover-Strips, Shur-Strips, Curi-Strips, Nichi-Strips, Cicagraf*, and *Suture Strips.*

INDICATIONS

Surgical tape closures are used to close wounds. In appropriate wounds, surgical tape closures have the following advantages over suture or staple closure—no suture scars, less skin reaction, greater resistance to wound infection, less need for anesthesia, no return visit needed for removal, may be used under casts and splints, less expensive than sutures or staples, and ease of application (Lammers & Trott, 2004). Surgical tape closures are indicated in the following situations:

1. To provide a noninvasive repair of a wound. Superficial, straight lacerations under little tension are the ideal wounds for surgical skin tapes.
2. To provide additional support to sutured or stapled wounds.
3. To provide wound stability and promote further healing after suture removal.
4. To approximate skin edges loosely on a wound too old to be sutured but gaping widely.
5. To hold skin flaps and grafts in place (Lammers & Trott, 2004).
6. To approximate wounds in skin that is compromised by long-term steroid use or peripheral vascular disease (Lammers & Trott, 2004).

CONTRAINDICATIONS AND CAUTIONS

1. Surgical skin tapes are not used in the following situations:
   a. Wounds under high skin stress, such as those over major joints
   b. Wounds that will become wet as a result of problems with hemostasis, perspiration, exudate, or ointment application
   c. Wounds that are infected
   d. Wounds that are surrounded by hair or skin abrasion
   e. Wounds that are irregular or over concave areas
2. Tapes should not be placed circumferentially around digits; digits should be wrapped in a semicircular or spiral fashion instead.
3. The tape should not be stretched during application; tape should be applied with only a small amount of tension to approximate wound edges.

EQUIPMENT

Surgical tape closures (available in widths from ⅛ to ½ in)
Skin adhesive such as tincture of benzoin (optional)
Transparent dressing (optional)
Forceps
Scissors

PATIENT PREPARATION
1. Anesthetize the area as indicated (see Procedures 135 and 136).
2. Cleanse the wound (see Procedure 134).
3. Provide tetanus prophylaxis as indicated.

PROCEDURAL STEPS
1. Maintain hemostasis using direct pressure.
2. Ensure a dry field; surgical tape closures do not adhere to moist skin.
3. Apply a skin adhesive to the wound margins and the surrounding skin (optional). Do not allow the adhesive to enter the wound, and do not use adhesive near the eye. Even with local anesthesia, there may be a brief episode of discomfort as the alcohol fumes from the adhesive evaporate. Allow the adhesive to dry and become tacky.
4. Cut the tapes to the desired length; allow for a 2- to 3-cm overlap on each side of the wound (Lammers & Trott, 2004). Remove the end tab from the paper backing of the strips.
5. Remove a tape from the backing by pulling it straight back with forceps; do not curl the tape backward during removal because this curls the tape and makes it more difficult to work with (3M Health Care, 1994).
6. Fresh wound (Figure 140-1):
   a. Place the first tape at the middle of the wound on one side only, approximate the wound edges as closely as possible (a second person may be required to assist), and apply the second half of the tape. Run your finger along the strip to help set the adhesive.
   b. Place additional tapes halfway between the previous tape and the wound edges. Continue to apply tapes until the wound is sufficiently closed but not totally occluded.
   c. Place supporting tapes horizontally across the tapes, approximately 1 inch from the wound; this is known as the ladder technique. The supporting tapes help prevent the ends of the tapes from curling and decrease skin stress at the tape ends.
7. Healing wound (after suture removal): Remove a few sutures at a time and replace them with tapes. (Apply tapes as described in step 6 above.)
8. If a tape needs to be repositioned after application, remove it by peeling both ends toward the wound.
9. A transparent dressing may be applied over the tapes for additional protection (3M, 2002).

AGE-SPECIFIC CONSIDERATIONS
1. Surgical skin tapes are useful in frightened children with suitable wounds.
2. Cover the skin tapes with a dry dressing to prevent small children and confused adults from picking at them. Do not use occlusive or adhesive bandages that encourage moisture formation.

COMPLICATIONS
1. Wound infection.
2. Impaired wound healing. Medications, such as steroids and hormones, and medical conditions, such as diabetes, uremia, malnourishment, and poor skin perfusion, contribute to poor wound healing.

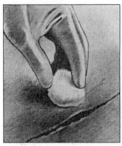

1. Clean and dry skin thoroughly, and remove any oils.

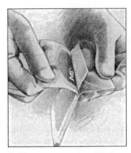

2. Remove card end tab from one end of card.

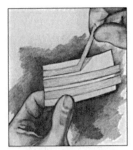

3. Grasp end of strip with fingers or fine forceps and lift straight forward from card using a slow motion.

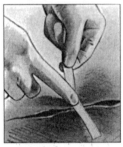

4. Appose skin edges with forceps.

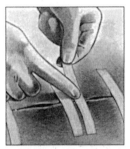

5. Place strips across wound, ensuring tension-less application. Divide the wound into sections, starting at the midpoint of the wound.

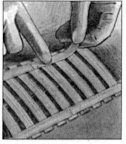

6. Set adhesive with light finger pressure by running along length of the strip.

FIGURE 140-1 Skin tape application technique. (Courtesy 3M Health Care. [1994]. *Professional adhesive closure education* [teacher's guide]. St. Paul, MN.)

3. Wound dehiscence if the strips loosen, fall off too early, or are improperly applied, or if there is poor patient compliance with wound care.
4. Blisters under the ends of the tapes from excessive skin tension. This complication can be avoided by use of supporting horizontal tapes across the tape tails and by not stretching the tapes during application. Wound swelling after tape application can also cause excessive skin tension.

PATIENT TEACHING

1. The wound must remain clean and dry. After 24 hours, you may shower with surgical tape closures in place but limit exposure to water and gently pat dry as soon as possible. The strips adhere better if exposure to water is limited (3M Health Care, 2002).
2. Do not apply any ointments or petroleum-containing products on the strips. The adhesive will dissolve, and the strips will fall off.
3. Trim the edges of the strips as they loosen and curl to prevent inadvertent removal.

4. Elevate the injured area as much as possible for the next 24 to 48 hours.
5. Report any signs of infection (redness, swelling, draining pus, fever) to your health care provider or return to the emergency department.
6. Remove strips if they have not fallen off after the prescribed number of days. For fresh wounds, see Procedure 142 for the recommended number of days.

REFERENCES

Lammers, R. L., & Trott, A. T. (2004). Methods of wound closure. In J. R. Roberts, & J. R. Hedges (Eds.), *Clinical procedures in emergency medicine* (4th ed., pp. 655-693). Philadelphia: Saunders.

3M Health Care. (1994). *Professional adhesive closure education (teacher's guide)*. St Paul, MN: Author.

3M Health Care. (2002). *3M Steri-Strip^TM adhesive skin closures: Commonly asked questions*. Retrieved October 19, 2006, at   http://www.multimedia.mmm.com/mws/mediawebserver. dyn?6666660Zjcr6IVs6AVs666_sMCOrrrrQ.

PROCEDURE 141

Skin Adhesive

Jean A. Proehl, RN, MN, CEN, CCRN, FAEN

Skin adhesive is also known as *tissue adhesive, wound glue, Dermabond (Ethicon)*, and *Indermil (Syneture)*.

INDICATION

Skin adhesive is used to close easily approximated, clean, traumatic or surgical lacerations. It is faster and less painful than suturing and may produce a better cosmetic outcome. It remains in place for 5 to 10 days before sloughing off. No removal is necessary.

CONTRAINDICATIONS AND CAUTIONS
(Ethicon, 2003; Syneture, 2003)

1. Skin adhesive is not suitable for high-tension wounds over joints unless they are immobilized.
2. Do not use in the presence of infection or contamination; on mucosal surfaces; on bites, jagged, stellate, or puncture wounds; or in dense hair.
3. Skin adhesive is contraindicated for patients with hypersensitivity to cyanoacrylate or formaldehyde.

4. Do not use in areas subjected to repetitive rubbing or washing, such as the hands, because the top layer of epidermis may peel off before healing is complete.
5. Some skin adhesives are low viscosity and may run off of the wound and fuse unintended areas together, such as eyelids, the practitioner's gloves, and so on. High-viscosity formulations decrease this risk and are easier to control during application.

EQUIPMENT
Forceps (optional)
Gauze sponges
Skin adhesive in an applicator

PATIENT PREPARATION
1. Administer tetanus prophylaxis as indicated.
2. If necessary, anesthetize the wound to facilitate cleansing (see Procedures 135 and 136).
3. Clean and irrigate the wound (see Procedure 134).
4. Establish hemostasis with direct pressure, and dry the area completely. Water accelerates the polymerization process; thus, skin adhesive should not be applied to wet wounds (Ethicon, 2003, Syneture, 2003).
5. *For deeper wounds, place subcutaneous sutures to help approximate the skin.
6. Position the area horizontally to prevent the skin adhesive from running onto adjacent tissue. If the wound is near the eye, position the wound slightly downhill from the eye and hold the eye closed with a gauze dressing.

PROCEDURAL STEPS
1. Prepare the applicator.
   a. *Dermabond:* Hold the applicator with the white tip up, and squeeze to crush the inner glass ampule. Invert the applicator and squeeze gently to start the flow of adhesive through the tip.
   b. *Indermil:* Hold the ampule upright, and twist the cap off. If desired, a blunt-tip applicator can be attached to the tip.
2. Approximate the wound with forceps or gloved fingers and evert the wound edges slightly. Excessive pressure may force the wound open and allow the adhesive to enter the wound. This should be avoided because the adhesive is not absorbed and can cause a foreign-body reaction.
3. *Apply the adhesive. The patient may feel warmth as the adhesive polymerizes.
   a. *Dermabond:* Gently apply a thin, even layer of adhesive to the wound edges and 0.5 cm beyond (Figure 141-1). Allow 30 seconds for the adhesive to dry between layers, and apply at least two thin layers in this fashion. Maintain wound-edge approximation manually or with forceps for 60 seconds after the last layer is applied. Full strength is achieved approximately 2.5 minutes after the last application.

---

*Indicates a portion of the procedure usually performed by a physician or an advanced practice nurse.

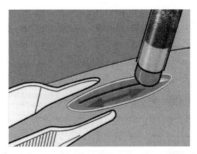

FIGURE 141-1 Apply the adhesive gently while approximating the wound edges. (Courtesy Ethicon, Inc., Somerville, NJ.)

    b. *Indermil:* Apply as minute drops or a very thin film along the edges of the wound. Maintain wound edge approximation with light pressure for 30 seconds to allow the adhesive to cure.
4. If the adhesive runs onto adjacent areas, it can be wiped off for the first 10 seconds. A petroleum-based ointment can be immediately applied to unintended areas of adhesive coverage to help promote dissolution.
5. Do not apply ointment to the area. No dressing is needed. If a dressing is preferred, wait at least 5 minutes to make sure the adhesive is no longer sticky before applying a dry, sterile dressing. Do not apply skin tapes or adhesive tape directly to the skin adhesive.

AGE-SPECIFIC CONSIDERATION

Skin adhesive is particularly useful in children because it is quicker and less painful than suturing. Also, a return visit for suture removal is not needed. A dressing may be helpful to keep children from picking at the adhesive.

COMPLICATION

Inadvertent adhesion to gloves, forceps, hair, or other skin surfaces. If this occurs, acetone or petroleum-based ointments can be used to loosen the adhesive. Peel off the film, but do not attempt to pull the skin apart.

PATIENT TEACHING

1. Report any signs of infection (e.g., redness, swelling, pus drainage, fever) or wound separation to your health care provider or return to the emergency department.
2. The skin adhesive will slough off the site in 5 to 10 days; no removal is needed. Do not scratch, rub, or pick at the adhesive. Do not apply ointment, cream, or tape to the adhesive.
3. Do not expose the wound to sunlight or tanning lamps while the adhesive is in place.
4. Do not swim or soak the wound. Showering and brief wetting of the wound are allowed (only after 48 hours for Indermil). To dry the wound, blot it with a towel instead of rubbing.

REFERENCES

Ethicon. (2003). *Dermabond Topical Skin Adhesive (2-octyl cyanoacrylate)*. Somerville, NJ: Author. Retrieved February 18, 2007, from http://www.dermabond.com/content/backgrounders/www.dermabond.com/www.dermabond.com/EPI.pdf

Syneture. (2003). *Indermil® Tissue Adhesive*. Norwalk, CT: United States Surgical.

PROCEDURE 142

Suture Removal

Maureen T. Quigley, MS, ARNP

INDICATION

To remove nonabsorbable suture material inserted for the purpose of wound approximation and primary healing. Adequate epithelialization of the wound is evidenced by a sturdy wound appearance, approximated edges, and evidence of healing. Timely suture removal is important to minimize scar formation. Removal of sutures is contingent on the integrity of the dermal closure and the degree of motion and healing properties of the particular area of the body. The dense vascularity and lack of tension on the face allows for quick, early healing and permits removal of sutures in only 3 to 5 days. Sutures on the trunk are left in place 6 to 7 days, and extremity sutures may remain for longer periods (Table 142-1).

TABLE 142-1
REMOVAL TIMES FOR SUTURES

Location	Time of Removal (Days)
Face	3-4 (adults)
	2-3 (children)
Scalp	5-7
Trunk	7
Lower extremity	8-10
Upper extremity	7-10
Extensor surface of joints	10-14
Delayed closure	8-12

CONTRAINDICATIONS AND CAUTIONS

1. To gain optimal cosmetic and functional results, sutures should be removed in a timely manner. The risk of infection at puncture sites, the development of epithelial tracts (characterized by epithelial growth in defect created by the suture), scarring, and the difficulty of suture removal is increased when sutures are left in longer than necessary. Premature suture removal predisposes the patient to wound disruption, delayed healing, and widening of the scar.
2. When the suture line is located in an area exposed to tensile stretch (e.g., joints), the sutures may be kept in place for up to 14 days, and thereafter the wound may require superficial support with skin tapes for an additional 5 to 7 days. Skin tape closures provide support and protection and can minimize scar widening.
3. Sutures with short ends are more difficult to remove.
4. Certain conditions interfere with wound healing. Populations at risk for impaired healing include those at the extremes of age, smokers, and those with diabetes, obesity, vascular disease, alcoholism, and immunosuppression, as well as those who have used steroids chronically. Deep wounds are at increased risk for infection and delayed wound healing.

EQUIPMENT

Scissors or suture removal scissors, No. 11 scalpel blade, or stitch cutter blade
Forceps
Gauze sponges
Normal saline solution
Antiseptic solution
Skin tape closures (optional)
(NOTE: Prepackaged kits containing some of the listed items are available.)

PROCEDURAL STEPS

1. The wound should be well visualized with proper lighting.
2. Cleanse sutures and the healed wound with antiseptic because it is impossible to avoid pulling a small portion of suture that has been outside the skin through the suture tract. Remove any crusting on the surrounding wound.
3. Grasp the knot of the suture with forceps with your nondominant hand and raise away from the skin.
4. Cut the suture distal to the knot and close to the skin surface on one side. This ensures that a contaminated suture is not drawn through the suture tract as the suture is withdrawn (Figure 142-1).
   a. If a vertical or horizontal mattress suture is in place, the suture must be cut on the side opposite the knot at a skin orifice (Figure 142-2).
   b. Running or continuous sutures (Figure 142-3) are removed by cutting every other loop. To determine that the ends are completely severed, gently lift the exposed ends away from skin (Perry & Potter, 2006).
5. Pull the suture out of the wound and discard.
6. Cleanse the wound with normal saline solution or an antiseptic solution.
7. Apply skin tape to wounds under tension or prone to separation (see Procedure 140).
8. Leave the suture line open to the air or apply a dressing as prescribed.

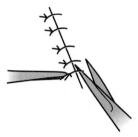

FIGURE 142-1 The suture should be removed by cutting the end away from the knot near the skin to prevent passage of the contaminated outer portion of the stitch back through the skin.

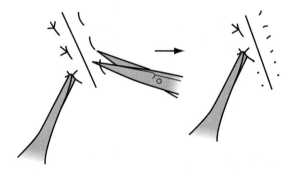

FIGURE 142-2 Removal of mattress sutures.

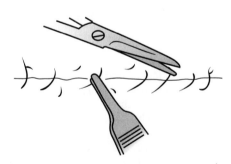

FIGURE 142-3 To remove a continuous suture, every other loop is cut.

AGE-SPECIFIC CONSIDERATION

Because children heal and form suture marks faster than adults, they may require earlier suture removal.

COMPLICATIONS

1. Wound infection
2. Widening of scar
3. Wound dehiscence
4. Retained suture

PATIENT TEACHING

1. Keep the wound clean and dry. Any crusted areas should simply be allowed to come off with usual soap and water cleansing. Do not pick at crusts or scabs.
2. Report any of the following signs and symptoms of wound infection: fever, increasing redness around the wound or on the extremity involved, red streaking, swelling, drainage of pus, increased pain or tenderness, or opening of the wound.
3. If the wound is in an area exposed to the sun, a sunscreen containing para-aminobenzoic acid is recommended for application to wound area because scars in the first 4 months redden to a greater extent than the surrounding skin (Lammers, 2004).

REFERENCES

Lammers, R. (2004). Principles of wound management. In J. R. Roberts, & J. R. Hedges (Eds.), *Clinical procedures in emergency medicine* (4th ed., pp. 623-654). Philadelphia: Saunders.

Perry, A., & Potter, P. (2006). *Clinical nursing skills and techniques* (6th ed.). St Louis: Mosby.

PROCEDURE 143

Staple Removal

Maureen T. Quigley, MS, ARNP

INDICATION

To remove skin staples inserted for the purpose of wound approximation and primary healing. Adequate epithelialization of the wound is evidenced by a sturdy wound appearance, approximated edges, and evidence of healing. Timely staple removal is important to minimize scar formation. Staple removal is performed under the same guidelines as skin sutures if healing is adequate (see Table 142-1).

CONTRAINDICATIONS AND CAUTIONS

1. To achieve optimal cosmetic and functional results, staples should be removed in a timely manner. There is a risk of infection at the puncture sites when staples are left in too long. Premature staple removal predisposes the patient to wound disruption, delayed healing, and widening of scar.
2. Generally, wound stapling and suturing have similar infection rates and wound healing. Staples should be removed promptly from patients who

scar more easily, because in this population, the scar formed by staples may be more prominent than that formed by sutures (Lammers & Trott, 2004).

3. Some conditions interfere with wound healing. Populations at risk for impaired healing include the elderly, smokers, and those with diabetes, obesity, vascular disease, and immunosuppression, as well as those who have used steroids on a long-term basis. Very deep and infected wounds may heal more slowly.

EQUIPMENT

Staple extractor (A variety of disposable skin stapler devices are on the market. Each stapler has its own specific staple extractor.)
Gauze sponges
Antiseptic solution
Normal saline solution
Skin closure strips (optional)

PROCEDURAL STEPS

1. Cleanse staples and healed wound with antiseptic solution. Remove any crusting on surrounding wound.
2. Place the lower tips of the staple extractor under the center of the staple (Figure 143-1).
3. Squeeze the extractor so that the center of the staple is depressed.
4. Lift the extractor and staple upward from the skin when both ends of the staple are visible.
5. After staple has been removed from skin, release handles of staple extractor, and dispose of staple in proper container.

AGE-SPECIFIC CONSIDERATION

For children, consider the use of a topical anesthetic prior to staple removal (see Procedure 135).

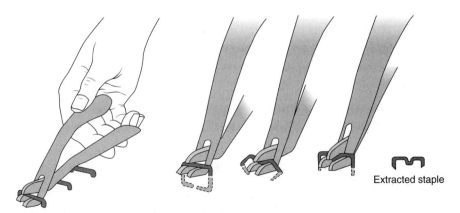

FIGURE 143-1 Technique for removing staples.

COMPLICATIONS
1. Wound infection
2. Scar widening
3. Wound dehiscence

PATIENT TEACHING
1. Keep your wound clean and dry. Any crusted areas should simply be allowed to come off with usual soap and water cleansing. Do not pick at crusts or scabs.
2. Report any of the following signs and symptoms of wound infection: fever, increasing redness around the wound or on the extremity involved, drainage of pus, increased pain or tenderness, or opening of the wound.
3. If the wound is in an area exposed to the sun, a sunscreen containing para-aminobenzoic acid is recommended for application to the wound area because scars in the first 4 months redden to a greater extent than the surrounding skin (Lammers & Trott, 2004).

REFERENCE
Lammers, R., & Trott, A. T. (2004). Methods of wound closure. In J. R. Roberts, & J. R. Hedges (Eds.), *Clinical procedures in emergency medicine* (4th ed., pp. 655-693). Philadelphia: Saunders.

PROCEDURE 144

Minor Burn Care

Joni Hentzen Daniels, MSN, RN, CEN, CCRN

Burn severity depends on the (1) extent, depth, and location of the burn injury; (2) age of the patient; (3) agents involved; (4) presence of inhalational injury, and (5) coexisting injuries or preexisting illness (Edlich, Bailey, & Long, 2006). This procedure only addresses the débridement and dressing of minor burns that may be managed on an outpatient basis. Minor burns, as defined by the American Burn Association (Edlich et al., 2006) and the American College of Surgeons (1999), are:
1. Partial-thickness and full-thickness burns covering less than 10% of body surface area (BSA) in patients younger than age 10 or older than age 50.

2. Partial-thickness and full-thickness burns covering less than 15% of BSA in other age groups that do not include the following mechanisms and do not present a serious threat of functional or cosmetic risk to:
   a. Eyes
   b. Ears
   c. Face
   d. Hands
   e. Genitalia
   f. Feet
   g. Perineum
   h. Overlying joints
3. Full-thickness burns covering less than 5% of BSA
4. No electrical injury (including lightning)
5. No chemical burns
6. No inhalational injury
7. No preexisting medical conditions that could complicate management, prolong recovery, or affect mortality
8. No concomitant trauma
9. No question of the reliability of the care giver or the home care environment

Methods used to assess percentage of BSA involved with burn management include the Rule of Nines (Figure 144-1) and the Lund and Browder burn chart (Figure 144-2). When small or irregular burns are being estimated, the patient's palmar surface is equal to about 1.25% of BSA (Bethel & Krisanda, 2004).

INDICATIONS

Minor burns managed on an outpatient basis requiring débridement and dressing to:
1. Minimize the potential for bacterial infection

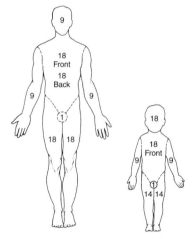

FIGURE 144-1 The Rule of Nines may be used to estimate body surface area burned. (From Bethel, C. A., & Krisanda, T. J. [2004]. Burn care procedures. In J. R. Roberts & J. R. Hedges [Eds.], *Clinical procedures in emergency medicine* [4th ed., p. 757]. Philadelphia: Saunders.)

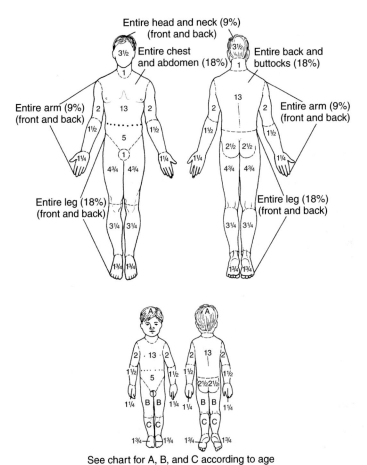

See chart for A, B, and C according to age

Age	Birth–1 yr	1–4 yr	5–9 yr	10–14 yr	15 yr	Adult
Head	19	17	13	11	9	7
Neck	2					
Ant trunk	13					
Post trunk	13					
R buttock	2½					
L buttock	2½					
Genitalia	1					
R U arm	4					
L U arm	4					
R L arm	3					
L L arm	3					
R hand	2½					
L hand	2½					
R thigh	5½	6½	8	8½	9	9½
L thigh	5½	6½	8	8½	9	9½
R leg	5	5	5½	6	6½	7
L leg	5	5	5½	6	6½	7
R foot	3½					
L foot	3½					

FIGURE 144-2 The Lund and Browder chart is a more accurate way to estimate body surface area burned than the Rule of Nines. (From Bethel, C. A., & Krisanda, T. J. [2004]. Burn care procedures. In J. R. Roberts & J. R. Hedges [Eds.], *Clinical procedures in emergency medicine* [4th ed., p. 752]. Philadelphia: Saunders.)

2. Prevent the conversion of a partial-thickness burn to a full-thickness burn
3. Promote spontaneous healing
4. Maximize patient comfort
5. Minimize cosmetic changes
6. Maintain optimal range of joint motion

CONTRAINDICATIONS AND CAUTIONS

1. Most burn units request that in the case of a patient with a major burn that requires admission, no débridement of the wound is performed in the emergency department. During the transfer, a dry sterile gauze dressing should be applied to isolated burns. In the case of large BSA involvement, a dry sterile sheet is recommended.
2. Current recommendations are to reserve the use of sterile saline soaks to partial-thickness burns of less than 10% of BSA. Moist dressings should not be used in any patient requiring transfer to a burn unit because of increased risk for both hypothermia and infection.
3. Cool saline may be used over the area initially to stop the burning process. Benefits of topical cooled fluids are:
   a. Inhibited lactate production and acidosis, thereby promoting catecholamine function and cardiovascular homeostasis
   b. Inhibited burn wound histamine release, which leads to blocked histamine-related increases in vascular permeability, minimizing edema formation
   c. Suppressed production of thromboxane (which has been implicated as the mediator of vascular occlusion and progressive dermal ischemia after burn injury)
4. Careful assessment must be made to determine whether, for any reason, admission of the patient is warranted.
5. The burn wound must be thoroughly cleaned and débrided before ointments or dressings are applied. If not, infection may be encouraged rather than avoided.
6. Ascertain that the patient or family has the financial, mental, and physical capabilities to follow aftercare instructions. If not, other arrangements or admission is required.

EQUIPMENT

Sterile gown, mask, and gloves
Sterile basin
Sterile towels
Sterile surgical instruments, such as fine-tipped scissors and forceps (with or without teeth)
Sterile normal saline solution for irrigation, warmed to body temperature, if possible (Many institutions use warm tap water.)
Mild soap, germicidal soap, chlorhexidine, or povidone-iodine
Mineral oil or petroleum ointments (for tar removal)
Sterile gauze dressings
Sterile (soft) surgical brush
Sterile gauze bandages
Adhesive tape

Burn dressing options:
   Sterile fine-mesh gauze
   1% Silver sulfadiazine (Silvadene)
   Silver dressings (Acticoat, Silverlon)
   Antibiotic ointment (Bacitracin, Polysporin)
   Nonadhering dressing (Adaptic)
   Transparent wound dressing (Op-Site, Tegaderm)
   Biobrane
   Bismuth tribromophenate gauze (Xeroform)

PATIENT PREPARATION

1. Remove jewelry from affected extremity/area (see Procedures 114 and 115).
2. Apply a moist sterile dressing to the wound as soon as possible to stop the burning process. Do not apply ice to the wound.
3. If chemicals are involved, consult the Poison Control Center before initiating wound débridement. Most chemicals require a minimum of 20 minutes of fluid irrigation; additional therapy may be necessary.
4. Administer tetanus prophylaxis as indicated.
5. Administer analgesia as prescribed.

PROCEDURAL STEPS
Wound Débridement

1. Arrange and organize on a sterile towel all supplies, instruments, and medications before initiating wound care.
2. Don a sterile gown, mask, and gloves.
3. Using sterile saline and a cleansing solution, begin to wash the injured area gently. It may be less painful to begin in the center of the burn and work toward the margin. Use sterile gauze dressings or a soft, sterile surgical brush. Maintain a circular motion, and attempt to create a moderate amount of suds or foam.
4. Rinse with sterile saline, and repeat as often as necessary until the wound is thoroughly cleaned.
5. If a blister is ruptured, débride the tissue. Initial management of intact blisters remains controversial, and research is inconclusive. Intact blisters are associated with less pain than débrided blisters (Bethel & Krisanda, 2004). Most recommend that blisters on the palms or soles be left intact (Edlich et al., 2006). Consult with the attending physician regarding the management of blisters. Blisters may be managed in several ways:
   a. The blister may be left intact, allowing underlying wounds to heal spontaneously.
   b. The blister fluid may be aspirated with a needle and syringe, leaving the overlying tissue (roof) in place.
   c. Large blisters may be débrided, whereas small ones remain intact.
6. Do not shave the affected area (Bethel & Krisanda, 2004).
7. Using fine-tipped scissors and forceps, elevate loose, devitalized tissue and remove it.
8. Cool tar with cold water to limit tissue damage (Edlich et al., 2006). Remove tar with mineral oil, petroleum ointments, 2% to 3% lanolin, or a nonpolar

solvent such as Medi-sol (Honari, 2004). Additional agents include sunflower oil, butter, and baby oil (Edlich et al., 2006). Multiple applications and time frames of 30 minutes to 2 hours may be expected.

9. Continue the above-listed procedures until the area is clean, moist, and pink.

Wound Dressing

Wound dressings are designed to absorb drainage, provide protection, isolate the wound from the environment, and decrease pain. Wound dressings are used to cover the topical agents applied to the burn wound. In some cases, such as the face, the topical agent may be applied in an open fashion, and no dressing is placed over the top. The other method is the closed method, in which a dressing and bandage are placed over the topical agent. The open method is easy, decreases risk of infection, and avoids difficult dressing maneuvers. However, the open method may increase discomfort and heat loss and increase cross-contamination, and it may not be practical for a working or active individual. The closed method may be more practical and comfortable, aid in débridement, and help prevent infection. Dressings may include fine mesh followed by layers of 4 × 4 gauze.

Silver Sulfadiazine

1. Using a sterile gloved hand or a sterile tongue blade, apply a thin ($\frac{1}{16}$-inch), smooth layer of cream over the area. Fine-mesh gauze may also be impregnated with the silver sulfadiazine, which is then cut to the appropriate size and placed over the wound. This may be less painful to the patient than rubbing the cream directly on the wound.

2. If using the closed method, cover with a sterile gauze dressing and bandage. When bandaging the hand, wrap each digit individually, or place a layer of dressing between adjacent skin surfaces. Anchor as necessary.

Silver Dressings

1. Cut the dressing to the shape and size of the burn.
2. Moisten the dressing with sterile water—do not use saline (Smith & Nephew, n.d.).
3. Allow the dressing to drain on a sterile absorbent surface for at least 2 minutes (Smith & Nephew, n.d.).
4. Apply the dressing to the wound surface, either side down. A transient stinging sensation is expected when the dressing is applied.
5. Cover the dressing with a moist absorbent dressing created by saturating gauze with sterile water and wringing out the excess. Alternately, commercial gel pads are available to maintain a moist environment.
6. Cover with a sterile gauze dressing and bandage, and anchor as necessary.
7. Silver dressings can remain in place for 3 to 7 days—consult the manufacturer's recommendations for the specific dressing.
8. The dressing should be inspected periodically to ensure that it remains moist (Smith & Nephew, n.d.)

9. Follow manufacturer's instructions, some silver dressings may not be used during Magnetic Resonance Imaging (MRI) or while patient undergoes radiation therapy treatment (Smith & Nephew, n.d.)

Antibiotic Ointment

1. Apply a thin layer of ointment to the wound, and place a piece of nonadhering dressing over the area.
2. Cover with a sterile gauze dressing and bandage, and anchor as necessary.

Transparent Wound Dressing or Bismuth Tribromophenate Gauze

1. Using sterile technique, apply the appropriate size of dressing directly to the burn.
2. Leave a small (½-in) margin that can adhere to the nonburned skin.
3. Apply a gauze pressure dressing and bandage.

Biobrane

Biobrane is a synthetic skin substitute that consists of a flexible silicone-nylon membrane and bonded collagen peptides.

1. Apply Biobrane directly over the clean wound.
2. Use surgical tape closures or a gauze bandage to hold the Biobrane in place.

AGE-SPECIFIC CONSIDERATIONS

Young children and debilitated elderly patients are at risk for nonaccidental burns; carefully evaluate the history of the burn incident for the possibility of abuse. The following injuries should be viewed suspiciously: cigarette burns, circumferential burns of the extremities or the perineum suggestive of immersion (splash marks are usually absent), and burns in the shape of an object, such as an iron. Admission may be indicated to ensure a safe environment while the circumstances surrounding the injury are investigated.

COMPLICATIONS

1. Infection
2. Loss of function
3. Damage to newly formed epithelium and slowed healing as a result of removing a dressing too vigorously
4. Localized skin irritation, itching, or rash secondary to a topical agent

PATIENT TEACHING

1. Keep the bandage clean. Do not wash dishes, swim, or shower. If a silver dressing is used, moisten the dressing as directed.
2. Elevate burned extremities above the level of the heart for 24 to 48 hours after the burn.
3. If the bandage requires changing, remove it carefully and reapply. If it sticks to the skin, soak it in lukewarm water. Remove and pat dry with a clean towel.
4. Do not break any blisters.

5. If cream or ointment is used: clean the area once or twice a day with warm soapy water. Reapply a thin layer of the prescribed topical agent, cream, or ointment. Do not use the same tongue blade or sterile utensil to remove the cream once it has touched the burn. Use a new sterile tongue blade each time you open the cream. Dress and bandage as instructed.

6. If a clear dressing or Biobrane is used: trim the edges as they loosen.

7. Return for follow-up appointments as instructed (usually within 24 hours).

8. Increase fluid and protein intake to promote healing.

9. Gently move burned extremities through their range of motion several times a day.

10. Report the following signs or symptoms:
    a. Increased pain, swelling, redness, foul odor, or red streaks from the wound
    b. Fever greater than 38° C (100.4° F)
    c. Numbness or swelling distal to a joint or inability to move the joint

11. To prevent hyperpigmentation and repeat injury once the burn is healed, limit exposure to the sun and use sunscreen on the area for the next 6 to 12 months.

REFERENCES

American College of Surgeons, Committee on Trauma. (1999). *Resources for optimal care of the injured patient.* Chicago: Author.

Bethel, C. A., & Krisanda, T. J. (2004). Burn care procedures. In J. R. Roberts, & J. R. Hedges (Eds.), *Clinical procedures in emergency medicine* (4th ed., pp. 749-772). Philadelphia: Saunders.

Edlich, R. F., Bailey, R. F., & Long, W. B. (2006). Thermal burns. In J. A. Marx, R. S. Hockberger, & R. M. Walls, et al. (Eds.), *Rosen's emergency medicine: Concepts and clinical practice* (6th ed., pp. 913-929). St Louis: Mosby.

Honari, S. (2004). Topical therapies and antimicrobials in the management of burn wounds. *Critical Care Nursing Clinics of North America, 16,* 1-11.

Smith & Nephew. (n.d.). *Acticoat∗3 antimicrobial dressing: Instructions for use.* Retrieved March 10, 2007, from http://wound.smith-nephew.com/us/Product.asp?NodeId=3287&Tab=5&Hide=

Escharotomy

Joni Hentzen Daniels, MSN, RN, CEN, CCRN

Escharotomies are not commonly performed in the emergency department but may be necessary in the critically burned patient before admission or transfer. Eschar is tough and rigid tissue that forms as a result of thermal or chemical burns. As edema forms in the injured extremity after the burn, the eschar restricts outward expansion of the tissue. The outcome is increased interstitial pressure that rises to the point that vascular flow is compromised (Edlich, Bailey, & Long, 2006). In short, the eschar behaves like a tourniquet. Incising the eschar allows return of flow and prevents further ischemic injury.

INDICATIONS

To decrease elevated intrathoracic or tissue pressure in the presence of:
1. Circumferential full-thickness burns to the chest, which mechanically constrict and compromise respirations.
2. Circumferential or electrical burns to the extremities causing loss of distal pulses, impaired capillary filling, paresthesias or motor weakness, cyanosis of distal uninjured skin, or tense edema with rigid muscle compartments (Bethel & Krisanda, 2004; Edlich et al., 2006) (Figure 145-1).
3. Loss of distal Doppler pulses (see Procedure 49) indicates the need for escharotomy of the extremity.
4. Tissue pressure exceeding 30 mm Hg, which indicates a need for escharotomy or fasciotomy (Bethel & Krisanda, 2004) (see Procedure 130).

CONTRAINDICATIONS AND CAUTIONS

1. Failure to perform emergency escharotomy may result in the inability to ventilate lung parenchyma, loss of neuromuscular function, or ischemic tissue injury (Edlich et al., 2006).
2. This procedure may cause significant blood loss in the patient already predisposed to hypovolemic shock or altered coagulation.
3. These new open wounds further predispose the patient to infection and sepsis.
4. Underlying tissues may be damaged if procedures are incorrectly performed.
5. If compartmental pressures do not decrease after escharotomy, a fasciotomy must be performed in the operating room.
6. Improper technique or locations of the incisions may damage nerves (Bethel & Krisanda, 2004).
7. Prophylactic antibiotics are strongly discouraged to prevent the development of resistant bacterial strains.

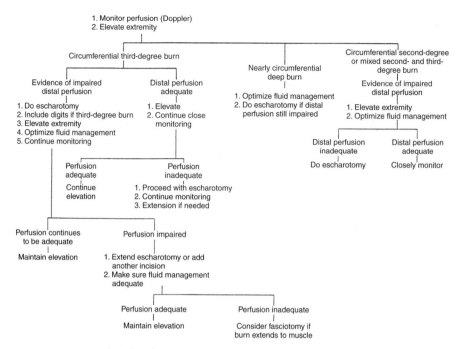

FIGURE 145-1 Algorithm for escharotomies of extremity burns. (From Demling, R. F., & Lalonde, C. [1989]. *Burn trauma* [p. 63]. New York: Thieme Medical Publishers.)

EQUIPMENT

Sterile gown, mask, and gloves for all team members

Local anesthetic infiltration (optional in deep, insensate burns)

Intracompartmental pressure monitor (may not be used in emergency situations)

Doppler to assess pulses

Sterile drapes

Sterile scalpel (coagulating or cutting device may be preferable)

Cautery, thrombin, and hemostats

Sterile dressing and bandages

Antimicrobial creams

PATIENT PREPARATION

1. Remove all constricting clothing and jewelry (see Procedures 114 and 115).
2. Elevate the burned extremity slightly above the level of the heart.
3. Administer analgesics and sedatives as prescribed.
4. Administer tetanus prophylaxis as indicated.
5. Place the patient in a supine anatomic position, unless contraindicated by other injuries or conditions.

PROCEDURAL STEPS

1. Drape below and around the surgical area.

2. *Anesthetize with local anesthetic infiltration or regional nerve block (see Procedures 135 and 136).
3. *Incise indicated areas:
   a. Chest: Along the anterior axillary aspects of the chest extending from the clavicle to the costal margin (Figure 145-2). Make a second incision transverse across the chest at the level of the diaphragm. Cut through the eschar but not into the subcutaneous tissue (Bethel & Krisanda, 2004). The incision should cause the eschar to gap, thus releasing pressure.
   b. Neck: Posteriorly and laterally to avoid major vessels in the neck.
   c. Upper extremities: Medial and lateral aspects of arms avoiding the radial nerve (Figures 145-3 and 145-4).
   d. Hands: Dorsal aspect of the hands and along the palmar crease (see Figure 145-4) and medial and lateral aspects of the digits (Figure 145-5).
   e. Legs: Midmedial and midlateral incisions; toes in a similar manner to the fingers (see Figure 145-3).
4. Reassess respiratory function and distal circulatory status.
5. *Apply direct pressure, cautery, clamps, or thrombin to all bleeding areas.
6. Reassess hematocrit, and consider blood administration if necessary.
7. Apply dressings to reduce the potential for infection. See Procedure 144 for dressing options.
8. Keep the affected extremities elevated, and monitor distal pulses frequently.

---

*Indicates portions of the procedure usually performed by a physician or an advanced practice nurse.

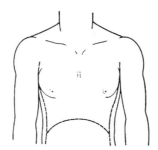

FIGURE 145-2 Chest escharotomy sites. (From Mlcak, R. P., & Buffalo, M. C. [2002]. Pre-hospital management, transportation and emergency care. In D. N. Herndon (Ed.), *Total burn care* [p. 69]. Philadelphia: Saunders.)

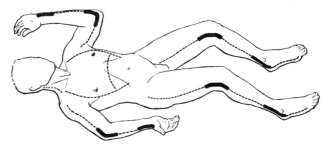

FIGURE 145-3 Extremity escharotomy sites. (From Davis, J. H., Foster, R. S., & Drucker, W. K. [1995]. *Surgery: A problem-solving approach* [2nd ed., p. 651]. St Louis: Mosby.)

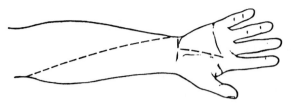

FIGURE 145-4 Arm and hand escharotomy sites. (From Edlich, R. F., Bailey, R. F., & Bill, T. J. [2002]. Thermal burns. In J. A. Marx, R. S. Hockberger, R. M. Walls, et al. (Eds.), *Rosen's emergency medicine: Concepts and clinical practice* [5th ed., p. 810]. St Louis: Mosby.)

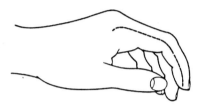

FIGURE 145-5 Escharotomy on a finger. (From Mlcak, R. P., & Buffalo, M. C. [2002]. Pre-hospital management, transportation and emergency care. In D. N. Herndon [Ed.], *Total burn care* [p. 69]. Philadelphia: Saunders.)

COMPLICATIONS
1. Wound infection
2. Sepsis
3. Blood loss
4. Nerve or vessel damage
5. Inadequate decompression may lead to tissue necrosis, myoglobinuria, renal failure, hyperkalemia, and acidosis (Bethel & Krisanda, 2004).

PATIENT TEACHING
1. This procedure will decrease the pain as it relieves the tissue pressure.
2. Care will be taken to help these wounds heal with as little scarring as possible.

REFERENCES
Bethel, C. A., & Krisanda, T. J. (2004). Burn care procedures. In J. R. Roberts, & J. R. Hedges (Eds.), *Clinical procedures in emergency medicine* (4th ed., pp. 749-772). Philadelphia: Saunders.

Edlich, R. F., Bailey, R. F., & Long, W. B. (2006). Thermal burns. In J. A. Marx, R. S. Hockberger, & R. M. Walls, et al. (Eds.), *Rosen's emergency medicine: Concepts and clinical practice* (6th ed., pp. 913-929). St Louis: Mosby.

Incision and Drainage

Margo E. Layman, MSN, RN, RNC, CN-A

Incision and drainage is also known as *I & D*.

INDICATIONS

1. To drain localized infections, such as sebaceous cysts, subungual abscesses, and carbuncles.
2. To remove foreign objects from soft tissue.

CONTRAINDICATIONS AND CAUTIONS

1. Patients with poor hygiene, malnutrition, diabetes, and immune deficiencies require careful techniques and follow-up.
2. Patients with bleeding disorders should be referred to a surgeon.
3. Consultation with a specialist should be considered for deep or anatomically complex abscesses and those on the hands, feet, or face.
4. Abscesses in some areas are close to major vessels and should be aspirated with a needle and syringe to rule out mycotic aneurysm before any attempt at I & D. The high-risk body areas for this are the anterior triangle of the neck (bordered by the sternocleidomastoid muscle, the mandible, and the anterior midline of the neck), supraclavicular fossa, deep axilla, antecubital space, groin, and popliteal space (Gutman, 2004).
5. Abscesses may be difficult to anesthetize adequately, and drainage in the operating room may be indicated (Gutman, 2004).

EQUIPMENT

Antiseptic solution
Irrigating solution (sterile saline)
Local anesthetic
Syringes and needles for local anesthetic and Irrigation
¼- or ½-in iodoform or plain sterile gauze packing
Sterile rubber bands or penrose drains
Sterile drapes
4 × 4 gauze dressings
Adhesive tape
Hydrogen peroxide (optional)
No. 11 scalpel
Hemostat (curved or straight)
Plain forceps
Surgical scissors
Cotton swabs
Culture collection supplies for aerobic and anaerobic specimens

PATIENT PREPARATION

1. Drape the area with waterproof drapes.
2. Clip the hair the area as indicated.
3. Cleanse the area with antiseptic solution with firm, circular scrubbing motions from the abscess outward.
4. *Anesthetize the area with local anesthetic (see Procedure 135). Intravenous analgesia and sedation may be necessary for large or deep abscesses (see Procedure 177).

PROCEDURAL STEPS

1. *Incise the periphery of the abscess cavity with the scalpel; purulent material is expressed immediately (Figure 146-1).
2. *Disrupt adhesions with a hemostat.
3. Obtain anaerobic and aerobic cultures from the drainage.
4. Cleanse the cavity with cotton swabs and then irrigate with sterile saline solution (see Procedure 134).
5. *Pack the wound loosely with plain or iodoform gauze strip leaving 1 cm of gauze exiting from the cavity. This packing keeps the wound open and permits drainage (Figure 146-2).
6. *Insert a sterile rubber band or penrose drain appropriate for size of abscess, allowing end to extrude from wound at least one centimeter. This keeps the wound open and permits drainage.
7. Apply a sterile dressing, and secure with adhesive tape.

AGE-SPECIFIC CONSIDERATION

Children may require sedation in addition to local anesthesia (see Procedure 177).

---

*Indicates portions of the procedure usually performed by a physician or an advanced practice nurse.

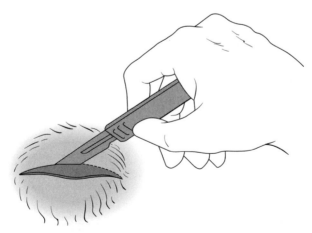

FIGURE 146-1 Incision of an abscess.

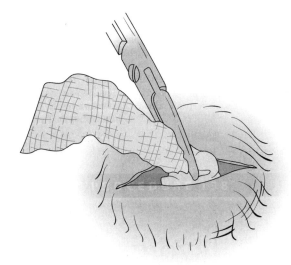

FIGURE 146-2 Gauze packing is packed loosely into the incised wound using a hemostat.

COMPLICATIONS

1. Reoccurrence of the abscess
2. Spread of the infection, especially in the perineal and rectal areas
3. Systemic infection or sepsis
4. Injury to nearby vessels or nerves
5. Scarring depending on size of abscess

PATIENT TEACHING

1. Leave dressing in place for 24 hours, unless it becomes soiled with excessive drainage; then it can be changed.
2. In 24 hours, remove the external dressing, and leave the packing in place.
3. Follow-up with the physician in 2 days to have packing or drain removed.
4. After packing or drain is removed, soak the site 20 to 30 minutes in warm water three to four times a day.
5. Continue to soak for 5 to 7 days or until the incision has healed. Redress the incision with a clean dressing after each soaking.
6. Watch for signs of ongoing or worsening infection, such as redness, swelling, draining pus, and fever.

REFERENCE

Gutman, S. J. (2004). Subcutaneous abscess incision and drainage. In E. F. Reichman, & R. R. Simon (Eds.), *Emergency medicine procedures* (pp. 812-820). New York: McGraw-Hill.

Thermoregulation

Measures to Reverse Hyperthermia

Daun A. Smith, RN, MSN, and
Jean A. Proehl, RN, MN, CEN, CCRN, FAEN

INDICATION

To lower body temperature to 39° C (102° F) or less through rapid cooling in patients whose temperatures are greater than 40.5° C (105° F). Hyperthermia may result from fever, heatstroke, metabolic disorders, thermoregulatory dysfunction, medications (e.g., malignant hyperthermia, neuroleptic malignant syndrome [NMS]), or drugs of abuse (cocaine, amphetamine derivatives) (Erickson & Prendergast, 2004). The best treatment is prevention—providing proper clothing, administering fluid and salt replacement, or moving to a cool, shady environment.

CONTRAINDICATIONS AND CAUTIONS

1. Cooling must be initiated immediately on the discovery of a hyperthermic state and must proceed rapidly. For a successful outcome, temperatures must be decreased to 39° C (102° F) or below within 1 hour of initiating treatment (Erickson & Prendergast, 2004).
2. Antipyretics are ineffective in lowering the body temperature and may result in additional complications, such as coagulopathy and hepatic damage (Erickson & Prendergast, 2004).
3. Initial diagnosis is often difficult. Early symptoms of significant heat illness are usually nonspecific (drowsiness, confusion, headache) and may be overlooked or attributed to other causes. The key to diagnosis is a history of a related incident (Schmidt & Nichols, 2005).
4. Do not sponge the patient with alcohol because it may be absorbed transcutaneously with resultant toxicity (Hadad Rav-Acha, Heled, Epstein, & Moran, 2004).

EQUIPMENT

Ice packs
Ice water
Spray or misting bottle
Large circulating fans
Bathtub or wash basin
Cooling blanket
Peritoneal lavage equipment
Temperature probe for continuous monitoring (rectal, bladder, or esophageal)

Cooled intravenous fluids (place the bags in an ice water slurry for 15 to 20 minutes)

PATIENT PREPARATION

1. Place the patient on high-flow oxygen because oxygen demand is increased in the hyperthermic state (see Procedure 25). Using *cool* aerosol mist may moderate body temperature and minimize fluid loss due to rapid respiratory rate.
2. Initiate an intravenous line to restore intravascular volume (see Procedure 60).
3. Initiate additional resuscitative efforts as indicated.
4. Place the patient on a cardiac monitor because nonspecific ST-segment changes, conduction disturbances, and ventricular arrhythmias have been reported during cooling (see Procedure 55).
5. Draw blood for complete blood count, potassium, sodium, phosphorus, calcium, magnesium, prothrombin time and partial thromboplastin time, blood urea nitrogen, glucose, creatinine, liver function tests, and creatine phosphokinase determinations (see Procedure 58).
6. Remove all of the patient's clothing.
7. Establish continuous temperature monitoring. Urinary bladder, rectal, or esophageal probes are options. Check the rectum for stool before placement of a rectal probe; if the probe is placed in feces, the reading is inaccurate.
8. Obtain a baseline 12-lead electrocardiogram (see Procedure 56).
9. Insert a urinary bladder catheter to monitor fluid output (see Procedure 104).

PROCEDURAL STEPS

A variety of modalities may be used for rapid cooling, depending on the patient's condition, the availability of resources, and the institutional protocols. The most effective are evaporative cooling or immersion in ice water (Erickson & Prendergast, 2004). Options include the following:

1. Evaporative cooling. Cover the patient with wet towels or spray the patient with water while circulating air around the patient with large fans to promote heat loss through evaporation. The latter method is preferred because of rapid heat loss, availability of supplies, and easy access to the patient.
2. Immersion in ice water is effective but logistically more difficult and adds the danger of injury or airway hazard because of the patient's altered mental status in circumstances where rescue is hampered. Also, while the body heat is transferred to the cooler water, the coolness may induce peripheral vasoconstriction that shunts blood flow to the body core lowering the rate of transfer. Sponging the patient with ice water may be tried initially. If initial cooling efforts are not rapidly effective, ice water immersion may be undertaken.
3. Cover the patient with a cooling blanket (controversial and slow) (see Procedure 151).
4. Apply ice packs to the neck, axilla, and inguinal area. Place a dry interface between the skin and the cold pack. Monitor the underlying skin for cold injury. This method is less effective than immersion in ice water.
5. Administer dantrolene as prescribed for malignant hyperthermia or NMS. Dantrolene is not effective in environmental hyperthermia.

6. Internal methods of cooling may be necessary in the patient with severe hyperthermia or who does not respond to external methods. Internal methods include cold peritoneal lavage (see Procedure 95), cold gastric lavage (see Procedure 99), and cardiopulmonary bypass (Vicario, 2006).
7. Stop cooling at 39° C (102.2° F) because the body temperature continues to drift downward, and hypothermia may result if cooling measures are continued beyond this point.

AGE-SPECIFIC CONSIDERATIONS

1. Both the elderly and the very young are at risk for classic hyperthermia because of decreased thermoregulatory functioning. The elderly have a relative inability to adapt to environmental temperatures, a decreased ability to perspire, and other chronic medical conditions that affect their ability to acclimate to warmer temperatures. Dependent elderly persons are at increased risk due to inadequate fluid intake, poor ability to make their needs known, and medicines that inhibit thermoregulation. Institutionalized elderly persons at facilities with high staffing ratios or staff shortage are especially at risk. The very young have a shorter stature, placing them closer to radiated heat from asphalt or cement; have fewer sweat glands; and are more easily dehydrated.
2. Young adults (e.g., athletes, outdoor laborers, military personnel) are at risk for exertional hyperthermia. Education on prevention and early treatment should be provided to leaders of such groups. During periods of unusual heat stress weather, public service announcements should be made regarding prevention, early treatment, and EMS access.
3. Patients taking psychotropic medicines and anticholinergics are at risk for impaired thermoregulation.

COMPLICATIONS

1. Violent shivering with rapid cooling, which may result in further heat production. Shivering can be controlled by the use of benzodiazepines (Erickson & Prendergast, 2004).
2. Hypotension
3. Acute renal failure
4. Metabolic acidosis
5. Increased serum potassium
6. Frostbite caused by ice packs
7. Rhabdomyolysis in severe exertional hyperthermia
8. Disseminated intravascular coagulation
9. Hypothermia from overly vigorous cooling
10. Aspiration (gastric lavage)

PATIENT TEACHING

Patients who have experienced hyperthermic episodes are predisposed to future recurrences. Instruct the patient on prevention strategies, as indicated by the cause of this episode:

- Awareness of environmental temperature and humidity
- The importance of staying in a cool environment
- Adequate fluid intake

- Avoiding extreme exertion during the hottest times of the day or in extreme weather
- Frequent rest breaks
- Proper conditioning

REFERENCES

Erickson, T., & Prendergast, H. (2004). Procedures pertaining to hypothermia. In J. R. Roberts, & J. R. Hedges (Eds.), *Clinical procedures in emergency medicine* (4th ed., pp. 1343-1357). Philadelphia: Saunders.

Hadad, E., Rav-Acha, M., Heled, Y., Epstein, Y., & Moran, D. S. (2004). Heat stroke: A review of cooling methods. *Sports Medicine, 34,* 501-511.

Schmidt, E. W., & Nichols, C. G. (2005). Heat-related illness. In A. B. Wolfson (Ed.), *Harwood-Nuss' clinical practice of emergency medicine* (4th ed., pp. 1757-1760). Philadelphia: Lippincott Williams & Wilkins.

Vicario, S. (2006). Heat illness. In J. Marx, R. S. Hockberger, & R. M. Walls (Eds.), *Rosen's emergency medicine: Concepts and clinical practice* (6th ed., pp. 2254-2267). St. Louis: Mosby.

PROCEDURE 148

Measures to Reverse Hypothermia

Daun A. Smith, RN, MSN, and
Jean A. Proehl, RN, MN, CEN, CCRN, FAEN

INDICATION

To increase the core temperature in patients with temperatures less than 35° C (95° F) because of a decrease in heat production, an increase in heat loss, a combination of both, or an impaired thermoregulatory system. Rewarming should continue until the patient's core temperature is 35° C (95° F).

CONTRAINDICATIONS AND CAUTIONS

1. Hypothermia creates myocardial irritability, so patients must be handled gently and procedures performed cautiously because stimulation may precipitate ventricular fibrillation. The risk is highest at temperatures below 29° C (85.2° F) (AHA, 2005; Chang, 2005).

2. With active external rewarming, patients may experience rewarming shock, which is evidenced by a decrease in blood pressure resulting from vasodilation in previously vasoconstricted extremities.

3. With active external rewarming, patients may experience a temperature afterdrop, which results from the shunting of cold blood from extremities to the core, which further chills the myocardium and increases the potential for ventricular fibrillation. This phenomenon occurs infrequently and appears to be of little clinical significance (Ulrich & Rathlev, 2004).

4. Medications must be used judiciously because most drugs have little effect on the hypothermic patient and may cause complications on rewarming because of delayed metabolism of drugs (e.g., metabolic alkalosis with sodium bicarbonate, hypoglycemia with insulin).

5. Skin should not be massaged or rubbed, and alcohol should not be used on the skin of hypothermic patients; these techniques increase vasodilation and move cold blood from the extremities to the core.

6. Attempts at defibrillation are usually unsuccessful until core temperature is above 28° to 30° C (82° to 86° F) (Chang, 2005). The American Heart Association suggests that with severe hypothermia, defibrillation should be attempted once and then active internal rewarming should be instituted (AHA, 2005).

EQUIPMENT

Cardiac monitor
Pulse oximeter
Warm intravenous (IV) solution (37.7° C [100° F])
IV fluid warmers
IV tubing
Warm normal saline for irrigation
Radiant warming lights
Heating pads
Hot water bottles
Forced air warming blanket
Cascade nebulizer or similar equipment to administer heated, humidified oxygen
Peritoneal lavage equipment
Urinary bladder catheter
Hemodialysis equipment
Cardiac bypass equipment
Gastric lavage equipment
Pleural lavage equipment
Hypothermia thermometer (capability to measure temperatures less than 34.4° C (94° F)

PATIENT PREPARATION

1. Remove the patient from the cold or wet environment. Remove all clothing, dry the patient, and place the patient on a stretcher covered with sheets or blankets to prevent heat loss via conduction. Long hair should be dried or positioned away from the patient's head.

2. Initiate resuscitation as indicated for the patient in cardiac arrest. Endotracheal intubation is necessary unless the patient is alert and has intact protective airway reflexes. Preoxygenate the patient before intubation to avoid dysrhythmias. Factors precipitating dysrhythmias during intubation are rough technique, hypoxia, and acid-base abnormalities (Chang, 2005; Erickson & Prendergast, 2004).
3. Establish continuous temperature monitoring. Urinary bladder, rectal, or esophageal probes are options. Check the rectum for stool before placement of a rectal probe; if the probe is placed in feces, the reading is inaccurate.
4. Apply the cardiac monitor for ongoing assessment during the rewarming procedures (see Procedure 55).
5. Obtain a baseline 12-lead electrocardiogram (see Procedure 56).
6. Perform a bedside blood glucose test (see Procedure 59). Obtain blood for complete blood count, arterial blood gases (uncorrected for temperature) (see Procedure 19), potassium, glucose, calcium, magnesium, prothrombin time and partial thromboplastin time, fibrinogen, fibrin split products, amylase, lipase, blood urea nitrogen, and creatinine determinations (see Procedure 58).

PROCEDURAL STEPS

There are three methods of rewarming: passive external rewarming (PER), active external rewarming (AER), and active core rewarming (ACR). The recommended rewarming methods are as follows (AHA, 2005; Ulrich & Rathlev, 2004):

Mild hypothermia	34° to 36° C (93.2° to 96.8° F)	PER, AER
Moderate hypothermia	30° to 34° C (86° to 93.2° F)	PER, AER (truncal areas only)
Severe hypothermia	Below 30° C (86° F)	ACR

Passive External Rewarming (PER)

1. Cover the patient with blankets to prevent heat loss from radiation and convection. Be sure to cover the head because a significant amount of heat is lost from an uncovered head.
2. If IV fluids are indicated, they should be warmed before administration to assist with rewarming and prevent further heat loss.

Active External Rewarming (AER)

The current recommendation is to heat only the thorax during AER of the moderately hypothermic patient and leave the extremities unheated to allow for the maintenance of peripheral vasoconstriction, thus preventing temperature afterdrop and rewarming shock (Chang, 2005).

1. Cover the patient with warm, electric blankets or a forced air warming blanket (see Procedures 150 and 151).
2. Place heated objects (e.g., heating pads, hot water bottles) in the groin or axilla or on the trunk.
3. Use overhead radiant warming lights (see Procedure 149).

Active Core Rewarming (ACR)

1. Infuse IV fluid warmed to 37.7° to 43° C (100° to 109° F) (see Procedure 75) (AHA, 2005). Warmed IV fluid alone is not enough to rewarm the patient; it must be used in conjunction with other therapies.
2. Administer warm, humidified oxygen via a cascade nebulizer or similar device. Warmed oxygen alone is not enough to rewarm the patient; it must be used in conjunction with other therapies. However, it should be begun immediately as it is quick and easy to set-up and pulmonary blood goes directly to the heart making this an important therapy.
3. Perform peritoneal lavage with fluid warmed to 40° to 45° C (105° to 113° F) to conduct heat directly through the intraperitoneal structures, posterior parietal peritoneum to the kidneys, and diaphragm to the heart and lungs. Two catheters may be inserted to allow concomitant infusion and drainage (see Procedure 95). Two liters are infused, allowed to dwell for 20 to 30 minutes, and then drained. Peritoneal dialysis exacerbates hypokalemia, and potassium supplementation of the dialysis fluid may be necessary (Erickson & Prendergast, 2004).
4. Initiate extracorporeal blood warming via continuous arteriovenous rewarming with a Level 1 fluid warmer (see Procedure 152) or cardiac bypass equipment in the operating room.
5. Perform warmed mediastinal or pleural irrigation via thoracotomy (usually performed in the operating room) (see Procedure 54).
6. Initiate hemodialysis with 40° to 45° C (104° to 113° F) fluid.
7. Perform warmed lavage of the stomach or rectum (see Procedure 99). Gastric and rectal lavage may deliver less heat than peritoneal lavage but are easier to perform. There is a risk of electrolyte imbalance and aspiration with gastric lavage (Erickson & Prendergast, 2004).

AGE-SPECIFIC CONSIDERATIONS

1. Infants are particularly susceptible to the development of hypothermia because of their lack of subcutaneous fat and larger body surface area–to–mass ratio, which allows for greater heat loss; because of their rapid metabolic rate; and because they are less able to regulate and generate their own heat. They may easily exhaust their glucose and glycogen stores when hypothermic so blood glucose should be monitored and supplemental glucose administered as indicated.
2. Elderly individuals have a lower metabolic rate and reduced muscle mass and subcutaneous tissue and have difficulty maintaining a normal body temperature when ambient temperatures fall. The aging process also lowers the ability to sense temperature changes; therefore, older individuals may not be aware of the need for countermeasures (i.e., warmer clothing, shelter) (Neno, 2005).

COMPLICATIONS

1. Ventricular fibrillation from rough handling or stimulation associated with procedures (AHA, 2005)
2. Rewarming shock associated with active external rewarming in severely hypothermic patients (AHA, 2005)

3. Burns as a result of heating devices in direct contact with the skin (which is poorly perfused in hypothermia) or using a warm air discharge hose under the patient's blankets without using the appropriate diffusion blanket (e.g., BAIR Hugger). Insensate patients, such as those with spinal cord injury, para/quadraplegia, or large burn or scar areas, will be unable to sense skin injury and may be relatively poikilothermic, poorly able to regulate their temperature with their skin, and very responsive to ambient temperature.
4. Complications of hypothermia include coagulopathies, pneumonia, pulmonary edema, thrombosis, decreased peripheral perfusion, and tissue ischemia (Erickson & Prendergast, 2004).

PATIENT TEACHING

Patients who have experienced accidental hypothermia should be instructed in how to prevent future episodes:

- Recognition of early symptoms (shivering, lethargy, confusion, loss of coordination)
- Appropriate clothing for the environment (including the importance of wearing a hat)
- Dangerous effects of alcohol and other intoxicants.

REFERENCES

American Heart Association (AHA). (2005). 2005 Guidelines for cardiopulmonary resuscitation and emergency cardiovascular care. *Circulation, 112,* IV.

Chang, A. K. (2005). Hypothermia. In A. B. Wolfson (Ed.), *Harwood-Nuss' clinical practice of emergency medicine* (4th ed., pp. 1749-1752). Philadelphia: Lippincott Williams & Wilkins.

Erickson, T., & Prendergast, H. (2004). Procedures pertaining to hypothermia. In J. R. Roberts, & J. R. Hedges (Eds.), *Clinical procedures in emergency medicine* (4th ed., pp. 1343-1357). Philadelphia: Saunders.

Neno, R. (2005). Hypothermia: Assessment, treatment, and prevention. *Nursing Standard, 19,* 47-52.

Ulrich, A. S., & Rathlev, N. K. (2004). Hypothermia and localized cold injuries. *Emergency Medicine Clinics of North America, 22,* 281-298.

Heat Lamp

Daun A. Smith, RN, MSN

INDICATIONS

1. To provide direct transfer of exogenous heat (active external rewarming) to a patient who is hypothermic. See Procedure 148 for further information on management of hypothermia.
2. To maintain body temperature and prevent hypothermia in patients undergoing resuscitation who are at high risk for hypothermia.

CONTRAINDICATIONS AND CAUTIONS

1. Frequent temperature assessment is necessary to identify hypothermia or hyperthermia that adversely affects oxygen consumption and metabolic function.
2. Caution must be exercised to avoid thermal burns to poorly perfused and vasoconstricted skin when using heat lamps.
3. External rewarming measures (e.g., heat lamps, warmed blankets, forced warm air units, water bottles) should be used in conjunction with active core rewarming measures (e.g., peritoneal lavage, warm intravenous fluids) in patients with core temperatures less than 30° C (86° F) (Erickson & Prendergast, 2004).

EQUIPMENT

Heat lamp
Light sheet or blanket
Measuring stick or tape

PATIENT PREPARATION

1. Remove any wet, frozen, or heavy clothing from the patient. Cover the patient with a light sheet or blanket for privacy.
2. Initiate cardiac monitoring because hypothermia may lower the threshold for dysrhythmias including ventricular fibrillation (see Procedure 55).

PROCEDURAL STEPS

1. Place the heat lamp over the thorax. If the heat lamp is focused only on the extremities, active external rewarming is not as effective.
2. Place the heat lamp at least 3 feet (0.91 meter) from the patient to avoid burns and skin irritation.
3. Duration of patient exposure to the heat lamp should be kept to a maximum of 5-minute intervals to avoid burns and skin irritation. Many lamps have a timer for this purpose.

AGE-SPECIFIC CONSIDERATIONS

1. Tables with thermostatically controlled overhead warming units are available for temperature resuscitation of the neonate. Be sure to follow the manufacturer's recommendations for correct positioning and shielding of the patient's sensor, to accurately servo-control the temperature and avoid error due to absorption of the radiant energy.
2. Neonates, infants, small children, and elders are at risk for iatrogenic hypothermia during resuscitative efforts; a heat lamp may be used to prevent hypothermia in these circumstances.

COMPLICATIONS

1. Temperature afterdrop (decreased core temperature when cold blood returns from the extremities)
2. Shock resulting from peripheral vasodilation with active external rewarming
3. Burns or skin irritation

PATIENT TEACHING

Patients who have experienced accidental hypothermia should be instructed in how to prevent future episodes:

- Recognition of early symptoms (shivering, lethargy, confusion, loss of coordination)
- Appropriate clothing for the environment (including the importance of wearing a hat)
- The dangerous effects of alcohol and other intoxicants

REFERENCE

Erickson, T., & Prendergast, H. (2004). Procedures pertaining to hypothermia. In J. R. Roberts, & J. R. Hedges (Eds.), *Clinical procedures in emergency medicine* (4th ed., pp. 1343-1357). Philadelphia: Saunders.

Forced Air Warming Blanket

Daun A. Smith, RN, MSN

A forced air warming blanket is also known as a *Bair Hugger®*.

INDICATION

To accomplish active external rewarming by passing heated air across the skin. Forced air rewarming is an effective method of active external rewarming. See Procedure 148 for further information on the management of hypothermia.

CONTRAINDICATIONS AND CAUTIONS

1. The patient's temperature should be monitored continuously or at least every 10 to 20 minutes.
2. When desired temperature goal is reached (37° C [98.6° F]), air temperature should be reduced or use of the warming blanket discontinued.
3. Patients with poor perfusion should be monitored closely during prolonged warming therapy because thermal injury may occur if heat is applied to poorly perfused areas. High temperatures should be avoided in this setting.
4. Active external rewarming is not recommended for severely hypothermic patients. See Procedure 148 for alternative warming methods.
5. Do not use the open hose end under ordinary blankets, it may cause burns. Always use the appropriate diffusing blanket from the manufacturer (Arizant Healthcare, 2005).
6. To avoid fires, be careful if oxygen is given to avoid accumulation under the blankets and use of cautery or other combustive sources.
7. Do not use a warming blanket over transdermal medication patches as increased drug delivery with adverse reactions may occur (Arizant Healthcare, 2005).

EQUIPMENT

Bath blanket
Forced air warming unit
Forced air warming blanket

PATIENT PREPARATION

Remove all clothing, sheets, and blankets from the top of the patient.

PROCEDURAL STEPS

1. Place the blanket with the perforated side toward the patient.
2. Insert the end of the hose of the forced air warming unit into the opening for the hose on the blanket, using a twisting motion to seat it securely (Figure 150-1).
3. Plug in the warming unit to a properly grounded power source.

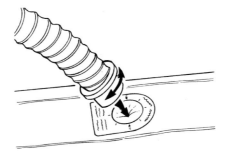

FIGURE 150-1 Insert the hose from the warming unit into the warming blanket. (Courtesy Mallinckrodt Medical Inc., Critical Care Division [1997], St. Louis, MO.)

4. Press the on button and select the appropriate temperature setting.
5. Place a bath blanket over the warming blanket to prevent warm air from escaping (Figure 150-2).
6. Assess the skin regularly for any sign of thermal injury.

AGE-SPECIFIC CONSIDERATIONS

1. Do not leave infants or small children unattended while a warming blanket is in use because of the risk of suffocation.
2. The very young and the elderly are at increased risk of thermal injury, monitor their skin carefully.

COMPLICATIONS

1. Thermal burns
2. Hyperthermia
3. Rewarming shock or temperature after drop secondary to peripheral vasodilation (in severely hypothermic patients)

PATIENT TEACHING

1. Recognize early signs of hypothermia (lethargy, incoordination, confusion).
2. Wear appropriate clothing for the weather.

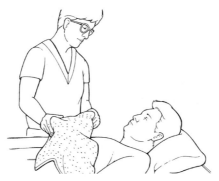

FIGURE 150-2 Cover the warming blanket with a bath blanket. (Courtesy Mallinckrodt Medical Inc., Critical Care Division [1997], St. Louis, MO.)

3. Drugs and intoxicants predispose to heat loss by vasodilation and a decreased perception of cold.

REFERENCE

Arizant Healthcare. (2005). *Bair Hugger Model 505 Temperature Management System: Operator's manual.* Eden Prairie, MN: Author. Retrieved February 17, 2007, from http://www.arizanthealthcare.com/arizant/manuals/200977C.pdf

---

PROCEDURE 151

Warm/Cool Water– Circulating Blankets

Daun A. Smith, RN, MSN

INDICATION

Warm/cool water–circulating blankets are used to actively rewarm hypothermic patients or to cool hyperthermic patients. Water is heated/cooled and pumped through coils in waterproof rubber or plastic mats that are placed under and/or over the patient.

See Procedure 148 for further information about the management of hypothermia and Procedure 147 for the management of hyperthermic patients.

CONTRAINDICATIONS AND CAUTIONS

1. Do not place any other heating sources between the patient and the warm/cool water–circulating blanket.
2. Prevent prolonged or excessive tissue pressure, especially over bony prominences, to prevent injury to hypothermic, poorly perfused skin.
3. The area between the patient and the blanket should be kept dry.
4. Active external rewarming is not recommended for severely hypothermic patients. Use alternative internal warming methods (see Procedure 148).

EQUIPMENT

Warming/cooling unit/console with blanket(s)
Sheets or bath blankets

Equipment to monitor temperature (rectal, skin, or esophageal probe for continuous monitoring is preferred)

PATIENT PREPARATION

1. Obtain baseline assessments of vital signs, level of consciousness, skin integrity and color, and initiate cardiac monitoring (see Procedure 55).
2. Moisturizing cream may be applied to the exposed skin.
3. Position the temperature probe (rectal, skin, or esophageal) per manufacturer's instructions if automatic mode will be used (see step 6 below).

PROCEDURAL STEPS

1. Check blanket and tubing for leaks or kinks.
2. Check water level in the warming/cooling console. Add sterile or distilled water if necessary.
3. Place one warming/cooling blanket under the patient with a bath blanket or sheet between the patient and the warming/cooling blanket. The tubing should be positioned toward the warming/cooling console.
4. Cover the patient with a bath blanket or sheet and a second warming/cooling blanket (if prescribed).
5. Connect the blanket tubing to the warming/cooling console and turn it on.
6. Choose manual or automatic mode. Temperature choice is governed by the mode chosen. In the manual mode, the selected temperature regulates the warmth or the coolness of the blanket. In automatic mode, the selected temperature is the desired patient temperature. Do not use a temperature probe when using the manual mode. In automatic mode, a temperature probe is required (Kelly, 2005).
7. Cover the hypothermic patient's head with a warm towel or blanket to prevent heat loss.
8. Assess vital signs, cardiac rhythm, and level of consciousness frequently (every 15 to 30 minutes or more often, as indicated by the patient's condition).
9. Turn the patient for skin assessment and care hourly (Kelly, 2005).

AGE-SPECIFIC CONSIDERATIONS

1. Young children and the elderly may have impaired thermoregulation and should be monitored closely during rewarming or cooling.
2. These devices are somewhat heavy and may impede respiratory effort when placed on the chest/abdomen of an infant or a small child.
3. The elderly are at increased risk for skin breakdown.

COMPLICATIONS

1. Inability to rewarm or cool the patient to the desired temperature
2. Skin breakdown
3. Hemodynamic instability and cardiac arrhythmias related to hypothermia
4. Hyperthermia or hypothermia
5. Thermal burns
6. Rewarming shock or temperature afterdrop secondary to peripheral vasodilation (in severely hypothermic patients)

PATIENT TEACHING

1. Patients who have experienced accidental hypothermia should be instructed about how to prevent future episodes:
   - Recognition of early symptoms (shivering, lethargy, confusion, loss of coordination),
   - Appropriate clothing for the environment (including the importance of wearing a hat),
   - The dangerous effects of alcohol and other intoxicants.
2. Patients who have experienced hyperthermic episodes are predisposed to future recurrences. Instruct the patient on prevention strategies, as indicated by the cause of this episode:
   - Awareness of environmental temperature and humidity
   - The importance of staying in a cool environment
   - . Drinking adequate fluids
   - Avoiding extreme exertion during the hottest times of the day or in extreme weather
   - Frequent rest breaks
   - Proper conditioning

REFERENCE

Kelly, E. M. (2005). External warming/cooling devices. In D. J. Lynn-McHale, & K. K. Carlson (Eds.), *AACN procedure manual for critical care* (5th ed., pp. 782-788). St Louis: Saunders.

PROCEDURE 152

Continuous Arteriovenous Rewarming

Daun A. Smith, RN, MSN

Continuous arteriovenous rewarming (CAVR) is a method of active internal rewarming. CAVR is similar to cardiopulmonary bypass in that it reinfuses warmed blood to the central circulation, thereby decreasing the risk of rewarming arrhythmias. However, CAVR does not require a bypass pump or heparinization. CAVR is accomplished by establishing a closed system in which blood flows from one of the patient's femoral arteries through an 8.5-Fr arterial catheter into a specially designed tubing, through the Level 1 fluid warmer (SIMS Level 1, n.d.) and back into the patient's opposite femoral vein via another 8.5-Fr catheter. CAVR can return a patient's temperature to 36° C in as little as 45 minutes (Schulman, 2005). See Procedure 148 for additional information about the management of hypothermia.

INDICATIONS

1. To rewarm hypothermic patients with a core body temperature of 30° C (86° F) or less and a systolic blood pressure greater than 60 to 80 mm Hg. A blood pressure of 60 mm Hg systolic is necessary to push blood through the system at a rate of 150 ml/min, which will keep the system open (SIMS Level 1 Inc., n.d.). However, other sources recommend a blood pressure of at least 80 mm Hg (Andreoni & Massey, 2001; Schulman, 2005).
2. To rewarm hypothermic patients and reverse hypothermia-induced coagulopathies.

CONTRAINDICATIONS AND CAUTIONS

1. Profound hypotension. It may be possible to maintain an adequate systolic blood pressure with intravenous (IV) fluids, blood products, or vasopressors.
2. CAVR is contraindicated in patients less than 90 lb (41 kg) (Schulman, 2005) because of the possibility that the large femoral catheter may occlude the vessels in a smaller person.
3. CAVR should not be used in the presence of femoral occlusive disease or compartment syndrome of the lower extremities because the large catheters could impede circulation to and from the legs.
4. Patients requiring CAVR should have constant hemodynamic and temperature monitoring (Schulman, 2005).
5. Remove all air from fluid bags and tubing before connecting them to the patient.
6. Use only the catheters provided in the rewarming kit. Other central catheters may be too small to sustain the flow rates needed (Schulman, 2005).
7. The maximum time for rewarming with CAVR is 3 hours to prevent clotting in the tubing (SIMS Level 1 Inc., n.d.)
8. Do not connect the Level 1 fluid warmer to the patient until the temperature of the device is at least 41° C (Schulman, 2005).
9. Do not add extensions, stopcocks, or other restrictive components to the tubing assembly because these may compromise blood flow (Schulman, 2005).
10. Do not close clamps in the system for more than 2 to 3 minutes because clotting may occur (SIMS Level 1 Inc., n.d.)

EQUIPMENT

Level 1 A/V rewarming kit (Figure 152-1)
Dressing materials for central venous and arterial line sites
1000 ml of normal saline IV fluid

AV-300 Disposable Set Components

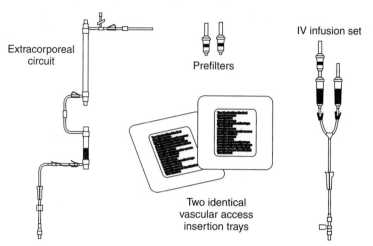

Extracorporeal
circuit

Prefilters

IV infusion set

Two identical
vascular access
insertion trays

FIGURE 152-1 Level 1 A/V rewarming kit. (Courtesy Level 1, Inc., Rockland, MA.)

PATIENT PREPARATION

1. *Obtain baseline vital signs. Initiate hemodynamic and core temperature monitoring.
2. Obtain baseline hemoglobin, hematocrit, coagulation studies, and arterial blood gases (see Procedures 19 and 58).
3. Place large-bore peripheral IV line for supplemental blood, IV fluid, or medication administration (see Procedure 60).
4. Minimize heat loss by using warm blankets, overhead heating lamps, or forced warm air heating blankets (see Procedures 150 and 151).

PROCEDURAL STEPS

Set Up the Level 1 Fluid Warmer (see Procedure 75 for more detailed information)

1. Push the bottom of the end of the heat exchanger into the socket labeled "1" (Figure 152-2).
2. Insert the heat exchanger into the guide. Slide the top socket, labeled "2," down over the top of the tube until it clicks.
3. Insert the filter/gas vent into its holder, labeled "3."
4. Plug in and press the ON button. The green SYSTEM OPERATIONAL indicator light on the display panel should be lit.
5. Ensure that all tubing connections are tight.

---

*Indicates portions of the procedure usually performed by a physician or an advanced practice nurse.

Prime Tubing

1. Attach the IV infusion set from the A/V rewarming procedural kit to the port just proximal to the heat exchanger.
2. Clamp the red arterial line off.
3. Spike the IV bag of saline and open the tubing clamp. Allow the infusion set, heat exchanger, filter assembly, and blue venous line to prime. Hold the filter/gas vent upside down until full. Gently tap the filter/gas vent against the chamber to dislodge any air bubbles. Return the filter to its holder, labeled "3."
4. Close the venous (blue) line clamp.
5. Open the arterial (red) line clamp. Allow saline to prime the arterial line, then close the arterial line clamp.

Establish Arterial and Venous Access

1. Use only the catheters included in the A/V rewarming kit.
2. See Procedure 65 for details.

Attach to the Patient

1. Ensure that the temperature of the Level 1 warmer has reached at least 41° C.
2. Close slide clamp to IV infusion set.
3. Connect arterial patient line (red tubing) to patient's arterial catheter and locate the ratchet clamp on the catheter.
4. Allow blood to flow completely through the tubing until it reaches the venous end of the line.
5. Close the venous patient line roller clamp A.
6. Gently tap filter/gas vent against cabinet to release any trapped air.

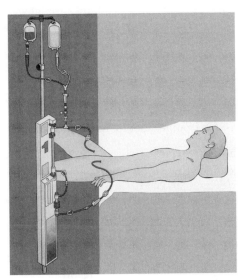

FIGURE 152-2 Assembly of tubing components for CAVR. See text for further details. (Courtesy Level 1, Inc., Rockland, MA.)

7. Attach the venous end of the line to the patient's venous catheter and open the roller clamp. Rewarming is now occurring.
8. Tape and anchor all catheters and lines to prevent kinking or dislodgment.
9. Dress catheter sites.
10. Monitor vital signs frequently during rewarming. Continuous temperature monitoring is recommended.

Transporting Patients During CAVR

CAVR must be interrupted during patient transport because the Level 1 fluid warmer does not have a battery and cannot function unless it is plugged into an electrical outlet. Interrupting the rewarming procedure during transport prevents the patient's blood from being cooled by exposure to ambient temperature.

1. Clamp the CAVR tubing at the arterial side and back flush with saline IV solution until clear. Clamp the arterial catheter.
2. Flush all of the patient's blood through the venous side of the tubing with normal saline solution and clamp the venous side.
3. Remove the tubing from the fluid warmer and place it in bed beside the patient.
4. To reestablish warming on arrival, reinsert the tubing into the fluid warmer and turn the warmer on. When the warmer reaches 37° C, open the arterial and venous clamps to restart the blood flow.

Troubleshooting

Patency difficulties in CAVR are usually due to low patient blood flow (systolic blood pressure less than 60 to 80 mm Hg) or kinks/clots in the tubing.

1. Monitor the tubing for kinking. Tape the arterial and venous ends of the tubing to the patient at the insertion site to prevent kinking when the patient is moved.
2. If the filter becomes clogged, clamp both the arterial and venous ends of the tubing. Remove the old filter. Attach the new filter at the arterial end first. Slowly and partially open the arterial clamp and allow the filter to prime completely. Close the arterial clamp. Attach the venous end of the tubing to the filter and place the filter back in its holder (labeled "3"). Open both arterial and venous clamps to reestablish blood flow.
3. Maintain the patient's systolic blood pressure with IV fluids, blood products, and vasopressors as prescribed.
4. See Procedure 75 for troubleshooting Level 1 alarms.

Discontinuing CAVR

CAVR may be discontinued when the patient's temperature has been stable at 36.5° C for 2 hours (Schulman, 2005).

1. Backflush saline IV solution into the arterial end of the catheter until the tubing is clear. Clamp the arterial catheter.
2. Flush the venous end of the catheter with saline IV solution until clear. Clamp the venous catheter.
3. The catheters may be left in place until the patient is stable. Do not remove the catheters until any coagulopathy has resolved.
4. When the catheters are removed, apply direct pressure to the sites for at least 15 minutes. Dress the sites and monitor for hematoma formation.

AGE-SPECIFIC CONSIDERATION

CAVR is contraindicated in patients weighing less than 90 lb (41 kg) (Schulman, 2005) because the size of the catheters may occlude the smaller blood vessels of these individuals.

COMPLICATIONS (Schulman, 2005)

1. Hematoma formation at catheter insertion sites
2. Impaired blood flow and loss of pulses to the lower extremities secondary to occlusion by vascular catheters
3. Clotting and occlusion of the filter
4. Kinking of tubing leading to decreased flow or clotting and occlusion
5. Insufficient blood flow secondary to hypotension
6. Persistent coagulopathy or hypothermia

PATIENT TEACHING

Patients who have experienced accidental hypothermia should be instructed about how to prevent future episodes:

- Recognition of early symptoms (shivering, lethargy, confusion, loss of coordination),
- Appropriate clothing for the environment (including the importance of wearing a hat),
- The dangerous effects of alcohol and other intoxicants.

REFERENCES

Andreoni, C., & Massey, D. (2001). Continuous arteriovenous rewarming: Rapid restoration of normothermia in the emergency department. *Journal of Emergency Nursing, 27*, 533-537.

Schulman, C. (2005). Continuous arteriovenous rewarming. In D. J. Lynn-McHale, & K. K. Carlson (Eds.), *AACN procedure manual for critical care* (5th ed., pp. 1004-1013). St Louis: Saunders.

SIMS Level 1, Inc. (n.d.). *A/V rewarming procedural kit: Gentilello technique* (product insert). Rockland, MA: Author.

Ophthalmic Procedures

Assessing Visual Acuity

Maureen T. Quigley, MS, ARNP

Assessing visual acuity is also known as the *vision test*, the *Henry F. Allen Preschool Test*, the *Snellen test*, the *Rosenbaum pocket screen*, and the *eye test*.

INDICATIONS

1. To assess the vision of patients presenting with ocular complaints
2. To document baseline visual acuity

CONTRAINDICATIONS AND CAUTIONS

1. Visual acuity testing should not precede treatment in patients whom have had chemical exposure to the eye. Copious saline irrigation should be performed immediately for all chemical exposures; tap water is usually the first available fluid which should be followed by a balanced salt solution buffered to a pH of approximately 7 (see Procedure 155). Visual acuity testing is performed after irrigation when chemical exposure occurs.
2. The abbreviations for right eye (oculus dexter; O.D.), left eye (oculus sinister; O.S.), and both eyes (oculi uterque; O.U.) are error prone and their use is discouraged by the Institute for Safe Medication Practices (ISMP, 2006).

EQUIPMENT

Snellen chart

or

Symbol chart such a tumbling "E" chart or a picture chart (for illiterate patients or preschool children)

or

Near-vision acuity chart (Figure 153-1)

Eye spoon, patch, or opaque card to cover the eye not being tested (optional)

Penlight (optional)

Marked distance of 20 or 10 feet for testing

Topical ophthalmic anesthetic (optional)

PATIENT PREPARATION

1. Instill a topical ophthalmic anesthetic (if prescribed) to increase the patient's comfort during the examination (optional).
2. Instruct the patient to occlude one eye during the vision test by using the eye spoon, patch, opaque card, or hand. Clean to remove copious discharge before visual acuity testing but after obtaining any necessary culture specimens. If there is discharge from the eye, use a disposable opaque card, and turn it over to the fresh surface when testing the other eye to prevent contamination. The patient should wash his or her hands after the procedure.

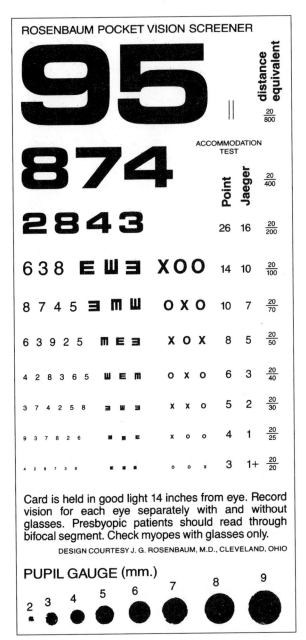

FIGURE 153-1 Rosenbaum pocket version screener for near-vision screening. This illustration is to scale and it, or a copy of it, may be used for assessment of visual acuity. (Courtesy Chiron Vision [1996], Claremont, CA.)

3. Instruct the patient not to apply excessive pressure when covering the eye because blurred vision may result.
4. Patients using a cupped hand should keep their fingers together to prevent a false reading caused by using binocular vision. The cupped hand may be a poor choice due to intentional or inadvertent peeking through the fingers.
5. Leave glasses or contact lenses in place during the examination if not contra-indicated by injury. When the patient's glasses or contact lenses are not available, document the results as "uncorrected visual acuity."

PROCEDURAL STEPS

1. Each eye is tested separately, with and without glasses.
2. Letters and objects are of a size that can be seen by the normal eye at a distance of 6 meters (20 feet) from the chart.
3. Letters appear in rows and are arranged so the normal eye can see them at distances of 9, 12, 15 meters (30, 40, 50 feet), and so forth.
4. A person who can identify letters of the size 6 at 6 meters (20 at 20 feet) is said to have 6/6 (20/20) vision.

Standard Method: Distant Visual Acuity

1. Sit or stand the patient at a marked distance of 20 feet from the standard Snellen chart with the chart positioned at eye level.
2. Test the vision of one eye at a time. Test the unaffected eye first to serve as a control.
3. Ask the patient to read the Snellen chart starting with the top line and working down until the letters are no longer legible.
4. Record the lowest line the patient is able to read, including the number of mistakes made on that line. For example, right eye, 20/20 means the patient can read the 20/20 line with no mistakes. Left eye, 20/25 –1 means the patient can read the 20/25 line with one mistake. Visual acuity is recorded as a fraction. The numerator represents the distance to the chart, and the denominator represents the distance from which a normal eye can read the lines. For example, 20/50 means that the patient can read at 20 feet what a person with 20/20 vision can read at 50 feet. If the patient is unable to read the first line of the Snellen chart at 20 feet, he or she may be placed at a distance of 10 feet from the chart and asked to read the lines. The acuity is then recorded as 10/50.
5. Repeat steps 3 and 4 for the opposite eye and for both eyes together.

Alternative Methods: Near Vision

1. Hand-held near-vision testing cards are commercially available when distance testing is not possible, such as the Rosenbaum near-vision chart. This is used for patients who are unable to stand (see Figure 153-1). The card is held 14 inches away from the patient. Attaching a 14-inch string to the card facilitates correct usage; however, patients may choose their own distance. The same procedure is used as for the Snellen chart testing.
2. If commercially prepared charts are unavailable, have the patient read a newspaper or another document with similarly-sized print and record the distance at which the patient is able to read the print.

3. Occasionally, patients who wear glasses or contact lenses carry the prescription in their wallet. This may serve as a gross baseline of visual acuity.
4. The pinhole method may be used to assess a refractive error when the patient's glasses or contact lenses are not available. The patient reads the Snellen chart while looking through pinholes in an opaque card. If the visual acuity improves, the decreased visual acuity may be attributed to a refractive error. When there is no improvement, causes other than refractive error should be considered.
5. If the patient is unable to read the top line of the Snellen chart (vision is less than 20/200 [6/60]), the following visual tests may be performed and recorded as follows:
   a. The patient can count the correct number of fingers at a measured distance. Counting fingers at ___ meters (___ feet).
   b. The patient can recognize hand motions at a measured distance and in a designated direction. Hand motion at ___ meters (___ feet).
   c. If the patient is unable to recognize hand motions, light perception is tested. Use a penlight and record whether the patient can determine the direction from which the light is coming. Light perception and projection.
      i. If the patient can determine which direction the light is coming from, record it as "light perception present."
      ii. If the patient is unable to recognize perceived light, record the visual acuity as "no light perception."

AGE-SPECIFIC CONSIDERATIONS

1. Use a symbol chart for illiterate patients or preschool children. Two symbol charts are available as pictures, such as Allen picture card or the Tumbling E test, with the letter E turned in four different directions. The patient is asked either to point a finger in the direction of the E bars or to identify the picture symbol printed on the chart. Follow the same procedure as for the Snellen chart.
2. Infants and young children can best be evaluated while sitting upright in the arms of their parents or caregivers.
3. Visual acuity testing for the preschool child may be inaccurate and is dependent on the cognitive development of the child. Generally, visual acuity reaches the adult level of 20/20 vision between ages 3 and 5.
4. To measure vision in infants more than 6 weeks old, assess their ability to fixate and follow a target. The human face works well as a target; in addition, brightly colored toys may be used (Olitsky & Nelson, 2004).
5. Snellen charts do not accurately test vision in older patients with complaints of faded objects and decreased vision with bright light (Miller & Magnante, 2004).

COMPLICATIONS

1. Injury causing edema or blepharospasm may prevent the patient from keeping the eyes open without manual assistance or medications to decrease pain or spasm.
2. Excessive tearing may blur the vision and affect the test results.

REFERENCES

Institute for Safe Medication Practices (ISMP). (2006). ISMP's list of error-prone abbreviations, symbols, and dose designations. Retrieved September 3, 2007, from http://www.ismp.org/Tools/errorproneabbreviations.pdf

Miller, D., & Magnante, P. (2004). Optics of the normal eye. In M. Yanoff (Ed.), *Ophthalmology* (2nd., pp. 59-67). St Louis: Mosby. Retrieved February 17, 2007, from URL:/das/book/view/60191306–2/1197/14.html/top

Olitsky, S., & Nelson, L. (2004). Disorders of the eye. In R. E. Behrman (Ed.), *Nelson textbook of pediatrics* (17th ed., pp. 2083-2126). Philadelphia: Saunders.

PROCEDURE 154

Contact Lens Removal

Margo E. Layman, MSN, RN, RNC, CN-A

INDICATIONS

1. To assist a patient who is unable to remove lenses prior to emergency surgery or sedation
2. To remove contact lenses in the presence of chemical irritants or foreign bodies
3. To remove contact lenses from a patient with an altered level of consciousness

CONTRAINDICATIONS AND CAUTIONS

1. Never use force to remove a lens. If you have difficulty, slide the lens onto the sclera and notify the physician.
2. Look for "lost" lenses in the upper cul-de-sac of the eye. This is their most common hiding place.
3. Do not replace the lens until a physician examines the patient's eyes.
4. If you suspect that your patient has a penetrating injury to the eye, do not manipulate the eye in any way.
5. If the eyes appear dry, instill several drops of sterile saline solution from a single-use dropper bottle and wait a few minutes before removing the lens to help prevent corneal damage.
6. Do not instill medications while the patient is wearing contact lenses. Contact lenses can combine chemically with the medication and cause eye irritation or lens damage.

7. Do not use saline solution with preservatives or tap water because they may damage the lenses.

EQUIPMENT

Contact lens storage case or two plastic specimen containers with lids
Contact lens soaking solution or sterile saline solution without preservatives
Suction cup or nasal suction bulb (optional)
Cotton balls
Towel

PATIENT PREPARATION

1. Place the patient in a supine or semi-Fowler's position.
2. Place a clean towel around the neck and across the chest.
3. Remove any glass particles with cellophane tape. Roll the tape so the adhesive is on the outside and gently touch it against the patient's closed eye to remove glass particles.
4. Gently remove blood, dirt, or makeup from the eyelids with a cotton ball moistened with saline solution.
5. Place several milliliters of sterile saline solution in each specimen container and label the containers left and right. If a contact lens case is used, place a few drops of saline solution in each compartment. Label the container(s) with the patient's name.

PROCEDURAL STEPS

Hard Lenses

1. Lubricate the eye with artificial tears.
2. Use one thumb to pull the patient's upper eyelid toward the orbital rim.
3. Place your other thumb on the lower lid, gently move the lids toward each other to trap the lens edge, and break the suction (Figure 154-1).
4. Cup your hand below the eye to catch the lens when it pops out.

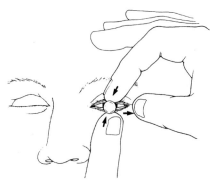

FIGURE 154-1 Removal of hard contact lenses. (From Novotny-Dinsdale, V. [1995]. Ocular emergencies. In S. Kitt, J. Selfridge-Thomas, J. A. Proehl, & J. Kaiser [Eds.], *Emergency nursing: A physiologic and clinical perspective* [2nd ed., p. 124]. Philadelphia: Saunders.)

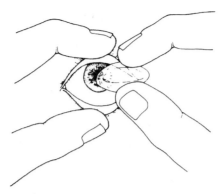

FIGURE 154-2 Removal of soft contact lenses. (From Novotny-Dinsdale, V. [1995]. Ocular emergencies. In S. Kitt, J. Selfridge-Thomas, J. A. Prohel, & J. Kaiser [Eds.], *Emergency nursing: A physiologic and clinical perspective* [2nd ed., p. 124]. Philadelphia: Saunders.)

5. Place the lens in an appropriate specimen container or contact lens case compartment.
6. Remove and care for the other lens by use of the same technique.
7. Examine the patient's eyes for redness or irritation.

Soft Lenses

1. Lubricate the eye with artificial tears.
2. Raise the upper eyelid with your index finger and hold it against the orbital rim.
3. Lightly place your thumb on the lower lid and pull it down.
4. Have the patient look up and slide the lens down gently with the index finger of your other hand.
5. Pinch the lens together with your thumb and index finger and lift it out of the patient's eye (Figure 154-2).
6. Place the lens in the appropriate specimen container or the contact lens case compartment.
7. Remove and care for the other lens using the same technique.
8. Examine the patient's eyes for redness or irritation.

Suction Cup Removal of Hard and Soft Lenses

1. Wet the suction cup with a drop of sterile saline solution.
2. Gently pull up the patient's upper eyelid with your index finger and pull the lower lid down with your thumb.
3. Press the suction cup gently to the center of the lens or squeeze nasal bulb syringe and gently place tip to center of lens and release slight suction to pull lens loose (Figure 154-3).
4. Pull the suction cup and the lens away from the eye in a straight line.
5. Place the lens in the appropriate specimen container or the contact lens case compartment.
6. Remove and care for the other lens using the same technique.
7. Examine the patient's eyes for redness or irritation.

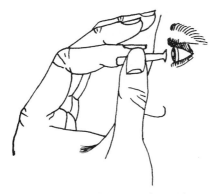

FIGURE 154-3 Removal of a contact lens with a suction cup.

COMPLICATIONS

1. Corneal damage can result from touching the cornea with the suction cup or attempting to remove dry lenses.
2. Corneal damage can occur if the lens is replaced in the wrong eye. Always label the containers and place the lenses in the proper containers or compartments.

PATIENT TEACHING

1. Watch for signs of eye irritation, such as purulent drainage, redness, or swelling.
2. Follow the usual cleaning procedures for lenses.

PROCEDURE 155

Eye Irrigation

Maureen T. Quigley, MS, ARNP

Eye irrigation is also known as *eye flushing*.

INDICATIONS

1. To dilute or remove chemicals from the eye and restore a normal pH
2. To remove foreign objects from the eye and help prevent ocular damage and vision loss after an eye injury
3. To relieve pain or burning that is usually associated with a foreign body or a chemical injury to the eye

CONTRAINDICATIONS AND CAUTIONS

1. Do not delay irrigation when a chemical exposure occurs. Irrigation should be initiated immediately and should be continued by caregivers before arrival at the emergency department. Until the causative agent is known, exposures should be presumed to be acid or alkaline substances (Brunette, 2006).
2. It is critical to identify the causative agent and to obtain an initial pH. In general, alkaline substances have a pH greater than 12 and acidic substances have a pH less than 2 (Brunette, 2006).
3. Lactated Ringer's solution is preferred over normal saline. The pH of lactated Ringer's is 6 to 7.5, which is closer to the pH of tears (7.1) than that of normal saline, which may range from 4.5 to 7 (MorTan, n.d.).
4. Use caution when a penetrating injury is present or suspected, and irrigate gently. Do not use a Morgan lens when there has been a penetrating injury or a ruptured globe is suspected or present.
5. Paper clips have been used as modified lid retractors; however, they may chip after twisting, causing metal fragments to enter the eye (Knoop, Dennis, & Hedges, 2004).
6. If a patient has contaminated his or her eye with a cyanoacrylate adhesive (e.g., Super Glue), evaluation by an ophthalmologist is recommended. Separation of glued eyelashes and gentle traction on the eyeball can be used, but the eyelids should not be forced open. Use of other agents to dissolve the adhesive is not recommended. Irrigation is not the first line of treatment.
7. An ophthalmology consultation may be necessary, depending on the type and the duration of the exposure as well as the clinical findings.

EQUIPMENT

Topical ophthalmic anesthetic
Sterile lactated Ringer's solution (1000-ml intravenous [IV] bag)
IV macrodrip tubing
18- or 20-G over-the-needle catheter with the stylet removed
or
Irrigation (Morgan) lens
Medi-Duct ocular fluid management system used with Morgan lens (optional)
Morgan lens delivery tubing (optional)
or
Syringe irrigating device
Basin
Tape (optional)
Gauze dressings or a commercially prepared eye patch
Towels or a patient gown
Tissues
Cotton-tipped applicators
Shampoo board or sink area (optional)
Desmarres retractor (Figure 155-1)
pH paper

PATIENT PREPARATION

1. Instill the prescribed topical ophthalmic anesthetic into the affected eye.

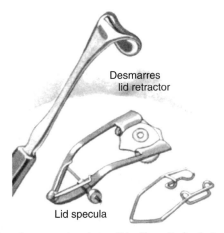

FIGURE 155-1 Devices for separating the eyelids. (From Fogle, J. A., & Spyker, D. A. [1990]. Management of chemical and drug injury to the eye. In L. M. Haddad & J. F. Winchester [Eds.], *Clinical management of poisoning and drug overdose* [2nd ed., p. 372]. Philadelphia: Saunders.)

2. If a chemical exposure has occurred, obtain a baseline pH measurement of the eye by placing pH paper in the conjunctival sac.
3. Another person may need to hold the eyelids open manually or with a retractor if an irrigating lens is not used.
4. Inform the patient that the eye irrigation may cause postnasal drip. Offer tissues for use as needed.
5. Use a gown or draped towels to protect the patient from excessive dampness during the procedure.
6. Position a basin or a large bag to catch the irrigant or position the patient over a sink. Using a shampoo board under the patient's head is another method to facilitate collection of the irrigant. Place the patient in a supine position. Place towels under the patient's neck to increase comfort. If the Medi-Duct fluid wicking drainage collector or shampoo boards are not readily available, treatment may begin with cooperative patients sitting and leaning over a sink or basin. There is an increased tendency for the irrigating lens to fall out in this position, especially if blinking occurs or flow is rapid.

PROCEDURAL STEPS
Manual Irrigation
1. Spike the IV tubing into the IV fluid and attach the catheter or irrigating syringe device and prime the tubing.
2. Use gauze pads to hold the eyelids open for irrigation if the patient is unable to do so. A lid retractor may be used to separate the eyelids and allow irrigation.
3. Direct the flow of the irrigant onto the conjunctiva from the inner to the outer canthus, avoid directing the stream directly onto the cornea, which can be harmful (Figure 155-2).
4. Instruct the patient to roll the eyes in all directions to ensure total eye irrigation.

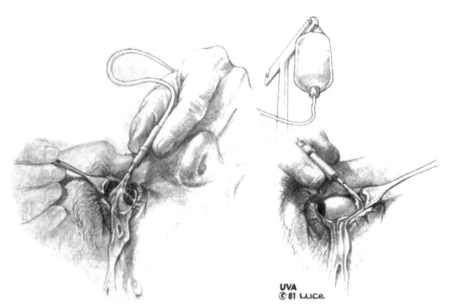

UVA
© 81 Luce

FIGURE 155-2 Irrigation using a Desmarres retractor. (From Fogle, J. A., & Spyker, D. A. [1990]. Management of chemical and drug injury to the eye. In L. M. Haddad & J. F. Winchester [Eds.], *Clinical management of poisoning and drug overdose* [2nd ed., p. 372]. Philadelphia: Saunders.)

5. For acidic exposure, irrigate with a minimum of 1000 ml of lactated Ringer's solution per eye. Acids (except hydrofluoric and heavy metal acids) are quickly neutralized by the proteins of the eye surface. After the eye is irrigated, acids cause no further damage (Knoop et al., 2004).

6. Irrigate alkaline injuries with a minimum of 2 L of lactated Ringer's or normal saline solution per eye over 1 hour. Extensive irrigation is required because alkaline substances, hydrofluoric acid, and heavy-metal acids can penetrate the cornea rapidly and continue to cause damage for days (Knoop et al., 2004).

7. Measure the pH of the eye at intervals during the irrigation by placing pH paper in the conjunctival sac. Continued irrigation is needed until the pH of the tear film is neutral, 7.5 to 8 (MorTan, n.d.). The normal conjunctival pH is 7.1 (MorTan, n.d.). If the pH remains alkaline, irrigation should be continued.

8. *Evert the eyelid and remove traces of alkali by using a wet cotton-tipped applicator to swab the fornices (Figure 155-3).

9. Check the patient's comfort level periodically. Instill additional ophthalmic anesthetic as necessary.

10. Recheck the conjunctival pH approximately 20 minutes after completion of irrigation and periodically as indicated to ensure that it remains in the normal range. Inadequate irrigation or improper swabbing of the fornices can cause delayed changes in the pH (Knoop et al., 2004).

---

*Indicates portions of the procedure usually performed by a physician or an advanced practice nurse.

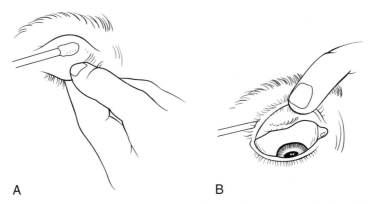

A   B

FIGURE 155-3 Eyelid eversion. **A,** Place cotton-tipped applicator at the midpoint of the eyelid. Have patient look downward and grasp eyelashes and pull downward. **B,** Pull the eyelid over the applicator to complete the lid eversion.

11. Obtain a baseline visual acuity level (see Procedure 153).
12. Prepare the patient for a corneal examination to determine the extent of the injury (see Procedure 156).

Irrigating or Morgan Therapeutic Lens

1. The irrigating lens fits onto the cornea like a soft contact lens and provides optimal continuous irrigation of the corneal surface while increasing patient comfort. The lens allows the patient to close the eyelids and decreases the risk of iatrogenic trauma often encountered during a difficult irrigation (Figure 155-4).
2. Spike the IV tubing into the IV fluid (lactated Ringer's is preferred), attach the Morgan lens, and prime. Ask the patient to look downward. Grasp the upper

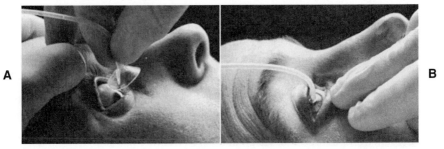

A   B

FIGURE 155-4 Placement of the Morgan lens for eye irrigation. **A,** Have the patient look downward, and then insert the lens under the upper lid. Have the patient look upward, and then retract the lower lid. **B,** For removal, have the patient look upward and then retract the lower lid, hold the position, and slide out the lens. (Courtesy of MorTan, Inc. [1996]. *Instructional chart for Morgan lens.* Missoula, MT: Author.)

eyelid and retract it upward. Holding the lens between the thumb and forefinger of your dominant hand, insert the upper portion of the lens under the upper eyelid with the IV fluid running. Ask the patient to look down. Retract the lower eyelid and place the lower portion of the lens onto the cornea. The insertion process is similar to that used to insert a contact lens.

3. Adjust the flow of IV fluid to a level tolerated well by the patient, and proceed with the continuous irrigation. A wide-open flow may create too much pressure and actually create more discomfort for the patient. Remind the patient to keep the eyes closed to ensure that the lenses stay in the eyes.

4. Tape the irrigation tubing to the patient's forehead to prevent accidental dislodgement of the lens (optional).

5. See steps 4 through 10 in the Manual Irrigation section of this procedure.

6. Remove the irrigation lens with the IV fluid running. Ask the patient to look upward, retract the lower lid, lift one side of the lens to break the suction, and gently slide the lens from the cornea.

AGE-SPECIFIC CONSIDERATIONS

1. Patients with chronic diseases, such as congestive heart failure or chronic obstructive lung disease, may need accommodations for positioning during irrigation. A supine position may not be tolerated.

2. The irrigating lens (Morgan lens) has been used without difficulty on infants and young children since the dimensions of the eye change little from infancy to adulthood (MorTan, n.d.).

COMPLICATIONS

1. Corneal or conjunctival abrasions may result from holding the eyelids open during the irrigation process.

2. Swelling or periorbital edema may occur after irrigation.

3. A fine punctate keratitis may result from direct irrigation onto the cornea (Knoop et al., 2004).

PATIENT TEACHING

1. Following irrigation, you may experience a burning sensation in the eyes similar to that which occurs after prolonged exposure to chlorinated water in a swimming pool. The sensation is self-limiting and usually subsides about 1 hour after tear production resumes.

2. Take analgesics as directed. A topical anesthetic cannot be used at home, because continued use prevents healing and may mask pain related to complications.

3. Return to the emergency department for increasing pain, decreasing vision, or other new symptoms. See an ophthalmologist as directed.

4. Use protective eyewear when appropriate to prevent future injuries.

5. Any functional decrease in vision of an eye (whether patched or medicated or by the injury or disease) causes monocularity to some extent with resultant loss of peripheral vision, inadequate depth perception due to loss of triangulation and a "blind spot." All of these effects can lead to injury and you should not drive, operate machinery, or perform other risky tasks until cleared by a physician.

REFERENCES

Brunette, R. (2006). Ophthalmology. In J. A. Marx, R. S. Hockberger, & R. M. Walls, et al. (Eds.), *Rosen's emergency medicine: Concepts and clinical practice* (6th ed., pp. 1044-1064). St Louis: Mosby.

Knoop, K. J., Dennis, W. R., & Hedges, J. R. (2004). Ophthalmologic procedures. In J. R. Roberts, & J. R. Hedges (Eds.), *Clinical procedures in emergency medicine* (4th ed., pp. 1241-1279). Philadelphia: Saunders.

MorTan, Inc. (n.d.). Frequently asked questions. Retrieved January 5, 2007, from www.morganlens.com/faq.html

PROCEDURE 156

Fluorescein Staining of Eyes

Maureen T. Quigley, MS, ARNP

Fluorescein staining of the eye is also known as an *ultraviolet examination*, a *Wood's lamp examination*, or a *black light examination*. Fluorescein reveals the area of epithelial defect by staining basement membrane, which may appear as yellow to the naked eye and glows green under ultraviolet light.

INDICATIONS

1. To diagnose blunt or penetrating eye injuries.
2. To evaluate suspected corneal abrasions, ulcers, foreign bodies, or infections of the eye. The exposed edge of epithelium created by the edge of a foreign body usually stains, rather than the entire foreign body.
3. To test for patency of the lacrimal drainage system. If the drainage system is patent, traces of fluorescein are present in the nasal secretions (Hurwitz, 2004).
4. To detect perforation of the eye with the Seidel test (Knoop, Dennis, & Hedges, 2004). A large amount of fluorescein is instilled into the eye, and the globe is examined for a stream of fluid leaking from the globe. The stream appears fluorescent blue or green, whereas the rest of the globe appears orange.

CONTRAINDICATIONS AND CAUTIONS

1. Penlight and funduscopic examination of the eye, as well as a presumptive diagnosis of corneal abrasion based on history, physical examination, and exclusion of other disorders should be done before fluorescein examination (Jacobs, 2006).

2. Measurement of visual acuity and visualization of the anterior segment and fundus may be impaired by prior use of fluorescein.

3. Soft contact lenses should be removed because the fluorescein stain may cause permanent tinting of the lens (see Procedure 154). Hard contact lenses are not affected by the dye.

4. With deep corneal disruption, the dye may enter the anterior chamber of the eye (Knoop et al., 2004). The dye is nontoxic, but it is difficult to flush out completely.

5. Use of sterile, individually wrapped fluorescein-impregnated strips is recommended rather than multiple-dose bottles of fluorescein stain, which increase the risk of contamination by organisms such as *Pseudomonas* (Knoop et al., 2004).

6. Some patients may develop a superficial punctuate keratitis after use of a topical anesthetic, but for many patients, examination is difficult without prior use of an anesthetic (Knoop et al., 2004).

7. Fluorescein staining of the conjunctiva is less sensitive in revealing true pathology than staining the cornea (Knoop et al., 2004).

8. Use of fluorescein is not recommended if penetration of the globe is evident since it may create problems with evaluation and surgical treatment (Thomas & Brown, 2006).

EQUIPMENT

Normal saline solution, artificial tears, or dextrose solution for the irrigant
Sterile fluorescein-impregnated strips
Light source: cobalt blue penlight, blue filter on slit lamp, or Wood's lamp
Patient gown or towel
Tissues
Emesis basin
Topical ophthalmic anesthetic (optional)

PATIENT PREPARATION

1. Remove glasses or contact lens (see Procedure 154).
2. Cover the patient's clothing with a gown or towel. Fluorescein is a dye and may permanently stain clothing.
3. Place the patient in either a seated or a supine position.
4. Provide tissues and instruct the patient to gently blot tears. This is especially important if the physician uses a topical anesthetic for the procedure, because additional corneal irritation may result.

PROCEDURAL STEPS

1. Instill two drops of the prescribed topical anesthetic into the affected eye or eyes if needed (optional).
2. Moisten the appropriate end of the fluorescein strip with saline or artificial tears.
3. After depressing the lower eyelid, gently place the moistened fluorescein impregnated paper strip into the conjunctival sac. Placement of a nonmoistened fluorescein strip may cause additional epithelial damage (Figure 156-1).
4. Instruct the patient to blink once, which distributes the dye over the ocular surface. An alternative method is to touch the moistened fluorescein strip

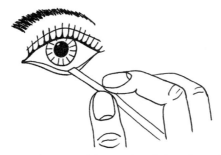

FIGURE 156-1 Placement of fluorescein strip into the conjunctival sac.

to the conjunctival sac and observe the flow of dye into the sac until an adequate amount is present to coat the corneal surface. Remove the strip and discard.

5. Instruct the patient to close the eyes for approximately 30 to 60 seconds. This promotes maximal distribution of the dye over the cornea by retaining tears within the eyelids.

6. Use the irrigant to remove excessive fluorescein dye. This enhances the contrast between the injured and the normal areas.

7. Dim the lights in the examination room.

8. *Use a cobalt blue penlight or black light source to inspect the corneal surface for epithelial defects, foreign bodies, or abrasions. Disrupted corneal surfaces are visualized as bright green under the blue light.

9. After the examination, irrigate the eye with saline solution or other irrigant to remove the fluorescein dye and prevent staining of either the clothing or the face. An emesis basin can be held close to the patient's cheek to catch the irrigant solution. This is optional and performed for aesthetic reasons only.

COMPLICATIONS

1. Although topical fluorescein is considered nontoxic, rare reactions, such as redness or swelling, have been reported when fluorescein solution was used. Use of fluorescein-impregnated strips removes this risk.

2. Soft contact lenses may be permanently stained by fluorescein.

PATIENT TEACHING

1. Yellowish-orange fluid may drain from your eyes or nose following the procedure.

2. Do not wear soft contact lenses for a few hours after fluorescein staining to prevent permanent staining of the lens.

3. No special directions are needed if you wear hard contact lenses.

---

*Indicates portions of the procedure usually performed by a physician or an advanced practice nurse.

REFERENCES

Hurwitz, J. J. (2004). The lacrimal drainage system. In M. Yanoff (Ed.), *Ophthalmology* (2nd ed., pp. 761-767). St Louis: Mosby.

Jacobs, D. S. (2006). Corneal abrasions and corneal foreign bodies. Retrieved January 7, 2007, from *UpToDate*, online version 14.3. www.uptodate.com

Knoop, K. J., Dennis, W. R., & Hedges, J. R. (2004). Ophthalmologic procedures. In J. R. Roberts, & J. R. Hedges (Eds.), *Clinical procedures in emergency medicine* (4th ed., pp. 1241-1279). Philadelphia: Saunders.

Thomas, S. H., & Brown, D. F. M. (2006). Foreign bodies. In J. A. Marx, R. S. Hockberger, & R. M. Walls, et al. (Eds.), *Rosen's emergency medicine: Concepts and clinical practice* (6th ed., pp. 859-879). St Louis: Mosby.

PROCEDURE 157

Ophthalmic Foreign Body Removal

Joni Hentzen Daniels, MSN, RN, CEN, CCRN

INDICATIONS

1. To remove a foreign body from the cornea or conjunctiva.
2. To prevent ocular damage or vision loss from a foreign body. Foreign bodies usually result from trauma, occupational injuries, or acts of nature, such as wind-blown objects or insects.

CONTRAINDICATIONS AND CAUTIONS

1. It is important to obtain a detailed description of the mechanism and circumstances of the injury. Find out the exact time of injury, the events leading to the injury, the description and composition of the foreign body, the distance it traveled to the eye, whether it was blown by the wind or propelled into the eye, the direction of travel, and the direction in which the eye was looking at the time of the injury.
2. A history providing material content of the foreign body is significant in management because some nonmagnetic foreign bodies may not be removed unless they are easily accessible. Siderosis (a rust brown or yellowish discoloration of the cornea, iris, or lens) may develop from steel and iron foreign bodies and may lead to chronic degenerative changes, such as visual field loss, cataracts, or open-angle glaucoma (Khaw, Shah, & Elkington, 2004).

Copper, bronze, and brass foreign bodies may cause chalcosis. Nonmetallic foreign bodies can be inert or toxic: glass, stone, and plastic can be tolerated for many years, with a rare reaction, as opposed to vegetable matter, which often results in a severe inflammatory reaction. Trauma involving vegetable matter (lash, thorn, wood, or soil) increases the possibility of infection, particularly fungal infection.

3. Plain radiographs, computed tomography (CT), or magnetic resonance imaging (MRI) may localize intraorbital foreign bodies. Plain films are helpful in the identification of opaque foreign bodies. CT is considered to be the gold standard for most foreign bodies, with the exception of dry wood. MRI is helpful in the identification of dry wood foreign bodies (Khaw et al., 2004). If an object is felt to be of metallic origin, MRI is contraindicated.

4. Patients with corneal foreign bodies often experience pain, a foreign body sensation, and tearing. Topical ophthalmic anesthetic facilitates the physical examination. The degree of pain relief afforded by the topical anesthetic can also assist in differentiating corneal injury from other types of acute eye pain (Brunette, 2006).

5. It is possible that patients may not remember the precipitating event, because the symptoms can be delayed or intermittent.

6. Obtain previous ophthalmic history: previously existing eye disease, surgery, and trauma, as well as vision before the presenting injury.

7. Do not apply pressure to the eye. Direct pressure should not be used to stop bleeding from or around the eye when a penetrating object is suspected or evident. Instruct the patient not to touch or rub the eye.

8. Unless contraindicated by other injuries, elevate the head of the bed to decrease intraocular pressure. Limit patient movement as much as possible.

9. If a foreign body is impaled in the eye, immobilize the object and patch both eyes to decrease ocular movement (see Procedures 159 and 161).

10. Contact lenses should be removed immediately in the presence of a foreign body (see Procedure 154).

11. Chemical injuries are considered penetrating and require immediate copious irrigation to prevent irreversible damage (see Procedure 155).

12. Abrasions or actinic injuries often mimic the sensation of an ocular foreign body, but they are easily diagnosed by the fluorescein examination (see Procedure 156).

13. If you are unable to locate an external foreign body despite patient complaints, consider the possibility of an intraocular or intraorbital foreign body. Symptoms suggestive of a penetrating injury include an irregular pupil, hyphema, lens opacification, hemorrhage, or prolapsed iris. Some intraocular foreign objects are toxic.

14. Paper clips have been used as modified lid retractors; however, they may chip after twisting, causing metal fragments to enter the eye (Knoop, Dennis, & Hedges, 2004).

15. Use of sharp instruments to remove ophthalmic foreign bodies should only be done by those with formal training.

EQUIPMENT

Topical ophthalmic anesthetic
Sterile fluorescein strip

Irrigation solution
Sterile cotton swabs
25- or 27-G needle or eye spud
3-ml syringe (or any size that is comfortable to hold)
Ophthalmoscope
Ultraviolet light
Penlight
Magnification source: loupe or slit lamp
Cycloplegic ophthalmic drops
Antibiotic ophthalmic drops or ointment
Lid retractor
Eye drill with bits (optional)

PATIENT PREPARATION

1. Assess and document visual acuity (see Procedure 153).
2. Place the patient in a seated or high Fowler's position.
3. Remove contact lens or lenses if present (see Procedure 154).
4. Anesthetize the affected eye with 1 or 2 drops of a topical ophthalmic anesthetic, as prescribed.
5. Apply the fluorescein stain as prescribed (see Procedure 156).

PROCEDURAL STEPS

1. A full eye examination should be performed. Use a penlight to examine the anesthetized corneal surface, lower fornix, conjunctiva, and upper-lid conjunctiva. Ask the patient to look in all directions. Vertical scratches suggest a foreign body trapped under the lid.
2. *Use a cotton swab to evert the upper eyelid (see Figure 155-3). Place the applicator in the middle of the upper lid and instruct the patient to gaze downward. Grasp the patient's eyelashes, pull downward, and then fold upward over the swab. Laying the swab shaft across the bridge of the nose adds support when everting the eyelid. While the eyelid is everted, use a moist cotton swab to sweep the upper fornix area and remove any debris.
3. Removal techniques vary once the foreign body is located. Options include the following:
   a. *Flush the eye with saline first, then remove the object with a commercial eye spud or 25-G needle (Brunette, 2006). Irrigation may dislodge the foreign body into the lower conjunctival sac where it can be removed with a moist cotton swab. This technique is helpful when there are multiple superficial foreign bodies.
   b. *Attempt to remove the foreign body by touching it gently with a moist cotton swab. Do not use a dry applicator or attempt prolonged dislodgment of the object, because additional epithelial damage may result.
   c. *Under a slit lamp or loupe magnification, embedded foreign bodies may be removed with a 27- or 25-G needle attached to a syringe, an eye spud, or a cotton swab. The syringe or cotton swab acts as a handle (Figures 157-1 and 157-2).

---

*Indicates portions of the procedure usually performed by a physician or an advanced practice nurse.

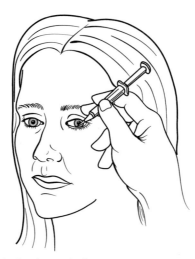

FIGURE 157-1 Removal of a foreign body using a syringe as a handle and a small gauge needle.

Ideally, use a slit lamp that has a chin rest to secure the head. The slit lamp provides adequate illumination, magnification, and a light focus point. The patient may also be asked to focus on the practitioner's ear to steady the eye. If a slit lamp is unavailable, instruct the patient to fix his or her gaze on a stationary object. Secure the patient's head against the examination chair headrest with your fingers, steadying your hand against the patient's face. Dim the room lights. Use a penlight to provide increased illumination to the eye. Magnification loupes may also be used.

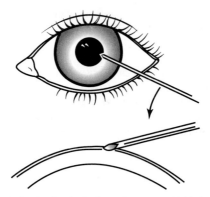

FIGURE 157-2 Removal of a foreign body from the cornea. Hold the syringe tangential to the foreign body and scrape gently away from the cornea. The side view demonstrates the thickness of the cornea relative to the beveled needle edge.

d. *When these methods are unsuccessful, an eye drill may be used to remove a visible foreign body.

4. *To prevent rust rings, completely remove any metallic foreign body particles. If removal is incomplete, the rust ring softens within 24 to 48 hours, facilitating easy removal (Knoop et al., 2004). Patients may be referred to an ophthalmologist for rust-ring removal.

5. *Magnetic removal is another method of extracting ferromagnetic foreign bodies. A magnet is placed on the handle of a sterile jeweler's forceps. The magnet attracts the foreign body, which is lifted or grasped from the cornea.

6. After removal of the foreign body, irrigate the eye with at least 10 ml of saline solution to remove any remaining traces of fluorescein or other particulate matter.

7. Instill prophylactic antibiotic ophthalmic drops or ointment as prescribed. Cycloplegics may also be prescribed to decrease ciliary muscle spasms and increase patient comfort.

8. Patch the affected eye (optional) (see Procedure 159).

AGE-SPECIFIC CONSIDERATIONS

1. Young children may require an immobilization device, such as a child restraint board to be evaluated effectively (see Procedure 191). An alternative method of examination is to have an assistant and parent sit facing each other, with the child positioned supine, with legs straddling the parent's waist. With the parent holding the child's extremities, the child's head is directed onto the assistant's lap, and the physician performs the examination. If these approaches fail, the evaluation should be performed under sedation in a monitored setting (see Procedure 177) or under general anesthesia. Avoid ketamine, which induces nystagmus and is thought to increase intraocular pressure.

2. In the elderly, eye and orbital trauma is frequently caused by falls, which may also cause other injuries, such as hip fractures. A fall could represent underlying cardiovascular disease, such as an arrhythmia or hypotension, which would necessitate further evaluation.

3. A child may be reluctant to provide a history of the injury if involved in behavior that was inappropriate.

COMPLICATIONS

1. Incomplete removal of a foreign body results in inflammation and delayed healing. Owing to the oxidation of iron, metallic foreign bodies create rust rings within hours. Rust rings cause continuing irritation of the eye.

2. Conjunctivitis may occur after the removal of a foreign body.

3. Use of a cotton swab, especially a dry one, may cause additional epithelial damage.

---

*Indicates portions of the procedure usually performed by a physician or an advanced practice nurse.

4. Pain after foreign object removal is common. Because topical anesthetics are contraindicated for ongoing use, a prescription for oral analgesia is often indicated.

PATIENT TEACHING

1. Do not touch or rub the injured eye.
2. Rest the uninjured eye, thus preventing involuntary movement of the injured eye.
3. Avoid reading or computer work. Television viewing is permitted at a distance of 10 feet or more. Fixed-gaze television watching limits the movement of the eye, as opposed to reading, which necessitates eye movement (Knoop et al., 2004).
4. The sensation of having a foreign body in the eye may return after the topical anesthetic wears off. A topical anesthetic cannot be used at home, because continued use prevents healing and may mask pain related to complications.
5. Use protective eyewear when appropriate to prevent future injuries.
6. A safe home environment/living arrangement is important after a serious eye injury.
7. Any functional decrease in vision of an eye (whether patched or medicated or by the injury or disease) causes monocularity to some extent with resultant loss of peripheral vision, inadequate depth perception due to loss of triangulation, and a "blind spot." All of these effects can lead to injury and you should not drive, operate machinery, or perform other risky tasks until cleared by a physician.

REFERENCES

Brunette, D. D. (2006). Ophthalmology. In J. A. Marx, R. S. Hockberger, & R. M. Walls, et al. (Eds.), *Rosen's emergency medicine: Concepts and clinical practice* (6th ed., pp. 1044-1065). St Louis: Mosby.

Khaw, P. T., Shah, P., & Elkington, A. R. (2004). Injury to the eye. *British Medical Journal, 328*(7430), 36-38. Retrieved January 1, 2007, from http://www.bmj.com/cgi/content/full/328/7430/36.

Knoop, K. J., Dennis, W. R., & Hedges, J. R. (2004). Ophthalmologic procedures. In J. R. Roberts, & J. R. Hedges (Eds.), *Clinical procedures in emergency medicine* (4th ed., pp. 1241-1279). Philadelphia: Saunders.

Instillation of Eye Medications

Maureen T. Quigley, MS, ARNP

INDICATIONS

1. To reduce the potential for secondary infection related to eye injury
2. To decrease pain related to eye irritation or injury
3. To provide treatment for an existing problem or infection
4. To assist in the examination of the eyes by anesthetizing the cornea or paralyzing the ciliary muscles, or both
5. To promote corneal reepithelialization

CONTRAINDICATIONS AND CAUTIONS

1. In the presence of penetrating injuries to the globe, do not instill medications without a physician's prescription.
2. Topical ocular steroids are usually used only on the order of an ophthalmologist because use of these medications can retard corneal epithelial wound healing and increase the risk of infection. Herpes simplex virus can worsen with use of topical ocular steroids. Use of topical ocular steroids should be avoided if a diagnosis has not been established (Brunette, 2006).
3. Caution should be used in instilling mydriatic, cycloplegic, or steroid drops because angle-closure glaucoma can be induced.
4. With its rich supply of nerve fibers, the eye is very sensitive and direct application of medication on the cornea should be avoided. Medication should be instilled in the less sensitive conjunctival sac (Perry & Potter, 2006).
5. If the medication is refrigerated, warm it in your hands and instill at room temperature.
6. Eye medications are absorbed rapidly into the anterior segment of the eye but can be absorbed systemically via the nasopharyngeal mucosa, potentially resulting in serious consequences. Systemic absorption can be minimized by applying pressure to the inner canthus of both eyes, causing occlusion of the puncta.
7. If multiple medications are prescribed, always instill drops before ointments.

EQUIPMENT

Gauze or tissues
Prescribed ophthalmic medication

PATIENT PREPARATION

1. Assess visual acuity (see Procedure 153) before instilling mydriatic medications. From a medicolegal standpoint, this documents that any decrease in vision is not a result of the medications (Knoop, Dennis, & Hedges, 2004).
2. Determine the patient's medication and significant ocular history, as well as history of allergies.
3. Place the patient in a supine position or in a sitting position with the head tilted back in a position of comfort.
4. Evaluate the eye for retained foreign matter.
5. Irrigate or remove the foreign matter from the eye (see Procedures 155 and 157).

PROCEDURAL STEPS
Instillation of Eye Drops

1. Instruct the patient to look up toward the top of his or her head. Remind the patient that drops will always fall vertically due to gravity; therefore, fix the open gaze vertically upward.
2. Gently pull the lower eyelid down or evert the lower lid by using a piece of gauze, a cotton swab, or a clean gloved finger with thumb or forefinger against the orbit. Never apply pressure on the eyeball.
3. Stabilize the dropper with the heel of your hand against the cheek, and instill a single drop into the conjunctival sac at the center of the lower lid (Figure 158-1). More than one drop at a time is not recommended because this increases tearing and decreases the concentration of the medication (Knoop et al., 2004).
4. Apply gentle pressure to the inner canthus of the eyes to occlude the puncta immediately when instilling eye drops that have the potential for systemic effects, such as atropine or β-blockers.
5. Have the patient close or blink the eyes gently to spread the medication.
6. If additional eye medications are prescribed, wait 5 to 10 minutes to improve absorption, and repeat steps 1 through 4. Always instill drops before ointment.

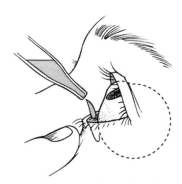

FIGURE 158-1 Instilling eye drops. (From J. A. Proehl & L. M. Jones [1998]. *Mosby's emergency department patient teaching guidelines* [p. J-3]. St. Louis: Mosby.)

Instillation of Eye Ointment

1. Instruct the patient to look up toward the top of his or her head.
2. Gently pull the lower eyelid down or evert the lower lid by using a piece of gauze or a cotton swab.
3. Spread a thin ribbon of ointment along lower eyelid on conjunctiva from the inner to the outer canthus.
4. Have the patient close or blink the eyes gently a few times to spread the medication.
5. The eyes should remain closed if an eye patch needs to be applied (see Procedure 159).

AGE-SPECIFIC CONSIDERATIONS

1. Have parent restrain infant or young child's head held in parent's lap when instilling eye medication.
2. If possible, instill eye medication when child or infant is sleeping.
3. Instill eye medication in restrained supine position at nasal aspect of eye(s) of young child or infant with tightly clenched eyes, so that medication flows into eyes when opened (Perry & Potter, 2006).
4. Older adults using β-blocker drops for glaucoma may have systemic effects if too much is used or the inner canthus is not tamponaded to minimize absorption.

COMPLICATIONS

1. Introduction of contaminated medication may result in an infection. Single-patient use of eye medications is recommended to prevent cross-contamination.
2. Trauma to the eye may result from movement of the patient's head during instillation.
3. Repeated use of topical anesthetics can result in epithelial damage to the cornea.
4. Temporary blurred vision may be a side effect of the medication or may result from the presence of ointment in the eye.
5. Systemically absorbed β-blocker drops can produce symptomatic bradycardia.

PATIENT TEACHING

1. Always wash your hands before instilling eye medications and do not allow the tip of the medication dropper or ointment to touch your eye or eyelashes.
2. Immediately apply gentle pressure to the inner corner of the eye to occlude the tear duct when instilling eye drops that have the potential for systemic effects such as atropine or β-blockers. Also, with systemically active medications, keep the drops no warmer than room temperature. Drops close to body temperature are not easily felt or counted when dropped into the eye and excessive dosage may only be noted when drops start running down the cheek
3. Do not rub your eyes or squeeze the lids together.
4. Some medications may make your eyes sensitive to light, so you may need to wear sunglasses.

5. Immediately report any increase in eye pain, purulent drainage, or visual problems.
6. If you wear contact lenses, do not wear them until their use is approved by your health care provider.
7. Topical anesthetics are not prescribed for ongoing use, because they may retard healing. During the time of anesthetic effect, do *not* touch or rub your eyes as you will not be able to correctly sense the pressure and may cause injury. If you have a strong urge to rub your eyes, sit on your hands to provide a distraction.
8. Some medications may affect vision, and you should not drive or perform activities that require sharp vision until you know how the medication affects your sight.
9. Do not "save" or share the eye medicine for any other person or eye problem. Discard leftover medications immediately at end of treatment.

REFERENCES

Brunette, R. (2006). Ophthalmology. In J. A. Marx, R. S. Hockberger, & R. M. Walls, et al. (Eds.), *Rosen's emergency medicine: Concepts and clinical practice* (6th ed., pp. 1044-1064). St. Louis: Mosby.

Knoop, K. J., Dennis, W. R., & Hedges, J. R. (2004). Ophthalmologic procedures. In J. R. Roberts, & J. R. Hedges (Eds.), *Clinical procedures in emergency medicine* (4th ed., pp. 1241-1279). Philadelphia: Saunders.

Perry, A. G., & Potter, P. A. (2006). *Clinical nursing skills and techniques* (6th ed.). St. Louis: Mosby.

PROCEDURE 159

Eye Patching

Maureen T. Quigley, MS, ARNP

The routine use of eye patches after simple corneal abrasions occurred previously under the assumption that it hastened healing and reduced pain; this has been proved false in multiple studies (Knoop, Dennis, & Hedges, 2004). Typically, hard patches or eye shields are used when the globe or cornea has been disrupted. This procedure addresses soft patches and eye shields or hard patches. Collagen shields and bandage contact lenses are beyond the scope of this procedure.

INDICATIONS

1. To avoid further injury after trauma to the eye(s), such as occurs in corneal abrasion, chemical damage, or ultraviolet light injuries. It may be useful to patch patients with large abrasions occupying more than half of the corneal surface for pain relief (Jacobs, 2006).
2. To protect the eye after administration of an anesthetic
3. To protect a dilated eye from bright light
4. To aid in resting the eye(s)
5. To protect an injured globe without applying any pressure to the eye, a metal eye shield or paper cup may be used. Injuries that require this type of protection may include hyphema, globe perforation, and protruding foreign objects imbedded in the globe, such as fishhooks or knives.
6. Pressure patching is used to hold the eyelid closed to facilitate healing of corneal defects to limit eyelid movement in an injured eye.

CONTRAINDICATIONS AND CAUTIONS

1. A visual acuity assessment (see Procedure 153) and *complete eye examination should be completed before patching.
2. Patching is contraindicated when corneal epithelial loss is the result of an infection. Patching an infected eye provides a dark, moist environment for bacterial growth (Knoop et al., 2004).
3. A pressure patch should never be applied to a patient who has a penetrating injury. Pressure applied to a globe that has anterior or posterior penetration can cause extrusion of the aqueous or vitreous humor, resulting in further injury to the eye. A protective cup should be used.
4. A pressure patch must be firm enough to keep the eyelid closed. A corneal abrasion may result if the patient is able to open the eye(s) under the patch, thereby scraping off new cells and further irritating the abraded area.
5. A patch should remain in place for no more than 24 hours. The patient is unable to monitor vision or discharge from the eye when a patch remains in place for a prolonged period, which may delay a diagnosis of infection. If needed, a new patch can be placed to reduce the risk of infection.
6. Avoid placing tape directly onto the eyebrow.
7. Black cloth "pirate patches" with elastic should not be used for corneal abrasions, because they are ineffective in keeping the eyelid down and can increase corneal edema (Jacobs, 2006).

EQUIPMENT

Eye patches (minimum of two per affected eye)
Metal eye shield (for selected injuries as noted above)
Tapeless eye shield (for long-term use)
Tape (1-in paper tape or nonallergenic tape)
Eye medications as prescribed

PATIENT PREPARATION

1. Place the patient in a supine position or seated with the head tilted back.

---

*Indicates portions of the procedure usually performed by a physician or an advanced practice nurse.

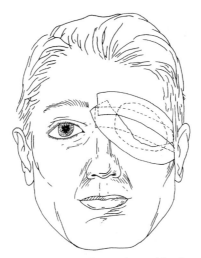

FIGURE 159-1 Eye patch taped in place.

2. Cleanse the skin around the eye to remove dirt, fluids, drainage, or residual eye medications.
3. Facial hairs may interfere with taping the patch and may need to be trimmed to anchor the tape securely.
4. Instill dilating (mydriatic) eye drops and antibiotic ointment, as prescribed (Knoop et al., 2004). Mydriasis relaxes ciliary muscle spasm. See Procedure 158.

PROCEDURAL STEPS
Soft Patches
1. Determine the number of eye pads needed according to the depth of the patient's eye socket:
   a. Ask the patient to close both eyes gently, and to keep them closed during entire procedure.
   b. Fold the first eye patch in half vertically and place it horizontally over the closed lid.
   c. Cover that patch with one or more flat eye patches to fill the eye socket.
2. Tape the patches, starting from the mid-forehead to the cheek and apply firm pressure to the lid. Several strips of tape are necessary. Slightly lifting the cheek before affixing the lower end of the tape will cause the weight of the cheek to exert a mild tension on the patch. Avoid placing tape near angle of the mandible because it may loosen with jaw movement. Skin preparations such as benzoin can be used to help the tape adhere to skin provided they are not used too close to the eye.
3. The tape should cover the entire eye patch to prevent slipping of the patch and movement of the eyelid (Figure 159-1). If the patient can blink, the patch should be reapplied.

Metal or Plastic Eye Shield

1. Stabilize any protruding objects with gauze dressings and tape.
2. Place a metal shield or a paper cup over the affected eye. The shield should contact the superior and inferior orbital rims but not touch the eyelid. The eye shield or cup may need to be cut to accommodate a protruding object (see Procedure 161).
3. Apply strips of tape to secure the shield so that movement or irritation from a foreign object is eliminated.
4. The uninjured eye is often patched with soft patches to minimize movement of the injured eye; patching one eye does not totally immobilize the globe because of conjugate eye movement.

AGE-SPECIFIC CONSIDERATIONS

1. Pediatric patients may be more receptive to eye patching if you tell them the patch is like what a pirate wears.
2. Elderly patients may benefit from assistance with routine ambulation after eye patch application.

COMPLICATIONS

1. Eye patches applied too tightly can result in increased ocular damage (e.g., central retinal artery occlusion).
2. Further trauma may occur to the injured eye from excessive lid motion under a loose eye patch.
3. Eyelashes trapped between the lids can cause corneal abrasion.

PATIENT TEACHING

1. Emphasize need for follow-up as directed.
2. Report any increase in eye pain or signs of infection, such as redness, swelling, or drainage.
3. Limit reading and computer work to help rest the injured eye because both eyes move together. Television viewing from a distance of 10 feet or more is acceptable because it promotes eye fixation (Knoop et al., 2004).
4. Patching affects depth perception, you may have difficulty walking up and down stairs and curbs. Any functional decrease in vision of an eye (whether patched or medicated or by the injury or disease) causes monocularity to some extent with resultant loss of peripheral vision, inadequate depth perception due to loss of triangulation, and a "blind spot." All of these effects can lead to injury and you should not drive, operate machinery, or perform other risky tasks until cleared by a physician.
5. Patching does not affect distance vision.
6. Use protective eyewear when appropriate to prevent future injuries.

REFERENCES

Jacobs, D. S. (2006). Corneal abrasions and corneal foreign bodies. Retrieved January 7, 2007, from *UpToDate*, online version 14.3. www.uptodate.com

Knoop, K. J., Dennis, W. R., & Hedges, J. R. (2004). Ophthalmologic procedures. In J. R. Roberts, & J. R. Hedges (Eds.), *Clinical procedures in emergency medicine* (4th ed., pp. 1241-1279). Philadelphia: Saunders.

Tonometry

Joni Hentzen Daniels, MSN, RN, CEN, CCRN

INDICATIONS

To assess intraocular pressure (IOP) under certain conditions:

1. Patients at risk of increased IOP include hypertensive and elderly patients, adult patients who have glaucoma, and patients who have diabetes or a history of retinal detachment.
2. Patients suspected of having acute angle-closure glaucoma. When a patient complains of acute aching pain in one eye, blurred vision (including "halos" around lights), and a red eye with a smoky cornea, and a fixed midposition pupil, IOP should be determined (Knoop, Dennis, & Hedges, 2004). Sometimes the only complaints may be nausea, vomiting, and headache, suggesting a flu rather than an eye disorder (Knoop et al., 2004).
3. Patients who have sustained blunt ocular injury. Acute increases in IOP are often seen in patients with hyphema (Knoop et al., 2004).
4. Patients who have iritis can develop both open- and closed-angle glaucoma, as well as steroid-induced glaucoma (Knoop et al., 2004).

CONTRAINDICATIONS AND CAUTIONS

1. Tonometry should not be performed if there is any question about the integrity of the globe. Application of pressure to the eye may lead to extrusion of contents and loss of vision.
2. For accurate determination of pressure, the patient must be completely relaxed. Patients who are unable to sustain a relaxed position because of anxiety, blepharospasm, uncontrolled coughing, or nystagmus cannot tolerate a satisfactory examination, and corneal injury may result when sudden movements occur during an examination (Knoop et al., 2004).
3. When corneal defects are present, tonometry is relatively contraindicated. An abraded cornea may suffer further injury if a tonometer is used (Knoop et al., 2004).
4. In the presence of eye infection, tonometry is relatively contraindicated. When possible, tonometry should be avoided in patients with active ocular and facial herpetic lesions as well as in those with acquired immune deficiency syndrome (Knoop et al., 2004). A tonometer with a covered tip, such as Tono-Pen XL or Schiøtz with a sterile, disposable covering, should be used to measure IOP in infected eyes.
5. There are multiple limitations with the use and accurate interpretation of the Schiøtz tonometer, which are beyond the scope of this discussion. Potential inaccuracies occur with differences in ocular rigidity between eyes, scleral rigidity, or extremes in corneal shapes or thickness (Ritch, 2003).

777

6. The Tono-Pen XL is useful in measurement of IOP in patients with scarred or irregular corneas. It is believed that readings in the normal range are accurate, but they may not be accurate in readings that are in high and low ranges, underestimating high-range IOPs, and overestimating IOPs in the low range (Ritch, 2003).

EQUIPMENT

Topical ophthalmic anesthetic

Tonometer (several types available) (Table 160-1)

Tonometers work on the physical principle that the force needed to deform a globe is directly related to the pressure within the globe. There are three basic types:

1. Indentation or high displacement tonometers determine IOP with a plunger that changes the shape of the cornea, making a measurable indentation, which displaces a significant volume of intraocular fluid. Conversion tables are used to estimate the original IOP from the indentation tonometric reading. An example is the Schiøtz tonometer, which is likely to be found in many emergency departments because of familiarity and relatively low cost.

2. Low-displacement or applanation tonometers measure IOP by using a force necessary to only flatten the cornea, which is converted to an IOP value. Examples include Goldmann, Perkins (portable), Draeger (portable), Maklakov, MacKay-Marg, and Tono-Pen XL (portable). The Goldmann applantation tonometer is considered the "gold standard" for IOP measurement (Ritch, 2003).

3. The noncontact tonometer applanates the cornea through a puff of air, measuring IOP without contact with the cornea. An example is the Keeler Pulsair device. The time needed to flatten the cornea is correlated with an estimated IOP. Noncontact tonometers are not useful when accurate readings are indicated; they are more helpful for screening purposes.

TABLE 160-1

COMPARISON OF DIFFERENT TONOMETRY DEVICES

	Devices			
	Schiøtz	**Goldmann**	**Tono-Pen**	**Pulsair**
Accuracy	Good	Excellent	Good	Good
Training	Minimal	Extensive	Minimal	Minimal
Difficulty	Simple	Complex	Simple	Simple
Cost	Low	Moderate	High	High
Position	Supine	Seated	Any	Any
Cross-contamination potential	Yes	Yes	No	No
Pediatric use	Difficult	Difficult	Simple	Simple
Portability	Yes	No	Yes	No

From Dieckmann, R., Fiser, D., & Selbst, S. (1997). *Illustrated textbook of pediatric emergency and critical care procedures* (p. 486). St Louis: Mosby.

PATIENT PREPARATION

1. Place the patient in a darkened room to help decrease ocular pain.
2. Place the patient in a supine (Schiøtz) or semirecumbent position. For the Tono-Pen XL, the patient can be in any position that permits the tonometer to be applied perpendicular to the corneal surface.
3. Instruct the patient not to blink or touch the eyes during the procedure.
4. Instill topical anesthetics or cycloplegics as prescribed. Anesthetics should be administered before cycloplegics.

PROCEDURAL STEPS

Schiøtz and Tono-Pen XL tonometers are discussed in this section. Review complete instructions provided by manufacturer. Other tonometers are rarely used in the emergency department and are beyond the scope of this procedure.

Schiøtz Tonometer (Figure 160-1)

1. Ask the patient to gaze at a fixed spot directly above the eyes.
2. *While the patient keeps both eyes wide open and fixed on an object, separate the eyelids. Be careful to apply direct pressure to the orbital rims instead

---

*Indicates portions of the procedure usually performed by a physician or an advanced practice nurse.

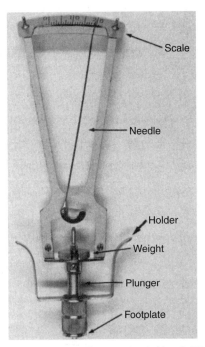

FIGURE 160-1 Schiøtz tonometer. (From Albert, D., & Jakobiec, F. [2000]. *Principles and practice of ophthalmology* [2nd ed., p. 2627]. Philadelphia: Saunders.)

Scale Reading	Plunger Load (g)			
	5.5	7.5	10	15
0	41	59	82	127
.5	38	54	75	118
1	35	50	70	109
1.5	32	46	64	101
2	29	42	59	94
2.5	27	39	55	88
3	24	36	51	82
3.5	22	33	47	76
4	21	30	43	71
4.5	19	28	40	66
5	17	26	37	62
5.5	16	24	34	58
6	15	22	32	54
6.5	13	20	29	50
7	12	19	27	46
7.5	11	17	25	43
8	10	16	23	40
8.5	9	14	21	38
9	9	13	20	35
9.5	8	12	18	32
10	7	11	16	30
10.5	6	10	15	27
11	6	9	14	25
11.5	5	8	13	23
12		8	11	21
12.5		7	10	20
13		6	10	18
13.5		6	9	17
14		5	8	15
14.5			7	14
15			6	13
15.5			6	11
16			5	10
16.5				9
17				8
17.5				8
18				7

FIGURE 160-2 Intraocular pressure table for use with the Schiøtz tonometer. (Courtesy J. Sklar Manufacturing Co., Inc., Long Island City, NY.)

of into the orbit to avoid obtaining an IOP reading that is falsely raised with pressure into the orbit (Knoop et al., 2004).

3. *Gently place the footplate of the tonometer onto the middle portion of the cornea in a position that allows free vertical movement of the plunger.

4. Fine movements on the scale indicate response to the ocular pulsations. The scale reading should be taken as the average between the extremes of these excursions. Extra weight should be added to the plunger when the scale reading is 5 or less (Knoop et al., 2004). The IOP is derived from the scale reading and the plunger weight using a conversion table (Figure 160-2). The same procedure is repeated in the other eye.

5. Normal IOP is 10 to 20 mm Hg. Consultation is indicated when IOP exceeds 20 mm Hg although treatment may not be indicated until pressure exceeds 30 mm Hg (Wightman & Hamilton, 2006).

---

*Indicates portions of the procedure usually performed by a physician or an advanced practice nurse.

TOP VIEW   SIDE VIEW

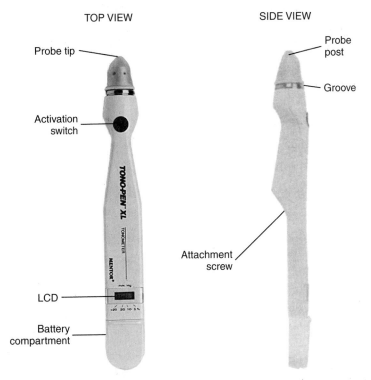

FIGURE 160-3 Tono-Pen diagram. (Courtesy Mentor O & O, Inc. [1993]. *Mentor Tono-Pen XL tonometer instruction manual* [p. 4]. Norwell, MA: Author.)

Tono-Pen XL (Figure 160-3)

1. Cover the probe tip of the calibrated Tono-Pen XL with a new Mentor Ocu-Film tip cover.
2. *Holding the Tono-Pen XL like a pencil, depress the activation switch briefly and then release.
3. When the Tono-Pen XL is available to take a measurement, a beep sounds, and a pattern (= = =) appears on the liquid crystal display.
4. *Touch the Tono-Pen XL unit to the cornea lightly and momentarily, and repeat several times.
5. When a valid reading is obtained, a click sounds, and a digital IOP measurement is exhibited.
6. A final beep is heard after four correct readings have been obtained. The average measurement with variability percentages appears on the liquid crystal display.

---

*Indicates portions of the procedure usually performed by a physician or an advanced practice nurse.

7. Normal IOP is 10 to 20 mm Hg. Consultation is indicated when IOP exceeds 20 mm Hg although treatment may not be indicated until pressure exceeds 30 mm Hg (Wightman & Hamilton, 2006).

AGE-SPECIFIC CONSIDERATIONS

1. Hand-held applanation tonometers and the Tono-Pen are helpful in assessment of children. The normal intraocular pressure in young children is underestimated by applanation tonometry, especially in children under 3 years of age under general anesthesia. The Tono-Pen correlates relatively well with applanation tonometry in children with IOP in the normal range, but it may underestimate elevated IOP.
2. Infants and young children may require examination under sedation (see Procedure 177) or general anesthesia for definitive evaluation of IOP.

COMPLICATIONS

1. Extrusion of the globe contents can occur during the examination if there is a penetrating injury to the globe.
2. Contaminated tonometers transmit infection. In addition to the more ordinary bacteria and viruses that can cause ocular infection, hepatitis B surface antigen can be detected from the tonometer tip after use on infected patients (Saw, Gazzard, & Friedman, 2003). The tip should be sterilized between patients. The CDC states "The tip can be cleaned with soap and water or with another cleansing agent suggested by the manufacturer and disinfected by soaking for at least 10 minutes in a solution containing 500 to 5000 ppm chlorine (e.g., a 1:100 to 1:10 dilution of household bleach) or in any commercial germicidal solution that is registered with the Environmental Protection Agency as a 'sterilant' and is compatible with the tonometer. The soaking time in commercial germicides necessary to achieve high-level disinfection (which includes inactivation of adenovirus type 8 and other viruses and bacteria that are pathogenic to the eye) varies by type and concentration of solution and should be indicated by the germicide manufacturer on the product label" (CDC, 1990). This process is not necessary with the Tono-Pen because a new Ocu-Film tip cover is used for each patient.
3. Corneal abrasions can be caused by movement of the eye during measurement of IOP with contact tonometers.

PATIENT TEACHING

1. Do not blink or touch your eyes during the examination.
2. Do not rub your eyes for at least 30 minutes after the examination.
3. Do not bend over, cough, blow your nose, or strain at stool (if IOP is elevated).

REFERENCES

Centers for Disease Control (CDC). (1990, Sept. 7). Epidemiologic notes and reports epidemic keratoconjunctivitis in an ophthalmology clinic—California. *MMWR, 39*(35), 598-601. Retrieved January 5, 2007, from http://www.cdc.gov/mmwr/preview/mmwrhtml/00001741.htm

Knoop, K. J., Dennis, W. R., & Hedges, J. R. (2004). Ophthalmologic procedures. In J. R. Roberts, & J. R. Hedges (Eds.), *Clinical procedures in emergency medicine* (4th ed., pp. 1241-1279). Philadelphia: Saunders.

Ritch, R. (2003). Assessing the treatment of angle closure. *Ophthalmology, 110,* 1867-1869. Retrieved January 2, 2007, from http://www.ophsource.org/periodicals/ophtha/article/PIIS016164200300719X/fulltext

Saw, S. M., Gazzard, G., & Friedman, D. S. (2003). Interventions for angle closure glaucoma: An evidence-based update. *Ophthalmology, 110,* 1869-1878. Retrieved January 2, 2007, from http://www.ophsource.org/periodicals/ophtha/article/PIIS0161642003005402/fulltext

Wightman, J. M., & Hamilton, G. C. (2006). Red and painful eye. In J. A. Marx, R. S. Hockberger, & R. M. Walls, et al. (Eds.), *Rosen's emergency medicine: Concepts and clinical practice* (6th ed., pp. 283-298). St Louis: Mosby.

PROCEDURE 161

Immobilization of an Ophthalmic Foreign Body

Joni Hentzen Daniels, MSN, RN, CEN, CCRN

INDICATION

To immobilize a foreign object penetrating the eye or periorbital region. Ophthalmic foreign bodies requiring stabilization most often include wooden and metallic fragments or shards (Thomas & Brown, 2006). Diagnosis is usually self-evident. Early diagnosis and treatment both minimize further damage to the eye and to minimize the risks associated with delayed sequelae (such as endophthalmitis) (Thomas & Brown, 2006).

CONTRAINDICATIONS AND CAUTIONS

1. Ophthalmic injuries are treated immediately after life-threatening conditions are stabilized.
2. Do not apply pressure to the eye. Direct pressure should not be used to stop bleeding from or around the eye when a penetrating object is suspected or evident.
3. The use of ophthalmic ointments is contraindicated because they may enter the globe and, in the case of anesthetic ointments, may have a prolonged effect.

4. Uncooperative patients should be examined under sedation or general anesthesia (see Procedure 177).

EQUIPMENT
Rigid eye shields
Gauze eye patches
4 × 4 gauze dressings
Fluffs
Roller bandages
Paper cups
Adhesive tape
Skin preparation material, such as alcohol or acetone

PATIENT PREPARATION
1. Instruct the patient not to touch or rub the eye.
2. Unless contraindicated by other injuries, elevate the head of the bed to decrease intraocular pressure.
3. Administer an antiemetic as prescribed to decrease nausea and vomiting if needed.
4. Administer tetanus immunization as indicated.
5. Maintain nothing per mouth (NPO) status in light of a possible operative intervention and ascertain when the patient had his or her last meal.
6. Obtain previous ophthalmic history: previous surgery and trauma, as well as vision before the presenting injury.
7. Key components of the history include the exact time of injury and events leading to the injury. Other important information include a description and composition of the foreign body, the distance it traveled to the eye, whether it was blown by the wind or propelled into the eye, the direction of travel, and the direction in which the eye was looking at the time of the injury (Khaw, Shah, & Elkington, 2004).

PROCEDURAL STEPS
1. Use a thick dressing to immobilize the foreign object. A variety of materials can be used, including a gauze dressing, fluffs, a paper drinking cup, or a paper cone.
2. Place the dressing around the foreign object to immobilize it and prevent further injury to the eye and surrounding structures. A hole may be cut in the center of the dressing, or the dressing can be arranged around the penetrating object to further immobilize it; the penetrating object should be in the center of the bandage.
3. Place a paper cup or other solid, lightweight object over the penetrating object. The paper cup should rest on the dressing. It should not place pressure on the eye or touch the penetrating object. With larger penetrating objects, it may be difficult or impossible to cover the end of the penetrating object with this type of protective bandage.
4. Patch or shield the uninjured eye to prevent movement in the injured eye (see Procedure 159). If rupture of the globe is suspected, be careful to apply a metal or plastic eye shield resting on the forehead and bony arch of the orbit.

AGE-SPECIFIC CONSIDERATIONS

1. Young children may require an immobilization device, such as a child restraint board, or sedation/anesthesia to be evaluated effectively (see Procedures 177 and 191).
2. In the elderly, eye and orbital trauma are frequently caused by falls, which may also cause other injuries, such as hip fractures. A fall could represent underlying cardiovascular disease, such as an arrhythmia or hypotension, which would necessitate further evaluation.
3. A child may be reluctant to provide a history of the injury if it involved behavior that was inappropriate.
4. A provider should consider abuse or neglect in the child or elderly person when a caregiver or parent seems unwilling to provide information about the injury.

COMPLICATIONS

1. Bacterial or fungal infection
2. Loss of vision or visual acuity
3. Penetration of sinuses or brain with concurrent risk of meningitis

PATIENT TEACHING

1. Do not touch or rub the injured eye.
2. Do not strain, cough, bend over, or lift heavy objects because pressure within the eye will be increased.
3. In some situations, both eyes may be patched to decrease eye movement.
4. Use protective eyewear when appropriate to prevent future injuries.
5. A safe home environment/living arrangement is crucial after a serious eye injury.
6. Any functional decrease in vision of an eye (whether patched or medicated or by the injury or disease) causes monocularity to some extent with resultant loss of peripheral vision, inadequate depth perception due to loss of triangulation, and a "blind spot." All of these effects can lead to injury and you should not drive, operate machinery, or perform other risky tasks until cleared by a physician.

REFERENCES

Khaw, P. T., Shah, P., & Elkington, A. R. (2004). Injury to the eye. *British Medical Journal*, *328*(7430), 36-38. Retrieved January 1, 2007, from http://www.bmj.com/cgi/content/full/328/7430/36.

Thomas, S. H., & Brown, D. M. (2006). Foreign bodies. In J. A. Marx, R. S. Hockberger, & R. M. Walls, et al. (Eds.), *Rosen's emergency medicine: Concepts and clinical practice* (6th ed., pp. 859-881). St Louis: Mosby.

Otic Procedures

Instillation of Ear Medications

Daun A. Smith, RN, MSN

INDICATION

To apply medicated solutions or suspensions (antibiotics, steroids, analgesics, or ceruminolytic agents) into the external auditory canal for otitis externa (swimmer's ear), otitis media, or cerumen accumulation.

CONTRAINDICATIONS AND CAUTIONS

1. Caution should be exercised to identify perforation of the tympanic membrane before instilling medications into the external auditory canal, because inadvertent introduction of foreign material into the middle ear may result in an infection.
2. Medications in suspension (oil based) do not absorb into ear wicks. Use ear wicks with medication in solution form only.
3. Ear medications should be single-patient use only.

EQUIPMENT

Otoscope
Ear wicks or cotton balls
Ear medication (antibiotic, analgesic, or ceruminolytic agent) as prescribed

PROCEDURAL STEPS

1. Place the patient on his or her side with the affected ear up.
2. Straighten and examine the external auditory canal. For an infant, gently pull the pinna down and back. For a child older than age 3 or an adult, pull the pinna up and backward (see Figure 164-1).
3. Clear any debris from the ear canal (see Procedures 164 through 166).
4. Warm the ear medication container by holding it in your hand or placing it in warm water for a short time.
5. Draw up only the amount of medication needed into the ear dropper. Do not return excess medication to the bottle.
6. Instill the correct number of drops along the side of the ear canal. To prevent contamination, do not allow the tip of the ear dropper to touch any part of the ear. Hold it about ½ inch above the ear canal.
7. Press firmly but gently on the tragus of the ear a few times. This helps the medication reach all portions of the canal.
8. Have the patient remain in the same position (with the affected ear up) for a few minutes.

9. Place a small piece of a cotton ball at the external auditory meatus for 15 minutes to help retain the medication when the patient is up. Do not press the cotton into the canal.
10. If an ear wick is to be used, see Procedure 163. Saturate the wick with a topical otic solution.

AGE-SPECIFIC CONSIDERATION

To straighten the external auditory canal of an infant, gently pull the pinna down and back; for a child older than 3 years of age or an adult, pull the pinna up and backward.

COMPLICATIONS

1. If cotton balls are used instead of an ear wick, disintegration may occur, and removal may be difficult. To avoid retention of pieces of cotton balls, place them only at the meatus.
2. Without an ear wick or a cotton ball, solutions or suspensions may extravasate from the ear canal.
3. Otic solutions frequently cause a burning or stinging sensation; suspensions are less painful.

PATIENT TEACHING

1. Report immediately ear pain, an edematous canal, tender ear cartilage, purulent drainage, or hearing loss.
2. If present, leave the ear wick in place for 48 to 72 hours. Repeat instillation of medication onto the ear wick three or four times daily or as directed.
3. Continuation of medication may be necessary after ear wick removal (approximately 10 days for antibiotics).
4. If an ear wick is not used, you may place a cotton ball at the external auditory meatus to prevent extravasation of the medication.

PROCEDURE 163

Ear Wick Insertion

Margo E. Layman, MSN, RN, RNC, CN-A

INDICATION

To allow continuous release of medication in the external ear canal and absorption of any excess secretions during the treatment of otitis externa.

CONTRAINDICATIONS AND CAUTIONS

1. If there are lacerations of the ear canal, an ear wick should not be inserted.
2. An ear wick could slip into the hole of a ruptured tympanic membrane.

3. Alcohol or acidic medications may cause a burning or stinging sensation.
4. If the ear canal is swollen shut, an ear wick cannot be inserted.

EQUIPMENT

Cotton, ½-in × ½-in selvedged gauze, or 2 × 10-mm compressed hydroxy-cellulose manufactured ear wick
Antibiotic/steroid cream
Prescribed ear drops with dropper
Cerumen spoon
Small metal suction tip
Small alligator forceps
Otoscope

PATIENT PREPARATION

Place the patient in semi-Fowler's position.

PROCEDURAL STEPS

1. Using an otoscope, check the external ear for redness or drainage.
2. Examine the internal ear with an otoscope.
3. Suction debris from the ear with the small metal suction tip, or remove debris gently with a cerumen spoon.
4. Irrigation may be necessary (after visualization of ear drum) before placement of ear wick to allow effective dispersal of medications to inflamed tissue. See Procedure 164.
5. Use a small alligator forceps to twist the ear wick in place in the canal. Follow the accompanying directions to insert a commercially prepared wick, or make a wick by wrapping cotton or selvedged gauze tightly around the tip of an alligator forceps, grasping the cotton or gauze with the forceps, and placing it in the ear canal. Antibiotic or steroid cream can be applied to gauze before wrapping.
6. Place the prescribed ear drops in the ear canal, taking care not to touch the dropper to the ear canal (Figure 163-1). Place drops along the side of the canal so that air is displaced as they flow. Cold drops may cause vertigo or nausea; this can be avoided by warming the medication slightly in your hands or by immersing the bottle in a cup of warm water for several minutes.
7. Place 1 or 2 additional drops on the ear wick to saturate it.

AGE-SPECIFIC CONSIDERATIONS

1. Place a small child in the supine position, restraining the knees, and holding the arms firmly against the head with the face turned left or right.
2. In small children, trim off one-fourth to one-third of a commercially prepared wick to help prevent it from falling out (Block, 2005).

COMPLICATIONS

1. The ear wick may adhere to the ear canal if it is not kept moist.
2. The ear wick may slip deeper into the canal. This could cause irritation of the tympanic membrane.

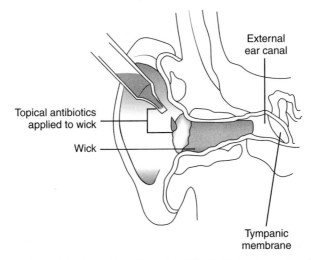

FIGURE 163-1 Ear wick in place. (From Block, S. L. [2005]. Otitis externa: Providing relief while avoiding complications. *Journal of Family Practice, 54*[8], 671.)

PATIENT TEACHING

1. Most ear wicks will spontaneously extrude in 12 to 36 hours (Block, 2005). If necessary, return in 24 to 48 hours to have ear wick removed or follow up with your physician to have it removed. Make sure the wick is moist before removing it.
2. Instill ear drops as instructed. Cold ear drops may cause dizziness or nausea. Warm the bottle between your hands or in a cup of warm water before instilling the drops.
3. Symptoms should subside in 1 or 2 days. If no improvement occurs or if symptoms worsen, contact your physician.
4. To prevent the ear wick from slipping, do not touch the ear, and do not place cotton in the ear canal over the wick, because the cotton will absorb all the drops.
5. Take oral pain medications as prescribed and apply a warm moist compress to ear for pain.
6. To prevent future infections, do not put foreign objects in the ear. Ear rinses used after swimming may be helpful. Avoid strong jets from showerheads going directly into the ears.

REFERENCE

Block, S. L. (2005). Otitis externa: Providing relief while avoiding complications. *Journal of Family Practice, 54*(8), 669-676.

Ear Irrigation

June F. Stacey, RN, BSN, CEN

INDICATIONS

1. To remove drainage, cerumen, or foreign bodies from the external auditory canal
2. To irrigate the external auditory canal with an antiseptic solution
3. To apply heat or cold to the external auditory canal

CONTRAINDICATIONS AND CAUTIONS

1. Irrigation is contraindicated if the tympanic membrane is perforated or potentially not intact, (secondary to injury, myringotomy tubes, or surgery) or in the presence of severe external otitis (Riviello, 2004).
2. Avoid extreme temperatures, which may cause pain, dizziness, nausea, and vomiting (Riviello, 2004).
3. If there is water-absorbent material in the ear, such as vegetable matter (e.g., beans), do not irrigate, because the material may swell and make removal more difficult (see Procedure 165) (Riviello, 2004).
4. Be careful not to abrade the ear canal with the irrigating device.
5. Discontinue the procedure and notify the physician if the patient experiences pain, vertigo, or nystagmus (Parshall, 2005).
6. Use caution with elderly and immunocompromised patients because irrigation may lead to malignant otitis externa (Riviello, 2005).
7. Do not attempt on an uncooperative patient or child who cannot be still or adequately restrained to perform the procedure safely (Forzley, 2003).
8. Referral to a specialist should be considered if the affected ear is the only hearing ear (Forzley, 2003).

EQUIPMENT

Otologic ear syringe (metal ear syringe)
or
60-ml syringe with an 18- or 20-G intravenous catheter sheath attached, or a butterfly, with the needle and wings removed, cut to leave approximately 1 in of tubing near the hub
or
Dental irrigating device (such as a Water-Pik) on low setting (A proper ear irrigating syringe is preferred to extemporized devices or a Water-Pik because it supplies a large volume at low pressure, rather than the high pressures of other devices.)
Irrigant—warm water, warm normal saline, or half-strength hydrogen peroxide

Basin to hold irrigant
Towels or waterproof pad
Emesis basin
Otoscope
Thermometer (optional)
Cotton balls or gauze dressings
Cotton-tipped applicators

PATIENT PREPARATION
1. Position the patient with the head tilted toward the affected ear.
2. Protect the patient's clothing with towels or a waterproof pad.

PROCEDURAL STEPS
1. Cleanse any discharge from the outer ear with a cotton-tipped applicator. Examine both ears with an otoscope before the procedure to establish a baseline. To examine the ear, pull the auricle of the ear up and outward to straighten the ear canal.
2. If a ceruminolytic is used, it should be instilled into affected ear(s) at least 10 minutes before attempting irrigation (Parshall, 2005).
3. Prepare the irrigation solution. Common irrigation solutions include tap water or a 1:1 solution of tap water and hydrogen peroxide. The solution should be at body temperature. If you drip some of the solution onto your inner wrist, it should be a comfortable temperature, or you can check the temperature with a thermometer.
4. Draw up the irrigation solution into the syringe and expel the air from the syringe.
5. Ask the patient to hold the emesis basin under the ear and against the neck.
6. Stress the importance of remaining still during the procedure.
7. Pull the auricle of the ear up and backward (Figure 164-1, A). Place the tip of the irrigating syringe at the opening of the ear canal. Do not occlude the opening of the ear canal, because this can cause excessive pressure, which could in turn lead to rupture of the tympanic membrane. Direct the fluid toward the posterior wall of the canal, not at the tympanic membrane (Figure 164-2). Visualize the perimeter of the canal as a clock face. For the left ear, direct the fluid toward 1 o'clock; for the right ear, direct the fluid toward 11 o'clock (Parshall, 2005).
8. Irrigate slowly to prevent build-up of pressure inside the canal. If a Water-Pik is used, special care must be taken to avoid excessive water pressure (Parshall, 2005).
9. After each irrigation, inspect the ear canal to assess the progress being made, or check the irrigation solution as it returns to the basin for cerumen or foreign bodies. If the irrigation is successful, the patient will generally report a relief of symptoms (Parshall, 2005).
10. Repeat the irrigation as needed, allowing the patient to rest between each irrigation if necessary.
11. If irrigation is not successful, ceruminolytic drops may be prescribed for several days and the patient referred for follow-up. Irrigation may be reattempted if cerumen impaction does not spontaneously resolve.

12. After irrigation, dry the outer ear with a cotton ball. The cotton ball may be left loosely in place for 5 to 10 minutes to absorb any excess moisture. Instillation of a drying agent such as isopropyl alcohol may be prescribed.

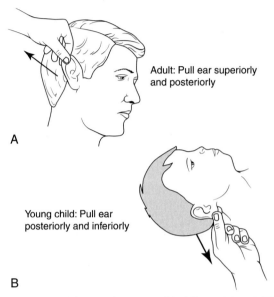

Adult: Pull ear superiorly and posteriorly

A

Young child: Pull ear posteriorly and inferiorly

B

FIGURE 164-1 Straightening the ear canal in **(A)** an adult and **(B)** a child.

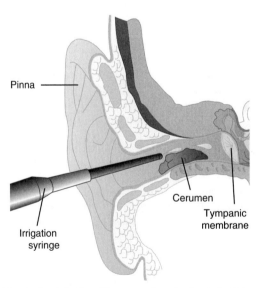

Pinna

Cerumen

Tympanic membrane

Irrigation syringe

FIGURE 164-2 Ear irrigation. The ear syringe is directed at the upper wall of the ear canal. (From Black, J., & Hawks, J. [2005]. *Medical-surgical nursing* [7th ed., p. 1984]. Philadelphia: Saunders.)

AGE-SPECIFIC CONSIDERATIONS

1. The ear canal in a child is small. Caution should be exercised to avoid totally occluding the canal during irrigation because excessive pressure within the ear canal may result.
2. To straighten the ear canal in a child younger than age 3, pull the ear down and outward (Figure 164-1, *B*).
3. Place the child in the supine position. If the child is uncooperative and all other appropriate control measures have failed, a child restraint board may be used to prevent movement (see Procedure 191).
4. Ill children may require ear irrigation if cerumen prevents visualization and assessment of the tympanic membrane, because this is a key component of the evaluation of a febrile child (Riviello, 2004).
5. A dental irrigation device should be used with caution in children because the jet stream is forceful. Use the lowest setting and aim toward the posterior wall of the ear canal. To decrease the child's fear, explain the procedure and demonstrate the device, allowing the child to feel the water on his or her hand and listen to the noise.
6. Do not use cool irrigant because dizziness or discomfort may result, especially in an older patient (Riviello, 2004).
7. Cerumen impaction is very common in the elderly, but care should be used as malignant otitis externa may result.
8. Caution should be used in the immunocompromised patient.

COMPLICATIONS

1. Vertigo, nausea, or pain during or after the procedure. Stop immediately if any of these symptoms occur. Allow the patient to rest until the symptoms resolve and then restart. Be sure gentle pressure is used. Aim at the posterior portion of the ear canal and use the proper irrigant temperature to help prevent recurrence of symptoms.
2. Rupture of the tympanic membrane with possible middle ear injury
3. Loss of hearing
4. Trauma or injury to the ear canal
5. Otitis externa

PATIENT TEACHING

1. Report any pain, nausea, dizziness, or loss of hearing as it occurs during the procedure.
2. Report any persistent pain, purulent drainage, vertigo, or fever (Riviello, 2004).
3. Cleanse the outer ears daily with a washcloth, soap, and water.
4. Do not place objects in your ears, especially cotton applicators that can impact cerumen. "Instrumentation" of the ear should only be done with direct vision by a competent practitioner.
5. Patients with unrelieved impactions, who are to return after a course of softening treatment, should be cautioned about a possible increased risk when driving and or performing hazardous tasks because of diminished hearing, attention, and possible dysequilibrium until the problem is resolved.

REFERENCES

Forzley, G. J. (2003). Cerumen impaction and removal. In J. L. Pfenning & G. C. Fowler (Eds.), *Procedures for primary care* (2nd ed., pp. 427-431). St Louis: Mosby.

Parshall, M. B. (2005). Ear irrigation. In J. Fultz & P. A. Sturt (Eds.), *Emergency nursing reference* (3rd ed., pp. 820-823). St Louis: Mosby.

Riviello, R. J. (2004). Otolaryngologic procedures. In J. R. Roberts & J. R. Hedges (Eds.), *Clinical procedures in emergency medicine* (4th ed., pp. 1287-1300). Philadelphia: Saunders.

PROCEDURE 165

Otic Foreign Body Removal

Daun A. Smith, RN, MSN

INDICATION

To remove a foreign body from the ear by means of water irrigation, suction, direct instrumentation, or magnet when digital removal has failed

CONTRAINDICATIONS AND CAUTIONS

1. Anatomical narrowing occurs at two separate points in the external auditory canal. Many objects become lodged at these points. Avoid pushing a foreign body beyond these narrowings during extrication attempts because damage to the ear may result (Figure 165-1).
2. The ear canal is sensitive, and instrumentation can be very painful. Conscious sedation or general anesthesia may be necessary as local anesthesia of the canal is traumatic to the patient and difficult to achieve (Riviello, 2004).
3. If the patient's history or physical examination (tinnitus, hearing loss, bleeding) suggests a tympanic membrane disruption, irrigation is contraindicated for foreign body removal (Riviello, 2004).
4. Irrigation of foreign bodies that have the potential to swell and become more firmly impacted when hydrated (e.g., vegetable matter) is contraindicated.
5. Live insects should be killed before removal is attempted. Instill mineral oil or alcohol into the ear to kill the insect. Another method is to irrigate with 2% lidocaine solution, which quickly kills the insect (Tami et al., 1992). Lidocaine may cause vertigo in patients with a perforated tympanic membrane (Riviello, 2004).
6. Miniature batteries lodged in the ear canal pose a special problem. In addition to a potential mechanical trauma, a chemical reaction may occur as a result of leakage of the battery contents. Tympanic membrane perforation, facial paralysis, or ossicular chain damage may result. Prompt otolaryngologic referral is crucial if the battery is not easily extracted (Riviello, 2004).

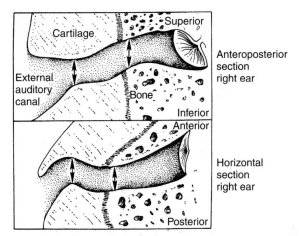

FIGURE 165-1 Horizontal and vertical cross sections of external ear canal showing points of anatomic narrowing. (From Thomas, S. H., & Brown, D. F. M. [2006]. Foreign bodies. In J. A. Marx, R. S. Hockberger, R. M. Walls, et al. [Eds.], *Rosen's emergency medicine: Concepts and clinical practice* [6th ed., p. 862]. St Louis: Mosby.)

7. Contralateral ear examination should be performed to rule out bilateral ear foreign bodies.
8. Instrumentation or direct irrigation onto the foreign body may cause it to move deeper into the canal toward the tympanic membrane.
9. If the foreign body cannot be easily removed, referral to an ear, nose, and throat specialist for removal under general anesthesia with an operating microscope is warranted. Repeated unsuccessful attempts at removal may injure the auditory canal.

EQUIPMENT
Various procedures may be used for removal of a foreign body from the ear. Some or all of the following equipment may be needed:
Adequate light source (otoscope or headlamp)
Ear speculum
Magnetized speculum (used for removal of metallic batteries)
Blunt right-angle hook, wire loops, cerumen curette, alligator or bayonet forceps (Figure 165-2)
Suction catheter (Frazier)
Suction setup
Schuknecht foreign body remover (a suction catheter that works well on smooth, round foreign bodies by conforming to their shape)
Irrigation equipment (20-ml syringe with flexible 18-G intravenous catheter or the tubing of a butterfly catheter with the needle removed) (Figure 165-3)
Fogarty biliary catheter

PATIENT PREPARATION
1. Sedate or restrain the patient as indicated (see Procedures 177 and 191).
2. Emphasize the importance of not moving during the procedure.

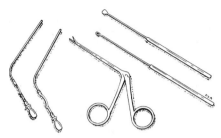

FIGURE 165-2 Instruments used for removal of foreign bodies from the external auditory canal (*left* to *right*): Frazier suction catheters, alligator forceps, wire loop, and ear curette. (From Votey, S., & Dudley, J. P. [1989]. Emergency ear, nose, and throat procedures. *Emergency Medicine Clinics of North America, 7*, p. 124.)

3. For irrigation, drape the patient with towels and place an emesis basin nearby for collection of the irrigation fluid.

PROCEDURAL STEPS

One or more of the following procedures may be necessary to remove a foreign body from the external auditory canal:

1. Instruments that grasp such as alligator forceps, loops, and curettes are used for easily visible and reachable objects such as erasers, small toys, crayons, or tissue (Kadish, 2005).
2. *Suction may be used for hard round objects (Kadish, 2005). Place the tip of the suction catheter on the foreign body and gently retract (Figure 165-4).

---

*Indicates portions of the procedure usually performed by a physician or an advanced practice nurse.

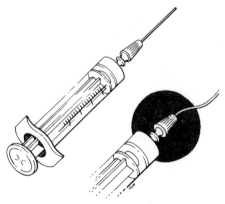

FIGURE 165-3 A flexible 18-G intravenous catheter attached to a 20-ml syringe *(left)* and a butterfly catheter with the needle cut off attached to a 20-ml syringe *(right)*. (From Votey, S., & Dudley, J. P. [1989]. Emergency ear, nose, and throat procedures. *Emergency Medicine Clinics of North America, 7*, p. 124.)

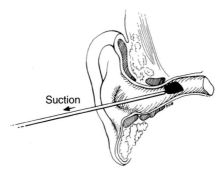

FIGURE 165-4 Use of Frazier suction catheter for removal of a foreign body in the external auditory canal. (From Votey, S., & Dudley, J. P. [1989]. Emergency ear, nose, and throat procedures. *Emergency Medicine Clinics of North America, 7*, p. 124.)

If using a Schuknecht foreign body remover, apply suction only after the catheter has conformed to the shape of the foreign body.

3. Irrigation is used for objects that are neither easily visualized nor removed by other measures. Irrigate the ear canal with lukewarm water to avoid stimulating the labyrinths. Direct the stream of fluid to the edge of the foreign body and attempt to force the fluid gently behind the foreign body and out the ear canal (see Procedure 164).

4. *Pass a right-angle hook (blunt ended) beyond the foreign body and gently retract.

5. *If removing a battery, observe the battery directly and insert a solid ferro-magnetic metallic speculum into the external auditory meatus. The object should move toward the speculum and can then be withdrawn.

6. *Insert a Fogarty biliary catheter past the foreign body, inflate the balloon, and retract the catheter, thus dislodging the foreign body.

7. *If removing a smooth round object, place a small drop of cyanoacrylate glue on the blunt end of a cotton-tipped swab. Straighten the ear canal with a slight traction (see Age-Specific Considerations item 4) to visualize the foreign object. Gently insert the blunt end of the swab into the ear canal to contact the object. The glue dries in 15 seconds, and the swab and object can both be removed. Mineral oil, alcohol, or acetone may be used to separate adherent edges if the glue comes in contact with the ear canal.

AGE-SPECIFIC CONSIDERATIONS

1. Otic foreign bodies are found most commonly in the younger pediatric population.

2. Toddlers consider any attempt to look into their ears as intrusive and threatening.

3. Occasionally, because of their age and inability to cooperate with the examination, young children may need sedation or general anesthesia. For their

---

*Indicates portions of the procedure usually performed by a physician or an advanced practice nurse.

safety, infants and toddlers should be restrained for otoscopic examination and foreign body removal. The small child can be held in the parent's lap. The parent can secure the child's arms by "hugging" the child. The child's head can then be turned with the ear to be examined tilted upward. If the child cannot be held securely in that manner, a mummy restraint or infant restraint board may be used (see Procedure 191).

4. In children who are younger than age 3, the pinna should be pulled down to straighten the ear canal. In children older than age 3, the ear canal is straightened in the same manner as an adult, by pulling up and back on the pinna (see Figure 164-1).

COMPLICATIONS

1. Blind attempts at foreign body removal may lead to complications, such as tissue trauma or pushing the foreign body farther into the ear canal. Direct visualization should always be used to remove foreign bodies from the ear.
2. Perforation of the tympanic membrane may occur as a complication of instrument use in the ear canal.
3. Topical antimicrobial therapy may be indicated if trauma is sustained to the epithelial tissue of the external canal during the procedure.
4. Part of the foreign body may be retained. Repeat direct observation after the foreign body has been removed to verify that no part of the object is retained.

PATIENT TEACHING

1. Do not attempt to remove foreign objects that are not readily visible or capable of being grasped easily.
2. Uncomplicated foreign body removal does not routinely require follow-up care unless there is evidence of otitis externa, injury to the external auditory canal or tympanic membrane, or retained foreign body. If drainage, fever, pain, or swelling occurs, seek medical attention.
3. Bleeding may occur as a result of damage caused by instrumentation.
4. Keep small objects away from small children to prevent recurrences.

REFERENCES

Kadish, H. (2005). Ear and nose foreign bodies: It's all about the tools. *Clinical Pediatrics, 44,* 665-670.

Riviello, R. J. (2004). Otolaryngologic procedures. In J. R. Roberts & J. R. Hedges (Eds.), *Clinical procedures in emergency medicine* (4th ed., pp. 1290-1292). Philadelphia: Saunders.

Tami, T. A., Crumley, R. L., & Mills, J. (1992). ENT emergencies: Disorders of the ear, nose, sinuses, oropharynx, and teeth. In C. E. Saunders & M. T. Ho (Eds.), *Current emergency diagnosis and treatment* (pp. 429-444). Norwalk, CT: Appleton-Lange.

Cerumen Removal

Daun A. Smith, RN, MS

INDICATION

To remove cerumen accumulation (partial occlusion of the ear canal) or impaction (complete occlusion of the ear canal with the tympanic membrane unable to be visualized) from the external auditory canal.

CONTRAINDICATIONS AND CAUTIONS

1. An accurate history should be taken to identify signs of infection or past problems with the ears that may indicate perforation of the tympanic membrane.
2. Irrigation is contraindicated in the presence of tympanic membrane perforation, tympanotomy tubes, or an intact tympanic membrane that has an atrophic region after perforation and suboptimal spontaneous healing.
3. Otitis externa is a relative contraindication to the removal of cerumen because irrigation may aggravate the condition. Otitis externa should be treated with antibiotic eardrops, and cerumen removal should be accomplished after the condition is resolved (Fox & Bartlett, 2001).
4. Hearing loss, tinnitus, and head noise have been linked to impacted cerumen, along with the potential for psychosocial disturbances. Conductive hearing loss may be caused by cerumen impaction and is often overlooked (Fox & Bartlett, 2001).
5. Use of a high-pressure irrigating device may result in tympanic membrane injury.

EQUIPMENT

Otoscope
Ceruminolytic agent (optional) (triethanolamine polypeptide [Cerumenex], or docusate sodium [Colace]) (Singer, Sauris, & Vicellio, 2000)
Low-pressure water irrigation equipment (including ear syringe, tubing, and basin)
or
High-pressure water irrigation equipment (including Water-Pik instrument, tubing, and basin)
Cerumen loop (metal or plastic)
Suction tip (optional)
Suction setup (optional)

PATIENT PREPARATION

1. Drape the patient with towels or absorbent padding to absorb excess irrigation fluid.

801

2. Advise the patient that sensations of dizziness are commonly experienced during irrigation.
3. The patient should be placed in a sitting or semi-Fowler's position with the head tilted toward the affected ear.

PROCEDURAL STEPS

1. Perform an otoscopic examination before and after cerumen removal. Gently pull the pinna up and back in adults (down and back in children younger than age 3) before inserting the otoscope (see Figure 164-1). Identify the cerumen plug and assess the integrity of the tympanic membrane. If the tympanic membrane is visible, cerumen removal is not necessary (Grossan, 2000).
2. If the tympanic membrane is intact, ceruminolytic agents may be used to penetrate the accumulation of cerumen and loosen the plug (see Procedure 162).
3. For irrigation, tilt the head 15 degrees toward the affected ear and position a basin to collect the fluid as it drains. Use lukewarm water to prevent dizziness and nystagmus (Riviello, 2004). Direct the flow of water to the edge of the cerumen, not directly onto the tympanic membrane (see Procedure 164).
4. *Removal of cerumen can also be performed with various sizes and shapes of suction tips (Figure 166-1). Wall or portable suction can then be applied through the suction tip, which is placed directly on the cerumen plug.
5. *A cerumen loop or curette (either metal or plastic) may be used to scrape and remove cerumen gently from the external auditory canal (Figure 166-2). Curettage should never be performed blindly.
6. If irrigation is used during the cerumen removal, gently dry the canal with a cotton-tipped applicator.

AGE-SPECIFIC CONSIDERATIONS

1. Cerumen impaction, accumulation, or both are common but often overlooked causes of conductive hearing loss in the elderly. Risk factors include hearing aids, overabundance of hairs in the ear canal, dry cerumen, and benign bony growths, such as osteophytes (Grossan, 2004).

---

*Indicates portions of the procedure usually performed by a physician or an advanced practice nurse.

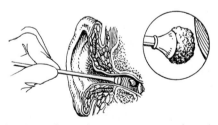

FIGURE 166-1 A suction tip can be used to remove cerumen from the ear canal. (From Harley, J. R. [1997]. Otic foreign body and cerumen removal. In M. C. Walsh-Sukys & S. E. Krug [Eds.], *Procedures in infants and children* [p. 351]. Philadelphia: Saunders.)

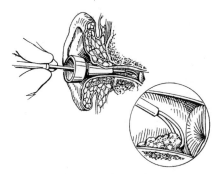

FIGURE 166-2 A curette or wire loop can be used to remove cerumen under visualization with an otoscope. (From Harley, J. R. [1997]. Otic foreign body and cerumen removal. In M. C. Walsh-Sukys & S. E. Krug [Eds.], *Procedures in infants and children [p. 351]*. Philadelphia: Saunders.)

2. Small children are apprehensive about an otoscopic examination. If necessary, the small child may be positioned in the parent's lap with the child's arms secured. The parent can accomplish this by "hugging" the child. The child's head can then be turned and held with the ear to be examined turned upward (see Procedure 191).

COMPLICATIONS

1. Otitis media may result from irrigation in the presence of a tympanic membrane perforation.
2. If cold water is used with irrigation, dizziness, nystagmus, and nausea may result.
3. Damage to the external canal can occur if the lining of the canal is scratched by the instruments used for cerumen removal.
4. Perforation of the tympanic membrane can result from blind instrumentation or from sudden movements of the patient.
5. Otitis externa may result if the ear canal is not dried after irrigation (Fox & Bartlett, 2001). "Swimmer's ear" drops (alcohol and glycerin) or a few drops of alcohol in the ear canal can displace water, drying and disinfecting the canal; some warmth will be noted briefly by the patient.

PATIENT TEACHING

1. Cerumen accumulation may cause hearing loss. Hearing loss may also be caused by sensorineural problems that result from damage to the eighth cranial nerve. A combination of conductive and sensorineural hearing loss may occur. Seek medical care promptly in the presence of hearing loss.
2. Cerumen impaction, dermatitis, and skin infections may result from self-treatment with cotton swabs or other objects. Avoid introducing objects into your ears.
3. Excessive ear hair may cause difficulty in manual removal of earwax and may require special attention to prevent cerumen build-up.
4. Hearing aids may increase wax production and impede the normal propulsive action of the ear cilia.

REFERENCES

Fox, A. & Bartlett, P. (2001). Nurse-led ear care: Training needs and the latest techniques. *Professional Nurse, 17,* 256-258.

Grossan, M. (2000). Safe effective techniques for cerumen removal. *Geriatrics, 55,* 80-86.

Riviello, R. J. (2004). Otolaryngologic procedures. In J. R. Roberts & J. R. Hedges (Eds.), *Clinical procedures in emergency medicine* (4th ed., pp. 1290-1292). Philadelphia: Saunders.

Singer, A. J., Sauris, E., & Viccellio, A. W. (2000). Ceruminolytic effect of docusate sodium: A randomized controlled trial. *Annals of Emergency Medicine, 36,* 228-232.

Nasal Procedures

Topical Vasoconstrictors for Epistaxis

Daun A. Smith, RN, MSN

INDICATION

To stop or slow anterior or posterior epistaxis. If topical vasoconstrictor therapy does not stop the bleeding, it may at least slow it and help provide a dry field for chemical or electrical cautery.

CONTRAINDICATIONS AND CAUTIONS

Topical vasoconstrictors may elevate the blood pressure and heart rate. Patients with cardiopulmonary problems or hypertension should be treated with caution.

EQUIPMENT

Headlamp
Nasal speculum
Atomizer (for medications not packaged in a spray bottle)
Topical vasoconstrictor, anesthetic, or both (e.g., phenylephrine hydrochloride, ephedrine, epinephrine, oxymetazoline)
Cotton swabs
Tissues

PATIENT PREPARATION

1. Place the patient in semi-Fowler's position or in a seated position in a dental chair.
2. Have patient blow his or her nose to expel clots and then apply firm, direct pressure by pinching the nares for a full 10 minutes.

PROCEDURAL STEPS

1. Place cotton swabs soaked with the topical vasoconstrictor in the nose for 5 to 10 minutes (Kucik & Clenney, 2005). Alternatively, have the patient spray the medication into each naris twice while inhaling through the nose (Van, 2004). The spray application may be repeated if the bleeding does not stop within a few minutes. Do not exceed the maximum safe dose of the medication.

2. *Examine both nares using a headlamp and a nasal speculum to verify that the bleeding has stopped.
3. Reassess heart rate and blood pressure after medication administration as indicated, especially for patients with cardiac disease.

AGE-SPECIFIC CONSIDERATIONS

1. Anterior nosebleeds are the most common among children. These usually result from cracks in the nasal lining because of exposure to abrupt temperature changes, dry heat, and nose picking.
2. In adults, anterior nosebleeds result from hypertension, coagulopathy, sinus disease, respiratory infections, allergies, and nasal steroid sprays.

COMPLICATIONS

1. Dizziness, tachycardia, dysrhythmia, nausea/vomiting, or hypertension
2. Topical therapy may fail to control bleeding and alternative therapies may be required (see Procedures 168 through 172).
3. Continued blood loss may result in hypovolemia and shock.

PATIENT TEACHING

1. For the next few days, avoid anything that may lead to more bleeding, such as heavy exercise or lifting, alcoholic beverages, hot drinks, aspirin, ibuprofen, blowing your nose, sneezing, or coughing. If you must sneeze, open your mouth to relieve the pressure.
2. Apply petroleum jelly or antibiotic ointment to the nares to decrease drying and scab formation.
3. Use a humidifier at home, especially in your bedroom at night.
4. Sleeping with extra pillows to raise the head may lessen likelihood of recurrence, ease stuffiness, and minimize post-nasal trickle.
5. Return to the emergency department or call your physician for any recurrence of bleeding that does not stop after 10 minutes of firmly pinching your nose. Emphasize that uninterrupted pressure must be held for 10 minutes or more without letting go, peeking, or dabbing; this will nearly always stop bleeding, and will certainly limit it en route to the hospital.

---

*Indicates portions of the procedure usually performed by a physician or an advanced practice nurse.

REFERENCES

Kucik, C. J., & Clenney, T. (2005). Management of epistaxis. *American Family Physician, 71*(2), 305-311.

Van, D. C. (2004). ENT emergencies: Disorders of the ear, nose, sinuses, oropharynx, & mouth. In C. K. Stone & R. Humphries (Eds.), *Current emergency diagnosis and treatment* (5th ed., pp. 626-653). New York: Lange Medical Books.

Electrical and Chemical Cautery for Epistaxis

Daun A. Smith, RN, MSN

INDICATION

To stop anterior epistaxis

CONTRAINDICATIONS AND CAUTIONS

1. Silver nitrate will not cauterize an actively bleeding area; hemostasis must be achieved first.
2. Septal damage or perforation may occur with overly aggressive electrocautery.
3. Silver nitrate reduces the blood supply to the area; bilateral use may cause septal necrosis.
4. If cautery is unsuccessful or rebleeding occurs within 72 hours, anterior packing is usually placed (see Procedures 169 and 171) (Riviello, 2004).
5. Electrocautery may be performed with a small battery-operated cautery unit or a larger electrosurgical unit. If the electrosurgical unit is used, a practitioner appropriately trained in the safe use of this modality should be responsible for ensuring that the patient is grounded and that other necessary safety precautions are taken.

EQUIPMENT

Headlamp
Nasal speculum
Frazier nasal suction tip
Silver nitrate sticks
Electrocautery
Cotton swabs
Antibiotic ointment
Topical or local anesthetic

PATIENT PREPARATION

1. Place the patient in a dental chair or in semi-Fowler's position on a stretcher.
2. Have the patient blow his or her nose to clear it of clots.
3. Attach grounding pad to the patient and take other appropriate electrical safety precautions if using a large electrosurgery unit.

PROCEDURAL STEPS

1. *Using headlamp and nasal speculum, locate the bleeding site.
2. Suction the area until the site is visualized and dry. The bleeding site must be dry for silver nitrate sticks to be effective.
3. *Anesthetize the nasal mucosa with a topical anesthetic for electrocautery (see Procedure 135).
4. *Coagulate the bleeding site with the silver nitrate sticks or electrocautery.
   a. Silver nitrate: Hold the stick in place for only 20-30 seconds.
   b. Electrocautery: Coagulate only a 1-mm area. The cautery damages and weakens tissue and may cause additional bleeding.
5. *After application of silver nitrate, dry the cautery site with cotton swabs to prevent the silver nitrate from spreading.
6. Apply antibiotic ointment to the cautery site to soften the crust formed by the cautery.

AGE-SPECIFIC CONSIDERATIONS

1. Anterior nosebleeds are the most common among children. These usually result from cracks in the nasal lining because of exposure to abrupt temperature changes, dry heat, and nose picking.
2. In adults, anterior nosebleeds result from hypertension, coagulopathy, sinus disease, respiratory infections, and allergies.

COMPLICATIONS

1. Cauterization can weaken the tissue and make future cauterization more harmful.
2. Burns may occur during cauterization with a large electrosurgery unit if appropriate grounding and other safety measures are not in place.
3. Continued blood loss may result in hypovolemia and shock.

PATIENT TEACHING

1. Avoid the following activities and substances for the next few days because they may lead to more bleeding: heavy exercise or lifting, alcoholic beverages, hot drinks, aspirin, ibuprofen, blowing your nose, sneezing, or coughing. If you must sneeze, open your mouth to relieve pressure.
2. Apply petroleum jelly or antibiotic ointment to the nares to decrease drying and scab formation.
3. Use a humidifier at home, especially in your bedroom at night.
4. Sleeping with extra pillows to raise the head may lessen likelihood of recurrence, ease stuffiness, and minimize post-nasal trickle.
5. Return to the emergency department or call your physician for any recurrence of bleeding that does not stop after 10 minutes of firmly pinching your nose. Emphasize that uninterrupted pressure must be held for 10 minutes or more without letting go, peeking, or dabbing; this will nearly always stop bleeding, and will certainly limit it en route to the hospital.

---

*Indicates portions of the procedure usually performed by a physician or an advanced practice nurse.

REFERENCE

Riviello, R. J. (2004). Otolaryngologic procedures. In J. R. Roberts, & J. R. Hedges (Eds.), *Clinical procedures in emergency medicine* (4th ed., pp. 1280-1316). Philadelphia: Saunders.

PROCEDURE 169

Anterior Packing for Epistaxis

Daun A. Smith, RN, MSN

INDICATION

To tamponade bleeding from the anterior nasal cavity

CONTRAINDICATIONS AND CAUTIONS

1. Nasal packing in sedated patients may lead to hypoxia (Riviello, 2004); monitoring of oxygen saturation is recommended.
2. Antibiotics may be prescribed because of the risk of toxic shock syndrome and sinusitis (Riviello, 2004; Sparacino, 2000).

EQUIPMENT

Headlamp
Swimmer's nose clip or respiratory nose clip (optional)
Topical anesthetic agent (e.g., lidocaine, pontocaine, cocaine)
Topical vasoconstricting agent (e.g., oxymetazoline, cocaine, phenylephrine)
Silver nitrate sticks
Atomizer (for medications not packaged in a spray bottle)
1-in-wide strips of plain gauze impregnated with antibiotic ointment or petroleum jelly
or
Hemostatic mesh (Gelfoam, Surgicel)
or
Commercially prepared nasal tampon (a variety of sizes and shapes are available)
Frazier nasal suction tip
Long bayonet forceps
Nasal speculum
Pharyngeal mirror

2 × 2 gauze pads
4 × 4 gauze pads
Tape
Cotton-tipped applicators

PATIENT PREPARATION

1. Place the patient in a dental chair or in semi-Fowler's position on a stretcher.
2. Cover the patient's clothing with a gown or towel and provide a basin.
3. Administer sedation as prescribed (see Procedure 177).

PROCEDURAL STEPS

1. Have the patient blow his or her nose to dislodge clots.
2. Apply swimmer's nose clip or have the patient pinch the nose for minimum of 5 minutes. If possible, manual pressure by the nurse allows time for calming, teaching, and demonstrates effective self-management by the patient; time the pressure by clock to reinforce unremitting pressure for an effective clotting period.
3. *With a headlamp, introduce a nasal speculum into the naris, and suction clotted blood from the nose to assess whether the patient has an anterior or posterior bleed (Figure 169-1).
4. *Anesthetize the area with cotton-tipped applicators soaked in a topical anesthetic or vasoconstrictive agent.
5. *Apply silver nitrate to cauterize the bleeding site (see Procedure 168).
6. *Pack the anterior nose.
   a. Vaseline gauze or hemostatic mesh: Pack the gauze/mesh loosely in accordion manner using bayonet forceps and allowing both ends to protrude anteriorly (Figure 169-2). Use a pharyngeal mirror to check for loose threads dangling into the nasopharynx which may gag the patient. The pack can then be held in place with a gauze dressing taped under the nose (a "mustache dressing") (Figure 169-3).
   b. Commercially prepared nasal tampon: If necessary, trim the tampon before insertion. Lubricate the tampon with antibiotic ointment or lubricant. Using bayonet forceps or gloved fingers, insert the tampon straight backward along the floor of the anterior cavity (Evans and Rothenhaus, 2005) (Figure 169-4). Two tampons may be needed; they should be inserted side by side (Riviello, 2004). The packing expands as it absorbs blood from the epistaxis, or it can be hydrated with sterile saline (Figure 169-5). The packing may be left in place for up to 3 days and should be rehydrated with 10 ml of saline or water 5 minutes prior to removal.

AGE-SPECIFIC CONSIDERATIONS

1. Anterior nosebleeds are the most common among children. These usually result from cracks in the nasal lining because of exposure to abrupt temperature changes, dry heat, and nose picking (Sparacino, 2000).

---

*Indicates portions of the procedure usually performed by a physician or an advanced practice nurse.

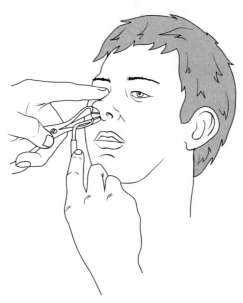

FIGURE 169-1   Nasal speculum in nose while clots are suctioned out.

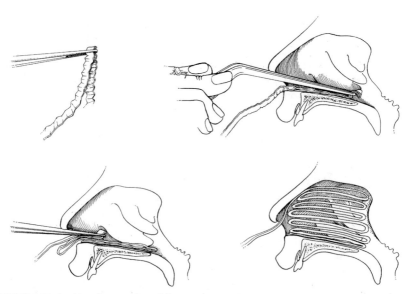

FIGURE 169-2   Accordion packing of the anterior nasal cavity with Vaseline gauze. (From Riviello, R. J. [2004]. Otolaryngologic procedures. In J. R. Roberts & J. R. Hedges [Eds.], *Clinical procedures in emergency medicine* [4th ed., p. 1305]. Philadelphia: Saunders.)

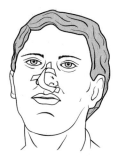

FIGURE 169-3 Packing taped in place with gauze under the nose.

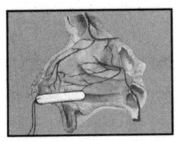

FIGURE 169-4 Merocel nasal tampon (compressed) inserted into the nose. (Courtesy Xomed Surgical Products, Inc., Jacksonville, FL.)

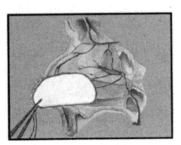

FIGURE 169-5 Merocel nasal tampon fully expanded after absorbing blood and/or saline. (Courtesy Xomed Surgical Products, Inc., Jacksonville, FL.)

2. In adults, anterior nosebleeds result from hypertension, coagulopathy, sinus disease, respiratory infections, allergies, nose picking, trauma, medications (aspirin, anticoagulants), and excessive dosage of topical nasal steroids (Kucik & Clenney, 2005).

COMPLICATIONS
1. Hypovolemia from blood loss
2. Inadequate hemostasis with recurrent hemorrhage

3. Airway obstruction from swelling or dislodgment of the packing
4. Hypoxia
5. Sinusitis
6. Toxic shock syndrome
7. Ethmoid fracture (Riviello, 2004)

PATIENT TEACHING

1. Do not remove the packing; see your physician or otolaryngologist for removal in 48 to 72 hours.
2. Avoid the following activities or substances for the next few days because they may lead to more bleeding: heavy exercise or lifting, alcoholic beverages, hot drinks, aspirin, ibuprofen, blowing your nose, sneezing, or coughing. If you must sneeze, open your mouth to relieve pressure.
3. The mouth may seem dry due to mouth-breathing and drinking extra fluids will be needed.
4. Sleeping with your head up on extra pillows may lessen recurrence, ease stuffiness, and minimize postnasal trickle.
5. Return to the emergency department or call your physician if you have recurrent bleeding, difficulty breathing, blood draining down the back of your throat, fever, malaise, or rash.

REFERENCES

Evans, J. A., & Rothenhaus, T. C. (2005). Epistaxis. In A. B. Wolfson (Ed.), *Harwood-Nuss' clinical practice of emergency medicine* (4th ed., pp. 185-190). Philadelphia: Lippincott Williams & Wilkins.

Kucik, C. J., & Clenney, T. (2005). Management of epistaxis. *American Family Physician, 71*(2), 305-311.

Riviello, R. J. (2004). Otolaryngologic procedures. In J. R. Roberts, & J. R. Hedges (Eds.), *Clinical procedures in emergency medicine* (4th ed., pp. 1280-1316). Philadelphia: Saunders.

Sparacino, L. L. (2000). Epistaxis management: What's new and what's noteworthy. *Lippincott's primary care practice, 4,* 498-507.

Posterior Packing for Epistaxis

Daun A. Smith, RN, MSN

INDICATION

To tamponade bleeding from the posterior nasal cavity. The most common site of posterior nosebleeds is from the lateral nasal branch of the sphenopalatine artery, which enters the nasal cavity behind the middle turbinate (Kucik & Clenney, 2005).

CONTRAINDICATIONS AND CAUTIONS

1. People aged 50 to 80 years with histories of cardiac and pulmonary disorders may develop problems (hyperventilation, hypoxia, and arrhythmias) because of compromised cardiac and pulmonary systems.
2. Baseline oxygenation with pulse oximetry should be established for patients with cardiopulmonary disease because hypoxia may result from nasal packing.
3. Patients with posterior packs should be admitted to the hospital (Riviello, 2004).
4. Supplemental oxygen and close observation may be needed. Sedatives and hypnotics should be minimized to avoid respiratory depression as the airway is partially obstructed.
5. Antibiotics are usually prescribed because of the risk of toxic shock syndrome (Riviello, 2004).
6. Posterior nasal gauze packs are rarely used because balloons provide an airway (see Procedure 171) and commercially prepared nasal tampons are easier to use and are less distressing to the patient.

EQUIPMENT

Headlamp
Topical anesthetic agent (e.g., lidocaine, tetracaine)
Topical vasoconstricting agent (e.g., oxymetazoline, phenylephrine)
Silver nitrate sticks
Frazier nasal suction tip
Long bayonet forceps
Nasal speculum
Pharyngeal mirror
Tongue blades
Cotton-tipped applicators

Pulse oximeter

Commercially prepared nasal tampon (a variety of sizes and shapes are available) coated with antibiotic ointment or lubricant

or

Posterior gauze pack supplies:

2 × 2 gauze pads

4 × 4 gauze pads

Dental roll

1-in-wide strips of plain gauze impregnated with antibiotic ointment or petroleum jelly

-0- silk suture

Urinary bladder catheter size 8 or 10

Straight medium hemostat or ring forceps

Tape

Umbilical clamp or 2-0 silk ties

PATIENT PREPARATION

1. Place the patient in a dental chair or in semi-Fowler's position on a stretcher.
2. Cover the patient's clothing and provide a basin.
3. Administer sedation as prescribed (see Procedure 177).
4. Monitor pulse oximetry, cardiac rhythm, and vital signs during the procedure (see Procedures 21 and 55).
5. Consider drawing baseline labs and obtaining IV access.

PROCEDURAL STEPS
Commercial Nasal Tampon

1. *If needed, trim the nasal tampon before insertion. Lubricate the tampon with antibiotic ointment or lubricant.
2. *Insert the nasal tampon along the floor of the nose (Figure 170-1). The packing expands as it absorbs blood from the epistaxis, or it can be hydrated with sterile saline (Figure 170-2). The packing may be left in place for up to 3 days and should be rehydrated with 10 to 15 ml of water for at least 5 minutes before removal.

---

*Indicates portions of the procedure usually performed by a physician or an advanced practice nurse.

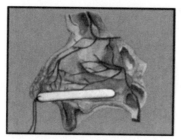

FIGURE 170-1 Merocel nasal tampon (compressed) for posterior epistaxis inserted into the nose. (Courtesy Xomed Surgical Products, Inc., Jacksonville, FL.)

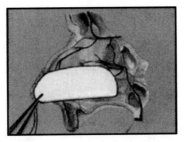

FIGURE 170-2 Merocel nasal tampon fully expanded after absorbing blood and/or saline. (Courtesy Xomed Surgical Products, Inc., Jacksonville, FL.)

Posterior Nasal Gauze Pack

1. Roll and cut to 1¾-in length a 4- × 4-in gauze and tie silk suture around the pack.
2. *Using cotton-tipped applicators, apply topical anesthetic or vasoconstrictor to the interior of the nose for 5 to 10 minutes.
3. *With a headlamp, introduce a nasal speculum into the naris, and suction clotted blood from the nose.
4. *Insert a urinary catheter through the nose into the nasopharynx. Then, with a hemostat, pull it out through the mouth (Figure 170-3).
5. *Tie two ties to the postnasal pack. Tie one to the end of the catheter, and pull the pack with the catheter through the mouth into the posterior nasopharynx. A bulge of the postnasal pack should be visible above the soft palate (Figure 170-4).
6. *If necessary, push the postnasal pack into place manually. A tongue blade or bite block can help prevent the uncooperative patient from biting you.

---

*Indicates portions of the procedure usually performed by a physician or an advanced practice nurse.

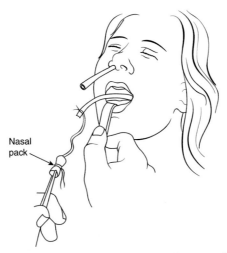

Nasal pack

FIGURE 170-3 Foley catheter threaded through the nose and gauze packing anchored to the end of the catheter and ready to pull into place.

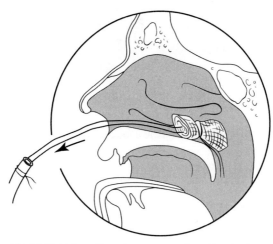

FIGURE 170-4 Posterior gauze nasal packing in place.

7. *Remove the catheter, and tie the suture ends protruding from the nose to a dental roll at the base of the nose with two ties applying traction. One tie protrudes through the mouth and should be taped to the cheek for use in removing the pack (Evans & Rothenhaus, 2005).
8. *Pack the anterior nose with gauze coated with antibiotic ointment or petroleum jelly using bayonet forceps and allowing both ends to protrude (see Procedure 169).
9. *Place the patient on low-flow humidified oxygen by face mask until packing is removed.

AGE-SPECIFIC CONSIDERATION
Posterior nosebleeds occur most often in the elderly and are associated with hypertension, atherosclerosis, and conditions that decrease platelets and clotting functions.

COMPLICATIONS
1. Hypovolemia from blood loss
2. Inadequate hemostasis with recurrent hemorrhage
3. Airway obstruction from swelling or dislodgment of postnasal pack
4. Hypoxia
5. Cardiac arrhythmias
6. Toxic shock syndrome
7. Ethmoid fracture (Riviello, 2004)
8. Hypertension as a result of the discomfort associated with posterior packing
9. Requirement of a replacement pack or surgical intervention if nasal packing fails

PATIENT TEACHING
1. You will be admitted to the hospital for close monitoring in case the pack does not control the bleeding or moves unexpectedly.

---

*Indicates portions of the procedure usually performed by a physician or an advanced practice nurse.

2. Do not remove the packing; your physician or otolaryngologist will remove it in 48 to 72 hours.
3. Avoid the following activities and substances for the next few days because they may lead to more bleeding: heavy exercise or lifting, alcoholic beverages, hot drinks, aspirin, ibuprofen, blowing your nose, sneezing, or coughing. If you must sneeze, open your mouth to relieve pressure.
4. The mouth may seem dry due to mouth-breathing and drinking extra fluids will be needed.
5. Sleeping with your head up on extra pillows may lessen recurrence, ease stuffiness, and minimize postnasal trickle.
6. Immediately report recurrent bleeding, difficulty breathing, blood draining down the back of your throat, fever, malaise, or rash.

REFERENCES

Evans, J. A., & Rothenhaus, T. C. (2005). Epistaxis. In A. B. Wolfson (Ed.), *Harwood-Nuss' clinical practice of emergency medicine* (4th ed., pp. 185-189). Philadelphia: Lippincott Williams & Wilkins.

Kucik, C. J., & Clenney, T. (2005). Management of epistaxis. *American Family Physician, 71*(2), 305-311.

Riviello, R. J. (2004). Otolaryngologic procedures. In J. R. Roberts, & J. R. Hedges (Eds.), *Clinical procedures in emergency medicine* (4th ed., pp. 1280-1316). Philadelphia: Saunders.

PROCEDURE 171

Balloon Catheters for Epistaxis

Daun A. Smith, RN, MSN

INDICATION
To tamponade anterior or posterior epistaxis

CONTRAINDICATIONS AND CAUTIONS
1. People aged 50 to 80 with a history of cardiac and pulmonary disorders may develop problems (hyperventilation, hypoxia, and arrhythmias) because of compromised cardiac and pulmonary systems. The potential for admission and need for observation increases proportionally.

2. Baseline oxygenation should be established with pulse oximetry for patients with cardiopulmonary disease because hypoxia may result from balloon catheter packing (Ho & Mansell, 2004).
3. Some balloons are filled with air and others with fluid; consult the manufacturer's directions for amount and substance to instill.

EQUIPMENT
Headlamp
Topical anesthetic (e.g., phenylephrine)
Silver nitrate sticks
Antibiotic ointment or petroleum jelly
Frazier nasal suction tip
Long bayonet forceps
Nasal speculum
4 × 4 gauze dressings
Cotton-tipped applicators
Intranasal balloon and syringe
Sterile water (for some products)
NOTE: A 12-Fr Foley catheter may also be used instead of a commercial balloon. If a Foley catheter is used, an umbilical clamp can be used to clamp off the catheter and hold it in place.
Pulse oximeter

PATIENT PREPARATION
1. Place the patient in a dental chair or in semi-Fowler's position on a stretcher.
2. Administer sedation as prescribed (see Procedure 177).
3. Monitor pulse oximetry, cardiac rhythm, and vital signs during the procedure (see Procedures 21 and 55).

PROCEDURAL STEPS
1. *With a headlamp, introduce a nasal speculum into the naris and suction clotted blood from the nose.
2. *Apply local anesthetic with cotton-tipped applicators.
3. *Coat the intranasal balloon per manufacturer's directions. Plain balloons are coated with antibiotic ointment or petroleum jelly; some balloons have a gel/mesh exterior that is premoistened by dipping in sterile water prior to insertion.
4. *Insert the intranasal balloon under direct vision with a headlamp.
5. *Instill air/fluid to about half of the posterior balloon's capacity (consult manufacturer's recommendations) and pull the balloon taut. Complete the inflation of the posterior balloon slowly while monitoring for pain. If the pain or downward deviation of the soft palate results, deflate the balloon until symptoms resolve (Riviello, 2004).

---

*Indicates portions of the procedure usually performed by a physician or an advanced practice nurse.

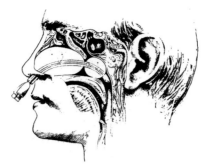

FIGURE 171-1 Epistaxis balloon in place. (Courtesy Xomed Surgical Products, Inc., Jacksonville, FL.)

6. *Inflate the anterior balloon slowly with air/fluid as recommended by the manufacturer. Deflate for adverse effects as described in step 5 (Figure 171-1).

7. Place a small piece of gauze between the catheter hub and the nose to help prevent skin breakdown (Kucik & Clenney, 2005).

COMPLICATIONS

1. Hypovolemia from blood loss
2. Inadequate hemostasis with recurrent hemorrhage
3. Airway obstruction from swelling, balloon dislodgment, or balloon overinflation
4. Hypoxia. Nasal balloons can cause a decreased PaO_2 as a result of nasopulmonary reflexes.
5. Sinusitis
6. Pressure necrosis of nasopharyngeal structures
7. Ethmoid fracture (Riviello, 2004)

PATIENT TEACHING

1. Do not remove or manipulate the balloon; see your physician or otolaryngologist for removal in 48 to 72 hours.
2. Avoid the following activities and substances for the next few days because they may lead to more bleeding: heavy exercise or lifting, alcoholic beverages, hot drinks, aspirin, ibuprofen, blowing your nose, sneezing, or coughing. If you must sneeze, open your mouth to relieve pressure.
3. The mouth may seem dry due to mouth-breathing and drinking extra fluids will be needed.
4. Sleeping with your head up on extra pillows may lessen recurrence, ease stuffiness, and minimize postnasal trickle.
5. Return to the emergency department or call your physician for recurrent bleeding, difficult breathing, blood draining down the back of your throat, fever, malaise, or rash.

---

*Indicates portions of the procedure usually performed by a physician or an advanced practice nurse.

REFERENCES

Ho, E. C., & Mansell, N. J. (2004). How we do it: A practical approach to Foley catheter posterior nasal packing. *Clinical Otolaryngology*, *29*, 750-757.

Kucik, C. J., & Clenney, T. (2005). Management of epistaxis. *American Family Physician*, *71*(2), 305-311.

Riviello, R. J. (2004). Otolaryngologic procedures. In J. R. Roberts, & J. R. Hedges (Eds.), *Clinical procedures in emergency medicine* (4th ed., pp. 1280-1316). Philadelphia: Saunders.

PROCEDURE 172

Nasal Foreign Body Removal

Daun A. Smith, RN, MSN

INDICATIONS

1. To remove a known nasal foreign body.
2. To rule out a foreign body in children or mentally compromised patients with foul, purulent nasal discharge or epistaxis. Unilateral nasal drainage is especially suggestive of a foreign body.

CONTRAINDICATIONS AND CAUTIONS

1. Beans or other vegetable matter should be removed as rapidly as possible because they swell as they absorb fluid.
2. If pushed farther into the nose, the object can be aspirated.

EQUIPMENT

Headlamp
Nasal speculum
Topical vasoconstrictor (e.g., cocaine, phenylephrine)
Topical anesthetic (e.g., lidocaine, tetracaine)
Cotton-tipped applicators
Miniature alligator forceps
Suction with No. 5 or No. 7 Frazier suction tip
Nasal packing
Hooked forceps

PATIENT PREPARATION

1. Place the patient in the Trendelenburg position.

2. Restrain the patient or use sedation if indicated (see Procedures 177 and 190).

PROCEDURAL STEPS

1. Anesthetize and decrease the swelling of the mucosa by spraying the nasal cavity with a nasal decongestant mixed with an anesthetic solution as prescribed.
2. *Using a headlamp and nasal speculum, attempt to visualize the foreign body.
3. If nasal swelling prevents visualization, spray the turbinates with topical vasoconstrictor (or use cotton-tipped applicators to apply the vasoconstrictor).
4. Ask patient to try to blow nose in an attempt to dislodge the foreign body (Kadish, 2005).
5. *Attempt to reach the foreign object with the tip of the suction catheter, hooked forceps, or miniature alligator forceps (Kadish, 2005).
6. *Remove mucus and debris with a small suction tip.
7. *After the swelling has decreased and the nasal debris is removed, use the hooked forceps, the miniature alligator forceps, or suction to retrieve the foreign body (Kadish, 2005).
8. *Apply nasal packing to control bleeding caused by irritation or manipulation if needed (see Procedure 169).
9. Apply an antibiotic ointment or petroleum jelly to the interior of the nose with cotton-tipped applicators.

COMPLICATIONS

1. Irritations and infection (including sinus infections) as a result of prolonged retention of a nasal foreign body
2. Perforation of the nasal canal as a result of manipulation of the foreign object
3. Airway obstruction if the foreign body is aspirated
4. Epistaxis

PATIENT TEACHING

1. Use a humidifier in your bedroom at night.
2. Do not place foreign objects in the nose, and keep items small enough to swallow, aspirate, or insert into body orifices away from children.
3. Use an antibiotic ointment or petroleum jelly in the interior of the nose for 2 to 3 days after foreign body removal.

---

*Indicates portions of the procedure usually performed by a physician or an advanced practice nurse.

REFERENCE

Kadish, H. (2005). Ear and nose foreign bodies: "It's all about the tools." *Clinical Pediatrics, 44,* 665-670.

Dental and Throat Procedures

Indirect Laryngoscopy

Garrett K. Chan, APRN,BC, PhD, CEN

INDICATIONS

1. To evaluate laryngeal or pharyngeal foreign body sensation
2. To evaluate hoarseness
3. To evaluate dysphagia

CONTRAINDICATIONS AND CAUTIONS

1. If possible, epiglottitis should be ruled out before attempting indirect laryngoscopy.
2. Indirect laryngoscopy has been almost replaced by the use of flexible fiber-optic laryngoscopes. Skillful use of a head mirror and light provides a wide field of view, light which is coaxial with vision, and more work space. Flexible or rigid endoscopy gives more detailed inspection, can be better directed, may allow railroading of a tube, possible video recording, and has less gagging with nasal passage but increases technical complexity and disinfection requirements and is difficult with increased secretions.

EQUIPMENT

Laryngeal mirror (size 3 to 6)
Gauze to grip tongue
Light source, such as a headlamp or head mirror
A method to prevent fogging (i.e., warming the mirror with warm water, an alcohol lamp, or an electric light bulb)
or
Antifogging solution (commercially available solution or soapy water can be used)
Topical anesthetic (e.g., lidocaine, Cetacaine, or aerosolized tetracaine)
Sedation (rarely needed)

PATIENT PREPARATION

1. Position the patient sitting upright with feet on the floor. Have the patient lean forward with the head in the sniffing position.
2. Place an emesis basin in the patient's hands.
3. *Anesthetize the pharynx as indicated by patient response and cooperation (see Procedure 135 for information on topical anesthetics).

---

*Indicates portions of the procedure usually performed by a physician or an advanced practice nurse.

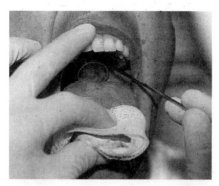

FIGURE 173-1 Grasp the tongue with a gauze dressing while elevating the upper lip with the middle finger. To prevent stimulation of the gag reflex, avoid touching the posterior pharynx or the tongue with the mirror. (From Riviello, R. J. [2004]. Otolaryngologic procedures. In J. R. Roberts & J. R. Hedges (Eds.), *Clinical procedures in emergency medicine* [4th ed., p. 1281]. Philadelphia: Saunders.)

PROCEDURAL STEPS

1. Have the patient protrude the tongue from the mouth as far as possible.
2. *Lay gauze over the tongue and then wrap it under the tongue.
3. *Grip the gauze-wrapped tongue between the thumb and the index finger of the nondominant hand and brace the middle finger against the teeth; then elevate the upper lip (Figure 173-1).
4. *Warm the mirror and test the temperature on your hand.
5. *Slide the mirror base down carefully, keeping it parallel to the tongue and without touching any tissue.
6. *Place the mirror with the back side against the uvula.
7. *Elevate the uvula and soft palate using one motion.
8. *Avoid touching the posterior tongue; this stimulation may result in gagging.
9. Instruct the patient to concentrate on breathing normally through the mouth with eyes open and focused on a distant fixed object.
10. *Direct the light onto the mirror.
11. *Examine the structures; look for pathology or a foreign body.
12. *Ask the patient to say "E." Observe the vocal cords as the epiglottis is displaced.

AGE-SPECIFIC CONSIDERATION

This procedure may not be possible in children because full cooperation and the ability to follow instructions are required for successful observation of the laryngeal structures.

COMPLICATIONS

1. Inability to perform the examination because of uncontrollable gagging
2. Burns from the laryngeal mirror if a warming method is used; nausea if soapy water is used

---

*Indicates portions of the procedure usually performed by a physician or an advanced practice nurse.

3. Contusions on the lips or the underside of the tongue from pressure application during the procedure

PATIENT TEACHING

1. Have nothing to eat or drink until the topical anesthetic is no longer active (approximately 1 hour).
2. Use caution when resuming oral intake. Begin slowly with sips of water.

PROCEDURE 174

Esophageal Foreign Body Removal

Joni Hentzen Daniels, MSN, RN, CEN, CCRN

The esophagus has three areas of narrowing: upper esophageal sphincter, which consists of the cricopharyngeus muscle; crossover of the aorta; and lower esophageal sphincter. These areas are where most esophageal foreign bodies become entrapped (Thomas & Brown, 2006). Structural abnormalities, including strictures, diverticula, and malignancies, increase the risk of foreign body entrapment, as do motor disturbances, such as scleroderma and achalasia. The oropharynx is well innervated, and patients can typically localize oropharyngeal foreign bodies; however, foreign bodies in the lower two thirds of the esophagus are poorly localized.

Two methods of removing a documented foreign body from the esophagus are described in this procedure: esophagoscopy and balloon-tipped catheter removal. Medications such as glucagon, nitroglycerin, nifedipine, and gas-forming agents are also used to remove esophageal foreign bodies in some cases.

ESOPHAGOSCOPY
Indications

1. This method provides direct visualization of the foreign body and the ability to evaluate the esophagus for pathology and allows control of the object during removal. Esophagoscopy is the preferred method of removal for sharp objects (e.g., bones, safety pins, and razor blades) and button batteries that may rapidly cause esophageal injury.
2. Esophagoscopy may also be used to rule out predisposing pathology or resultant complications (Munter & Heffner, 2004). An emergency physician does not usually perform esophagoscopy; a specialist is consulted.

Contraindications and Cautions

Sharp, pointed objects (e.g., toothpicks, bones) may require removal in the operating room.

Equipment

Endoscopic equipment
Suction setup
Pulse oximeter
Topical anesthetic
Emergency airway and resuscitative equipment

Patient Preparation

1. Establish venous access for medication administration (see Procedure 60).
2. If the object poses a high risk for esophageal perforation, prophylactic antibiotics should be administered intravenously before the endoscopy (Munter & Heffner, 2004).
3. Consider endotracheal intubation if the airway is at risk for compromise (see Procedures 8 through 11).
4. Place the patient in a Trendelenburg, lateral decubitus position.
5. Assess vital signs and oxygen saturation, and continue to monitor them frequently throughout the procedure (see Procedures 21 and 55).
6. *Administer a topical anesthetic as prescribed to control gagging.
7. Administer sedatives and analgesics as prescribed.
8. Have suction assembled and turned on at the patient's head.

Procedural Steps

1. *Intubate the esophagus with the endoscope.
2. *Visualize the foreign body.
3. *Push the foreign body into the stomach; grasp it and remove it through the scope; or grasp it and remove it with the scope as a unit.
4. *Evaluate the esophagus for preexisting pathology or trauma induced by the foreign body.
5. *Dilate the esophagus as necessary.

BALLOON-TIPPED CATHETER
Indications

This technique is used for removal of coins and other nonobstructing, smooth, blunt foreign bodies in cooperative patients who have ingestions of a short (24- to 48-hour) duration (Munter & Heffner, 2004; Thomas & Brown, 2006). This technique has a high success rate in pediatric patients who have ingested coins—96% in one series of 337 patients (Harned, Strain, Hay, & Douglas, 1997).

Contraindications and Cautions

1. Esophageal perforation or aspiration may occur.
2. There is no direct visualization of either the object or the esophagus and no direct control of the object.

---

*Indicates portions of the procedure usually performed by a physician or an advanced practice nurse.

3. This procedure cannot be used in the presence of a total obstruction because the catheter must be able to pass distal to the foreign body.
4. This procedure should not be used with sharp, irregularly shaped objects, because damage to the esophagus or balloon rupture may occur (Munter & Heffner, 2004).
5. The patient must be cooperative during this procedure; sedation may be necessary.
6. This procedure is not suitable for patients in respiratory distress or with symptoms of perforation (Thomas & Brown, 2006).

Equipment

Fluoroscopy equipment (optional)
Suction setup
Foley or Fogarty catheter, 8 Fr to 26 Fr
Water-soluble lubricant
5 to 10 ml of normal saline solution or a contrast agent to inject into the balloon
10-ml syringe
Laryngoscope
Magill forceps
Emergency airway and resuscitative equipment

Patient Preparation

1. Place the patient in the deep Trendelenburg (30-degree) position on a fluoroscopy table (if fluoroscopy is to be used).
2. Assess vital signs and oxygen saturation, and continue to monitor them frequently throughout the procedure.
3. Administer a local anesthetic as prescribed to control gagging.
4. Administer sedatives and analgesics as prescribed.
5. Have suction assembled and turned on at the patient's head.

Procedural Steps

1. Sedate the patient as indicated (see Procedure 177).
2. Inflate the catheter balloon to ensure that it expands evenly. Lubricate the catheter with a water-soluble lubricant.
3. *Insert the catheter through the nose or mouth until the balloon is distal to the foreign body.
4. Slowly inflate the balloon with saline solution or a contrast agent (fluid is preferred because it is less compressible than air). Stop the inflation immediately if the patient complains of increased pain; reposition the balloon and attempt inflation again.
5. *With smooth, steady traction, withdraw the catheter until the foreign body enters the patient's mouth. If significant resistance is encountered, stop and consider another modality.

---

*Indicates portions of the procedure usually performed by a physician or an advanced practice nurse.

6. *Grasp the object with Magill forceps if the patient does not expel it.
7. Repeat radiographic assessment to rule out multiple foreign bodies.
8. If the foreign object is not retrieved, the object may have passed into the stomach; assess foreign body location with fluoroscopy or radiography.

Age-Specific Considerations

1. The balloon-tipped catheter technique is frequently used for small children who have swallowed coins. Sedation and/or a patient restraint board may be necessary to hold the child still during the procedure (see Procedure 191).
2. No more than 5 ml of fluid should be used to inflate a catheter in children (Munter & Heffner, 2004).

Complications

1. Esophageal rupture may be caused by erosion due to the foreign body, puncture by the foreign body, or iatrogenic trauma from the procedures used to remove the foreign body.
2. Esophageal fistula may develop.
3. Button batteries may lead to esophageal necrosis and death if not removed promptly.
4. Aspiration of saliva, vomit, or the foreign body may occur during removal.
5. If the foreign object cannot be removed in the emergency department, surgical intervention may be necessary.

Patient Teaching

1. Immediately report fever, difficulty swallowing, and shortness of breath, swelling of the neck, chest pain, abdominal pain, vomiting, or blood in the stool or vomit.
2. Advance the diet slowly as tolerated or as directed.
3. If the object was pushed into the stomach, return for follow-up radiographs if the object does not pass in the stool within 4 to 7 days.
4. Prevention tips:
   • Avoid alcohol while eating.
   • Take small bites and chew food well.
   • Place nothing but food in the mouth.
   • Check meat for bones, especially if you have dentures.
   • Small toys and hard candy should be out of the reach of children younger than age 3.
   • Do not talk, laugh, or run with food in your mouth.

---

*Indicates portions of the procedure usually performed by a physician or an advanced practice nurse.

REFERENCES

Harned, R. K., II, Strain, J. D., Hay, T. C., & Douglas, M. R. (1997). Esophageal foreign bodies: Safety and efficacy of Foley catheter extraction of coins. *American Journal of Roentgenology, 168,* 443-446.

Munter, D. W., & Heffner, A. C. (2004). Esophageal foreign bodies. In J. A. Marx, R. S. Hockberger, & R. M. Walls, et al. (Eds.), *Rosen's emergency medicine: Concepts and clinical practice* (6th ed., pp. 775-993). St Louis: Mosby.

Thomas, S. H., & Brown, D. F. M. (2006). Foreign bodies. In J. A. Marx, R. S. Hockberger, & R. M. Walls, et al. (Eds.), *Rosen's emergency medicine: Concepts and clinical practice* (6th ed., pp. 859-881). St Louis: Mosby.

PROCEDURE 175

Tooth Preservation and Replantation

K. Sue Hoyt, RN, PhD, FNP, APRN,BC, CEN, FAEN

INDICATION

To preserve and replant a tooth that has been avulsed from the socket (Figure 175-1)

CONTRAINDICATIONS AND CAUTIONS

1. Patients who are unresponsive or are combative, or have compromised airways are unable to facilitate preservation of teeth by replacing them in the socket. Replantation should not be attempted because of risk of aspiration.
2. If the bone and soft tissue are too traumatized to support the tooth, replantation should not be attempted.
3. If the location of the avulsed tooth is not known, there should be an attempt to locate it in the mouth and pharynx. Radiographs should be considered if there is a possibility that a tooth could have been forced into the bone, swallowed, or aspirated.
4. The treatment of an avulsed tooth is divided into 10 categories, depending on the specific clinical conditions associated with that particular avulsed tooth, which include the physiologic status of the periodontal ligament (PDL) fibers, the stage of development of the root apex, the type of storage environment, and the length of extraoral time (Table 175-1). Maintenance of the PDL fibers' vitality, rather than the length of extraoral time, is key to the success of the replanted tooth (Krasner, 1995).
5. The critical links in the prereplantation stage are as follows (Krasner, 1995):
   a. Storage of the avulsed tooth in a physiologic medium until replantation.

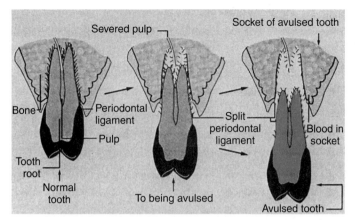

FIGURE 175-1 Anatomy of tooth avulsion. (From Krasner, P. [1990]. Treatment of tooth avulsion by nurses. *Journal of Emergency Nursing, 16,* 31.)

   b. Replenishment of the depleted cellular nutrients of the PDL cells.

   c. Protection of the root PDL cells from trauma, especially crushing.

6. Avulsed teeth should be placed in a pH-balanced cell preservative that reconstitutes PDL cells in a cushioned container (e.g., the basket device found in commercial preparations of Hanks solution, such as Save-A-Tooth) that permits atraumatic tooth retrieval. Before reimplantation, teeth that have been avulsed for more than 20 minutes need to remain in a cell preservative for at least 30 minutes to rehydrate the periodontal ligament cells.

7. Storage in media such as gauze or hard containers is contraindicated.

8. If the patient has other, more serious injuries, the tooth can remain in Hanks solution until reimplantation can be accomplished.

9. When a cell preservative is not available, cold milk is the best alternative storage medium. The osmolality and availability of milk are more conducive

TABLE 175-1
TREATMENT CATEGORIES OF AVULSED TEETH

Category 1	Mature apex, less than 15 min extraoral time
Category 2	Mature apex, 15 min to 24 hr extraoral time, reconstituting storage media
Category 3	Mature apex, 15 to 360 min extraoral time, nonreconstituting but wet storage media
Category 4	Mature apex, 120 min or less extraoral time, dry storage
Category 5	Mature apex, 120 min or longer extraoral time, dry storage
Category 6	Immature apex, less than 15 min extraoral time
Category 7	Immature apex, 15 min to 24 hr extraoral time, reconstituting storage media
Category 8	Immature apex, 15 to 360 min extraoral time, nonreconstituting but wet storage media
Category 9	Immature apex, 120 min or less extraoral time, dry storage
Category 10	Immature apex, 120 min or longer extraoral time, dry storage

From Krasner, P. (1995). New philosophy for the treatment of avulsed teeth. *Oral Surgery, Oral Medicine, Oral Pathology, and Oral Radiology Endodontics, 79,* 619.

to maintaining the vitality of the periodontal ligament than is saline solution or tap water. Ideally, the avulsed tooth is placed in a container of milk that is packed in ice (Perry, 2006).

10. If milk or cell culture media are not available immediately, saliva is an acceptable alternative (Perry, 2006).

11. The neurovascular supply to the tooth is disrupted during avulsion of a tooth. Timely reimplantation may enable some return of the neurovascular supply. Often, avulsions lead to hypoxia, which causes pulpal necrosis. As a result, the pulp of most replanted teeth needs to be removed (root canal therapy) immediately or within 1 week of replantation.

EQUIPMENT

Solution for tooth storage—Hanks solution (commercially available as Save-A-Tooth emergency tooth-preserving system, made by Biological Rescue Producers, Inc., Pottstown, Pennsylvania)

Sterile normal saline

2×2 gauze or dental pads

Emesis basin

Tonsil-tip suction

Dental mirror (optional)

Coe-Pak periodontal dressing (optional)

PATIENT PREPARATION

1. Cleanse the mouth with a gentle rinse of normal saline to remove debris, blood, and dirt.

2. Elevate the head of the stretcher, unless contraindicated, to help prevent the patient from swallowing blood, which may precipitate nausea.

3. Administer tetanus prophylaxis as indicated.

PROCEDURAL STEPS

1. Control hemorrhage in the mouth.

2. Inspect socket for blood clots or bone fragments. Gently suction as needed, avoiding sharp scraping, which can result in injury to the periodontal ligament or attachment fibers.

3. If the tooth is obviously dirty, gentle soaking in the preservation fluid helps loosen particles. Do not scrub the tooth, which damages remaining periodontal ligament fibers, which would make successful reattachment less likely.

4. The tooth should be gently removed by lifting the basket out of the container without using forceps, which could damage the PDL cells.

5. The tooth should be carefully held by the crown and not by the root so that the periodontal ligament cells are not damaged further.

6. *Local anesthesia may be needed before replantation can be accomplished. See Procedure 135.

7. *If the avulsed tooth is classified in treatment category 1 (mature apex, less than 15 minutes extraoral time), flush the socket with a physiologic solution. For avulsed teeth in all other categories, consult a dentist.

---

*Indicates portions of the procedure usually performed by a physician or an advanced practice nurse.

8. *The tooth should be placed in the socket with the clinician's thumb slowly, with firm pressure. If the position of the replanted tooth does not seem certain, the tooth should be removed and placed in a balanced solution, and the patient should be referred to a dentist.

9. *The replanted tooth should be splinted in place to adjacent teeth for a maximum of 2 weeks. A variety of methods can be used for stabilization, including Erich arch bars, stainless steel wire that is affixed to the teeth with an enamel bonding acrylic agent, an acrylic by itself, or a periodontal surgical splint, such as Coe-Pak, which is a zinc oxide–eugenol preparation. (Benko, 2004). Application of an arch bar is not recommended by the nondentist.

10. A dentist should see the patient within 24 hours.

11. Antibiotic administration following tooth replantation is generally recommended, although efficacy has not been proved (Perry, 2006).

AGE-SPECIFIC CONSIDERATIONS

1. Avulsed primary teeth in children are not replanted because they may fuse to alveolar bone, causing craniofacial abnormalities or infection or they may interfere with eruption of secondary teeth (Benko, 2004).

2. Generally, immature permanent teeth have a better chance for survival than do older teeth (Benko, 2004).

3. When no satisfactory history of trauma is reported, domestic violence or abuse should be considered.

COMPLICATIONS

1. Pain from reinsertion of tooth
2. Infection
3. Loss of tooth
4. Improper alignment of replanted tooth
5. Ankylosis of replanted tooth to the bone. In children, this can cause facial deformity.

PATIENT TEACHING

1. Mouth protection during recreation and sports activities is recommended.
2. Consume a liquid or soft diet for the duration indicated by the dentist.
3. Loss of the replanted tooth is possible not only early after reimplantation but also several years later.

---

*Indicates portions of the procedure usually performed by a physician or an advanced practice nurse.

REFERENCES

Benko, K. (2004). Emergency dental procedures. In J. R. Roberts, & J. R. Hedges (Eds.), *Clinical procedures in emergency medicine* (4th ed., pp. 1317-1340). Philadelphia: Saunders.

Krasner, P. (1995). New philosophy for the treatment of avulsed teeth. *Oral Surgery, Oral Medicine, Oral Pathology, and Oral Radiology Endodontics, 79,* 616-623.

Perry, M. (2006). Head, neck and dental emergencies. *Annals of the Royal College of Surgeons of England, 82*(2), 246-247.

Medication Administration

Nitrous Oxide Administration

Jean A. Proehl, RN, MN, CEN, CCRN, FAEN

Nitrous oxide combined with oxygen is also known as *laughing gas, Nitronox,* and *Entonox.*

NOTE: *The use of nitrous oxide in the manner described herein is usually considered analgesia and anxiolysis, not sedation. Consult your institutional protocols to determine whether sedation guidelines apply to nitrous oxide use in your setting.*

INDICATIONS

1. To provide rapid-onset (2 to 6 minutes), quickly reversible (2 to 5 minutes) analgesia for 30 minutes or less. Nitrous oxide may be used to relieve pain associated with trauma, renal colic, myocardial infarction, minor surgical procedures, wound care, diagnostic procedures, and reduction of fractures and dislocations.
2. To relieve the anxiety associated with painful conditions and procedures

CONTRAINDICATIONS AND CAUTIONS

1. When used for analgesia in the emergency setting (versus anesthesia in the operative setting), the gas mixture should be fixed at 50% nitrous oxide to 50% oxygen. For altitudes above 3500 feet, a 65% nitrous oxide to 35% oxygen mixture is recommended because the lower partial pressure of the nitrous oxide at higher altitudes does not provide adequate analgesia.
2. The patient should always self-administer the gas to prevent oversedation. Therefore, the patient must be cooperative and able to follow instructions. The mask or mouthpiece should never be strapped to or held on the patient's face.
3. Nitrous oxide causes drowsiness and should not be used in patients with altered levels of consciousness or head injuries, or those who are heavily sedated or intoxicated. Patients who have received opioids should be individually evaluated for suitability before receiving nitrous oxide.
4. Nitrous oxide occasionally causes nausea and vomiting, so caution is indicated with recent ingestion of food or fluids.
5. The gas mixture contains 50% oxygen (35% at high altitude); therefore, it does not supply enough oxygen for patients who have pulmonary edema and may suppress the hypoxic respiratory drive in a patient who has chronic obstructive pulmonary disease.

6. Nitrous oxide collects in dead air spaces and can expand the preexisting pockets of air associated with pneumothorax, otitis media, perforated viscus, bowel obstruction, air embolism, and decompression sickness.

7. Nitrous oxide should not be used during early pregnancy, because it has been associated with fetal defects and spontaneous abortion.

8. A scavenger system to dispose of exhaled gas protects health care providers who administer nitrous oxide. Studies involving operating room and dental personnel have associated long-term exposure to nitrous oxide with psychomotor impairment and congenital malformations, as well as spontaneous abortion in exposed women and sexual partners of exposed men. Possible association with bone marrow suppression, cancer, liver disease, and renal disease has also been reported.

9. A mask is preferred to facilitate disposal of exhaled gas. If the patient is unable to use a mask because of facial trauma or other conditions, a mouthpiece may be used in place of a mask.

10. Nitrous oxide has abuse potential. The unit should be kept in a secure area. A pop-off demand valve is available; the valve can then be locked up with the narcotics.

11. A fail-safe valve should be incorporated into the system to prevent administration of 100% nitrous oxide if the oxygen supply is interrupted.

12. A nurse or physician should be present at all times during nitrous oxide administration in the hospital setting unless institutional policies are in place specifying other qualified personnel who may monitor the patient.

EQUIPMENT

Nitrous oxide and oxygen tanks connected to a blender preset to deliver 50% nitrous oxide and 50% oxygen (65% nitrous oxide and 35% oxygen at altitudes above 3500 feet) with demand valve and scavenger (Figure 176-1). (Units are also available for use in the prehospital environment and for nitrous oxide supplied by pipeline.)

Mask or mouthpiece

Wall suction and suction connection tubing

Pulse oximeter

NOTE: In countries other than the United States, nitrous oxide may be available in a single-tank mixture known as *Entonox.*

PATIENT PREPARATION

1. Assess and document vital signs.
2. Initiate pulse oximetry monitoring (see Procedure 21).
3. Instruct the patient to do the following:
   a. Form a tight seal with the mask or mouthpiece and take slow, deep breaths. A sucking sound will be heard when the demand valve is tripped—this is expected.
   b. Exhale into the mask or mouthpiece so that the exhaled gas is removed by the scavenger.
   c. Avoid unnecessary conversation to limit exhalation of nitrous oxide into the room.
   d. Discontinue use if nausea, light-headedness, or other side effects occur.

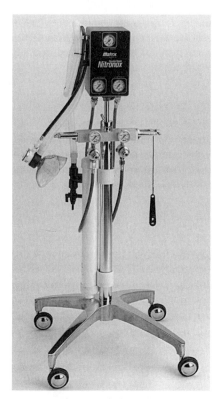

FIGURE 176-1 Nitronox nitrous oxide unit with demand valve and scavenger system. Nitrous and oxygen tanks not shown. (Courtesy Matrx Medical, Inc., Orchard Park, NY.)

PROCEDURAL STEPS

1. Turn on the nitrous oxide and oxygen tanks by opening the cylinder valves with a wrench. Check that the mixture pressure is within the safe level per manufacturer's specifications (30 to 35 psi for Nitronox by Matrx Medical, Inc. [1996]). Do not use the unit if the mixture pressure is not within the safe level. Check the pressure of each cylinder, and replace any cylinder with a pressure less than 300 psi (see Procedure 26).
2. Connect the scavenger to the wall suction and turn the suction on. Turn the ball valve lever on the scavenger tube to the ON position. Adjust the suction to 30 to 60 L/min.
3. Attach mask or mouthpiece to the demand valve.
4. Allow the patient to inhale the gas for 3 or 4 minutes before beginning any procedures. Some patients may require up to 6 minutes for adequate induction.
5. Monitor pulse oximetry continuously, and document it frequently (i.e., every 5 minutes) throughout the procedure.
6. As the patient becomes relaxed, he or she will be unable to create an adequate amount of negative pressure to trip the demand valve. This prevents excessive sedation.

7. When the patient drops the mask or mouthpiece, position or hold it so that the exhaled gas can be taken up by the scavenger.
8. Allow the patient to resume gas inhalation when he or she is able to hold the mask or mouthpiece.
9. Nitrous oxide administration is usually limited to a maximum of 30 minutes.
10. Assess and document vital signs and pulse oximetry.
11. When the procedure is completed, turn off the suction and nitrous and oxygen tanks. Clear the lines by blowing forcefully through the small holes on the back of the demand valve until all pressure gauges read zero. If the oxygen line bleeds before the nitrous line, you will not be able to remove the nitrous. Open and close the oxygen line and try again.
12. Monitor pulse oximetry and heart rate for 5 to 15 minutes after procedure.

NOTE: Some sources recommend that the patient receive supplemental oxygen for a period of time after receiving nitrous oxide to counteract the effects of diffusion hypoxia caused by the diffusion of nitrous oxide from the arterial blood into the alveoli, which dilutes alveolar oxygen levels. Research has demonstrated that diffusion hypoxia does not occur in healthy subjects after self-administration of nitrous oxide analgesia (Holcomb, Erdmann, & Corssen, 1976; Nieto & Rosen, 1980; Stewart, Gorayeb, & Pelton, 1986).

AGE-SPECIFIC CONSIDERATION

Nitrous oxide can be used by children and elderly patients as long as they can cooperate and self-administer the nitrous oxide as described previously. The mask should never be held on the patient's face.

COMPLICATIONS

1. Side effects are unusual but may require termination of nitrous oxide administration. Side effects may include vomiting, shortness of breath, excitement, drowsiness, confusion, and light-headedness.
2. Propping or holding the mask against the patient's face may result in excessive sedation. The patient must hold the mask to prevent overdosage.
3. Aspiration may occur if the patient vomits with the mask in place.
4. The Nitronox unit has a mixer pressure whistle alarm that sounds if there is a disruption in gas pressures resulting in a low oxygen concentration. Discontinue use immediately and notify the manufacturer (Matrx, 1996).

PATIENT TEACHING

1. Report immediately any uncomfortable sensations during nitrous oxide use.
2. Keep conversation to a minimum, and exhale into the mask or mouthpiece.

REFERENCES

Holcomb, C., Erdmann, W., & Corssen, G. (1976). The significance of diffusion hypoxemia. *Southern Medical Journal, 69,* 1282-1284.

Matrx Medical, Inc. (1996). *Instructions Nitronox hospital model.* Orchard Park, NY: Author.

Nieto, J., & Rosen, P. (1980). Nitrous oxide at higher elevations. *Annals of Emergency Medicine, 9,* 610-612.

Stewart, R. D., Gorayeb, M. J., & Pelton, G. H. (1986). Arterial blood gases before, during, and after nitrous oxide administration. *Annals of Emergency Medicine, 15,* 1177-1180.

Sedation

Andrew A. Galvin, APRN,BC, CEN

Sedation is also known as *conscious sedation* and *moderate sedation*. The current term for sedation is *procedural sedation and analgesia* (*PSA*). PSA encompasses a continuum that ranges from minimal sedation to general anesthesia, with distinct criteria for each level (Bahn, 2005).

INDICATIONS

To allay patient fear, anxiety, and pain and to improve the patient's ability to cooperate during painful therapeutic, diagnostic, or surgical procedures. Procedural sedation is the administration of sedatives or dissociative agents (with or without analgesics) which will allow the patient to tolerate painful or unpleasant procedures while maintaining normal cardiorespiratory function and independent airway control (ACEP, 2005; Bahn, 2005).

NOTE: The Joint Commission (formerly the Joint Commission on Accreditation of Healthcare Organizations) standards specifically address sedation practices; consult the current standards and your institutional policy for up-to-date requirements and recommendations.

ABSOLUTE CONTRAINDICATIONS

1. Hemodynamic or respiratory instability that requires immediate intervention
2. Refusal of a competent patient
3. Allergy to drug class

CONTRAINDICATIONS AND CAUTIONS

If any of the following conditions are present, use of sedation must be approached with caution. Consult with the physician about the risks and plan for sedation before medication administration. An anesthesia consultation may be indicated.

1. Intoxicated with central nervous system depressants
2. Neurologically impaired
3. Concurrent shock or myocardial infarction
4. Adrenal insufficiency or long-term steroid use (premedicate with intravenous steroid)
5. Moderate-to-severe liver or renal insufficiency
6. Pregnancy
7. Monoamine oxidase inhibitor use within the previous 2 weeks
8. Any condition that could make intubation difficult (e.g., facial or neck trauma, large tongue, short neck, congenital malformation of upper airway structures)
9. ASA Patient Physical Status Classification greater than Class 2 (Table 177-1)

TABLE 177-1

AMERICAN SOCIETY OF ANESTHESIOLOGISTS' PHYSICAL STATUS CLASSIFICATION SYSTEM

Class	Description	Suitability for Sedation
P1	Normal healthy patient	Excellent
P2	Mild systemic disease; well-controlled chronic condition	Generally good
P3	Severe systemic disease; poorly controlled chronic condition; acute illness such as pneumonia	Intermediate
P4	Severe systemic disease that is a constant threat to life	Poor
P5	Moribund patient who is not expected to survive without the operation	Extremely poor

From American Society of Anesthesiologists. (n.d.) *ASA physical status classification system.* Retrieved February 17, 2007, from http://www.asahq.org/clinical/physicalstatus.htm; and Doyle, L. (2006). Pediatric procedural sedation and analgesia. *Pediatric Clinics of North America, 53,* 279–292.

EQUIPMENT

Oral and nasopharyngeal airways (appropriate size for patient)

Suction equipment

Supplemental oxygen source, oxygen cannula, and mask (appropriate size for patient)

Bag-mask (appropriate size for patient)

Cardiac monitor (if indicated by patient's condition)

Blood pressure monitoring equipment

Pulse oximeter

Crash cart with defibrillator

Reversal agent(s) for medications to be administered (naloxone, nalmefene, and/or flumazenil)

PATIENT PREPARATION

1. Establish intravenous access (see Procedure 60). Intravenous access must be continuously maintained to provide a method of administering sedatives and initiating corrective action for adverse effects. For other routes of medication administration, you must have the ability to obtain intravenous access immediately (ASA, 2002).
2. Initiate pulse oximetry monitoring (see Procedure 21). Initiate end tidal CO_2, cardiac, and blood pressure monitoring as indicated (see Procedures 24 and 55).

PROCEDURAL STEPS

1. *Before the administration of sedatives, complete a preanesthesia assessment, with documentation, to include at least the following (ASA, 2002):
   a. Past and present medical history

---

*Indicates portions of the procedure usually performed by a physician or an advanced practice nurse.

    b. Drug allergies or sensitivities

    c. Current medications, tobacco, ethanol, or illicit drug use

    d. Last oral intake (liquid and solid)

    e. Previous anesthesia or sedation experience

    f. Patient physical status classification (see Table 177-1)

    g. Results of relevant diagnostic studies

    h. Plan (choice) of anesthesia

2. Assess baseline physiologic status of patient including, but not limited to, the following:

    a. Blood pressure

    b. Heart rate

    c. Respiratory rate and status

    d. Level of consciousness

    e. Pulse oximetry

    f. Cardiac rhythm (optional)

    g. End-tidal CO_2

    h. Skin color and temperature

    i. Ability to communicate

3. Have the following available in the procedure area before the administration of any medications: an emergency cart with defibrillator, suction, airway management devices, and reversal agents for the medications being administered.

4. Have supplemental oxygen and suction immediately available.

5. Establish provisions for backup personnel who are experts in airway management and cardiopulmonary resuscitation in the event that complications arise.

6. Maintain a sedation checklist to complete all requirements and record frequently monitored physiologic parameters. Documentation should include the following (AORN, 2002):

    a. Dosage, route, time, and effects of medications

    b. Type and amount of fluids administered

    c. Any interventions and the patient's response

    d. Any untoward reaction and interventions

7. Monitor the patient carefully from the administration of the medications until recovery. The nurse monitoring the patient should have no other responsibilities during or after the procedure that will interfere the nurse's ability to adequately monitor the patient (AORN, 2002; ASA, 2002; ENA & ACEP, 2005).

8. During the procedure, document the following physiologic parameters at regular intervals (usually every 5 to 15 minutes, consult your institutional policy) (ASA, 2002):

    a. Respiratory rate

    b. Oxygen saturation

    c. Heart rate

    d. Blood pressure (unless it will interfere with sedation such as in a pediatric patient)

    e. Level of consciousness

    f. Cardiac rhythm (optional)

    g. End-tidal CO_2

9. After the procedure, document the patient's level of consciousness, vital signs, and pulse oximetry every 15 minutes until he or she has recovered. Recovery is indicated by stable vital signs and oxygen saturation and alert and oriented state (or return to baseline mental status). Before discharge, the patient should be able to sit and ambulate (age appropriate) and tolerate oral fluids (ASA, 2002).

SAMPLE QUALIFICATIONS FOR ADMINISTERING AND MONITORING SEDATION

The nurse monitoring the patient must be competent in the use of resuscitation and monitoring equipment and should be able to interpret the data obtained (AORN, 2002; ENA, ACEP, 2005). This includes the ability to identify, rescue, and support a patient who slips into deep sedation and who may not be able to maintain a patent airway and adequate ventilation without assistance. Education in and demonstration of these competencies may be accomplished via the following:

1. Advanced cardiac life support (ACLS)
2. Basic life support (BLS)
3. Training in the recognition of the cardiovascular and respiratory side effects of sedatives as well as the variability of patient response
4. Training in airway management
5. Emergency nursing pediatric course (ENPC) or pediatric advanced life support (PALS) for sedation of children
6. Knowledge of the pharmacology of the medications administered

AGE-SPECIFIC CONSIDERATIONS

1. Consider dosage reduction in the elderly and chronically ill.
2. When selecting the medications for a pediatric patient, consider the nature of the procedure (painful or nonpainful), the desired onset and duration of action, and the route of administration. In children, moderate sedation may not be adequate, and deep sedation may be the goal. Careful monitoring is indicated.

COMPLICATIONS

1. Respiratory depression or apnea
2. Increase in untoward side effects with the dose and the number of different agents used
3. Paradoxical excitement occasionally caused by some drugs instead of the desired effect
4. Side effects as related to specific drug administered
5. Airway obstruction
6. Cardiopulmonary impairment

PATIENT TEACHING

1. Stay with a responsible adult for 12 hours after the procedure.
2. Do not drive an automobile or operate dangerous machinery for at least 6 to 12 hours. Children should not climb stairs unassisted, ride bikes, or play on playground equipment.
3. Return to the emergency department or call an ambulance for difficulty in breathing, pale or gray skin, or difficulty arousing.

4. Call the physician if vomiting is persistent and fluids do not stay down.

REFERENCES

American College of Emergency Physicians (ACEP). (2005). Clinical policy for procedural sedation and analgesia in the emergency department. *Annals of Emergency Medicine, 31,* 663-677.

American Society of Anesthesiologists (ASA). (2002). Practice guidelines for sedation and analgesia by non-anesthesiologists. *Anesthesiology, 96,* 1004-1017.

American Society of Anesthesiologists (ASA). (n.d.) *ASA physical status classification system.* Retrieved February 17, 2007, from http://www.asahq.org/clinical/physicalstatus.htm.

Association of Operating Room Nurses (AORN). (2002). Recommended practices for managing the patient receiving moderate sedation. *AORN Journal, 75,* 642-652.

Bahn, E. L. (2005). Procedural sedation and analgesia: A review and new concepts. *Emergency Medicine Clinics of North America, 23,* 503-517.

Doyle, L. (2006). Pediatric procedural sedation and analgesia. *Pediatric Clinics of North America, 53,* 279-92.

Emergency Nurses Association (ENA) & American College of Emergency Physicians (ACEP). (2005). Delivery of agents for procedural sedation and analgesia by emergency nurses: *Joint ENA/ACEP Statement.* Retrieved January 29, 2007, from http://www.ena.org/about/position/ACEP/ProceduralSedation.asp.

PROCEDURE 178

Peripheral Nerve Stimulator

Patricia Kunz Howard, PhD, RN, CEN

Peripheral nerve stimulator is also known as *twitch monitor* or *train of four (TOF) stimulator.*

INDICATION

To assess the level of neuromuscular blockade for patients who require chemical paralysis. TOF is the most commonly used peripheral nerve stimulation; it delivers four low-frequency (2 to 4 Hz) pulses for a duration of 2 seconds at 0.5-second intervals. The response is graded based on the number of muscle contractions (twitches) observed after the stimulus is delivered.

CONTRAINDICATIONS AND CAUTIONS

1. There are no absolute contraindications for TOF monitoring; however, patients with physiologic paralysis or degenerative neuromuscular disorders

may not have normal muscle contractions in response to peripheral nerve stimulation.

2. Diaphoresis may impede electrode contact altering the muscle response to stimulation.
3. Low batteries may result in less than desired stimulus magnitude.
4. Significant edema or previous nerve damage may produce an altered muscle response.
5. Administer analgesia before starting TOF testing.

EQUIPMENT

Peripheral nerve stimulator
Two electrodes (pediatric size preferred)
Two lead wires

PATIENT PREPARATION

Select the site for electrode placement; the ulnar nerve is the preferred site. The posterior tibial nerve is an acceptable site if the ulnar nerve is not an option.

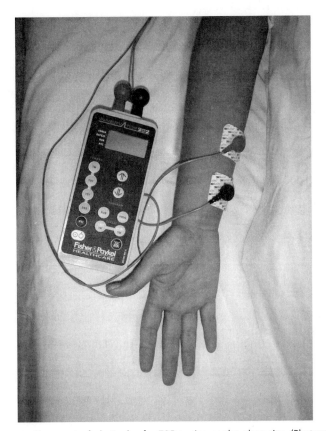

FIGURE 178-1 Placement of electrodes for TOF testing at the ulnar site. (Photograph courtesy of P. Howard).

TABLE 178-1
ELECTRODE SITES AND RESPONSE ELICITED

| Nerve Stimulated | Electrode Placement | | Muscle Innervated | Expected Response |
	Negative (Black)	Positive (Red)		
Ulnar	Anterior wrist over the head of the ulna	3 to 5 cm proximal to the negative electrode (in line with the little finger)	Adductor pollicis	Flexion-adduction of the thumb
Posterior tibial	Both electrodes are placed behind the medial malleolus in the groove adjacent to the Achilles tendon	3 to 5 cm proximal to the negative electrode	Flexor hallucis brevis	Plantar flexion of the great toe
Facial	2 cm lateral to the outer canthus of the eye and proximal to the tragus of the ear	1 cm distal to the negative electrode	Orbicularis oculi	Eyelid twitching
Peroneal*	Lateral to the neck of the fibula and posterior to the lateral malleolus	3 to 5 cm proximal to the negative electrode	Peroneal muscles (longus or brevis)	Dorsiflexion of the foot

*Limited data exist regarding the reliability of the peroneal site for TOF monitoring (Rowlee, 1999).

PROCEDURAL STEPS

1. Apply electrodes at the selected site (Figure 178-1 and Table 178-1).
2. Attach the peripheral nerve stimulator leads to electrodes. The negative (black) electrode should be placed most distal when using the ulnar nerve site (UNC, 2005).
3. Turn the peripheral nerve stimulator on and set the mA at 10.
4. Push the TOF button and observe for the expected movement (see Table 178-1). Obtain the baseline TOF level by increasing the threshold (amplitude) by increments of 10 mA (to a maximum of 30) until four distinct muscle contractions are observed. If the expected muscle contractions are not seen at 30 mA, check the connections, electrode placement, electrode moisture, and batteries.
5. After neuromuscular blocking agents (NMBA) are initiated, TOF should be assessed every hour until the desired level of block is obtained and then re-assessed at least every 4 hours and more often if titration is required. See Table 178-2 for TOF responses indicating the degree of neuromuscular blockade present; adequate paralysis is indicated by one or two twitches. Common clinical practice for patients receiving NMBA and sedation is to use 80 mA for ongoing TOF monitoring.
6. Document TOF response indicating number of twitches out of four (i.e., ¼ for one twitch), the site, and the mA used.

AGE-SPECIFIC CONSIDERATION

Neonatal electrodes may need to be used with pediatric patients.

COMPLICATIONS

1. Skin breakdown (change electrode site daily).
2. Inadequate response to stimulus (low batteries, improper electrode placement, or poor connections [dry electrodes]).
3. If a facial site is used, facial contractions may be distressing to family members.

TABLE 178-2
TRAIN OF FOUR RESPONSE

Train of Four Response	Approximate Percentage of Receptors Blocked by Agent
Four contractions	0% to 75%
Three contractions	75%
Two contractions	80%
One contraction	90%
No contraction	100%

Adapted from Jones, S. K. (2003). An algorithm for train-of-four monitoring in patients receiving neuromuscular blockade. *Dimensions of Critical Care Nursing, 22*(2), 50–57.

PATIENT TEACHING

Describe rationale for use of peripheral nerve stimulation to family members. Explain to families that the muscle contractions (twitches) observed are not painful (Rowlee, 1999).

REFERENCES

Jones, S. K. (2003). An algorithm for train-of-four monitoring in patients receiving neuromuscular blockade. *Dimensions of Critical Care Nursing, 22*(2), 50-57.

Rowlee, S. C. (1999). Monitoring neuromuscular blockade in the intensive care unit: The peripheral nerve stimulator. *Heart & Lung, 28*(5), 352-362.

University of North Carolina Hospitals (UNC). (2005). Nerve stimulation peripheral. *Nursing Procedure Manual (revised September 2005)*. Retrieved May 16, 2006, from www.unchealth-care.org/site/Nursing/nurspractice/procedures/procedures/proceduren3.pdf/

PROCEDURE 179

Streptokinase Administration

Teresa L. Will, MSN, RN, CEN

Streptokinase is also known as *SK, STK, Streptase,* or *Kabikinase.* In the United States, it has been replaced by other fibrinolytics and therapies and is rarely used.

INDICATIONS

To lyse thromboses in the presence of:

1. Acute myocardial infarction (AMI) diagnosed by the following:
   a. Typical ischemic chest pain lasting at least 30 minutes and less than 12 hours and which is unresponsive to sublingual nitroglycerin *and*
   b. ST segment elevation of more than 1 mm in two of the three inferior leads (II, III, aVF), two of the six precordial leads (V_1 through V_6); or lateral leads I and aVL *or*
   c. New-onset bundle-branch block
2. Pulmonary embolism diagnosed by angiography or lung scan, involving obstruction of blood flow to a lobe or multiple segments, with or without unstable hemodynamics

3. Deep vein thrombosis
4. Arterial thrombosis or embolism
5. Occlusion of arteriovenous cannulae

ABSOLUTE CONTRAINDICATIONS

1. Active internal bleeding
2. Recent (within 2 months) cerebrovascular accident or intracranial or intraspinal surgery
3. Intracranial neoplasm
4. Severe uncontrolled hypertension
5. History of allergic reactions to streptokinase (Astra USA, 1994)

CAUTIONS

Caution in the use of streptokinase is indicated in the presence of events or conditions that alone or combined may increase the risk of streptokinase therapy and include the following:
1. Previous treatment with streptokinase or exposure to *Streptococcus* infection in the past 6 months (this could result in the formation of antibodies and create resistance to the drug)
2. Recent (within 10 days) major surgery, obstetrical delivery, or organ biopsy
3. Recent (within 10 days) gastrointestinal bleeding
4. Recent (within 10 days) trauma, including cardiopulmonary resuscitation
5. Recent (within 10 days) puncture of subclavian or internal jugular vessel
6. Hypertension: systolic blood pressure greater than 180 mm Hg or diastolic blood pressure greater than 110 mm Hg
7. High likelihood of left-sided heart thrombus (e.g., mitral stenosis with atrial fibrillation)
8. Subacute bacterial endocarditis
9. Hemostatic defects, including those secondary to severe hepatic or renal disease
10. Pregnancy
11. Age greater than 75 years
12. Cerebrovascular disease
13. Diabetic hemorrhagic retinopathy
14. Septic thrombophlebitis or occluded arteriovenous cannula at a seriously infected site
15. Current treatment with oral anticoagulants
16. Any other condition in which bleeding constitutes a significant hazard or would be particularly difficult to manage because of its location

EQUIPMENT

Streptokinase vial (1,500,000 international units)
Normal saline (NS) or dextrose 5% in water (D_5W) solution for reconstitution, 5 ml NS or D_5W solution for further dilution, 40 to 90 ml
Syringes: two 5 ml and one 50 ml
18-G needles
Catheter plug (also known as click lock, PRN adapter, heparin or saline lock)
Intravenous (IV) infusion pump and tubing

PATIENT PREPARATION

1. Perform a thorough assessment, including:
   a. 12-lead electrocardiogram (see Procedure 56)
   b. Complete history and physical examination, including time of onset of chest pain
   c. Review of selection criteria for streptokinase therapy
2. Establish continuous cardiac monitoring (see Procedure 55).
3. Establish IV access with a minimum of two to three sites using 18- to 20-G catheters. The use of a double-lumen peripheral IV catheter may reduce the number of punctures (see Procedure 60).
4. Provide routine AMI care as prescribed, which may include but is not limited to the following (Antman et al., 2004):
   a. Oxygen
   b. Aspirin, chewable
   c. Nitroglycerin, sublingual or IV
   d. IV narcotic analgesia
   e. IV β-blocker
   NOTE: Heparin, if prescribed, will be given after streptokinase administration. See step 7 under Procedural Steps.
5. Administer pretreatment corticosteroids or diphenhydramine as prescribed.
6. Obtain laboratory studies, including the following:
   a. Cardiac markers (myoglobin, troponin, creatine kinase–MB)
   b. Chemistry profile
   c. Electrolyte profile
   d. Prothrombin time (PT), partial thromboplastin time (PTT)
   e. Complete blood count with platelets

PROCEDURAL STEPS

1. Mix streptokinase for administration. In some institutions, the pharmacy prepares the streptokinase solution.
   a. Add 5 ml of NS or D_5W solution for injection slowly to the streptokinase vial, directing the fluid stream against the side of the vial rather than into the powder. Roll and tilt the vial gently to mix the contents. To prevent further foaming, *do not shake the vial.*
   b. Withdraw the reconstituted solution from the vial slowly, and dilute carefully to a total volume as listed in Table 179-1.
2. When diluting the 1,500,000 international units infusion bottle (50 ml), as in the AMI dose, follow the same procedure as in step 1a, but after the initial reconstitution, the drug can be further diluted in the same vial with an additional 40 ml of NS or D_5W.
3. Assemble IV tubing. An in-line IV filter size 0.8 micron or larger may be used.
4. Because streptokinase contains no preservatives, it must be reconstituted just before use. It may be stored up to 8 hours at 2° to 8° C (36° to 46° F) if necessary.
5. Because of the limited availability of compatibility information, no other medications should be added to the container of streptokinase.
6. Administer the loading dose and initiate the maintenance dose as outlined in Table 179-1. Note that there is no loading dose for use with AMI.

TABLE 179-1
RECOMMENDED DOSAGES FOR IV STREPTOKINASE

Indication	Vial Size	Total Solution Volume (ml)	Infusion Rate
Acute myocardial infarction	1,500,000 international units	45	Infuse 45 ml within 60 min
Pulmonary embolism	1,500,000 international units	90	Loading dose 250,000 international units/hr Infuse 30 ml/hr for 30 min Maintenance infusion 100,000 international units/hr Infuse 6 ml/hr
Deep vein thrombosis	1,500,000 international units	45 (use when a more concentrated solution is desired)	Loading dose 250,000 international units Infuse 15 ml/hr for 30 min Maintenance infusion 100,000 international units/hr Infuse 3 ml/hr

Data from Astra USA. (1994). *Streptase (streptokinase) prescribing information.* Westborough, MA: Author.

7. Anticoagulation with heparin sodium may or may not be required after streptokinase administration (Astra USA, 1994). If heparin sodium is used intravenously, a bolus dose is not administered, and the continuous heparin infusion is begun only after the PTT falls to 2 times the normal control value. This can take several hours to occur after the conclusion of the streptokinase infusion. Therefore, the PTT should be monitored every 2 hours to determine when it falls in that range. Subcutaneous heparin may be administered in lieu of IV heparin (GUSTO, 1993).

PATIENT MANAGEMENT

1. Monitor cardiac rhythm and neurologic status continuously.
2. Monitor patient for signs and symptoms of allergic response, which can vary from a low-grade fever to an anaphylactic reaction. For a mild-to-moderate reaction, the physician may prescribe a corticosteroid and an antihistamine, but the streptokinase infusion may be continued. For a severe allergic reaction, the streptokinase infusion should be stopped and anaphylaxis treatment initiated.
3. Assess and document the vital signs every 5 to 10 minutes during streptokinase infusion. Be alert for a precipitous drop in blood pressure. Decrease the rate of streptokinase infusion if hypotension occurs. Hypotension may require volume replacement, pressor therapy, or both.

4. Monitor and document clinical signs of reperfusion, which include cardiac arrhythmias, resolution of chest pain, and normalization of the ST segments. The arrhythmias seen are the same as those seen in many patients having an MI and may include ventricular tachycardia, ventricular fibrillation, sinus bradycardia, accelerated idioventricular rhythm, and heart block. Any arrhythmias that occur are treated following Advanced Cardiac Life Support (ACLS) guidelines.

5. Assess for signs of bleeding complications and coronary artery reocclusion (e.g., recurrence of chest pain or ST segment elevation) every 15 minutes during the infusion and every 2 hours thereafter until 2 hours after the heparin is discontinued.

6. Document the time the chest pain resolves and the time the streptokinase infusion ends.

7. Monitor the PTT every 2 hours. When the PTT falls to less than two times the normal control, a continuous heparin infusion may be initiated.

8. Institute thrombolytic bleeding precautions, which include the following:
   a. Avoid the use of automatic blood pressure cuffs if possible.
   b. Avoid unnecessary arterial and venous punctures. All puncture sites should be compressed manually for a minimum of 10 minutes for venous punctures and 20 minutes for arterial punctures. Apply pressure dressings after discontinuation of lines and after vessel puncture.
   c. Use a heparin or saline lock for blood draws, and consolidate blood draws when possible.
   d. Monitor all puncture sites and the gingivae for bleeding.
   e. Use a draw sheet to move and position the patient to avoid contusions. Instruct the patient to request assistance when changing positions.
   f. Observe for frank blood, and test urine, stools, and emesis for occult blood.
   g. Avoid intramuscular injections.
   h. Monitor hemoglobin and hematocrit for evidence of acute blood loss.

COMPLICATIONS

1. Bleeding should be expected to occur after streptokinase therapy. The goal is to avoid significant bleeding through careful screening and observation of precautions pertaining to thrombolytic therapy bleeding. Careful monitoring and prompt treatment are critical in minimizing the effects of bleeding if it does occur. Types of bleeding seen with streptokinase therapy include the following:
   a. Intracranial
   b. Gastrointestinal
   c. Genitourinary
   d. Epistaxis
   e. Retroperitoneal
   f. Venous and arterial puncture sites
   g. Femoral artery catheter
   h. Gingival
   i. Ecchymosis
   Intracranial bleeding is the most serious form of bleeding that can occur after thrombolytic therapy. Although intracranial bleeding is rare (less than 1%),

it is so potentially devastating that care must be taken to exclude patients at risk for intracranial hemorrhage and to recognize and treat changes in neurologic status without delay.

PATIENT TEACHING

1. Request assistance when moving.
2. Report any bleeding, although some minor bleeding and bruising are normal.
3. Report any changes in chest pain or other symptoms immediately.

REFERENCES

Antman, E. M., Anbe, D. T., Armstrong, P. W., Bates, E. R., Green, L. A., & Hand, M., et al. (2004). ACC/AHA guidelines for the management of patients with ST-elevation myocardial infarction: Executive summary: A report of the ACC/AHA Task Force on Practice Guidelines (Committee to Revise the 1999 Guidelines on the Management of Patients With Acute Myocardial Infarction). *Circulation, 110*, 588-636.
Astra USA. (1994). *Streptase (streptokinase) prescribing information.* Westborough, MA: Author.
GUSTO. (1993). An international randomized trial comparing four thrombolytic strategies for acute myocardial infarction. *New England Journal of Medicine, 329*, 673-682.

PROCEDURE 180

TNK-tPA Administration for Acute Myocardial Infarction

Ruth Altherr Rench, MS, RN, FAHA, and *Teresa L. Will, MSN, RN, CEN*

TNK-tPA is also known as *tissue plasminogen activator, TNK, tenecteplase,* or *TNKase.*

INDICATION

To lyse thromboses in the presence of acute myocardial infarction diagnosed by the following:

1. Chest discomfort or related symptoms lasting for at least 15 minutes and less than 12 hours and that are unresponsive to sublingual nitroglycerin. (Pollack, Diercks, Roe, & Peterson, 2004)
   and

2. ST-segment elevation of more than 1 mm in one of the following locations: two of the three inferior leads (II, III, aVF), two of the six precordial leads (V_1 through V_6), or lateral leads I and aVL.
    or
3. New-onset bundle-branch block.

Treatment should begin as soon as possible after the onset of symptoms.

CONTRAINDICATIONS

1. Active internal bleeding
2. Any history of cerebrovascular accident
3. Recent (within 2 months) intracranial or intraspinal surgery or trauma
4. Intracranial neoplasm, arteriovenous malformation, or aneurysm
5. Known bleeding disorder
6. Severe uncontrolled hypertension

CAUTIONS

Cautions or relative contraindications to the use of TNK-tPA are those events or conditions that either in isolation or combination may increase the potential risk of TNK-tPA therapy and include the following:

1. Recent major surgery
2. Cerebrovascular disease
3. Recent gastrointestinal or genitourinary bleeding
4. Recent trauma
5. Recent puncture of subclavian, internal jugular, or other noncompressible vessel
6. Uncontrolled hypertension: systolic blood pressure greater than or equal to 180 mm Hg or diastolic blood pressure greater than or equal to 110 mm Hg
7. High likelihood of left-sided heart thrombus (e.g., mitral stenosis with atrial fibrillation)
8. Acute pericarditis
9. Subacute bacterial endocarditis
10. Hemostatic disorders, including those secondary to severe hepatic and renal disease
11. Pregnancy
12. Diabetic hemorrhagic retinopathy or other hemorrhagic ophthalmic conditions
13. Septic thrombophlebitis or occluded arteriovenous cannula at seriously infected site
14. Age greater than 75 years
15. Current treatment with oral anticoagulants (e.g., warfarin sodium)
16. Recent administration of glycoprotein (GP) IIb/IIIa inhibitors
17. Any condition in which bleeding constitutes a significant hazard or would be particularly difficult to manage because of its location

EQUIPMENT

50-mg TNK-tPA kit (contains one 50-mg vial of TNK-tPA powder, one 10-ml vial of sterile water, and one 10-ml syringe with TwinPak dual-cannula device)

10-ml syringe for flush

10 ml of normal saline

Intravenous (IV) starting equipment

IV catheter plug (also known as PRN adapter, heparin or saline lock, buffalo cap)

PATIENT PREPARATION

1. Perform a thorough assessment, including:
   a. 12-lead electrocardiogram (see Procedure 56)
   b. Complete history and physical examination, including time of onset of chest pain
   c. Review of selection criteria for TNK-tPA therapy
2. Establish continuous cardiac monitoring (see Procedure 55).
3. Establish IV access with a minimum of one to two sites using 18- to 20-G catheters (see Procedure 60). The use of a double-lumen peripheral IV catheter may reduce the number of punctures.
4. Provide routine acute myocardial infarction care as prescribed, which may include but is not limited to the following (Antman et al., 2004):
   a. Oxygen therapy
   b. Aspirin, chewable
   c. IV unfractionated heparin bolus 60 units/kg (maximum of 4000 units) and continuous infusion 12 units/kg/hr (maximum 1000 units/hr)
   d. Oral and/or IV β-blocker therapy
   e. IV nitroglycerin
   f. IV narcotic analgesia
5. Obtain laboratory studies, including:
   a. Cardiac markers (myoglobin, troponin, creatine kinase–MB)
   b. Chemistry profile
   c. Electrolyte profile
   d. Prothrombin time, partial thromboplastin time
   e. Complete blood count with platelets

TNK-tPA RECONSTITUTION

1. Reconstitute TNK-tPA using a 50-mg vial.
   a. Remove the shield assembly from the supplied 10-ml syringe with TwinPak dual-cannula device and aseptically withdraw 10 ml of sterile water for injection, from the supplied diluent vial using the red hub cannula syringe filling device. Do not use bacteriostatic water. NOTE: Do not discard the shield assembly.
   b. Inject the entire contents of the syringe (10 ml) into the TNK-tPA vial, directing the diluent stream into the powder. Slight foaming upon reconstitution is not unusual; any large bubbles will dissipate if the product is allowed to stand undisturbed for several minutes.
   c. Gently swirl until contents are completely dissolved. DO NOT SHAKE. The reconstituted preparation results in a colorless to pale yellow transparent solution that contains TNK-tPA at 5 mg/ml.
2. Once reconstituted, the TNK-tPA solution (5 mg/ml) may be used for direct administration. Determine the appropriate dose of TNK-tPA using Table 180-1 and withdraw this volume (in milliliters) from the reconstituted vial with the syringe. Any unused solution should be discarded.

TABLE 180-1
TNKase DOSING INFORMATION

Patient Weight (kg)	TNKase (mg)	Volume TNKase to be Administered (ml)
Less than 60	30 mg	6
60-69	35 mg	7
70-79	40 mg	8
80-89	45 mg	9
90 or greater	50 mg	10

Modified from Genentech. (2004). *TNKase (tenecteplase, recombinant) prescribing information.* San Francisco: Author.

3. Once the appropriate dose of TNK-tPA is drawn into the syringe, stand the shield vertically on a flat surface (with green side down) and passively recap the red hub cannula. Remove the entire shield assembly, including the red hub cannula, by twisting counterclockwise. NOTE: The shield assembly also contains the clear-ended blunt plastic cannula; retain for split-septum IV access.
4. Once reconstituted, TNK-tPA solution may be stored for 8 hours at 2° to 30° C (36° to 86° F). After 8 hours, any unused portion should be discarded.
5. The reconstituted TNK-tPA is not light sensitive, and no special handling is required. Unreconstituted TNK-tPA may be sensitive to light and therefore should be stored in its carton until use.
6. TNK-tPA is not compatible with other medications; flush the IV line with normal saline before and after TNK-tPA bolus is delivered through any IV line containing other medications or solutions other than normal saline, or use a separate IV line for TNK-tPA administration.

ADMINISTRATION OF TNK-tPA FOR ACUTE MYOCARDIAL INFARCTION
Procedural Steps
1. Visually inspect the product for particulate matter and discoloration before administration. TNK-tPA may be administered as reconstituted at 5 mg/ml.
2. Precipitation may occur when TNK-tPA is administered in an IV line containing dextrose. Dextrose-containing lines should be flushed with a saline-containing solution before and after single-bolus administration of TNK-tPA.
3. Reconstituted TNK-tPA should be administered as a single IV bolus over 5 seconds. Flush IV line with normal saline to ensure complete dose delivery.
4. Although the supplied syringe is compatible with a conventional needle, the supplied syringe is designed to be used with needleless IV systems. See Table 180-2 for information applicable to the IV system in use.

Patient Management for Acute Myocardial Infarction
1. Continuously monitor the cardiac rhythm and neurologic status.
2. Assess and document vital signs and status for clinical signs of reperfusion, bleeding complications (e.g., neurologic checks), and signs of coronary artery reocclusion (e.g., recurrence of chest pain or ST-segment elevation)

TABLE 180-2
IV SYSTEM COMPATIBILITY

System in Use	Instructions
Split-septum IV system	1. Remove the green cap. 2. Attach the clear-ended blunt plastic cannula to the syringe. 3. Remove the shield and use the blunt plastic cannula to access the split-septum injection port. 4. Because the blunt plastic cannula has two side ports, air or fluid expelled through the cannula exits in two sideways directions; direct away from face or mucous membranes.
Luer-Lok system	Connect the syringe directly to the IV port.
Conventional needle	Attach a large-bore needle, e.g., 18-G (not supplied in TNKase kit), to the syringe's universal Luer-Lok.

Modified from Genentech. (2004). *TNKase (tenecteplase, recombinant) prescribing information.* San Francisco: Author.

every 15 minutes during TNK-tPA infusion and every 2 hours thereafter until 2 hours after heparin is discontinued. Clinical signs of reperfusion may include cardiac dysrhythmias, resolution of chest pain, and resolution of ST-segment elevation. These signs may indicate that TNK-tPA has been successful; however, absence of these signs does not indicate that TNK-tPA has failed. The dysrhythmias seen are the same as those seen in many myocardial infarction patients and may include accelerated idioventricular rhythm, sinus bradycardia, ventricular tachycardia, ventricular fibrillation, and heart block. Any dysrhythmias that occur are treated according to Advanced Cardiac Life Support (ACLS) guidelines.

3. Document the time the chest pain resolves.
4. Maintain heparin infusion and monitor the partial thromboplastin time to maintain it at 1.5 to 2 times the control. Heparin may be continued for 24 to 72 hours until time of cardiac catheterization or other diagnostic tests.
5. Institute thrombolytic bleeding precautions as described subsequently.

THROMBOLYTIC BLEEDING PRECAUTIONS

1. Avoid the continuous use of automatic blood pressure cuffs if possible. If automatic blood pressure cuffs are used, monitor them carefully to ensure that they are not repeatedly inflating to high pressures, which may cause underlying bruising and bleeding into the extremity.
2. Avoid unnecessary arterial and venous punctures. Puncture sites should be compressed manually for a minimum of 10 minutes for venous punctures and 20 minutes for arterial punctures. Apply pressure dressings after discontinuation of lines and vessel punctures.
3. Use a saline or heparin lock for blood draws, and consolidate blood draws.
4. Monitor all puncture sites and the gingivae for evidence of bleeding.
5. To avoid contusions, use a draw sheet to move and position the patient. Instruct the patient to request assistance in changing positions.
6. Observe for frank blood, and test urine, stools, and emesis for occult blood.
7. Avoid intramuscular injections.

8. Monitor hemoglobin and hematocrit for evidence of acute blood loss.
9. Suggest the use of antecubital or femoral sites for placement of central lines if needed.

COMPLICATIONS

1. Almost all adverse reactions attributable to TNK-tPA therapy are due to bleeding that occurs after TNK-tPA therapy. Bleeding should be expected to occur during and after TNK-tPA infusion. The goal is to prevent serious bleeding through careful screening and by observation of thrombolytic bleeding precautions. Thorough assessment and prompt treatment are also critical to minimize the effects of bleeding when it does occur. Most bleeding can be divided into two categories: surface bleeding and internal bleeding. Examples of the types of bleeding seen with TNK-tPA include the following:
   - Intracranial. Intracranial bleeding is the most serious form of bleeding that can occur after thrombolytic therapy. Although intracranial bleeding is rare (less than 1%) (Genentech, 2000), it is so potentially devastating that care must be taken to exclude patients at risk for intracranial hemorrhage and to recognize and treat changes in neurologic status without delay.
   - Gastrointestinal
   - Genitourinary
   - Epistaxis
   - Retroperitoneal
   - Venous arterial puncture
   - Femoral artery catheter sites
   - Gingival
   - Ecchymosis
2. In addition, cholesterol embolization has been reported in patients treated with all types of thromobolytic agents. Cholesterol embolization is rare, can be lethal, and is also associated with vascular procedures (e.g., cardiac catheterization, vascular surgery) and anticoagulation.

PATIENT TEACHING

1. Ask for assistance before moving.
2. Report any bleeding.
3. Report any change in or recurrence of symptoms immediately.

REFERENCES

Antman, E. M., Anbe, D. T., Armstrong, P. W., Bates, E. R., Green, L. A., & Hand, M., et al. (2004). ACC/AHA guidelines for the management of patients with ST-elevation myocardial infarction: Executive summary: A report of the ACC/AHA Task Force on Practice Guidelines (Committee to Revise the 1999 Guidelines on the Management of Patients With Acute Myocardial Infarction). *Circulation, 110*, 588-636.

Genentech. (2000). *TNKase (tenecteplase, recombinant) prescribing information.* San Francisco: Author.

Pollack, C. M., Diercks, D. B., Roe, M. T., & Peterson, E. D. (2004). 2004 American College of Cardiology/American Heart Association guidelines for the management of patients with ST-elevation myocardial infarction: Implications for emergency department practice. *Annals of Emergency Medicine, 45*, 363-376.

tPA Administration for Acute Myocardial Infarction or Pulmonary Embolus

Ruth Altherr Rench, MS, RN, FAHA, and *Teresa L. Will, MSN, RN, CEN*

tPA is also known as *tissue plasminogen activator, TPA, r-tPA, alteplase,* or *Activase.*

INDICATIONS

To lyse thromboses in the presence of:
1. Acute myocardial infarction diagnosed by:
   a. Chest discomfort or related symptoms lasting for at least 15 minutes and less than 12 hours and that are unresponsive to sublingual nitroglycerin (Pollack, Diercks, Roe, & Peterson, 2004), *and*
   b. ST-segment elevation of more than 1 mm in one of the following locations: two of the three inferior leads (II, III, aVF), two of the six precordial leads (V_1 through V_6), or lateral leads I and aVL, *or*
   c. New-onset bundle-branch block
   Treatment should begin as soon as possible after the onset of symptoms.
2. Acute massive pulmonary embolus in which there is either obstruction of blood flow to a lobe or multiple lung segments or when accompanied by unstable hemodynamics. The diagnosis should be confirmed by objective means, such as pulmonary angiography, or noninvasive procedures, such as lung scanning. Pulmonary embolism should be considered in patients who present with acute onset shortness of breath, any unexplained hemodynamic deterioration, or hypoxia (Goldhaber, 2005).

CONTRAINDICATIONS

1. Active internal bleeding
2. Any history of cerebrovascular accident
3. Recent (within 2 months) intracranial or intraspinal surgery or trauma
4. Intracranial neoplasm, arteriovenous malformation, or aneurysm
5. Known bleeding disorder
6. Severe uncontrolled hypertension

CAUTIONS

Cautions or relative contraindications to the use of tPA are those events or conditions that in either isolation or combination may increase the potential risk of tPA therapy and include the following:

1. Recent major surgery
2. Cerebrovascular disease
3. Recent gastrointestinal or genitourinary bleeding
4. Recent trauma
5. Recent puncture of subclavian, internal jugular, or other noncompressible vessel
6. Uncontrolled hypertension: systolic blood pressure greater than or equal to 180 mm Hg or diastolic blood pressure greater than or equal to 110 mm Hg
7. High likelihood of left-sided heart thrombus (e.g., mitral stenosis with atrial fibrillation)
8. Acute pericarditis
9. Subacute bacterial endocarditis
10. Hemostatic disorders, including those secondary to severe hepatic and renal disease
11. Pregnancy
12. Diabetic hemorrhagic retinopathy or other hemorrhagic ophthalmic conditions
13. Septic thrombophlebitis or occluded arteriovenous cannula at seriously infected site
14. Age greater than 75 years
15. Current treatment with oral anticoagulants (e.g., warfarin sodium)
16. Any condition in which bleeding constitutes a significant hazard or would be particularly difficult to manage because of its location

EQUIPMENT

100-mg tPA kit (contains one 100-mg vial of tPA powder, one 100-ml vial of sterile water, and one double-sided transfer device)
Two 20-ml syringes
25 ml of normal saline (NS) or dextrose 5% in water (D_5W)
Intravenous (IV) starting equipment
IV catheter plug (also known as PRN adapter, heparin or saline lock, buffalo cap)
Volumetric IV pump and tubing (vented tubing preferred)

PATIENT PREPARATION

1. Perform a thorough assessment, including:
   a. 12-lead electrocardiogram (see Procedure 56)
   b. Complete history and physical examination, including time of onset of chest pain
   c. Review of selection criteria for tPA therapy
2. Establish continuous cardiac monitoring (see Procedure 55).
3. Establish IV access with a minimum of two or three sites using 18- to 20-G catheters (see Procedure 60). The use of a double-lumen peripheral IV catheter may reduce the number of punctures.

4. Provide routine acute myocardial infarction care as prescribed, which may include but is not limited to the following (Antman, 2004):
   a. Oxygen therapy
   b. Aspirin, chewable
   c. Oral and/or intravenous β-blocker therapy
   d. IV nitroglycerin
   e. IV narcotic analgesia
5. Obtain laboratory studies, including
   a. Cardiac markers (myoglobin, troponin, creatine kinase–MB)
   b. Chemistry profile
   c. Electrolyte profile
   d. Prothrombin time (PT), partial thromboplastin time (PTT)
   e. Complete blood count with platelets

ACCELERATED INFUSION (90 MINUTES) FOR ACUTE MYOCARDIAL INFARCTION
tPA Reconstitution

NOTE: tPA is available in 50-mg and 100-mg vials. This procedure describes use of the 100-mg vial. The reconstitution is different for the 50-mg vial. Refer to the package insert for information.

1. Reconstitute tPA using a 100-mg vial.
   a. Insert one end of the transfer device into the vial containing the diluent. Hold the tPA vial upside-down, and insert the other end of the transfer device into the center of the stopper. Invert the vials.
   b. After transferring the sterile water, gently swirl or invert the vial to mix the contents. Do not shake. If foaming occurs, let the vial stand for 2 to 5 minutes so the foam dissipates.
2. Assemble IV tubing without the use of an in-line filter. An in-line filter is not used because it can trap the tPA molecule and prevent it from reaching the patient. Vented pump tubing must be used to administer the solution directly from the 100-mg vial.
3. Once reconstituted, the tPA solution (1 mg/ml) may be used for direct administration. Although it may be further diluted with either NS or D_5W, most institutions prefer 1:1 dilution for ease of calculation and to limit fluids.
4. Hang the vial with vented tubing for direct infusion, or transfer the contents of the vial to an IV bag, bottle, or volume control chamber.
5. Set up infusion pump with the IV tubing and prime the tubing with the tPA solution, being careful not to discard any of the solution.
6. Once reconstituted, tPA solution may be stored for 8 hours at 2° to 30°C (36° to 86°F). After 8 hours, any unused portion should be discarded.
7. The reconstituted tPA is not light sensitive, and no special handling is required. Unreconstituted tPA may be sensitive to light and therefore should be stored in its carton until use.
8. tPA is not compatible with other medications; use a separate IV line for tPA administration.

Procedural Steps

1. Bolus dose:
   a. Withdraw 15 mg from the tPA bag or vial, and administer over 1 to 2 minutes, *or*
   b. Administer the 15-mg bolus by setting the infusion pump at 450 ml/hr to deliver 15 ml over 2 minutes. NOTE: Careful attention to pump programming is warranted if this option is chosen; some institutions prohibit bolus administration via this method.
2. After the bolus has infused, set the infusion pump at 100 ml/hr to deliver 50 mg over the first 30 minutes (see step 6 for patients weighing less than 67 kg).
3. At the end of 30 minutes, decrease the IV rate to 35 ml/hr and continue until the infusion is complete. *Remember to decrease the rate at the end of the first 30 minutes.*
4. When the pump alarm sounds indicating the vial is empty, hang 25 ml of NS, or D_5W solution, and continue to infuse at the same rate until the pump alarm sounds that the infusion is complete. This step ensures that the complete dose has been administered. After the full dose has been infused, convert the tPA line to a heparin or saline lock to use for blood draws.
5. The tPA dosing described here is based on the U.S. Food and Drug Administration–recommended dose of 100 mg, which is given over a 90-minute period (Table 181-1).
   NOTE: A 3-hour infusion dose of tPA is also considered acceptable and is described more fully in the tPA prescribing information.
6. If a patient weighs 67 kg or less, administer a dose to the patient based on a milligram per kilogram schedule. The total dose approved by the U.S. Food and Drug Administration is 1.25 mg/kg, and the total tPA dose should never exceed 100 mg. Table 181-2 lists specific doses and infusion rates.
7. It is generally accepted that a loading dose of heparin should be administered and a continuous infusion started before the end of the tPA administration period. The PTT is then maintained at 1.5 times the control to prevent reocclusion.

Patient Management for Acute Myocardial Infarction

1. Continuously monitor the cardiac rhythm and neurologic status.
2. Assess and document vital signs and status for clinical signs of reperfusion, bleeding complications (e.g., neurologic checks), and signs of coronary artery

TABLE 181-1

ACCELERATED 90-MINUTE tPA INFUSION FOR ACUTE MYOCARDIAL INFARCTION (tPA CONCENTRATION 1 MG/ML)

	Dose (mg)	Pump Rate (ml/hr)
Bolus (over 2 min)	15	450
First 30 min	50	100
Next 60 min	35	35
Total dose	100	

Data from Genentech. (2005). *Activase (alteplase, recombinant) prescribing information.* San Francisco: Author.

TABLE 181-2

WEIGHT-BASED tPA DOSAGE CALCULATION CHART FOR ACUTE MYOCARDIAL INFARCTION (tPA CONCENTRATION 1 MG/ML)

Weight (kg)	15-mg Bolus (ml)	30-minute Infusion Rate (ml/hr) 0.75 mg/kg	60-minute Infusion Rate (ml/hr) 0.5 mg/kg	Total Dose (mg)
41	15	62	20.5	66.5
42	15	63	21	67.5
43	15	64	21.5	68.5
44	15	66	22	70
45	15	68	22.5	71.5
46	15	69	23	72.5
47	15	70	23.5	73.5
48	15	72	24	75
49	15	74	24.5	76.5
50	15	75	25	77.5
51	15	76	25.5	78.5
52	15	78	26	80
53	15	80	26.5	81.5
54	15	81	27	82.5
55	15	82	27.5	83.5
56	15	84	28	85
57	15	86	28.5	86.5
58	15	87	29	87.5
59	15	88	29.5	88.5
60	15	90	30	90
61	15	92	30.5	91.5
62	15	93	31	92.5
63	15	94	31.5	93.5
64	15	96	32	95
65	15	98	32.5	96.5
66	15	99	33	97.5
67	15	100	33.5	98.5
Over 67	15	100	35	100

Data from Genentech. (2005). *Activase (alteplase, recombinant) prescribing information.* San Francisco: Author.

reocclusion (e.g., recurrence of chest pain or ST-segment elevation) every 15 minutes during tPA infusion and every 2 hours thereafter until 2 hours after heparin administration is discontinued. Clinical signs of reperfusion may include cardiac arrhythmias, resolution of chest pain, and resolution of ST-segment elevation. These signs may indicate that tPA has been successful; however, absence of these signs does not indicate that tPA has failed. The arrhythmias seen are the same as those seen in many myocardial infarction patients and may include accelerated idioventricular rhythm, sinus bradycardia, ventricular tachycardia, ventricular fibrillation, and heart block. Any arrhythmias that occur are treated according to Advanced Cardiac Life Support (ACLS) guidelines.

3. Document the time the chest pain resolves.

4. Be sure to turn down the tPA infusion and document the time at exactly 30 minutes into the infusion or 60 minutes into the infusion, depending on whether the accelerated 90-minute infusion or the 3-hour infusion is used.
5. Monitor the tPA infusion closely to ensure that it is infusing at the correct rate.
6. Maintain heparin infusion and monitor the PTT to maintain it at 1.5 to 2 times the control. Heparin may be continued for 24 to 72 hours until time of cardiac catheterization or other diagnostic tests.
7. Institute thrombolytic bleeding precautions as described subsequently.

DOSING AND ADMINISTRATION FOR PULMONARY EMBOLUS
Procedural Steps
1. Reconstitute the tPA as described above under Myocardial Infarction.
2. The recommended dose of tPA for pulmonary embolus is 100 mg over 2 hours. Administer via volumetric pump at 50 ml/hr.
3. Heparin therapy should be instituted near the end or immediately after the tPA infusion when the PTT returns to twice normal or less.

Patient Management for Pulmonary Embolus
1. Monitor the cardiac rhythm and pulmonary and neurologic status continuously.
2. Assess and document vital signs, pulmonary status, and neurologic status, and check for evidence of bleeding every 15 minutes during tPA infusion and every 2 hours thereafter until the patient is stable.
3. Monitor the tPA infusion closely to ensure that it is infusing at the correct rate.
4. Institute heparin therapy when PTT returns to twice normal or less.
5. Repeat baseline laboratory and diagnostic tests to assess results of treatment.
6. Institute thrombolytic bleeding precautions as described subsequently.

THROMBOLYTIC BLEEDING PRECAUTIONS
1. Avoid the continuous use of automatic blood pressure cuffs if possible. If automatic blood pressure cuffs are used, monitor them carefully to ensure that they are not repeatedly inflating to high pressures, which may cause underlying bruising and bleeding into the extremity.
2. Avoid unnecessary arterial and venous punctures. Puncture sites should be compressed manually for a minimum of 10 minutes for venous punctures and 20 minutes for arterial punctures. Apply pressure dressings after discontinuation of lines and vessel punctures.
3. Use a saline or heparin lock for blood draws, and consolidate blood draws.
4. Monitor all puncture sites and the gingivae for evidence of bleeding.
5. To avoid contusions, use a draw sheet to move and position the patient. Instruct the patient to request assistance in changing positions.
6. Observe for frank blood, and test urine, stools, and emesis for occult blood.
7. Avoid intramuscular injections.
8. Monitor hemoglobin and hematocrit for evidence of acute blood loss.
9. Suggest the use of antecubital or femoral sites for placement of central lines if needed.

COMPLICATIONS

1. The only adverse reactions attributable to tPA therapy are primarily due to bleeding that occurs after tPA therapy. Bleeding should be expected to occur during and after tPA infusion. The goal is to prevent serious bleeding through careful screening and by observation of thrombolytic bleeding precautions. Thorough assessment and prompt treatment are also critical to minimize the effects of bleeding when it does occur. Most bleeding can be divided into two categories: surface bleeding and internal bleeding. Examples of the types of bleeding occurring with tPA include the following:
   - Intracranial
   - Gastrointestinal
   - Genitourinary
   - Epistaxis
   - Retroperitoneal
   - Venous arterial puncture
   - Femoral artery catheter sites
   - Gingival
   - Ecchymosis
   - Intracranial bleeding is the most serious form of bleeding that can occur after thrombolytic therapy. Although intracranial bleeding is rare (less than 1%) (Genentech, 2005), it is so potentially devastating that care must be taken to exclude patients at risk for intracranial hemorrhage and to recognize and treat changes in neurologic status without delay.
2. In addition, rarely, cholesterol embolization has been reported in patients treated with all types of thrombolytic agents. Cholesterol embolization can be lethal and is also associated with vascular procedures (e.g., cardiac catheterization, vascular surgery) and anticoagulation.

PATIENT TEACHING

1. Ask for assistance before moving.
2. Report any bleeding.
3. Report any change in or recurrence of symptoms immediately.

REFERENCES

Antman, E. M., Anbe, D. T., Armstrong, P. W., Bates, E. R., Green, L. A., & Hand, M., et al. (2004). ACC/AHA guidelines for the management of patients with ST-elevation myocardial infarction: Executive summary: A report of the ACC/AHA Task Force on Practice Guidelines (Committee to Revise the 1999 Guidelines on the Management of Patients With Acute Myocardial Infarction). *Circulation, 110*, 588-636.

Genentech. (2005). *Activase (alteplase, recombinant) prescribing information.* San Francisco: Author.

Goldhaber, S. Z. (2005). Pulmonary embolism. In D. P. Zipes, et al. (Eds.), *Braunwald's heart disease: A textbook of cardiovascular medicine*, Vol. 2 (7th ed., pp. 1789-1806). Philadelphia: Saunders.

Pollack, C. M., Diercks, D. B., Roe, M. T., & Peterson, E. D. (2004). 2004 American College of Cardiology/American Heart Association guidelines for the management of patients with ST-elevation myocardial infarction: Implications for emergency department practice. *Annals of Emergency Medicine, 45*, 363-376.

tPA Administration for Acute Ischemic Stroke

Ruth Altherr Rench, MS, RN, FAHA, and *Teresa L. Will, MSN, RN, CEN*

tPA is also known as *tissue plasminogen activator, TPA, r-tPA, alteplase,* and *Activase.* Acute ischemic stroke is one type of cerebrovascular accident (CVA).

INDICATIONS

tPA is indicated for the management of acute ischemic stroke in adults to improve neurologic recovery and reduce the incidence of disability when the following situations exist:

1. Identification of a focal neurologic deficit indicates a probability of acute ischemic stroke.
2. Treatment can be initiated within 3 hours after stroke symptom onset.
3. Intracranial hemorrhage is excluded by a cranial computed tomography (CT) scan or other diagnostic imaging method sensitive for the presence of hemorrhage.
4. Intravenous tPA, when used with rigorous adherence to eligibility criteria has been shown to have the same beneficial outcomes as the outcomes documented in the NINDS trial in 1996. Further analysis of the NINDS data confirmed the validity of the original trial results. IV tPA is recommended for patients with acute ischemic stroke who meet the eligibility requirements and is prescribed by a physician with a clearly defined protocol, a knowledgeable team, and an institutional commitment (AHA, 2005).

CONTRAINDICATIONS

1. Evidence of intracranial hemorrhage on pretreatment evaluation
2. Suspicion of subarachnoid hemorrhage
3. Recent intracranial surgery, serious head trauma, or recent previous stroke
4. History of intracranial hemorrhage
5. Uncontrolled hypertension at time of treatment (e.g., greater than 185 mm Hg systolic blood pressure or greater than 110 mm Hg diastolic blood pressure)
6. Seizure at the onset of stroke
7. Active internal bleeding
8. Intracranial neoplasm, arteriovenous malformation, or aneurysm
9. Known bleeding diathesis including but not limited to the following:
   a. Current use of oral anticoagulants (e.g., warfarin sodium) with prothrombin time (PT) greater than 15 seconds
   b. Administration of heparin within 48 hours preceding the onset of stroke with an elevated activated partial thromboplastin time (aPTT) at presentation
   c. Platelet count less than 100,000/mm^3

CAUTIONS

The following are cautions for using tPA to treat acute ischemic stroke. In these situations, the risk of treatment with tPA may be increased and should be weighed against the anticipated benefits.

1. Patients with severe neurologic deficit at presentation who have an increased risk of intracranial hemorrhage
2. Patients with major early infarct signs on a cranial CT scan
3. Events or conditions that alone or combined may increase the risk of tPA therapy include:
   a. Recent major surgery
   b. Cerebrovascular disease
   c. Recent gastrointestinal or genitourinary bleeding
   d. Recent trauma
   e. Recent puncture of subclavian, internal jugular, or other noncompressible vessel
   f. Hypertension: systolic blood pressure 180 mm Hg or higher or diastolic blood pressure 110 mm Hg or higher
   g. High likelihood of left-sided heart thrombus (e.g., mitral stenosis with atrial fibrillation)
   h. Acute pericarditis
   i. Subacute bacterial endocarditis
   j. Hemostatic disorders including those secondary to severe hepatic and renal disease
   k. Pregnancy
   l. Diabetic hemorrhagic retinopathy or other hemorrhagic ophthalmic conditions
   m. Septic thrombophlebitis or occluded arteriovenous cannula at seriously infected site
   n. Age greater than 75 years
   o. Current treatment with oral anticoagulants (e.g., warfarin sodium)
   p. Any condition in which bleeding constitutes a significant hazard or would be particularly difficult to manage because of its location

EQUIPMENT

One 100-mg tPA kit (contains one 100-mg vial of tPA powder, one 100-ml vial of sterile water, and one double-sided transfer device)

Two 20- to 30-ml syringes

25 ml normal saline (NS) or dextrose 5% water (D_5W) solution

Intravenous (IV) catheter plug (also known as PRN adapter, heparin lock or saline lock, buffalo cap)

Volumetric IV pump and tubing (vented tubing required if administering solution directly from the 100-mg vial)

20-ml syringe with needle for discard solution

PATIENT PREPARATION

1. Provide critical care measures as prescribed, which may include but are not limited to:
   a. Oxygen therapy
   b. 12-lead electrocardiogram (see Procedure 56)

    c. Continuous cardiac monitoring (see Procedure 55)

    d. Establishment of IV access with a minimum of two to three sites using 18- to 20-G catheters (see Procedure 60)

    e. Complete history and physical examination, including time of stroke symptom onset

    f. Review of selection criteria for tPA therapy

2. Do not administer heparin or aspirin for the first 24 hours after tPA treatment for acute ischemic stroke.

3. Obtain laboratory studies, including the following:

    a. Chemistry profile

    b. Electrolyte profile

    c. Prothrombin time (PT), partial thromboplastin time (PTT)

    d. Complete blood count with platelets

4. Monitor blood pressure every 15 minutes

5. Administer medications as ordered to maintain systolic blood pressure at 185 mm Hg or less and diastolic blood pressure at 110 mm Hg or less

PROCEDURAL STEPS

NOTE: tPA is available in 50-and 100-mg vials. This procedure describes use of the 100-mg vial. The reconstitution is different for the 50-mg vial. Refer to the package insert for information.

1. Reconstitute tPA using a 100-mg vial.

    a. Insert one end of transfer device into the vial containing diluent. Hold the tPA vial upside-down, and insert the other end of the transfer device into the center of the stopper. Invert the vials.

    b. After transferring the sterile water, gently swirl or invert the vial to mix the contents. Do not shake. If foaming occurs, let the vial stand for 2 to 5 minutes so foam dissipates.

2. Assemble IV tubing without the use of an in-line filter. An in-line filter is not used because it can trap the tPA molecule and prevent it from reaching the patient. Vented pump tubing must be used to administer the solution directly from the 100-mg vial.

3. Once reconstituted, the tPA solution (1 mg/ml) may be used for direct administration. Although it may be further diluted with either NS or D_5W, most institutions prefer 1:1 dilution for ease of calculation and to limit fluids.

4. Withdraw any tPA to be discarded and the bolus dose (Table 182-1).

5. Hang the vial with vented tubing for direct infusion or transfer the contents of the vial to an IV bag, bottle, or volume control chamber.

6. Set up infusion pump with the IV tubing, and prime the tubing with the tPA solution, being careful not to discard any of the solution.

7. Once reconstituted, tPA solution may be stored for 8 hours at 2° to 30° C (36° to 86° F). After 8 hours, any unused portion should be discarded.

8. The reconstituted tPA is not light sensitive, and no special handling is required. Unreconstituted tPA may be sensitive to light and therefore should be stored in its carton until use.

9. tPA is not compatible with other medications; use a separate IV line for tPA administration.

TABLE 182-1

WEIGHT-BASED tPA DOSAGE CALCULATION CHART FOR ACUTE ISCHEMIC STROKE
(tPA CONCENTRATION 1 MG/ML)

Weight (kg)	Bolus Over 1 min (ml)	1-Hour Infusion Rate (ml/hr)	Total Dose 0.9 mg/kg (mg)	Unused/Discard Quantity (mg)
41	3.7	33.2	36.9	63.1
43	3.9	34.8	38.7	61.3
45	4.1	36.5	40.5	59.5
47	4.2	38.1	42.3	57.7
49	4.4	39.7	44.1	55.9
51	4.6	41.3	45.9	54.1
53	4.8	42.9	47.7	52.3
55	5	44.5	49.5	50.5
57	5.1	46.2	51.3	48.7
59	5.3	47.8	53.1	46.9
61	5.5	49.4	54.9	45.1
63	5.7	51	56.7	43.3
65	5.9	52.6	58.5	41.5
67	6	54.3	60.3	39.7
69	6.2	55.9	62.1	37.9
71	6.4	57.5	63.9	36.1
73	6.6	59.1	65.7	34.3
75	6.8	60.7	67.5	32.5
77	6.9	62.4	69.3	30.7
79	7.1	64	71.1	28.9
81	7.3	65.6	72.9	27.1
83	7.5	67.2	74.7	25.3
85	7.7	68.8	76.5	23.5
87	7.8	70.5	78.3	21.7
89	8	72.1	80.1	19.9
91	8.2	73.7	81.9	18.1
93	8.4	75.3	83.7	16.3
95	8.6	76.9	85.5	14.5
97	8.7	78.6	87.3	12.7
99	8.9	80.2	89.1	10.9
100 or greater	9	81	90	10

Data from Genentech. (2005). *Activase (alteplase, recombinant) prescribing information.* San Francisco: Author.

10. tPA dosing for acute ischemic stroke is always based on patient weight (see Table 182-1). The U.S. Food and Drug Administration–recommended total dose is 0.9 mg/kg. Never exceed 90 mg for the total dose of tPA for acute ischemic stroke (Genentech, 2005).
    a. Administer 10% of the total dose as an IV bolus over 1 minute.
    b. Administer the remainder of the dose as a continuous infusion over 1 hour.

PATIENT MANAGEMENT

1. Continuously monitor the patient's condition, cardiac rhythm, and neurologic status. Assess and document vital signs, neurologic status, and bleeding every 15 minutes for the first 2 hours after starting the tPA infusion, then every 30 minutes for 6 hours, then every hour for 16 hours.
2. Monitor the tPA infusion closely to ensure it is infusing at the correct rate.
3. Do not give heparin, aspirin, or warfarin sodium for 24 hours after the tPA infusion. If heparin or any other anticoagulant is indicated after 24 hours, it is recommended that a CT scan be performed to rule out intracranial hemorrhage first.
4. Administer medications as ordered to maintain blood pressure at less than or equal to 185/110 mm Hg.
5. Institute thrombolytic bleeding precautions, which include the following:
   a. Avoid the use of automatic blood pressure cuffs if possible.
   b. Avoid unnecessary arterial and venous punctures. All puncture sites should be compressed manually for a minimum of 10 minutes for venous punctures and 20 minutes for arterial punctures. Apply pressure dressings after discontinuation of lines and vessel punctures.
   c. Use a saline or heparin lock for blood draws, and consolidate blood draws.
   d. Monitor all puncture sites and the gingivae for evidence of bleeding.
   e. To avoid contusions, use a draw sheet to move and position the patient. Instruct the patient to request assistance in changing positions.
   f. Observe for frank blood, and test urine, stools, and emesis for occult blood.
   g. Avoid intramuscular injections.
   h. Monitor hemoglobin and hematocrit for evidence of acute blood loss.
   i. Suggest the use of antecubital or femoral sites for placement of central lines if needed.
6. Observe for signs of intracranial hemorrhage, such as any acute neurologic deterioration, new headache, acute hypertension, or nausea and vomiting. If intracranial hemorrhage is suspected, discontinue the tPA infusion and obtain an emergency CT scan.

COMPLICATIONS

The only adverse reactions attributable to tPA therapy are due to bleeding that occurs after tPA therapy. Cholesterol embolization has been reported but is a rare complication. Bleeding should be expected to occur during and after tPA infusion. The goal is to prevent serious bleeding through careful screening and by observation of thrombolytic bleeding precautions. Thorough assessment and prompt treatment are also critical to minimize the effects of bleeding when it does occur. Most bleeding can be divided into two categories: surface bleeding and internal bleeding. Examples of the types of bleeding seen with tPA include the following:

1. Intracranial
2. Gastrointestinal
3. Genitourinary
4. Epistaxis
5. Retroperitoneal

6. Venous or arterial puncture
7. Femoral artery catheter sites
8. Gingival
9. Ecchymosis

   Intracranial bleeding is the most serious form of bleeding that can occur after thrombolytic therapy. It is so potentially devastating that care must be taken to exclude patients at risk for intracranial hemorrhage and to recognize and treat changes in neurologic status without delay.

PATIENT TEACHING

1. Ask for assistance before moving.
2. Report any bleeding.
3. Report any changes in symptoms immediately.

REFERENCES

Genentech. (2005). *Activase (alteplase, recombinant) prescribing information.* San Francisco: Author.

American Heart Association (AHA). (2005). Guidelines for cardiopulmonary resuscitation and emergency cardiovascular care. Part 9: Adult stroke. *Circulation, 112*(suppl IV), IV-111–IV-120.

PROCEDURE 183

Reteplase Administration for Acute Myocardial Infarction

Teresa L. Will, MSN, RN, CEN

Reteplase recombinant is also known as *Retavase, recombinant plasminogen activator, RPA,* and *rPA.*

INDICATIONS

To lyse thromboses in the presence of acute myocardial infarction (AMI) diagnosed by:

1. Typical ischemic chest pain lasting for at least 30 minutes and less than 12 hours and which is unresponsive to sublingual nitroglycerin.

2. ST-segment elevation of more than 1 mm in one of the following locations: two of three inferior leads (II, III, aVF), two of six precordial leads (V_1 through V_6), or two of four lateral leads (I, aVL, V_5, V_6) *or*
3. New-onset bundle-branch block, *or*
4. Tall R waves in V_1 and V_2 with ST depression consistent with true posterior AMI where findings are acute changes.

CONTRAINDICATIONS (PDL BioPharma, 2006)

1. Active internal bleeding
2. Any history of cerebrovascular accident
3. Recent (within 2 months) intracranial or intraspinal surgery or trauma
4. Intracranial neoplasm, arteriovenous malformation, or aneurysm
5. Known bleeding disorder
6. Severe uncontrolled hypertension

CAUTIONS

Cautions or relative contraindications to the use of reteplase are those events or conditions that either in isolation or combination may increase the potential risk of reteplase therapy, including the following (PDL BioPharma, 2006):

1. Recent major surgery
2. Cerebrovascular disease
3. Recent gastrointestinal or genitourinary bleeding
4. Recent trauma
5. Recent puncture of subclavian, internal jugular, or other noncompressible vessel
6. Hypertension: systolic blood pressure greater than or equal to 180 mm Hg or diastolic blood pressure greater than or equal to 110 mm Hg
7. High likelihood of left-sided heart thrombus (e.g., mitral stenosis with atrial fibrillation)
8. Acute pericarditis
9. Subacute bacterial endocarditis
10. Hemostatic disorders, including those secondary to severe hepatic and renal disease
11. Pregnancy
12. Diabetic hemorrhagic retinopathy or other hemorrhagic ophthalmic conditions
13. Septic thrombophlebitis or occluded arteriovenous cannula at seriously infected site
14. Advanced age
15. Current treatment with oral anticoagulants (e.g., warfarin sodium)
16. Any condition in which bleeding constitutes a significant hazard or would be particularly difficult to manage because of its location

EQUIPMENT

Reteplase administration kit (contains two vials of reteplase 10.8 units each and two vials of sterile water for injection, two dispensing pins, two 10-ml syringes, and two 20-G needles)

Intravenous (IV) starting equipment

IV catheter plug (also known as PRN adapter, heparin or saline lock, buffalo cap)

PATIENT PREPARATION

1. Perform a thorough assessment including:
   a. 12-lead electrocardiogram (see Procedure 56).
   b. Complete history and physical examination including time of onset of chest pain.
   c. Review of selection criteria for thrombolytic therapy.
2. Establish continuous cardiac monitoring (see Procedure 55).
3. Establish IV access with a minimum of two or three sites using 18- to 20-G catheters (see Procedure 60). The use of a double-lumen peripheral IV catheter may reduce the number of punctures.
4. Provide routine AMI care as prescribed, which may include but is not limited to the following (Antman et al., 2004):
   a. Oxygen therapy
   b. Aspirin, chewable
   c. IV nitroglycerin
   d. IV narcotic analgesia
   e. IV β-blocker therapy
   f. Heparin therapy
5. Obtain laboratory studies, including:
   a. Cardiac markers (myoglobin, troponin, creatine kinase–MB)
   b. Chemistry profile
   c. Electrolyte profile
   d. Prothrombin time (PT), partial thromboplastin time (PTT)
   e. Complete blood count with platelets

PROCEDURAL STEPS

1. Reconstitute a 10-unit/10-ml dose of reteplase (PDL BioPharma, 2006):
   a. Use the 10-ml syringe with attached needle to withdraw 10 ml of supplied diluent, sterile water for injection.
   b. Remove the needle from the syringe, and discard the needle. Remove the protective cap from the Luer-Lok port of the dispensing pin, and connect the syringe to the dispensing pin.
   c. Insert the spike of the dispensing pin into the vial of reteplase. Transfer 10 ml of sterile water for injection through the dispensing pin into the vial of reteplase.
   d. With the dispensing pin and syringe still attached to the vial, swirl the vial gently to dissolve the reteplase. Do not shake. Foaming after reconstitution is common; let the vial stand for several minutes if necessary to dissipate any large bubbles.
   e. Withdraw 10 ml of reconstituted reteplase back into the syringe. A small amount of solution remains in the vial because of overfill.
   f. Detach the syringe from the dispensing pin, and attach the sterile 20-G needle if needed for injection.
2. Administer the 10-ml bolus of reteplase over 2 minutes. No other medications should be infusing through the IV line or the line must be flushed before reteplase administration. Flush the line again after reteplase administration.

3. The second bolus of 10 units of reteplase must be administered 30 minutes after the first bolus. Repeat steps 1 and 2 for the second bolus.
4. Heparin and aspirin should be administered concomitantly.

PATIENT MANAGEMENT FOR ACUTE MYOCARDIAL INFARCTION

1. Continuously monitor the cardiac rhythm and neurologic status.
2. Assess and document vital signs and status for clinical signs of reperfusion, bleeding complications (e.g., neurologic checks), and signs of coronary artery reocclusion (e.g., recurrence of chest pain or ST-segment elevation) every 15 minutes for the first 2 hours after administration of the first reteplase bolus, then every 2 hours thereafter until 2 hours after heparin is discontinued. Clinical signs of reperfusion include cardiac dysrhythmias, resolution of chest pain, and resolution of ST-segment elevation. These signs may indicate the fibrinolytic has been successful; however, absence of these signs does not indicate the fibrinolytic has failed. The dysrhythmias seen are the same as those seen in many myocardial infarction patients and may include accelerated ventricular rhythm, sinus bradycardia, ventricular tachycardia, ventricular fibrillation, and heart block. Any dysrhythmias that occur are treated following Advanced Cardiac Life Support guidelines (ACLS).
3. Document the time the chest pain resolves.
4. Do not forget to give the second bolus of reteplase at precisely 30 minutes after the first dose. Remember to flush the line completely before and after the reteplase administration so that reteplase does not mix with other medications. Heparin and reteplase are incompatible when combined in solution (PDL BioPharma, 2006).
5. Maintain heparin infusion and monitor PTT levels closely. The patient may be on heparin for 24 to 72 hours until time of cardiac catheterization or other diagnostic tests.
6. Institute bleeding precautions, including the following:
   a. Avoid the use of automatic blood pressure cuffs if possible.
   b. Avoid unnecessary arterial and venous punctures. Puncture sites should be compressed manually for a minimum of 10 minutes for venous punctures and 20 minutes for arterial punctures. Apply pressure dressings after discontinuation of lines and vessel punctures.
   c. Use a saline or heparin lock for blood draws, and consolidate blood draws.
   d. Monitor all puncture sites and the gingivae for evidence of bleeding.
   e. To avoid contusions, use a draw sheet to move and position the patient. Instruct the patient to request assistance in changing positions.
   f. Observe for frank blood, and test urine, stools, and emesis for occult blood.
   g. Avoid intramuscular injections.
   h. Monitor hemoglobin and hematocrit for evidence of acute blood loss.
   i. Suggest the use of antecubital or femoral sites for placement of central lines if needed.

COMPLICATIONS

1. The major adverse reactions attributable to reteplase therapy are due to bleeding that occurs after therapy. Bleeding should be expected to occur

during and after reteplase infusion. The goal is to prevent serious bleeding through careful screening and by observation of bleeding precautions. Thorough assessment and prompt treatment are also critical to minimize the effects of bleeding when it does occur. Most bleeding can be divided into two categories: surface bleeding and internal bleeding. Examples of the types of bleeding seen with reteplase include the following:

   a. Intracranial
   b. Gastrointestinal
   c. Genitourinary
   d. Epistaxis
   e. Retroperitoneal
   f. Venous or arterial punctures
   g. Femoral artery catheter sites
   h. Gingival
   i. Ecchymosis

2. Intracranial bleeding is the most serious form of bleeding that can occur after fibrinolytic therapy. Although intracranial bleeding is rare (less than 1%), it is so potentially devastating that care must be taken to exclude patients at risk for intracranial hemorrhage and to recognize and treat changes in neurologic status without delay (PDL BioPharma, 2006). The effective half-life of reteplase is 13 to 16 minutes. In the event of serious bleeding, the second reteplase bolus should not be given, and heparin should be stopped immediately (PDL BioPharma, 2006). Heparin effects can be reversed by protamine.

3. Arrhythmias may be associated with reperfusion and should be treated with standard antiarrhythmic therapy as needed.

4. Rare side effects that have been reported include:
   a. Allergic reaction (PDL BioPharma, 2006)
   b. Nausea, vomiting (PDL BioPharma, 2006)
   c. Fever, hypotension (PDL BioPharma, 2006)
   d. Cholesterol embolization (PDL BioPharma, 2006)

PATIENT TEACHING

1. Ask for assistance before moving.
2. Report any bleeding.
3. Report any change in symptoms immediately.

REFERENCES

Antman, E. M., Anbe, D. T., Armstrong, P. W., Bates, E. R., Green, L. A., & Hand, M., et al. (2004). ACC/AHA guidelines for the management of patients with ST-elevation myocardial infarction: Executive summary: A report of the ACC/AHA Task Force on Practice Guidelines (Committee to Revise the 1999 Guidelines on the Management of Patients With Acute Myocardial Infarction). *Circulation, 110*, 588-636.

PDL BioPharma, Inc. (2006). *Retevase (Reteplase recombinant) prescribing information.* Fremont, CA: Author. Retrieved December 20, 2006, from http://www.retavase.com

High-dose Steroids for Spinal Cord Injury

Daun A. Smith, RN, MSN

INDICATION

High-dose steroids are an option for spinal cord–injured patients with motor and/or sensory deficits. Although the mechanism of action is yet unknown, research has shown that high-dose steroid therapy using methylprednisolone sodium succinate within 8 hours of a spinal cord injury improved motor function and response to pinprick and light touch (Bracken et al., 1990). Further research showed that if methylprednisolone was begun 3 to 8 hours after injury and continued for 48 hours, treatment was likely to improve neurologic outcomes (Bracken, Shepard, & Collins, 1997).

CONTRAINDICATIONS AND CAUTIONS

1. Methylprednisolone therapy must be initiated within 8 hours of injury to have any positive neurologic effects in spinal cord–injured patients (Bracken et al., 1990).
2. Although methylprednisolone has been shown to be compatible with many medications, compatibility should be checked before infusing methylprednisolone with any medication.
3. Methylprednisolone is available in two forms: methylprednisolone sodium succinate and methylprednisolone acetate. Only methylprednisolone sodium succinate may be given intravenously.
4. Not all physicians endorse this treatment for spinal cord–injured patients.

EQUIPMENT

Methylprednisolone sodium succinate, 4 g
Normal saline solution (for intravenous [IV] use), 250 ml
IV infusion pump and tubing

PATIENT PREPARATION

1. Maintain spinal alignment as indicated.
2. Initiate IV access (see Procedure 60).
3. Assess baseline neurologic status, including motor and sensory levels.

PROCEDURAL STEPS
Preparation of the Infusion

1. Withdraw enough fluid from the bag of normal saline to account for the volume of medication to be added and the manufacturer's overfill of the IV fluid bag (contact pharmacy or manufacturer for specific information).

TABLE 184-1
DOSING OF METHYLPREDNISOLONE[1]

Patient Weight (kg)	Loading Dose (30 mg/kg)	Rate of Loading Dose in ml/hr for 15 min only		Maintenance Dose Per Hour (5.4 mg/kg/hr)	Maintenance Dose (Rate in ml/hr for 23 hours)
30	900 mg/56 ml	225		162	10
35	1050 mg/66 ml	262		189	12
40	1200 mg/75 ml	300		216	14
45	1350 mg/84 ml	338		243	15
50	1500 mg/94 ml	375		270	17
55	1650 mg/103 ml	412	45 minute interval	297	19
60	1800 mg/113 ml	450	without medication	324	20
65	1950 mg/122 ml	488	between loading	351	22
70	2100 mg/131 ml	525	dose and maintenance	378	24
75	2250 mg/141 ml	562	dose	405	25
80	2400 mg/150 ml	600		432	27
85	2550 mg/159 ml	638		459	29
90	2700 mg/169 ml	675		486	30
95	2850 mg/178 l	712		513	32
100	3000 mg/188 ml	750		540	34

[1]Table reflects preparation of methylprednisolone as a 16-mg/ml solution. Loading dose rate is in ml/hr; total loading dose is run in over 15 minutes. Then the infusion is stopped for 45 minutes before the maintenance infusion is initiated.

2. Mix and add 4 g of methylprednisolone sodium succinate to the prepared 250-ml IV bag (this provides a concentration of 16 mg/ml).

Loading Dose

1. A loading dose of 30 mg/kg is given over 15 minutes.
2. Prime the tubing with the prepared mixture before starting the infusion.
3. Infuse the loading dose at the appropriate rate for the patient's weight (Table 184-1). *The rate is in ml/hr, but infuse it at the loading dose rate for only 15 minutes.*
4. After the loading dose has infused, turn off the methylprednisolone for 45 minutes, and run IV fluid at a keep-open rate.

Maintenance Dose

1. Over the next 23 hours, infuse the above-prepared solution at a rate to provide a dose of 5.4 mg/kg per hour (see Table 184-1).
2. If treatment is initiated 3 to 8 hours after injury, continue the infusion for 27 hours at the 5.4-mg/kg per hour rate (see Table 184-1).

AGE-SPECIFIC CONSIDERATIONS

1. Studies have not yet addressed either the pediatric or the geriatric populations.
2. If it is necessary to restrict IV fluids, mix the solution in a more concentrated form and recalculate infusion rates based on the new concentration.

COMPLICATIONS

1. Impaired wound healing
2. Gastrointestinal bleeding
3. Infection
4. Hyperglycemia
5. Hypertension
6. Hypokalemia
7. Thrombocytopenia

PATIENT TEACHING

1. Report any signs of infection.
2. Report any signs of gastrointestinal bleeding.
3. Results of the steroid infusion are not dramatic; however, even small gains in neurologic status can make a difference in postinjury function.

REFERENCES

Bracken, M. B., Shepard, M. J., & Collins, W. F., et al. (1990). A randomized controlled trial of methylprednisolone or naloxone in the treatment of acute spinal cord injury. *New England Journal of Medicine, 322,* 1405-1411.

Bracken, M. B., Shephard, M. J., & Holford, T. R., et al. (1997). Administration of methylprednisolone for 24 or 48 hours or tirilazad mesylate for 48 hours in the treatment of acute spinal cord injury. *Journal of the American Medical Association, 277*(20), 1597-1604.

Administration of Methotrexate for Ectopic Pregnancy

Daun A. Smith, RN, MSN

INDICATION

To cause resorption or spontaneous tubal abortion of an ectopic pregnancy (Kirchner, 2000) in selected patients. Methotrexate is an antineoplastic agent (folic acid antagonist) that interferes with DNA synthesis, particularly affecting cells that are dividing or multiplying rapidly. Inclusion criteria for the use of methotrexate are:

1. Hemodynamic stability
2. Ultrasound findings consistent with ectopic pregnancy
    a. Absence of intrauterine gestational sac
    b. Unruptured ectopic mass less than 3.5-cm diameter
3. A patient able and willing to comply with follow-up monitoring
4. Lack of contraindications to methotrexate therapy
5. Lack of fetal cardiac motion
6. β-human chorionic gonadatropin (βhCG) level less than 5000 international units per liter (Murray, Baakdah, Bardell, & Tulandi, 2005; Tenore, 2000)
7. White blood cell count less than 1500 cells/ml
8. No immune compromise (Lipscomb, 2006)

CONTRAINDICATIONS AND CAUTIONS

1. Contraindications to methotrexate include:
    a. Pregnancy
    b. Lactation
    c. Alcoholism
    d. Chronic liver disease
    e. Immune deficiencies
    f. Blood dyscrasias
    g. Hypersensitivity to methotrexate (Karch, 2006).
2. Because of the cytotoxicity and teratogenic properties of methotrexate, health care personnel administering the drug should:
    a. Not handle the drug if pregnant
    b. Wear nitrile gloves and protective gowns
    c. Follow the facility's protocols for handling and disposal of methotrexate (Wallemaco et al., 2006).

PATIENT PREPARATION

1. Diagnostic testing to rule out other etiologies and to establish baseline values (βhCG, ultrasound, liver and kidney function tests, CBC)
2. Offer bereavement counseling and support

PROCEDURAL STEPS

1. Single-dose methotrexate therapy is given intramuscularly (50 mg/m² of body surface area) (Walling, 2000). *Body surface area is calculated with the following equation or with a nomogram (Figure 185-1):

$$BSA \ (m^2) = \Big([Height(cm) \times Weight(kg)]/3600 \Big)^{\frac{1}{2}}$$

Alternately, a multiple-dose regimen may be used and consists of methotrexate (1 mg/kg of body weight) alternating with leucovorin (0.1 mg/kg of body weight) for up to four doses of each agent (Walling, 2000).
2. Serial βhCG measurements should be assessed daily or weekly until no longer detectable (Loseau & Potter, 2005).
3. If βhCG levels do not decrease, a second course of methotrexate may be given.
4. Follow up also consists of laboratory assessment of liver function tests, blood counts, and creatinine to monitor for untoward effects of methotrexate (Shima, 2002).

COMPLICATIONS

1. Side effects related to methotrexate (Tenore, 2000):
   a. Nausea
   b. Vomiting
   c. Urinary frequency
   d. Mild diarrhea
   e. Abnormal liver function
   f. Bone marrow suppression
2. Treatment failure (as evidenced by lack of decrease in βhCG)
3. Abdominal pain (resulting from tubal abortion or tubal rupture)

PATIENT TEACHING (Ohio Reproductive Medicine, 2006; Proehl & Jones, 1998)

1. Do not drink beverages containing alcohol.
2. Do not take vitamins containing folic acid.
3. Avoid gas-forming foods.
4. Avoid nonsteroidal antiinflammatory painkillers.
5. Avoid sexual intercourse or strenous activity because it may cause fallopian tube rupture.
6. Prevent conception for 3 months after treatment with methotrexate to prevent possible birth defects.

---

*Indicates portions of the procedure usually performed by a physician or an advanced practice nurse.

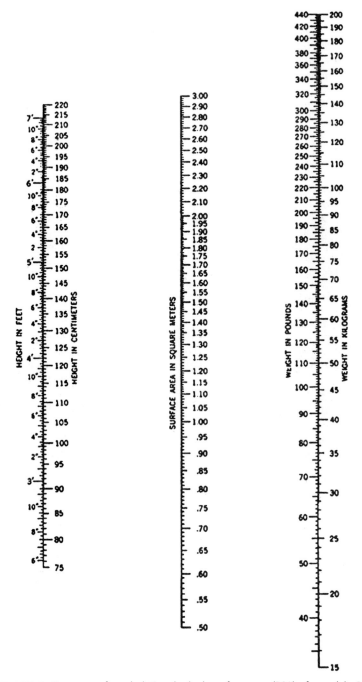

FIGURE 185-1 Nomogram for calculating the body surface area (BSA) of an adult. Position a straight-edge from the location of the patient's height to the location of the patient's weight; the BSA appears where the straight-edge crosses the center column.

7. Notify your physician or return to the emergency department for:
   a. Severe abdominal pain
   b. Dizziness, fainting
   c. Heavy vaginal bleeding
   d. Severe nausea and vomiting
   e. Fever with temperature above 38.3° C (101° F)
8. Scheduled follow-up care and diagnostic tests

REFERENCES

Karch, A. M. (2006). *Lippincott's nursing drug guide*. Philadelphia: Lippincott Williams & Wilkins.

Kirchner, J. (2000). Methotrexate in the treatment of ectopic pregnancy. *American Family Physician, 61*(7), 2228-2229.

Lipscomb, G. (2006). Ectopic pregnancy. In R. E. Rakel & E. T. Bope (Eds.), *Conn's current therapy* (pp. 1230–1232). Philadelphia: Saunders.

Loseau, A., & Potter, B. (2005). Diagnosis and management of ectopic pregnancy. *American Family Physician, 72*(9), 1707-1714.

Murray, H., Baakdah, H., Bardell, T., & Tulandi, T. (2005). Diagnosis and treatment of ectopic pregnancy. *Canadian Medical Association Journal, 173*(8), 905-912.

Ohio Reproductive Medicine. (2006, January 3). *Treatment of abnormal pregnancy with methotrexate*. Retrieved July 21, 2006, from www.ohiorepromed.com/_ppt/info-methotrexate.grosskinsky.doc.pdf

Proehl, J. A., & Jones, L. M. (1998). Methotrexate for ectopic pregnancy. *Mosby's emergency department patient teaching guides*. St Louis: Mosby.

Shima, T. L. (2002). Ectopic pregnancy. *Topics of Emergency Medicine, 24*(4), 12-20.

Tenore, J. L. (2000). Ectopic pregnancy. *American Family Physician, 61*(4), 1080-1088.

Wallemaco, P. E., Capron, A., Vanbinst, R., Boeckmans, E., Gillard, J., & Favier, B. (2006). Permeability of 13 different gloves to 13 cytotoxic agents under controlled dynamic conditions. *American Journal Health-System Pharmacology, 63*, 547-556.

Walling, A. D. (2000). Single-dose methotrexate therapy for ectopic pregnancy. *American Family Physician, 62*(2), 427.

Miscellaneous Procedures

Drug and Alcohol Specimen Collection

Reneé Semonin Holleran, RN, PhD, CEN, CCRN, CFRN, CTRN, FAEN

INDICATIONS

1. To identify whether the patient is intoxicated by a drug or alcohol
2. To obtain evidence in a criminal case
3. As required by an employer for job-related injuries
4. To obtain laboratory data for a differential diagnosis for an altered mental status or specific signs and symptoms, such as the following (Ohio Chapter of the International Association of Forensic Nurses, 2002; Kerrigan & Goldberger, 2006):
   a. Slurred speech
   b. Dizziness
   c. Confusion
   d. Blurred vision
   e. Anxiety
   f. Euphoria
   g. Hallucinations
   h. Amnesia/memory impairment
   i. Lack of muscle coordination
   j. Hyperthermia
5. To help determine a cause of death and the manner of a patient's death

CONTRAINDICATIONS AND CAUTIONS

1. Life-threatening conditions should be managed before evidence collection.
2. Blood or body fluid specimen collection for evidence in an alleged crime generally requires patient consent or a court order. Each emergency department should have protocols that govern the collection of blood and/or urine for alcohol and drug screening. Some states have laws or regulations that stipulate that specimens can be obtained without the patient's consent in specified circumstances, such as a motor vehicle crash resulting in serious injury or death.
3. Collection of blood/urine for alcohol or drug screening for an alleged crime without patient permission may be considered assault and battery.
4. If the patient is exhibiting altered mental status, always rule out organic causes for the patient's behavior, signs, and symptoms. Hypoglycemia, shock, traumatic brain injury, and drug interactions are only a few of the conditions that can cause signs and symptoms similar to those of drug and alcohol intoxication.

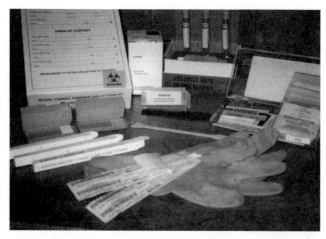

FIGURE 186-1 Example of a commercial forensic evidence kit with several containers for biological, physical, and trace evidence. (From V. Lynch [Ed.], [2006]. *Forensic nursing*, [p. 102]. St Louis: Mosby.)

EQUIPMENT

Most states have a specific kit that is used for the collection of blood/urine for legal purposes (Figure 186-1). These kits may be stored in the emergency department or supplied by the law enforcement agency requesting the test.

The following lists an example of the contents of an alcohol/drug determination kit:

Nonalcohol disinfectant

One 10-ml blood tube containing sodium fluoride and potassium oxalate

Two 7-ml blood tubes containing EDTA

Two 40-ml plastic screw-cap containers

One instruction sheet

Two police evidence seals for resealing kit box after collection of evidence

One biohazard bag for transportation of specimens

PATIENT PREPARATION

1. If not covered by state law/regulation or court order, obtain patient consent according to institutional policy.
2. Ensure that the law-enforcement agency requesting the test has explained the procedure and the patient's rights before the blood or urine is collected.
3. The law enforcement officer should witness the collection of the specimens whenever possible.
4. For all specimen collection, in order to ensure evidence security use the four Ws (Kerrigan & Goldberger, 2006):
   a. Who handled the evidence?
   b. What was handled?
   c. Why was it handled?
   d. Where it was located at all times?

PROCEDURAL STEPS

1. For blood specimens:
   a. Clean the skin with a nonalcohol disinfectant.
   b. Draw blood as per Procedure 58.
   c. Label the evidence with the patient's name, area of collection, date, time, and the person collecting the evidence. In some cases, the label must be placed across the stopper of the blood tube.
2. For urine specimens:
   a. Have the patient place the specimen in a urine cup. For legal specimens, the patient is usually monitored during urination or placed in an area where no water or other fluid is available with which the specimen can be diluted.
   b. The more urine, the better, but at least 30 ml is required. Some drug screens require at least 100 ml of urine.
   c. For some legal samples, the temperature of the urine must be taken and documented as soon as the specimen is received. In this case, the patient's temperature should also be taken and documented.
3. Follow and document chain of custody procedures carefully.
4. Blood and urine may require refrigeration if they are not immediately transported by law enforcement or taken to the laboratory.
5. If the specimen must be sent to a laboratory, the laboratory should provide directions for packaging, chain-of-custody maintenance, temperature control, and shipment.
6. Provide the toxicologist with information concerning the suspected drugs, the time the drugs were ingested, how they were ingested, and if the patient has been given any medications in the emergency department.

AGE-SPECIFIC CONSIDERATION

Minors require parental/legal guardian permission for specimen collection unless institutional or state laws or regulations stipulate otherwise.

COMPLICATIONS

1. If only legal specimens are requested and no medical screening examination is performed, the patient may not be appropriately evaluated and could suffer serious injury or even death.
2. If the specimens are not appropriately collected and handled, they may be considered contaminated and ruled inadmissible.
3. If the chain of custody is not preserved and documented, the evidence may be ruled inadmissible.

PATIENT TEACHING

1. Provide the patient with information related to the law enforcement agency that requested the specimens for follow up regarding legal procedures.
2. Instruct the patient/family when to return to the emergency department or call 911 for problems related to alcohol or drug intoxication.
3. Refer the patient/family to the appropriate agency for substance abuse counseling as indicated.

REFERENCES

Kerrigan, S., & Goldberger, B. A. (2006). Forensic toxicology. In V. Lynch (Ed.), *Forensic Nursing* (pp. 123-139). St Louis: Mosby.

Ohio Chapter of the International Association of Forensic Nurses. (2002). *The Ohio Adolescent and Adult Sexual Assault Nurse Examiner Training Manual.* Columbus: Author.

PROCEDURE 187

Preservation of Evidence

Reneé Semonin Holleran, RN, PhD, CEN, CCRN, CFRN, CTRN, FAEN

Evidence is something legally submitted to a court of law as a means of determining the truth related to an alleged crime (Doyle, 2001). The sources of evidence are the victim, the suspect, and the scene of the crime (Burgess, 2000). The patient's body, hospital supplies used to care for the patient, documentation, and the emergency department itself can be sources of evidence in a criminal investigation (Saferstein, 2006). Every emergency department should have a protocol for evidence collection and preservation. The most common types of evidence collected include clothing; bullets; hairs; fibers; blood stains; fragments of materials, such as paint, glass, and wood; dirt; or plants.

INDICATIONS

1. To properly preserve, document, and maintain the chain of custody for evidence that has been collected from the victim of an alleged crime or a suspected perpetrator. Evidence should be collected for (Lynch, 1995; Saferstein, 2006):
   a. A medicolegal case or when there is a treatment situation with legal implications
   b. Suspicious deaths
   c. Crime-related injuries: child maltreatment, sexual assault
   d. Motor vehicle crashes
2. To properly store evidence so that it may not be altered.
3. See specific procedures on collection of evidence for drug and alcohol testing (Procedure 186), sexual assaults (Procedure 188), and bite marks (Procedure 189).

CONTRAINDICATIONS AND CAUTIONS

1. Medical interventions may destroy evidence. Emergency care providers should recognize and preserve evidence whenever possible. For example, placing paper bags over the hands of gunshot victim can help preserve trace evidence of gunpowder and identify whether it is a self-inflicted wound (Figure 187-1). Also, try not to cut through bullet or knife holes in clothing.
2. Some evidence may be misinterpreted or assumptions made that an injury is self-inflicted. The role of the emergency care provider is one of observation, collection, labeling, storing, and maintaining chain of custody, not interpretation (Lynch, 1995). For example, do not describe bullet wounds as per your interpretation of "entrance" and "exit." Instead, limit your documentation to objective information, such as wound location, size, and appearance.
3. In order to ensure good evidence collection, emergency care providers should possess accurate knowledge about what may or may not be evidence. Emergency departments should have protocols that indicate when evidence should be collected.
4. If photographic evidence is being collected, photographs should be taken before any treatment, whenever possible. A consent form must be obtained prior to taking evidentary photographs. When the patient is unable to give consent, parents, guardians, or other representatives of the patient may provide consent (Saferstein, 2006).
5. All evidence must be properly collected, identified, and stored. The chain of custody must be maintained or the evidence may not be admissible in a court of law.
6. Do not handle bullets with forceps, because scratches on the bullet may interfere with ballistics analysis.

EQUIPMENT

Sterile gloves

Evidence collection kit (Kits are available for specific crimes, such as sexual assault or driving under the influence of alcohol. See Procedures 186 and 188 for specific information.)

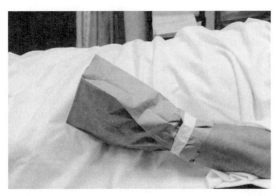

FIGURE 187-1 Hands should be covered with paper bags to preserve evidence. (Photo courtesy of R.A. De Jarnette.)

Suitable containers and sample contents if an evidence collection kit is not available (Containers need to be puncture resistant or tamper evident and prevent exposure to blood and body fluids.)

Glass or plastic vials for foreign objects, like bullets or rocks, sharp objects

Paper bags for clothing

Cardboard boxes for larger items, like boots or heavy coats

Envelopes for fingernail cuttings or scrapings, hair combings or pluckings

Evidence tape (provides tamper-evident seal)

Camera and film (instant camera with close-up capability or high-resolution digital camera)

Metric ruler (rigid)

Labels

Locked box or area where evidence can be stored until law enforcement assumes custody

PATIENT PREPARATION

1. Obtain consent for evidence collected based on institutional policy.
2. Obtain and document history related to the incident or alleged crime.

PROCEDURAL STEPS

1. Identify the indication for evidence collection and consult with law enforcement if you have any questions about what to collect. DNA profiling can be performed on saliva, bone, soft tissue, hair with roots, nasal secretions, blood or blood stains, semen or semen stains, vaginal secretions, skin and sweat, vomit, feces, and properly stored urine (Doyle, 2001).
2. Obtain the appropriate evidence collection kit (e.g., sexual assault kit) (see Procedure 188).
3. Obtain patient consent for evidence collection according to institutional policy. Note that in some cases, such as homicide or suicide, consent may not be required from the patient for evidence collection. Refer to your state laws and regulations.
4. Check the patient's clothing for the following and collect clothing as appropriate. If in doubt, collect the item.
   a. Blood
   b. Semen
   c. Gunshot residue
   d. Hair
   e. Dirt
   f. Debris
5. Change gloves often to prevent cross contamination (Ohio Chapter of the International Association of Forensic Nurses, 2002).
6. Do not perform wound care until injuries have been photographed.
7. Place all collected evidence in appropriate, separate containers. Each article of clothing should be placed in an individual bag or envelope. Avoid placing evidence from multiple victims on the same surface to prevent accidental transfer of vital evidence.
8. Wet evidence should always be dried before packaging. Evidence should always be placed in a paper bag. If you need to submit blood-soaked clothing, place the paper bags in open plastic bags to prevent exposure to

blood and fluids. Notify the receiving law enforcement officer that it should be removed from the plastic and allowed to dry in a secure evidence room as soon as possible.

9. Label all evidence with:
   a. Patient's name
   b. Source of collection
   c. Date
   d. Time
   e. Person collecting the evidence

10. Evidence should be sealed with evidence tape. Never lick envelopes or use staples. Licking envelopes may contaminate the evidence with your saliva and DNA.

11. A professional forensic photographer is preferred for evidentiary photography. However, photographs taken by emergency nurses are often helpful.
   a. Take a wide-angle picture of the victim to establish identity.
   b. Clearly label each picture with the date, time, patient's name, photographer's name, and location on victim's body (for close-ups).
   c. Include a rigid measuring device when taking close-up pictures of wounds or other small areas. If such a device is not available, a coin can be included in the photograph to provide a frame of reference for size.
   d. Film, negatives, photographs, photographic memory cards, or computer discs must be safely stored in a secure area until retrieved by law enforcement.

12. Document the evidence collection procedure. A checklist may useful to ensure that all of the steps have been correctly followed (Johnson, 2003). Document any interventions that may have interfered with evidence collection, for example, cutting off clothing.

13. Place evidence in a locked, secured area. Maintain chain of custody and only release the evidence to the appropriate law enforcement agency.

14. Notify the appropriate law enforcement agency per institutional protocols.

15. Complete the chart and ensure that all pertinent documentation is completed, including a list of what was given to the law enforcement agency, the name of the receiving officer, and the date and time that the evidence was released.

AGE-SPECIFIC CONSIDERATIONS

1. For every infant death, all clothing, including soiled diapers, should be saved for the medical examiner.

2. Consider abuse or neglect as a cause of a child's or elderly patient's injury, and collect and document evidence.

3. There are conditions that mimic abuse and/or neglect and these must be carefully differentiated when examining a patient to avoid false accusations. For example, coining—which may be performed to relieve pain—can leave marks that may be misconstrued for patterned bruising (LaSala & Lynch, 2006).

COMPLICATIONS

1. Essential medical interventions may interfere with evidence collection and preservation.
2. The chain of custody may be violated, interfering with the admissibility of the evidence.
3. Evidence stored in an inappropriate container may be altered or ruled inadmissible.

PATIENT TEACHING

1. Provide the patient/family with the appropriate legal agency to follow-up with regarding legal procedures.
2. Provide information about care specific to the injuries that the patient sustained.

REFERENCES

Burgess, A. (2000). *Violence through a forensic lens*. King of Prussia, PA: Nursing Spectrum.

Doyle, J. S. (2001). *Evidence collection handbook from the Kentucky State Police*. Retrieved October 8, 2006, from www.firearmsID.com, last updated 2005.

Johnson, M. (2003). Child sexual abuse. In D. Thomas, L. Bernardo, & B. Herman (Eds.), *Core curriculum for pediatric emergency nursing* (pp. 585-592). Boston: Jones and Bartlett Publishers.

LaSala, K. B., & Lynch, V. (2006). Child abuse and neglect. In V. Lynch (Ed.), *Forensic nursing* (pp. 249–270). St Louis: Mosby.

Lynch, V. (1995). Clinical forensic nursing. *Critical Care Nursing Clinics of North America, 7*, 489-507.

Ohio Chapter of the International Association of Forensic Nurses. (2002). *The Ohio adolescent and adult sexual assault nurse examiner training manual*. Columbus, Ohio: Author.

Saferstein, R. (2006). Evidence collection and preservation. In V. Lynch (Ed.), *Forensic nursing* (pp. 101-122). St Louis: Mosby.

Sexual Assault Examination

Reneé Semonin Holleran, RN, PhD, CEN, CCRN, CFRN, CTRN, FAEN, SANE

INDICATIONS

1. To provide the physical and psychosocial assessment and management for the survivor of sexual assault (ENA, 2007)
2. To provide nonjudgmental documentation of the history of the crime
3. To collect, preserve, and document forensic evidence
4. To prevent some of the physical and psychological health risks that may be associated with the sexual assault
5. To prepare documentation so that expert testimony can be given in a court of law

CONTRAINDICATIONS AND CAUTIONS

1. Consult state laws and regulations. In some states, sexual assault is a felony and must be reported to law enforcement authorities even if the victim decides she/he is not interested in talking to the police. Also, some states have procedures that allow evidence to be collected and held anonymously by the state crime laboratory for a period of time while the victim decides whether or not to report the assault.
2. Improper interventions may destroy or alter potential evidence. If sexual assault is suspected, every effort should be made to collect according to local law enforcement requirements.
3. Improper or incomplete evidence collection, preservation, and documentation may result in evidence that is inadmissible in a court of law. Survivors of sexual assault are best served by a sexual assault nurse examiner (SANE) (Ledray, 2006; Ledray, Faugno, & Speck, 1997). SANEs are specially trained in evidence collection and management as well as in documentation and testimony related to sexual assault. Employment of SANEs in emergency departments is highly recommended (ENA, 2007).
4. Survivors of sexual assault should be triaged as emergent and taken to a private area for assessment as soon as they present to the emergency department.
5. Emergency care providers should receive additional training approved by the International Association of Forensic Nurses (IAFN) before performing pediatric sexual assault examinations (ENA, 2007; IAFN, 2002).
6. Research has demonstrated that the standardized collection of evidence contributes to easier identification of the perpetrator, improved testimony

The author wishes to acknowledge Linda A. Hutson, RN, SANE for her contribution to this procedure in the third edition of this text.

in court, and eventual conviction. Each state has its own legal definitions of sexual assault, and evidence should be collected according to state protocol. State protocols should comply with IAFN guidelines (U.S. Department of Justice, 2004).

7. See Procedure 186 and your local laboratory/crime lab procedures if testing for "date rape" or other drugs is indicated.

EQUIPMENT

Sexual assault kit. Where available, use the kit specific to your jurisdiction. The following contents are in the State of Ohio Rape Kit (Ohio Chapter of the International Association of Forensic Nurses, 2002):

History and consent forms
Swabs
Glass slides and slide holders
Fingernail scraper
Paper sheet
Paper bags for evidence storage
Sterile saline or sterile water
Comb
Tweezers
Scissors
Filter paper
Envelopes
Labels
Evidence tape
Blood tubes
Urine tubes
Speculum
Wood's lamp (black light)
Camera
Colposcope
Toiletries
Change of clothing

PATIENT PREPARATION

1. Perform a primary and secondary assessment to identify any life-threatening injuries that must be managed before evidence collection can begin. In critical situations, the forensic evidence may need to be collected in the operating room or critical care unit. A protocol should be developed and approved jointly by the medical and SANE staff for the management of these patients.

2. Explain the procedures to the patient and have the victim sign the consent forms for evidence collection and photographs. Also have the victim sign consent for release of evidence to law enforcement.

3. The sexual assault examination should be carried out in a private area. Many emergency departments have specific rooms used only for sexual assault patients (Figure 188-1). A patient advocate should be called to talk to the survivor. Some patients may request that a family member or friend accompany them during the examination. The patient's request should be honored to encourage their attempts to regain control.

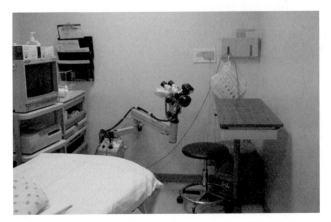

FIGURE 188-1 Sexual assault examination room. (Courtesy R. A. DeJarnette.)

PROCEDURAL STEPS

1. Document the history of the assault using a standard form (Figure 188-2). If the patient has showered or changed clothing since the assault, document this and collect evidence regardless. It is suggested that the history be taken with law enforcement present if they have not already interviewed the patient to decrease the need to repeat the history of the assault multiple times. Take pictures of obvious injury at this time. Also take an orientation picture of the victim at this time. Label all pictures per protocol.

2. Unfold the paper sheet on the floor and have the patient remove all clothing. Be sure to give the patient a gown for cover and have her/him sit on the stretcher. At this time, observe the victim for signs of injury, such as bruising, bleeding, swelling, redness, or bite marks. Collect all pertinent clothing worn during or immediately after the assault. Do not shake the clothing, and place each item in a separate paper bag. Seal with evidence tape.

3. Collect oral swabs regardless of the history given. Make a smear with a swab on a slide. Allow the swabs to air dry or place in a swab dryer. When the swab is dry, place it in an envelope and seal with evidence tape.

4. Collect hair standards. Allow the patient to pull 10 to 15 strands of hair from various spots on the head with gloved hands. Place the hairs in an envelope, seal with evidence tape, and label. (Protocols vary and may allow cutting or pulling hairs).

5. Scrape/swab under the patient's fingernails. If there are broken nails, cut a piece of the nail and place in the envelope, seal with evidence tape, and label.

6. Scan the patient's body with the Wood's lamp to identify any dried semen or saliva stains. Different fluids fluoresce under black light. Any areas that fluoresce should be swabbed. If the area is dry, use a moistened swab (water or saline) to sample. If the area if moist, use a dry swab. Air dry the swabs and place them in an envelope, seal with evidence tape, and label. Swab injured areas only after a photograph has been taken.

7. Place the patient in the lithotomy position. Comb through the patient's pubic hair several times with an envelope or a paper towel under the patient's buttocks. If there is an area of matted hair, cut the area out with scissors

THE UNIVERSITY HOSPITAL
CENTER FOR EMERGENCY CARE
EVIDENTIARY REPORT FOR REPORTED SEXUAL ASSAULT

SXASLT

Patient Name_____

Date_____ Sex_____ Age_____

S.W.

Police _____ Badge# _____ District/Agency _____

I voluntarily consent to this examination and the gathering of potential evidence including photographs of injured areas. In some cases, this may include the use of a magnifying camera called a colposcope to document internal vaginal injuries.

I authorize the hospital to release this record and all evidence collected to the police.

SIGNATURE _____

TUH-412, Rev. 9/99, Page 1 of 2

S

Date of Exam:_____Time of Exam:_____Hours Since Assault :_____LNMP: _____

Bath/Shower: Yes____ No ____Douche: Yes____ No ____ Urinated: Yes_____ No _____ Defecated: Yes _____ No _____

Changed Clothes: Yes __ __ No _____ Smoked/Ate: Yes _____ No _____ Mouthwash/Brushed Teeth: Yes _____ No _____

History as stated by patient: Patient's description of pertinent details of the assult: (oral, rectal vaginal, penetration: digital, penile, foreign objects), (oral contact), (ejaculation location, if known by the patient):

A

N

E

PHYSICAL EVIDENCE OF EXTRA-GENITAL TRAUMA: (Include all details of trauma—tears, lacerations, abrasions, ecchymosis, redness, bitemarks, presence of blood or other secretions.):

Photos Taken _____

Signature_____

Legend: T—tear, E—eechymosis, A—abrasion, R—redness, S—swelling

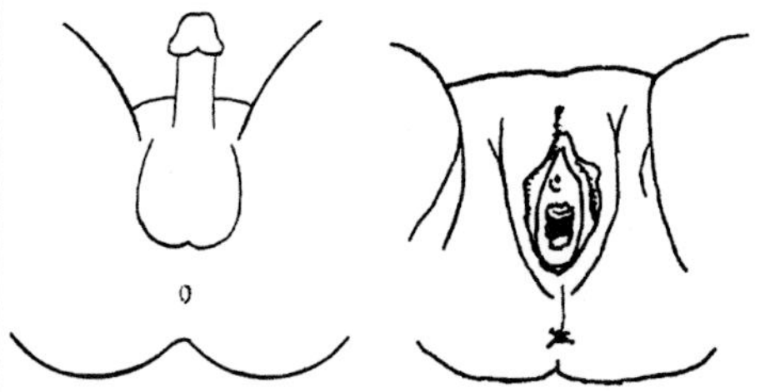

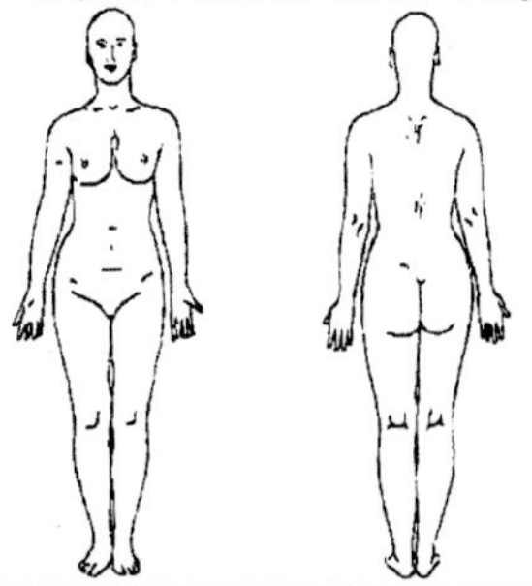

White - Medical Records, Yellow - Billing; Pink -SS; Goldenrod -Police

FIGURE 188-2 Sexual assault form. (Courtesy University Hospital, Center for Emergency Care, Cincinnati, OH.).

SXASLT

THE UNIVERSITY HOSPITAL
CENTER FOR EMERGENCY CARE
EVIDENTIARY REPORT FOR REPORTED SEXUAL ASSAULT

TUH-412, Rev. 9/99, Page 2 of 2

S

GENITAL EXAM: (Describe any trauma. Use common English terms): Trauma Visible: Yes ___ No ____

Labia Majora: _____

Labia Minora: _____

Posterior Fourchette: _____

Hymen: _____

Vagina _____

Cervix _____

A

Penis _____

Scrotum: _____

Rectal Exam: _____

c̄-with   s̄-without   NTN-no trauma noted   o-none   N/A-not applicable

N

E

EVIDENCE COLLECTION: (Collect and initial items below. Use stamped labels to seal envelopes. Use evidence tape to seal paper bags, blood and urine tubes. Collector dates and initials all labeled specimen envelopes; discard unused envelopes.)

Initial:

_____ **A. Clothing** Flouresce each item and place any stained clothing in a separate paper bag sealed with label and evidence tape.
_____   Articles submitted: _____
_____ **B. Saline swab of fluorescing body stains** (examine in dark room using Wood's lamp):
_____   Location _____
_____ **C. Tampons/Pads** (Dry and place in envelope - never in plastic)
_____ **D. Clipped Fingernails** (only if blood or tissue present or freshly broken)
_____ **E. Foreign Material** (e.g., burrs, grass, twigs)
_____ **F. Oral Swab** (roof of mouth and lower gum line) (four dry and smear)
_____ **G. Loose hair on body**
_____ **H. Bite Mark Swabs**
_____ **I. Combed Pubic Hair**
_____ **J. 10-15 pulled pubic hairs** from four different quadrants
_____ **K. 10-15 pulled head hairs** from various areas of head
_____ **L. Vaginal Swabs** (at least four dry)-smear
_____ **M. Rectal Swab** (four dry)-smear
_____ **N. Penile Swab** (four dry)
_____ **O. Other evidence:** _____
_____ **P. Photographs:** (Use ruler in photo to document size) # _____
_____ **Q. Colposcopy Exam**
_____ **R. #** _____ **Blood/Urine Tubes**

S
A
N
E
/
S
W

Examiner's Signature:_____ Initials: _____ Print Last Name: _____

Number of Evidence Parcels Secured: _____ Initials/Signature _____

Evidence Released By: _____ Date: _____ Time: _____

Evidence Released To: _____ Badge #: _____ Unit: _____

FIGURE 188-2 Sexual assault form.

and place it in the envelope. Place comb in the envelope with the hair. Seal with evidence tape and label. If there is no pubic hair, document that on the envelope.

8. With a gloved hand, the patient should pull 10 to 15 stands of pubic hair. Place these in an envelope, seal with evidence tape, and label. Refer to your state protocol for the required amount.

9. *For female patients: Inspect the genital area, photograph all injuries, and explain the speculum examination. Colposcopic photography may be performed at this time. Insert the speculum (plastic is recommended to provide better photography). Collect four swabs from the vaginal vault and cervix. Collect any foreign objects. If a tampon/pad is present, collect, dry, and seal in the kit. Make a slide from one of the swabs, dry, and seal in a labeled envelope. Allow the speculum to air dry and place in the evidence envelope.

10. *For male patients: Inspect the genital area, and photograph all injuries using the colposcope. Moisten four swabs with saline or water. Swab the glans and shaft of the penis. Make a slide, dry, and place in the labeled evidence envelopes.

11. *Examine the anal area for injury, and photograph all injuries. Collect four anal swabs regardless of the assault history. Make a smear with one of the swabs on a slide. Place this swab in a labeled evidence envelope.

12. Collect blood standard on filter paper provided in the kit. Wear gloves, label the filter paper, wipe patient's finger with alcohol, perform a fingerstick, and place a drop of blood on each circle. Dry and place in the envelope. Alternatively, some jurisdictions require a tube of blood be drawn from the patient.

13. *Complete the assault history form (see Figure 188-2) documenting sites of injury and your findings during the examination. One set of photographs should be given to law enforcement with the kit. One set of photographs should be kept with the medical record.

14. Administer sexually transmitted infection (STI) prophylaxis and pregnancy prophylaxis as prescribed and indicated. Explain to the patient about the need for follow up with these treatments.

15. Make sure that all evidence is sealed correctly and that your documentation is completed according to protocol. The sealed completed kit and documentation should be immediately surrendered to a law enforcement officer to maintain chain of custody. If you are unable to give your kit to law enforcement immediately, a locked, secured cabinet should be available for storage until law enforcement retrieves the kit. It is critical to maintain the chain of custody with all evidence and documentation.

AGE-SPECIFIC CONSIDERATIONS

1. Pediatric sexual assault survivors should be evaluated only by those trained to care for pediatric patients (ENA, 2007).

---

*Indicates portions of the procedure usually performed by a physician or an advanced practice nurse if a SANE is not available.

2. Postmenopausal women may incur vaginal tears and lacerations because of thinner skin due to hormonal changes.

COMPLICATIONS

1. The patient may decline specific parts of the sexual assault examination. Document "the patient declines" as indicated.
2. Improper collection or handling of the evidence or a break in the chain of custody could cause the evidence to be inadmissible in a court of law.
3. Patients may experience nausea and vomiting from the STI and/or pregnancy prophylaxis. Discuss this with the patient and offer suggestions for successful completion of the medication regimen. Written discharge instructions should be given to the victim so that the victim or a family member can review it at a later time. Because of the traumatic circumstances of the assault, victims may not comprehend the instructions at the time of discharge. Provide a phone number for any follow-up questions.
4. STI and pregnancy prophylaxis may not be effective. It is imperative that the patient be instructed about follow-up care.
5. Male survivors of sexual assault tend to suffer more physical injuries and should be carefully examined so a life-threatening injury is not missed (Burgess, 2000).

PATIENT TEACHING

1. The patient/family should receive clear instructions about the side effects of any medications given or prescribed. Antiemetics should be offered if pregnancy prophylaxis ("morning after" therapy) is prescribed.
2. The patient/family should be instructed about the importance of follow-up medical care. They should be given information about repeat STI testing and pregnancy testing because the specimens collected during this examination can diagnose preexisting conditions only, not infection or pregnancy that results from the assault.
3. The patient/family should be advised about local HIV and hepatitis testing and risks to the victim.
4. Provide information about sexual assault survivor advocacy groups and counseling opportunities.
5. Provide information regarding costs associated with the sexual assault exam and treatment and availability of victims' reparation funding as made available under state regulations and resources. This is generally available to victims who cooperate with law enforcement personnel (U.S. Department of Justice, 2004).

REFERENCES

Burgess, A. W. (2000). *Violence through a forensic lens.* King of Prussia, PA: Nursing Spectrum.
Emergency Nurses Association (ENA). (2007). *Sexual assault and rape victims (position statement).* Des Plaines, IL: Author. Retrieved March 11, 2007, from http://www.ena.org/about/position/
International Association of Forensic Nurses (IAFN). (2002). *Sexual assault nurse examiner standards of practice.* Pitman, NJ: Author.

Ledray, L. (2006). Sexual assault. In V. Lynch (Ed.), *Forensic nursing* (pp. 279-291). St Louis: Mosby.

Ledray, L., Faugno, D., & Speck, P. (1997). Efficacy of SANE evidence collection: A Minnesota study. *Journal of Emergency Nursing, 23*, 182-186.

Ohio Chapter of the International Association of Forensic Nurses. (2002). *The Ohio adolescent and adult sexual assault nurse examiner training manual.* Columbus: Author.

U.S. Department of Justice, Office of Violence Against Women. (2004). *A national protocol for sexual assault medical forensic examinations.* NCJ 206554, Washington, D.C.: Author.

PROCEDURE 189

Collection of Bite Mark Evidence

Ruth L. Schaffler, RN, PhD, ARNP, CEN

Bite marks are often found in cases of sexual assault, child or elder abuse, and homicide (Pretty & Hall, 2002). Screening for abuse is a priority during triage (Sekula, 2005), and many of these bite marks can be identified while patients are in the emergency department. Prompt assessment of these injuries is essential for collection of DNA evidence and bite mark patterns for forensic analysis. Scientific evidence may be more reliable than individual testimony in criminal trials so collection of evidence can be crucial.

INDICATIONS

1. To obtain samples of saliva residue remaining on the patient's skin. It is nearly impossible to bite without leaving traces of saliva. More than 80% of the general population secrete substances in body fluids (e.g., saliva, perspiration, semen, and vaginal secretions) that identify their major blood type as well as other laboratory-detectable factors (e.g., gram-negative and gram-positive bacteria, hepatitis B virus, and human immunodeficiency virus [HIV]). In addition, teeth are excellent sources of DNA material (Pretty & Sweet, 2001).
2. To obtain a sample of the patient's saliva as a control for comparison to skin samples
3. To obtain blood samples from the patient as a comparison to samples obtained from the skin, if appropriate
4. To obtain blood samples for baseline testing for bloodborne pathogens (e.g., HIV)

5. To photograph wounds identified or suspected of being bite marks. The pattern of the biting edges are believed to be unique to the biter (Sweet & Pretty, 2001) and can be captured in a photograph.
6. To collect, preserve, and surrender specimens according to local chain-of-custody protocols
7. To document the original appearance of the patient, as well as all history, interventions, or pertinent observations. Identifiable patterns of injury should be documented with a diagram and photograph. If bite marks are incurred during the commission of a crime, law enforcement personnel and a forensic odontologist should be involved as soon as possible. For names and locations of forensic odontologists, contact the American Academy of Forensic Sciences, 410 North 21st, Suite 203, Colorado Springs, CO 80904-2798; telephone (719) 636-1100; fax (719) 636-1993. The American Board of Forensic Odontology, Inc. (ABFO) is located at the same address or can be contacted through their website at http://www.abfo.org.

CONTRAINDICATIONS AND CAUTIONS

1. DNA degrades over time, so evidence should be collected as soon as possible after the bite occurs (ABFO, 2006).
2. Saliva swabbings of the bite mark site should be obtained whenever possible. Interventions such as washing of the area destroy or alter potential evidence that could be sufficient to prove the identity of the attacker. Emergency personnel should be aware of forensic considerations to avoid loss of potentially valuable evidence, thus complicating criminal investigations.
3. Bite marks may be accompanied by contusions, abrasions, lacerations, ecchymosis, petechiae, avulsion, indentations, erythema, or punctures. Fingernail scratches may indicate a struggle with an assailant.
4. Bites can be located on any body part. Among males, most bites occur on the arms and shoulders while the breast and legs are more common sites among females (Freeman, Senn, & Arendt, 2005). Because there is usually no eyewitness, a thorough inspection is necessary to look for bite marks. If one bite is present, others should be suspected as well. Look for representative patterns caused by the contact of teeth on the skin. Note the shape, color, and size of the wound(s).
5. Photograph the wound before treatment or sample collection is begun. It is important to determine whether the bite mark has been affected by cleaning, contamination, change in position, or lividity.
6. Forensic proof is very influential when a case goes to trial (Giannelli, 2005). Improper collection, preservation, or labeling of specimens may result in the evidence being inadmissible in a court of law. Maintain chain-of-custody protocols for all evidence and photographic materials. Mishandled evidence may be reason for dismissal of a case against a suspected perpetrator (Evans & Stagner, 2003).
7. Deceased persons should be refrigerated, but not embalmed, until evidence can be collected.

EQUIPMENT

Sterile gloves
Distilled water or sterile water

Sterile cotton swabs for collecting samples and controls

One sterile No. 10 envelope or sterile test tube for each area swabbed (essential to avoid evidence contamination)

Lavender-topped blood collection tubes

1 × 1 gauze squares

Nonflexible metric ruler or scale; ABFO No. 2 scale is preferred (Lightning Powder Co., Eugene, OR)

Camera (black and white and color film [35 mm], digital, video, or other nondistorting model for close-up views)

PATIENT PREPARATION

1. Obtain and document a thorough history and description of the bite mark(s). Ask conscious patients if they were bitten or if they bit anyone. A suspect may have been bitten by the victim as well and may have identifiable bite marks that can be examined for evidence.
2. Document interventions that may interfere with evidence or produce other wounds, such as venipuncture or defibrillation.
3. Do not clean wounds until after photographs and samples are taken.
4. Obtain a written consent for photographs and evidence collection according to institutional policy.

PROCEDURAL STEPS
Photographing Bite Marks

Forensic photography is a specialty. The information supplied here is offered to assist with evidence collection when a specially trained photographer is not available. Law enforcement personnel should be involved with these cases as soon as possible, and they can determine the need for photography. Nurses who take evidentiary photographs may be required to testify in court and have their photography skills and training questioned by a defense attorney. Generally, it is preferable to have an experienced photographer or forensic dentist take the pictures (ABFO, 2006).

1. Place the area to be photographed on a firm flat surface.
2. Place the ABFO No. 2 scale or an equivalent right angle as close to the bite mark as possible and on the same plane adjacent to the wound. The most critical photographs should be taken in such a way as to avoid distortion. A flexible ruler, such as a cloth tape measure, conforms to the body contours and distorts the dimensions of the bite in the photograph. Video or digital imaging can be used in addition to conventional photography (ABFO, 2006).
3. Color film or black and white film may be used. If color film is used, verify the accuracy of the color.
4. Off-angle lighting using a pointflash should be used whenever possible (Ramsland, 2005). A light source perpendicular to the bite site can be used in addition to off-angle lighting; however, care should be taken to prevent light reflection from obliterating bite mark details (ABFO, 2006).
5. Position the camera so that it is perpendicular to the bite mark. This is especially important if the bite is on a rounded surface, such as an extremity, a shoulder, or a breast (Figure 189-1).

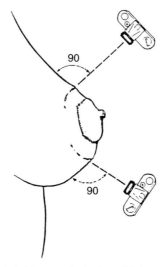

FIGURE 189-1 The camera is held perpendicular (at a 90-degree angle) to the bite mark when a forensic photograph is taken. (Courtesy P. F. Hampl.)

6. Take photos with and without the scale from a close distance to show that there are no wound areas under the ruler.
7. Photograph wounds from several angles both before and after cleaning the area. Include close-up views from several angles as well as photos orienting the relationship of the bite mark to the rest of the body. Change the lighting to show contours and shadows.
8. Take several pictures because this may be the only opportunity to photograph evidence.

Collecting Swabs

1. To prepare the bite mark site for evidence collection, use a double-swab technique (Sweet et al., 1997). Wet a cotton swab with distilled or sterile water, shake off the excess, and moisten the tissues surrounding the bite using a circular motion from the periphery toward the center. Discard this swab.
2. Using a dry swab, rotate the tip over the moistened skin so that the sample from the bite area is equally distributed on the surface of the swab. Avoid contamination with blood.
3. Using the same two-swab technique, obtain a control sample by swabbing at least a 1× 1-in site that has not been bitten.
4. Air dry the swabs thoroughly.
5. Place each of the sample and control swabs in separate sterile No. 10 envelopes or sterile test tubes that are appropriately labeled with the name of the patient, site of the sample, date, time, and name of the collector.
6. Collect a saliva sample by having the patient chew on a 1-inch square of gauze for 1 minute.
7. Air dry the gauze thoroughly and place it in a sterile envelope. Caution: Do not contaminate the gauze during the process of drying, which may

take 1 full day. Seal the envelope with tape; do not lick the glue on the flap (P. F. Hampl, personal communication, 1997).

8. Collect blood samples as needed (see Procedure 58). This may include fresh or dried blood on the skin as well as venipuncture.

COMPLICATIONS

1. A bite mark may not be recognized. The clarity and shape of a bite mark may change in a relatively short time in both living and dead victims (ABFO, 2006).
2. Incisions, punctures, or other wounds made in close proximity to the bite mark during medical treatment may alter or destroy evidence.
3. Improper collection or preservation of evidence or a break in the chain of custody may result in the evidence being declared inadmissible during legal proceedings.

PATIENT TEACHING

1. Follow up with law enforcement regarding legal proceedings and the possible need for additional photographs at a later date (e.g., after bruising is well developed).
2. Report any signs of infection (redness, swelling, pain or tenderness, draining pus) to your primary care provider.

REFERENCES

American Board of Forensic Odontology (ABFO). (2006). *ABFO bitemark methodology guidelines.* Retrieved November 27, 2006, from http://www.abfo.org/htm

Evans, M., & Stagner, P. (2003). Maintaining the chain of custody: Evidence handling in forensic cases. *AORN, 78*(4), 563-569.

Freeman, J., Senn, D., & Arendt, D. (2005). Seven hundred seventy eight bite marks: Analysis by anatomic location, victim and biter demographics, type of crime, and legal disposition. *Journal of Forensic Science, 50*, 1436-1443.

Giannelli, P. (2005). Forensic science. *Journal of Law, Medicine & Ethics, 33*, 535-544.

Pretty, I., & Hall, R. (2002). Forensic dentistry and human bite marks: Issues for doctors. *Hospital Medicine, 63*, 476-482.

Pretty, I., & Sweet, D. (2001). A look at forensic dentistry: Part 1: The role of in the determination of human identity. *British Dental Journal, 190*, 359-366.

Ramsland, K. (2005). *Bite marks as evidence to convict: How it's done.* Retrieved November 27, 2006, from http://crimelibrary.com/forensics/bitemarks/6.html

Sekula, L. K. (2005). The advanced practice forensic nurse in the emergency department. *Topics in Emergency Medicine, 27*, 5-14.

Sweet, D., & Perry, I. (2001). A look at forensic dentistry—Part 2: Teeth as weapons of violence: Identification of bitemark perpetrators. *British Dental Journal, 109*, 416-418.

Sweet, D., & Lorente, M., Lorente, J. A., Valenzuela, A., Villanueva, E. (1997). An improved method to recover saliva from human skin: the double swab technique. *Journal of Forensic Science, 42*, 320-322.

Application of Restraints

Teresa L. Will, MSN, RN, CEN,
and *Jean A. Proehl, RN, MN, CEN, CCRN, FAEN*

The Joint Commission (TJC) and the Centers for Medicaid and Medicare Services (CMS) have specific requirements, restrictions, and regulations regarding restraint use, which are updated regularly. States may also have specific laws and regulations pertaining to restraint use. Health care institutions in the United States must follow all current laws, requirements, restrictions, and regulations. This procedure will focus on the actual application of restraints, not the requirements for restraint use and documentation. Consult your institution's restraint committee, CMS, and TJC regulations for current information (CMS, DHHS, 2006; TJC, 2007).

INDICATIONS

Restraint may be indicated because the patient is a danger to self or others or to protect the cognitively impaired patient from interfering with therapy that is medically necessary. The patient should be carefully assessed to determine whether other, less restrictive measures will control the behavior. Examples of less restrictive alternatives include:

- Verbal intervention
- Environmental modifications
- Diversional activity
- Family or patient sitter presence
- Security presence
- Show-of-force

CONTRAINDICATIONS AND CAUTIONS

1. Restraints should be used only after less-restrictive measures have failed. Restraints should never be used for convenience or because staffing is inadequate. An assessment process must be used to identify and prevent potential behavioral risk factors.
2. Review your institutional policy and procedure regarding restraint use, paying particular attention to:
   a. Required components of physician/nurse practitioner orders for restraints
   b. Indications for restraint application
   c. Identification of personnel who may place restraints
   d. Observation and assessment of patients in restraints and documentation of same
   e. Guidelines for removal of restraints
   f. Guidelines for renewal of restraint orders

3. Restraints should not be used as fall prevention. Numerous devices are available to alert staff when patients are attempting to get out of bed. The use of restraints may actually increase the incidence of falls and patient injury.

4. Side rails are also considered restraint in some circumstances (CMS, DHHS, 2006; TJC, 2007).

5. Use only approved restraint devices. Gauze rolls, sheets, tape, and so on, are not intended to be used for restraint and have been associated with patient injury and death.

6. Avoid applying restraints to injured extremities whenever possible.

7. Beware of statements or actions that may escalate a violent patient. Paranoia and hostility are common reactions in a variety of medical conditions, when a patient is under the influence of drugs or alcohol, and when a patient is being treated against his or her will. Speak slowly and in a calm, low voice. Emphasize that violent behavior cannot be tolerated and that if the patient is unable to control the behavior, the team will help him/her control the behavior to prevent injury to self or others.

8. Position yourself cautiously when dealing with a combative or violent patient.
   a. Stand to the side of the patient to protect your vulnerable zone. Never stand in front of the patient.
   b. Stand more than an arm's length from the patient to protect yourself from a patient who lunges or kicks.
   c. Never turn your back on the patient, and never precede the patient into a room.
   d. Always place yourself, not the patient, closest to the door to allow a means of escape. However, avoid standing so you "trap" the patient in the room.
   e. Stethoscopes worn around the neck, neck ties, jewelry, and scissors can all be used by the patient as weapons to hurt you. Be aware of what is on your body and in your pockets when caring for violent or potentially violent patients.

9. After restraints are discontinued, remove them from the room or lock them to the stretcher so that they cannot be used by the patient to harm self or others.

10. If the patient is in locked restraints, do not leave the patient unattended. Keep the key readily accessible to caregivers at the bedside, especially during emergencies, including fire alarms.

11. Patients in handcuffs per law enforcement should be attended and monitored by a law enforcement officer.

12. Leather cuffs and belts cannot be adequately cleaned in the event of blood or body fluid contamination. They have largely been replaced by nylon or vinyl devices.

EQUIPMENT

Numerous devices are available; always consult the manufacturer's instructions for application instructions. Some devices commonly used in the emergency department include:

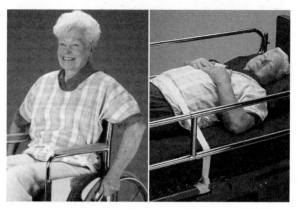

FIGURE 190-1 Vest restraint; Posey jackets and vests. (Courtesy of the Posey Company, Arcadia, CA.)

Vest Restraint (Figure 190-1)

Also known as Posey jacket or vest. For patients who require less restrictive restraint methods, a vest restraint may be adequate to remind the patient not to get out of the chair or bed. If used while the patient is in bed, all side rails should be up and any gap between split side rails covered as described below. A vest restraint is not appropriate for patients exhibiting violent, assaultive behavior. Follow the manufacturer's recommendations for application and tying this device as these restraints have caused strangulation when applied inadequately or not in compliance with the manufacturer's directions.

Soft Limb Restraints, Locked or Unlocked (Figures 190-2 and 190-3)

Used to prevent patients from pulling on IV lines, catheters, and so on. Stronger versions are used for patients who are combative and striking or kicking out at others. A quick release knot should be used to tie the restraint to the stretcher or bed frame (not the side rails).

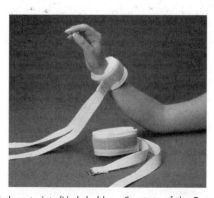

FIGURE 190-2 Soft limb restraint. (Limb holders. Courtesy of the Posey Company, Arcadia, CA.)

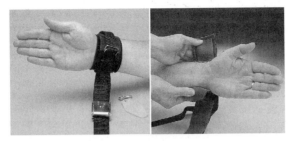

FIGURE 190-3 Nylon limb restraint with double hook and loop closure. (Twice-as-Tough Cuff-Keylock; courtesy of the Posey Company, Arcadia, CA.)

Nylon, Vinyl, or Leather Limb Restraints (Figure 190-4)

Used for patients who are extremely combative or violent. These restraints are used for patients who are displaying aggressive assaultive behavior and present a danger to themselves or others. These restraints are used only as a last resort and for the minimal amount of time necessary for the patient to control his/her behavior. These are typically used for four-point restraint.

Cloth Straps

Cloth straps secured with Velcro or other wide belt-like closures may be used across the patient's chest, hips, or knees if the patient continues to thrash and struggle when all extremities are restrained. Neither sheets nor tape should be used because both are difficult to release quickly in an emergency.

PATIENT PREPARATION

1. If possible, undress the patient. At a minimum, attempt to remove the patient's belt and shoes to prevent their use as weapons.
2. Attempt voluntary restraint application, but do not bargain with the patient. Be prepared with adequate personnel to safely hold the patient down and apply restraints if necessary.

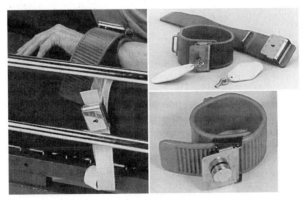

FIGURE 190-4 Locking vinyl limb restraint. (E.D. Security Cuffs. Courtesy of the Posey Company, Arcadia, CA.)

3. The patient should receive a thorough medical examination. Completion of the examination may need to be deferred until restraints have been applied if the patient is violent or combative. Consider the use of pharmacologic agents if the patient continues to struggle and fight after restraints have been applied.

4. Consider obtaining alcohol and toxicology panels. Rule out organic and neurologic causes for the behavior, especially in the elderly.

PROCEDURAL STEPS

1. Ideally, four or five people should assist in the application of restraints to a violent, assaultive patient. One person should be assigned to the head and one to each extremity. Holding the patient's head to the side with pressure on the forehead and mandible helps decrease the movement of the patient's body.

2. Apply all devices in accordance with manufacturer's directions.

3. Apply extremity cuffs snugly to prevent escape. To ensure that the cuff is not too tight, you should be able to insert one finger between the cuff and the patient's skin. Secure the restraints to the stretcher frame and never the side rails. Leave only enough slack to position the extremity safely.

   a. Full four-point arm and leg restraints should be used in patients who are a serious danger to self or others.

   b. Two-point restraints using an upper and lower extremity on opposite sides may be employed for less agitated patients or as an intermediate step when restraints are removed after the violent assaultive behavior has resolved. This prevents the patient from removing restraints, flipping off the stretcher, or tipping the stretcher over in an attempt to stand. For patients who are attempting to pull out tubes or lines, restraining both hands is appropriate.

   c. If there is one hand unrestrained, locking cuffs should be used on all other restrained extremities to prevent self release.

   d. One-point restraint is not a safe option for patients with violent or assaultive behavior.

4. Consider a strap across the chest, hips, and knees in addition to four-point restraints to protect a patient from injury if the patient continues to thrash about. Be careful not to restrict chest excursion and impair ventilation with straps placed across the chest.

5. Position the restrained on his or her side or supine, with the head of the bed slightly elevated. Because restrained patients often are under the influence of drugs, alcohol, or both, suction and airway equipment should be readily available.

6. If necessary, apply restraint cuffs while the patient is on the floor. In this case, place the cuffs on the extremities while the patient is on the floor. Then, lift the patient to the stretcher in the prone position with assistance from a belt placed around the waist. This decreases the patient's ability to struggle while being transferred to the stretcher.

7. Search the patient thoroughly and remove all objects from pockets after applying restraints. Remove the patient's shoes and remove or loosen any constricting clothing.

8. Observe the patient as per institutional policy.

9. Obtain a written order for restraints if not previously obtained. Refer to your institution's policy regarding the requirements for restraint orders.
10. Reassess the patient per institutional policy.
11. Restraint keys should be readily available to caregivers. A quick-release knot should be used for all restraints that are tied.
12. A debriefing with the patient and staff should occur after restraints are discontinued from the patient who was restrained because of violent or assaultive behavior. This debriefing should focus on the events that led to restraint and how future episodes of restraint could be avoided.

AGE-SPECIFIC CONSIDERATIONS

1. Therapeutic holding, comforting of children, and restraint associated with procedures (IV arm boards, and so on) are not considered restraint (TJC, 2007).
2. Requirements for time limits in the restraint of children are more restrictive. The order should not exceed 2 hours for children and adolescents aged 9 to 17. The order should not exceed 1 hour for children under age 9 (TJC, 2007).
3. Risks of restraint in the geriatric population include injury, death from strangulation, decline in functional status, altered skin integrity, sequelae of immobilization, and emotional desolation.

COMPLICATIONS

1. Circulatory compromise or altered skin integrity of restrained extremities
2. Respiratory compromise related to positioning or aspiration of vomitus
3. Vulnerability of the restrained patient to attack or abuse by other patients or family members. Close observation is warranted to ensure patient safety.
4. Compromised patient dignity, privacy, comfort, and rights
5. Injury to staff or patient during application of restraints

REFERENCES

Centers for Medicare & Medicaid Services (CMS), Department of Health & Human Services (DHHS). (2006). *Medicare and Medicaid programs; Hospital conditions of participation: Patients' rights*, 42 CFR Part 482 (2006). Retrieved March 1, 2007, from http://a257.g.akamaitech.net/7/257/2422/01jan20061800/edocket.access.gpo.gov/2006/pdf/06-9559.pdf

The Joint Commission (TJC). (2007). *2007 Comprehensive accreditation manual for hospitals. The official handbook (CAMH)*. Oakbrook Terrace, IL: Joint Commission Resources.

Preparing and Restraining Children for Procedures

Daun A. Smith, RN, MSN

INDICATIONS

1. All children need some form of preparation for a procedure to secure cooperation and in consideration of emotional well-being. This preparation should be performed in a manner appropriate to the child's developmental level.
2. Restraint may be indicated to facilitate examination or to perform interventions.
3. Positioning means to put the child in a position needed for a procedure; securing or restraining involves the use of physical, manual, or pharmacologic means to maintain the position (Pearch, 2005).

CONTRAINDICATIONS AND CAUTIONS

1. Administration of sedatives and/or analgesics may be the most appropriate method of restraining a child for a procedure that is painful or takes more than just a few minutes (see Procedure 177).
2. Infants release tension by gross motor activity; limiting this movement with physical restraint increases anxiety.
3. Preschoolers view restraint as a form of punishment.
4. Restraining a child for a procedure can cause feelings of powerlessness, anxiety, or anger.
5. Alternatives to physical restraint should be explored first (e.g., diversional activities) (Pearch, 2005).
6. Restraints should be kept to a minimum, both in the amount of restraint and in the length of time applied. The form of restraint chosen should be the least restrictive to accomplish the purpose (Pearch, 2005).
7. Whenever possible, the child should be restrained manually because this method provides human contact.
8. A child should never be restrained to accomplish a sexual assault examination. The child should be sedated or anesthetized if he or she is unable to cooperate with this examination.

PATIENT PREPARATION

All patient preparation for procedures should take place according to the child's developmental level and age-specific fears, concerns, and approaches.

Infants (birth to 18 months)
Fears
1. Separation from parents
2. Stranger anxiety after 6 months

Approaches
1. Encourage parental presence.
2. Use touch, voice, and non-nutritive sucking (pacifiers) to distract the infant.
3. Restrain the infant only as much and as long as is needed to accomplish the procedure. Infants cope with anxiety by movement; restraints increase anxiety. However, holding a young infant's flailing arms together and gently placing them on the child's chest may help the child calm down. Swaddling works in a similar fashion for neonates.
4. Return the infant to the parents immediately after the procedure for comforting and soothing.

Toddlers (18 months to 3 years)
Fears
1. Separation from parents
2. Strangers
3. Pain

Approaches
1. Toddlers learn through sensorimotor experiences. Let them handle equipment whenever possible.
2. Toddlers have limited coping abilities and need to be told that it is all right to cry. Allow them to keep a familiar object with them (e.g., blanket, stuffed animal).
3. Toddlers have limited language skills. Use simple, nonmedical language. Whenever possible, use their words for objects, body parts, and functions.
4. At this age, there is little conception of time. Toddlers need a brief explanation immediately before the procedure.
5. Some procedures (e.g., physical examination) can be accomplished with the child sitting on a parent's lap.

Preschool (3 to 5 years)
Fears
1. Body mutilation
2. The dark
3. Pain
4. The unknown
5. Loss of control

Approaches
1. Preschoolers learn through words, sight, motor, touch, and hearing. Let them play with equipment when possible. Focus your explanations on what they will hear, see, smell, and feel.

2. Preschoolers have a vivid imagination, which facilitates learning but also increases their fears. Clarify misconceptions and explain procedures in clear, simple language. Explain the procedure immediately before it occurs, so that the child does not have time to imagine the worst.
3. At this age, children want to please you. Praise all their efforts, whether successful or unsuccessful.
4. Preschoolers ask why continuously but are usually satisfied with clear, simple explanations.
5. Assure the child that this procedure is not a punishment for some imagined misbehavior.
6. Cover wounds, even injection sites, with a dressing or bandage.
7. Encourage parental presence.
8. Distract, encourage, and reward with colorful toys, crayons, or stickers.

School Age (6 to 11 years)
Fears
1. Loss of body parts
2. Disability
3. Loss of control

Approaches
1. The school-aged child wants to cooperate and to be seen as an adult. Praise all efforts to cooperate.
2. Abstract concepts are not understood. Encourage questions and clarify misconceptions.
3. Regression is not uncommon; be nonjudgmental.
4. The school-aged child understands rules and time limits. The child can be bribed or bargained with. Explain what needs to be done, and set time limits for cooperation (then allow a break if the procedure is not yet finished). Offer simple choices (e.g., which arm for the injection). Be careful not to offer a choice when there is no choice (e.g., "Can I give you this injection now?").
5. Peers are important. Allow for privacy so that a child does not have to be seen in a compromised situation (e.g., crying) in front of peers.

Adolescence (12 to 18 years)
Fears
1. Loss of control
2. Changes in body image

Approaches
1. Allow for privacy.
2. Encourage questions, clarify misconceptions, and explain carefully.
3. Be honest.
4. Accept any regression nonjudgmentally.
5. Peers are important to adolescents. Allow for privacy so that the child is not seen in a compromised situation (e.g., crying) in front of peers.

PROCEDURAL STEPS
Equipment
Child restraint board
Sheet, blanket, pillowcase
24%-25% sucrose solution (neonate)
1-ml syringe (neonate)
Pacifier

Oral Sucrose for Neonatal Analgesia (Thompson, 2005; Zempsky et al., 2004)

1. Administer sucrose solution, 0.01 to 2 ml into infant's mouth.
   a. By syringe, administer up to 1 ml into each cheek, *or*
   b. Allow infant to suck sucrose from nipple or pacifier.
2. Sucrose should be administered no more than 2 minutes before the start of the procedure.
3. Provide pacifier for non-nutritive sucking.

Mummy Restraint (Parnell, 2002)

1. Fold down one corner of a sheet to form a triangle (Figure 191-1).
2. Place the infant or child on the sheet with his or her head on the middle of the folded edge.
3. Bring one side of the sheet firmly down across the child's shoulder and torso, and tuck securely under the opposite side of the body.
4. Fold the bottom corner of the sheet up. This secures the child's feet.

Mummy restraint (body restraint)

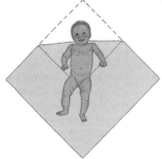

A restraint can be made from a sheet folded into a square of the appropriate size for the infant. Start by folding the top corner under the infant's shoulders and aligning the head with the folded edge.

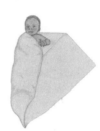

Fold one point of the sheet across the child and tuck it firmly behind his back.

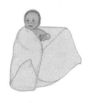

Fold the bottom corner of the sheet up to cover and restrain the infant's feet.

Fold the remaining corner over the child and tuck firmly behind his back.

FIGURE 191-1 Mummy restraint with a sheet. (From James, S. R., Ashwill, J. N., & Droske, S. C. [Eds.], [2002]. *Nursing care of children: Principles and practice* [2nd ed., p. 360]. Philadelphia: Saunders.)

5. Bring the other side of the sheet down snugly across the remaining shoulder and across the torso, and tuck snugly under the infant.
6. The mummy restraint can be modified by tucking the sheet over each ipsilateral arm and under the child's body, leaving the chest exposed. Adhesive tape over the arms and chest makes this more secure.
7. Monitor respiratory status and distal neurovascular status during the procedure, to be certain that the restraint is not too tight.
8. Remove the child as soon as the procedure is completed.

Child Restraint Board (Olympic Medical, Seattle, WA)

A restraint board, also known as a papoose board, consists of a solid back, with nylon or cloth wrappings and Velcro fastenings. Three sizes are available: regular (ages 2 to 6), large (ages 6 to 12), and extra large (teenagers and adults).

1. Place the board on a solid surface (stretcher, bed) where the procedure is to be performed. Open the Velcro straps.
2. Place a sheet folded into a triangle over the board with the wide part of the triangle placed where the child's head will be.
3. Place the child in a supine position on the board with his or her arms at each side.
4. Wrap the child mummy-fashion with the sheet to facilitate secure restraint with the Velcro fasteners.
5. Place the wrappings snugly around the child, securing them with the Velcro fasteners (Figure 191-2).
6. Monitor respiratory status and distal neurovascular status during the procedure to be certain that the restraint is not too tight.
7. Remove the child as soon as the procedure is completed.

Pillowcase Restraint

This restraint can be used for a toddler, preschooler, or small, school-aged child (ENA, 2004).

1. Slide a pillowcase up both arms behind the child to the axillae.
2. Have the child lie supine on the pillowcase. This restrains both arms with minimal restraint of the rest of the child's body.

COMPLICATIONS

1. Hypoventilation, vomiting, aspiration

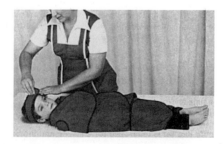

FIGURE 191-2 Child immobilized on a restraint board. (Courtesy Olympic Medical, Seattle, WA.)

2. Distal neurovascular compromise
3. Mistrust, fear
4. Soft tissue bruising
5. Choking and transient desaturation with sucrose solution administration (Thompson, 2005)

PATIENT TEACHING

1. Give age-appropriate explanations for the restraint and procedure.
2. Compliment the child on the positive aspects of his or her cooperation.
3. Reassure the child and the parents.

REFERENCES

Emergency Nurses Association (ENA). (2004). *Emergency nursing pediatric course* (3rd ed.). Des Plaines, IL: Author.

Parnell, D. N. (2002). Application of nursing principles to pediatrics. In J. W. Ashwill & S. C. Droske (Eds.), *Nursing care of children: Principles and practice* (2nd ed., pp. 430–485). Philadelphia: Saunders.

Pearch, J. (2005). Restraining children for clinical procedures. *Paediatric Nursing, 17*(9), 36-38.

Thompson, D. G. (2005). Utilizing an oral sucrose solution to minimize neonatal pain. *Journal for Specialists in Pediatric Nursing, 10*(1), 3-10.

Zempsky, W. T., & Cravero, J. P. Committee on Pediatric Emergency Medicine and Section on Anesthesiology and Pain Medicine. (2004). Relief of pain and anxiety in pediatric patients in emergency medical systems. *Pediatrics, 114*, 1348-1356.

PROCEDURE 192

Decontamination

Andrew A. Galvin, APRN,BC, CEN

BACKGROUND INFORMATION

Decontamination is defined as the reduction or removal of chemical (or biologic) agents so that they are no longer hazards (Hurst, 1997). Decontamination can be further classified as personal (self-decontamination), casualty (decontamination of patient), or personnel (decontamination of noncasualties). Emergency medical services (EMS) and emergency departments (EDs) may be responsible for decontaminating single or multiple patients after industrial incidents or intentional terrorist activities. It is imperative that hospitals actively participate with their communities and emergency medical agencies in designing and implementing aggressive and comprehensive disaster planning. It is preferred that patients be decontaminated upwind from the immediate area as quickly and completely as possible, before arriving at the ED (Houston, 2005; Lepler & Lucci, 2004). However, panicked patients may bypass EMS and arrive at the door of the ED. The Joint Commission (TJC) and the Occupational Safety and Health Administration (OSHA) require that hospitals train for and prepare for the possibility of a chemical, biological, or nuclear event. Because the ED is the gateway to the hospital, it is the most vulnerable area.

Decontamination is a physical skill that requires considerable and repetitive hands-on training (Houston, 2005). This procedure is intended to provide general guidance only and should be used with institutional and local protocols. Resources for current information are listed at the end of the procedure.

INDICATIONS

The primary goals of decontamination are prevention of agent absorption by the patient and protection of the health care workers and hospital facility from contamination (Lepler & Lucci, 2004). Decontamination remains the first line of defense against nuclear, biologic, or chemical (NBC) agents.

Whether one or many patients are exposed, the following questions should be considered:

1. What is the substance (if known)?
2. What are the risks to yourself and others?
3. When did contamination occur, and is it by a rapid-acting substance?
4. Where outside of the hospital can you effectively decontaminate patients?
5. How can this safely and efficiently occur during high-volume hours or during seasonal patient census fluctuations?

CONTRAINDICATIONS AND CAUTIONS

1. An external, free-standing decontamination unit is recommended for the ED (Schultz & Koenig, 2006).
2. It is vitally important that the rescuers are not contaminated themselves. The appropriate personal protection equipment (PPE) should be used. Careful observation for signs and symptoms of contamination among health care workers is paramount. Even with PPE, once someone touches a patient, they are contaminated. Chemical agent detectors may be used by staff wearing PPE (CDC, 2003).
3. It is imperative that all entry points into the hospital are secure; individuals will require an initial screening in order to determine whether or not they may have been contaminated.
4. Radiation survey instrumentation should be used before and after decontamination to measure radiation levels on nuclear exposure victims (CDC, 2003). All ED personnel should know how to contact their facility's radiation safety officer (Schultz & Koenig, 2006).
5. Establish three separate Zones (Hot, Warm, & Cold) if patients have not been decontaminated before arriving in the ED. Potentially injured patients are initially evaluated in the Hot Zone, where the patient is undressed and only immediate life-saving procedures such as airway and breathing interventions are performed. The patients will be decontaminated in the Warm Zone. Finally, the Cold Zone is considered contaminant free.

6. Do not taste, smell, or touch anything.
7. Minimize the number of staff performing decontamination.
8. Do not transfer the patient to another facility if you can provide the necessary care. Transfer of patients can result in transfer of contamination (Treat, Williams, Furbee, Manly, Russell, & Stamper, 2001).

EQUIPMENT
Staff Personal Protective Equipment
Full-face shield
Chemical-resistant suit with hood
Chemical-resistant gloves
Waterproof chemical-resistant rubber boots
Air-purifying respirator or self-contained breathing apparatus

Patient Identification and Belongings
Waterproof triage tags
Small and large plastic bags
Permanent marker/labels

Cleaning Supplies
Mild soap
Sponges
Long-handled brushes
Buckets
Water source
Hoses with gentle flow, controlled nozzles
or
Shower with multiple heads
Drain
Plastic pallets for fall prevention

Patient Privacy
Gowns
Towels, blankets, or sheets
Portable modesty screens

Miscellaneous
Duct tape
Scissors
Traffic cones

PREPARATION (USDHHS, 2001)
1. Establish a Hot Zone where contaminated patients are identified and undressed.
2. Establish a decontamination area (Warm Zone).
3. First aid and treatment takes place in a Cold Zone inside of the hospital.
4. Assign staff to each zone (with appropriate PPE in the Hot and Warm Zones). Most biological agents are not effectively transmitted from person to person. Because of this, standard contact precautions using gloves, masks/face

shields, and gowns are often sufficient enough to protect health care workers from becoming affected (Lepler & Lucci, 2004). There are exceptions, of course, and certain agents can be communicated via respiratory routes, such as smallpox and pneumonic plague. These agents will require extra respiratory precautions.

5. Notify institutional administration, who should in turn notify the local public safety officials (health department, law enforcement, fire, and EMS), the Federal Bureau of Investigation, the Federal Emergency Management Administration, and the Centers for Disease Control and Prevention (Richards, Burstein, Waeckerle, & Jutson, 1999).
6. Maintain a log of all persons decontaminated.
7. The patient must have his or her clothing removed and bagged, have any physical agent removed via gentle brushing, blotting, and/or irrigation, and then be decontaminated with copious irrigation. A sponge, along with simple soap and water, will decontaminate most chemical or biologic threats (USDHHS, 2001).

PROCEDURAL STEPS

1. With known biologic or radioactive agents, wet the patient down from top to bottom using copious amounts of water before undressing. This prevents the agent from re-aerosolizing. With unknown or chemical agents, strip patients before wetting down because wetting clothing further contaminates skin. If mustard is the substance, blot (do not rub) first to remove liquid. Attempts should be made to remove all clothing as soon as possible. Remember that pantyhose can maintain a large amount of contaminate close to the skin and cover a large area. Eighty percent of contamination should be removed with clothing.
2. Remove or cut clothing head to toe and front to back. Keep clothing away from face during removal to prevent inhalation and eye contamination. All clothing and valuables should be placed in a prelabeled plastic resealable bag. Label with the following information: name, date of birth, and date, time, and type of contaminate, if known. Hospital security or police should handle this as evidence if possible. Law enforcement agencies will determine whether or not clothing and valuables are needed as evidence. If this material is released to law enforcement agencies, they will be responsible for decontamination of bag contents. If not needed for evidence, valuables may be released to patient on discharge, according to hospital policy (after decontamination).
3. Wet the patient from top to bottom. Have patient stand with arms and legs apart. Soap and water is best, but do not wait. Using a large amount of water immediately is better than waiting for soap.
4. Maintain patient modesty at all times. Beware of the public and press who may be observing decontamination activities.
5. After thorough wet down, cover patient with gown, sheet, or blanket.
6. Assume that all patients in the Hot Zone are contaminated.
7. Leave contaminated equipment in Hot Zone until the situation is deemed over.
8. After all patients are decontaminated, contact hospital environmental services to begin clean-up.
9. After removing PPE, health-care providers should shower immediately with soap and water.

AGE-SPECIFIC CONSIDERATIONS
Pediatric and elderly patients are more prone to hypothermia, so pay close attention to preserving body temperature.

COMPLICATIONS
1. Patients refusing to be decontaminated must remain isolated in the Hot Zone.
2. If exposed to contaminated patient before PPE, staff must be decontaminated.
3. Limit the number of health care providers on the decontamination team to prevent any further contamination.
4. Be watchful for contamination of yourself and your peers.
5. Ensure that nonconfined water run-off does not flow into clean areas.
6. If run-off flows into storm drainage, notify the proper authorities.
7. If run-off goes into sewer system, notify receiving waste water treatment facility.

PATIENT TEACHING
1. Continually explain the purpose and steps of decontamination.
2. Continually reinforce the rationale for PPE for health care workers.
3. Reassure and calm patients.
4. Provide information regarding follow-up care if the patient is discharged.

REFERENCES
Centers for Disease Control and Prevention (CDC). (2003). *Interim guidelines for hospital response to mass casualties from a radiological incident.* Available at http://www.bt.cdc.gov/radiation/pdf/MassCasualtiesGuidelines.pdf

Houston, M. (2005). Decontamination. *Critical Care Clinics, 21,* 653-672.

Hurst, C. (1997). Medical aspects of chemical and biological warfare. In F. R. Dsidell, E. R. Takafuji, & D. R. Frans (Eds.), *Textbook of military medicine* (pp. 351–358). Washington, DC: TMM Publications.

Lepler, L., & Lucci, E. (2004). Responding to and managing casualties: Detection, personal protection, and decontamination. *Respiratory Care Clinics of North America, 10*(Part 1), 9-22.

Richards, C., Burstein, J., Waeckerle, J., & Jutson, H. (1999). Emergency physicians and biological terrorism. *Annals of Emergency Medicine, 34,* 183-190.

Schultz, C. H., & Koenig, K. L. (2006). Weapons of mass destruction. In J. A. Marx, R. S. Hockberger, R. M. Walls, et al. (Eds.), *Rosen's emergency medicine: Concepts and clinical practice* (6th ed., pp. 3021–3032). St Louis: Mosby.

Treat, K., Williams, J., Furbee, P., Manly, W., Russell, F., & Stamper, C. (2001). Hospital preparedness for weapons of mass destruction incidents: An initial assessment. *Annals of Emergency Medicine, 34,* 562-565.

U.S. Department of Health and Human Services (USDHHS), Agency for Toxic Substances and Disease Registry (Version 2001). *Managing hazardous materials incidents: Volume II-Hospital emergency departments: A planning guide for the management of contaminated patients.* Retrieved september 11, 2007 from http://www.atsdr.cdc.gov/MHMI/mhmi-v2-3. pdf

Additional Resources Regarding NBC Agents
Centers for Disease Control and Prevention: www.cdc.gov
Federal Emergency Management Agency: www.fema.gov
Poison Center: 1-800-222-1222.

Preparation for Interfacility Ground or Air Transport

Reneé Semonin Holleran, RN, PhD, CEN, CCRN, CFRN, CTRN, FAEN

INDICATIONS

To prepare a patient for transport to another facility. Transfer may be necessary in the following situations:
1. When personnel, technology, and procedures are not available at the referring facility (Warren, Fromm, Orr, Rotello, Horst, & ACCCM, 2004)
2. Based on local or state protocols related to regional care of particular patient groups (e.g., trauma patients, neonatal patients, stroke patients, burn patients)
3. Per patient and/or family request

CONTRAINDICATIONS AND CAUTIONS

1. There is no contraindication for patient transfer; however, the referring facility must ensure that the patient is transported in a safe vehicle by skilled and competent transport care providers or, if the referring facility staff will accompany the patient, that they are educated about the type of transport vehicle being used and the care the patient requires during transport.
2. A combative, violent patient must be transported with caution and may require sedation, analgesia, and/or neuromuscular blockade before and during transport by air or ground to ensure patient and transport crew member safety.
3. Weather may prohibit safe transport by either air or ground.

EQUIPMENT

Equipment needs are dictated by the patient's condition and current or potential interventions.

PATIENT PREPARATION

1. A patient with an extreme fear of flying may require sedation for transport.
2. Patients with motion sickness may require antiemetics or sedatives for transport.

---

*Indicates portions of the procedure usually performed by a physician or an advanced practice nurse.

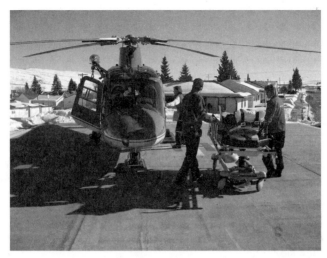

FIGURE 193-1 Example of a crew unloading a helicopter after transport. (Courtesy R. Linsler.)

PROCEDURAL STEPS

1. Identify an indication for transport. Transport decisions should be based on local protocols and hospital or facility agreements and should be conducted in accordance with Consolidated Omnibus Reconciliation Act (COBRA) and Emergency Medical Treatment and Active Labor Act (EMTALA) requirements (Frew, 1995; Mitchiner & Yeh, 2002; NHTSA, 2006).
2. Decide which mode of transportation is appropriate for patient transport. Several factors influence this decision, including the following:
    a. Health care systems (e.g., trauma systems)
    b. Facility agreements
    c. Weather at the referring and receiving destinations
    d. Condition of the patient and the equipment required for care during transport
    e. Distance to the referring facility
    f. Location of the patient (e.g., rural, urban)
3. *Contact a physician at the receiving facility to accept the patient.
4. Contact the receiving facility and ensure that the referring facility has agreed to accept the patient.
5. *Obtain consent from the patient or family as required by institutional or local protocols.
6. Perform any critical interventions that the patient may require before transport (e.g., airway management, immobilization of the cervical spine, initiation of vasoactive drugs).
7. Prepare copies of all current medical records, radiology studies, and laboratory results for transfer with the patient.
8. Remove all valuables from the patient and give to family members when possible.
9. Allow the patient to see the family and significant others.

10. Check to see if a family member may accompany the patient and, if allowed, prepare the family for transport. If the family may not accompany the patient, provide written directions to the receiving facility. Obtain contact telephone numbers for the family including cell phone numbers of those in transit.
11. Empty all containers before transport (e.g., urinary drainage bags, gastric contents, chest drainage units), and document output.
12. Provide sedation, analgesia, or antiemetics as indicated.
13. Contact the receiving nursing staff and provide pertinent patient information.
14. Provide patient care follow up to the referring facility as soon as possible.
15. Provide information to the patient's family about the patient during the transport.

SAFETY

1. Be aware of the potential safety hazards related to the transport vehicle (Holleran, 2003).
2. Never approach a running vehicle (helicopter or ambulance) unless signaled by the transport team.
3. Always approach the transport vehicle from the front, in view of the pilot or driver.
4. Protect hearing and vision by wearing earplugs and eye protection when approaching aircraft.
5. Learn to load and unload specific transport vehicles safely (Figure 193-1).
6. Always secure or remove loose objects (e.g., a stretcher mattress, oxygen tanks, gravel) around a helicopter landing area.

AGE-SPECIFIC CONSIDERATIONS

1. Ensure that a pediatric patient is placed in the appropriate safety device for transfer (e.g., pediatric board or age- and weight-appropriate safety seat).
2. When possible, allow a caregiver to accompany the child during transport.
3. Obtain any advance directives related to patient care during transport.

COMPLICATIONS

1. Risk of a vehicle crash during transport
2. Changes in patient condition that cannot be managed during the transport
3. Loss of communication with medical control during transport
4. Effects of changes in altitude during air medical transport could place the patient at risk for such problems as vomiting and aspiration or developing a pneumothorax
5. Increase in risk of a malfunction of equipment that cannot be fixed or replaced during transport

PATIENT TEACHING

1. Explain to the patient about the mode of transport he or she will be placed in for transfer (e.g., noise, where they will be placed, safety precautions).
2. When possible, introduce the patient to the entire transport team, including the pilot or driver.

3. Explain why family members may or may not accompany the patient during transport.

REFERENCES

Frew, S. A. (1995). *Patient transfers: How to comply with the law* (2nd ed). Dallas: American College of Emergency Physicians.

Holleran, R. S. (2003). *Air and surface patient transport: Principles and practice* (3rd ed). St. Louis: Mosby.

Mitchiner, J., & Yeh, C. (2002). The Emergency Medical Treatment and Active Labor Act: What emergency nurses need to know. *Nursing Clinics of North America, 37,* 19-34.

National Highway Traffic Safety Administration (NHTSA). (2006). *Guide to interfacility patient transfer.* Washington, DC: Author, DOTH 810599.

Warren, J., Fromm, R. E., Orr, R., Rotello, L. V., & Horts, M., & American College of Critical Care Medicine (ACCCM). (2004). Guidelines for the inter-and intrahospital transport of critically ill patients. *Critical Care Medicine, 32*(1), 256-262.

Index